T0200062

# Advance Praise For
## Management of Adults With Traumatic Brain Injury

"Drs. Arciniegas, Zasler, Vanderploeg, and Jaffee have edited an outstanding book on traumatic brain injury for clinicians. The authors of the chapters are internationally recognized experts in brain injury medicine, rehabilitation psychology, neuropsychiatry, and neuroscience. They provide an evidence-informed and practical guide for health care professionals. The chapter authors also give excellent clinical advice in the management of the cognitive, emotional, behavioral, and somatic impairments that frequently accompany TBI. This manual is unique in that it is both comprehensive and concise. It is essential reading for health care professionals who manage these persons."

*Robert E. Hales, M.D., M.B.A., Joe P. Tupin Endowed Chair, Distinguished Professor of Clinical Psychiatry, UC Davis School of Medicine; Editor-in-Chief, Books, American Psychiatric Publishing*

"This manual edited by Arciniegas and colleagues represents a contemporary and relatively complete treatment of the cognitive, emotional, behavioral, and sensory motor disorders associated with a spectrum of traumatic brain injuries. The contributing authors provide practical guidance on medical evaluation and neuropsychological assessment, while also discussing the treatment of those disorders that follow from traumatic injuries to the brain. This volume should be of benefit both to the seasoned practitioner and those just beginning their journey into the assessment and treatment of some of the most complex central nervous system disorders known to man."

*John T. Povlishock, Ph.D., Professor and Chair, Department of Anatomy and Neurobiology, and Director, Commonwealth Center for the Study of Brain Injury, Virginia Commonwealth University; Editor-in-Chief, Journal of Neurotrauma*

"This volume is a virtual encyclopedia of useful information on TBI, addressing a wide range of topics from posttraumatic behavioral disturbances and cognitive deficits to head injury in athletes and military personnel. As a guide for the clinician and researcher, this book provides a comprehensive, accessible, and practical resource."

*Jeffrey L. Cummings, M.D., Sc.D., Director, Lou Ruvo Center for Brain Health, Camille and Larry Ruvo Chair for Brain Health, Cleveland Clinic*

"Finally, we have a manual focused on the practical clinical management of patients with TBI, written by the world's leading investigators and clinicians in traumatic brain injury. Dr. Arciniegas and colleagues have edited a book which fills an important niche in the TBI literature. The clinical focus of each chapter, including a summary of key clinical points at the end, makes this an essential reference for every clinician who is involved in the care of patients with TBI."

*Robert G. Robinson, M.D., Emeritus Paul W. Penningroth Professor and Chair, Department of Psychiatry, Carver College of Medicine, University of Iowa*

"A clearly written, comprehensive overview of the varied day-to-day information medical professionals need to care for individuals with brain injury . . . . With content spanning from assessment and diagnosis to pharmacologic and nonpharmacologic treatment approaches, the manual is a "must have" for all brain injury professionals!"

*Flora Hammond, M.D., Professor and Chair of Physical Medicine and Rehabilitation, Indiana University School of Medicine, and Chief of Medical Affairs, Rehabilitation Hospital of Indiana*

"This well-referenced, well-organized book covers a broad range of relevant and important topics, [providing] a rich focus on emotional and behavioral disturbances. It also covers important special topics such as concussion injury, forensic issues, and TBI in late life, which have received insufficient attention in the literature."

*Jeffrey S. Kreutzer, Ph.D., ABPP, FACRM, Rosa Schwarz Cifu Professor of Physical Medicine and Rehabilitation, and Professor of Neurosurgery and Psychiatry, Virginia Commonwealth University–Medical Center; Director, Virginia Commonwealth TBI Model System of Care*

"*Management of Adults with Traumatic Brain Injury* is a comprehensive and accessible resource for clinicians and researchers. Step-by-step information . . . will ensure that the practices of those who are new to the field, as well as those with a long history of working with individuals with TBI, are up to date and evidence-informed. It also promises to be an invaluable teaching tool for rehabilitation and medical educators."

*Lisa A. Brenner, Ph.D., Associate Professor of Psychiatry, Neurology, and Physical Medicine and Rehabilitation, University of Colorado Denver, School of Medicine*

# MANAGEMENT OF
# Adults With
# Traumatic
# Brain Injury

# MANAGEMENT OF
## Adults With
## Traumatic
## Brain Injury

*Edited By*

David B. Arciniegas, M.D.

Nathan D. Zasler, M.D.

Rodney D. Vanderploeg, Ph.D.

Michael S. Jaffee, M.D.

*Managing Editor*

T. Angelita Garcia, M.B.A.

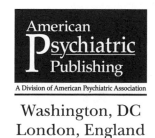

American Psychiatric Publishing

A Division of American Psychiatric Association

Washington, DC
London, England

**Note:** The authors have worked to ensure that all information in this book is accurate at the time of publication and consistent with general psychiatric and medical standards, and that information concerning drug dosages, schedules, and routes of administration is accurate at the time of publication and consistent with standards set by the U.S. Food and Drug Administration and the general medical community. As medical research and practice continue to advance, however, therapeutic standards may change. Moreover, specific situations may require a specific therapeutic response not included in this book. For these reasons and because human and mechanical errors sometimes occur, we recommend that readers follow the advice of physicians directly involved in their care or the care of a member of their family.

Books published by American Psychiatric Publishing (APP) represent the findings, conclusions, and views of the individual authors and do not necessarily represent the policies and opinions of APP or the American Psychiatric Association.

Purchases of 25–99 copies of this or any other American Psychiatric Publishing title may be made at a 20% discount; please contact Customer Service at appi@psych.org or 800-368-5777. For purchases of 100 or more copies of the same title, please e-mail us at bulksales@psych.org for a price quote.

Copyright © 2013 American Psychiatric Association
ALL RIGHTS RESERVED

Manufactured in the United States of America on acid-free paper
17   16   15   14   13        5   4   3   2   1
First Edition

Typeset in ITC New Baskerville and Avenir LT STD.

American Psychiatric Publishing
A Division of American Psychiatric Association
1000 Wilson Boulevard
Arlington, VA 22209-3901
www.appi.org

**Library of Congress Cataloging-in-Publication Data**
Management of adults with traumatic brain injury / edited by David B. Arciniegas ... [et al.]. – 1st ed.
      p. ; cm.
   Includes bibliographical references and index.
   ISBN 978-1-58562-404-1 (pbk. : alk. paper)
   I. Arciniegas, David B. (David Brian), 1967- II. American Psychiatric Association.
   [DNLM: 1.  Brain Injuries–therapy. 2.  Neuropsychiatry–methods. 3.  Rehabilitation–psychology.  WL 354]
   617.4'81044–dc23
                              2012044002

**British Library Cataloguing in Publication Data**
A CIP record is available from the British Library.

*For Debbie*

The inspiration and vision for this book belong to Deborah Warden, M.D., who nurtured it through its initial developmental phases.

Dr. Warden assumed responsibility as National Director of the Defense and Veterans Brain Injury Center (DVBIC) in July 2001, just two months prior to 9/11. Under her adroit and prescient leadership from 2001 through 2007, Dr. Warden was instrumental in raising the awareness of concussion and traumatic brain injury among our military service members and Veterans. She ushered the care of these individuals, who put themselves in harm's way while serving their country, into the twenty-first century through groundbreaking research, case management, practice guidelines, and educational initiatives. Her work is a shining example of the power of military, federal, and civilian collaboration.

Dr. Warden is an outstanding scientist, a compassionate clinician, and an invaluable mentor. She is a true friend to all of us who care for persons and families affected by traumatic brain injuries.

# CONTENTS

Contributors. . . . . . . . . . . . . . . . . . . . . . . . xv
Preface . . . . . . . . . . . . . . . . . . . . . . . . . xxi
Acknowledgments . . . . . . . . . . . . . . . . . . xxv

## PART I
### INTRODUCTION

## Chapter 1

Overview of Traumatic Brain Injury . . . . . . . . . . 3
*Erin D. Bigler, Ph.D.*
*William L. Maxwell, Ph.D., Sc.D.*

## PART II
### Assessment

## Chapter 2

Medical Evaluation. . . . . . . . . . . . . . . . . . . . . . 35
*David B. Arciniegas, M.D.*

## Chapter 3

Neuropsychological Assessment . . . . . . . . . . . 73
*Rodney D. Vanderploeg, Ph.D.*

# PART III
## MANAGEMENT

### *Posttraumatic Cognitive Impairments*

# Chapter 4

## Disorders of Consciousness . . . . . . . . . . . . . . 103
*John Whyte, M.D., Ph.D.*
*Joseph T. Giacino, Ph.D.*

# Chapter 5

## Cognitive Impairments . . . . . . . . . . . . . . . . 131
*David B. Arciniegas, M.D.*
*Kimberly L. Frey, M.S.*
*Thomas W. McAllister, M.D.*

### *Posttraumatic Emotional and Behavioral Disturbances*

# Chapter 6

## Disorders of Mood and Affect . . . . . . . . . . . 167
*Ricardo E. Jorge, M.D.*
*David B. Arciniegas, M.D.*

# Chapter 7

## Anxiety Disorders . . . . . . . . . . . . . . . . . . 195
*Jesse R. Fann, M.D., M.P.H.*
*Matthew Jakupcak, Ph.D.*

# Chapter 8

## Posttraumatic Stress Disorder . . . . . . . . . . . 213
*Jan E. Kennedy, Ph.D.*
*Michael S. Jaffee, M.D.*
*Douglas B. Cooper, Ph.D.*

# Chapter 9

Posttraumatic Psychosis. . . . . . . . . . . . . . . . 239

*Perminder S. Sachdev, M.B.B.S., M.D., Ph.D.*

# Chapter 10

Aggressive Disorders. . . . . . . . . . . . . . . . . 259

*Stuart C. Yudofsky, M.D.*
*Jonathan M. Silver, M.D.*
*Karen E. Anderson, M.D.*

# Chapter 11

Apathy . . . . . . . . . . . . . . . . . . . . . . . . . 283

*Robert van Reekum, M.D.*
*Emma van Reekum, B.S.*

# Chapter 12

Substance Use Disorders . . . . . . . . . . . . . . . 303

*Jennifer Bogner, Ph.D.*

### *Posttraumatic Somatic Problems*

# Chapter 13

Headache. . . . . . . . . . . . . . . . . . . . . . . . 323

*Robert L. Ruff, M.D., Ph.D.*
*Ronald G. Riechers II, M.D.*
*Mark F. Walker, M.D.*
*Suzanne Ruff, Ph.D.*

# Chapter 14

Seizures and Epilepsy. . . . . . . . . . . . . . . . . 345

*Lauren Frey, M.D.*

# Chapter 15

Sleep and Fatigue . . . . . . . . . . . . . . . . . . . . 371

*Sandeep Vaishnavi, M.D., Ph.D.*
*Una McCann, M.D.*
*Vani Rao, M.D.*

# Chapter 16

Posttraumatic Sensory Impairments . . . . . . . 395

*Nathan D. Zasler, M.D.*

## PART IV
### SPECIAL TOPICS

# Chapter 17

Traumatic Brain Injury in Late Life . . . . . . . . 423

*William C. Walker, M.D.*
*David X. Cifu, M.D.*

# Chapter 18

Athletes and Sports-Related Concussion . . . 443

*Christopher M. Bailey, Ph.D.*
*Michael A. McCrea, Ph.D.*
*Jeffrey T. Barth, Ph.D.*

# Chapter 19

Military Personnel and Veterans With
Traumatic Brain Injury. . . . . . . . . . . . . . . . . 461

*Kimberly Meyer, M.S.N.*
*Michael S. Jaffee, M.D.*

# Chapter 20

Persistent Symptoms After a Concussion . . . 475

*Jonathan M. Silver, M.D.*
*Thomas Kay, Ph.D.*

# Chapter 21

Forensic Issues and Traumatic Brain Injury. . . 501

*Robert P. Granacher Jr., M.D., M.B.A.*

Appendix A: Suggested Readings. . . . . . . . . 529

Appendix B: Relevant Web Sites . . . . . . . . . 533

Index . . . . . . . . . . . . . . . . . . . . . . . . . . . . 537

*Color Plates appear as an insert*

# Contributors

**Karen E. Anderson, M.D.**
Assistant Professor, Departments of Psychiatry and Neurology, University of Maryland School of Medicine, Baltimore, Maryland

**David B. Arciniegas, M.D.**
Beth K. and Stuart C. Yudofsky Chair in Brain Injury Medicine; Executive Director, Beth K. and Stuart C. Yudofsky Division of Neuropsychiatry; Professor of Psychiatry and Physical Medicine & Rehabilitation, Baylor College of Medicine; and Senior Scientist and Medical Director for Brain Injury Research, TIRR Memorial Hermann, Houston, Texas

**Christopher M. Bailey, Ph.D.**
Assistant Professor and Neuropsychologist, Department of Neurology, Case Western Reserve University School of Medicine, Neurological Institute, University Hospitals Case Medical Center, Cleveland, Ohio

**Jeffrey T. Barth, Ph.D.**
John Edward Fowler Professor, Director, Brain Injury and Sports Concussion Institute, Neurocognitive Assessment Laboratory, Department of Psychiatry and Neurobehavioral Sciences, Department of Neurological Surgery, University of Virginia School of Medicine, Charlottesville, Virginia

**Erin D. Bigler, Ph.D.**
Professor, Department of Psychology and Neuroscience Center, Brigham Young University, Provo; and Adjunct Professor, Department of Psychiatry, University of Utah School of Medicine, Salt Lake City, Utah

**Jennifer Bogner, Ph.D.**
Psychologist, Associate Professor, and Vice-Chair of Research, Department of Physical Medicine and Rehabilitation, Division of Rehabilitation Psychology, Ohio State University, Columbus, Ohio

**David X. Cifu, M.D.**
National Director, Veterans Health Administration, Physical Medicine and Rehabilitation Program Office, Herman J. Flax, MD Professor and Chairman, Virginia Commonwealth University School of Medicine, Physical Medicine and Rehabilitation, Richmond, Virginia

**Douglas B. Cooper, Ph.D.**
Research Director, Defense and Veterans Brain Injury Center (DVBIC), Department of Neurology, San Antonio Military Medical Center, Fort Sam Houston, Texas

**Jesse R. Fann, M.D., M.P.H.**
Professor, Department of Psychiatry and Behavioral Sciences, Adjunct Professor, Department of Rehabilitation Medicine, University of Washington School of Medicine, and Adjunct Professor, Department of Epidemiology, University of Washington School of Public Health, Seattle, Washington

**Kimberly L. Frey, M.S.**
Director, Speech Department, Craig Hospital, Englewood, Colorado

**Lauren Frey, M.D.**
Assistant Professor, Department of Neurology, University of Colorado Anschutz Medical Campus, Aurora, Colorado

**Joseph T. Giacino, Ph.D.**
Director of Rehabilitation Neuropsychology, Spaulding Rehabilitation Hospital; Associate Professor, Department of Physical Medicine and Rehabilitation, Harvard Medical School, Boston, Massachusetts

**Robert P. Granacher Jr., M.D., M.B.A.**
Clinical Professor of Psychiatry, Lexington Forensic Neuropsychiatry, University of Kentucky College of Medicine, Lexington, Kentucky

**Michael S. Jaffee, M.D.**
Past National Director, Defense and Veterans Brain Injury Center; Associate Professor of Neurology, Uniformed Services University of the Health Sciences, Bethesda, Maryland; Adjunct Professor of Neurology and Psychiatry, University of Texas Health Sciences Center, San Antonio, Texas

**Matthew Jakupcak, Ph.D.**
Deployment Health Services, VA Puget Sound Health Care System, and Assistant Professor, Department of Psychiatry and Behavioral Sciences, University of Washington School of Medicine, Seattle, Washington

**Ricardo E. Jorge, M.D.**
Associate Professor, Department of Psychiatry, Roy J. and Lucille A. Carver College of Medicine, University of Iowa, Iowa City, Iowa

**Thomas Kay, Ph.D.** *(deceased)*
Director of Neuropsychology, Carmel Psychological Associates, Carmel, New York

**Jan E. Kennedy, Ph.D.**
Neuropsychologist and Senior Scientific Director, Defense and Veterans Brain Injury Center, Wilford Hall Medical Center, Lackland Air Force Base, San Antonio, Texas

**William L. Maxwell, Ph.D., Sc.D.**
Senior Lecturer in Human Anatomy, Department of Anatomy, University of Glasgow, Glasgow, Scotland, United Kingdom

**Thomas W. McAllister, M.D.**
Millennium Professor of Psychiatry and Neurology, Vice Chair for Neuroscience Research, and Director, Section of Neuropsychiatry, Department of Psychiatry, Dartmouth-Hitchcock Medical Center, Lebanon, New Hampshire

**Una McCann, M.D.**
Professor, Department of Psychiatry; Director, Anxiety Disorders Program; Co-Director, Center for Interdisciplinary Sleep Research and Eduction, Johns Hopkins School of Medicine, Baltimore, Maryland

**Michael A. McCrea, Ph.D.**
Professor and Director of Brain Injury Research, Departments of Neurosurgery and Neurology, Medical College of Wisconsin, Milwaukee, Wisconsin

**Kimberly Meyer, M.S.N.**
Defense and Veterans Brain Injury Center (DVBIC) National Headquarters, Rockville, Maryland

**Vani Rao, M.D.**
Associate Professor, Department of Psychiatry; Director, Neuropsychiatry Fellowship Program; Medical Director, Brain Injury Program, Johns Hopkins University and School of Medicine, Baltimore, Maryland

**Ronald G. Riechers II, M.D.**
Medical Director, Polytrauma Team, Louis Stokes Cleveland Department of Veterans Affairs Medical Center, Neurology Service; Assistant Professor, Department of Neurology, Case Western Reserve University, Cleveland, Ohio

**Robert L. Ruff, M.D., Ph.D.**
Neurology Service Chief, Neurology and Polytrauma Services, Louis Stokes Cleveland Veterans Affairs Medical Center, Cleveland, Ohio

**Suzanne Ruff, Ph.D.**
Health Psychology and Polytrauma Services, Louis Stokes Cleveland Department of Veterans Affairs Medical Center, Cleveland, Ohio

**Perminder S. Sachdev, M.B.B.S., M.D., Ph.D.**
Scientia Professor of Neuropsychiatry and Co-Director, Centre for Healthy Brain Ageing, School of Psychiatry, University of New South Wales; Director, Neuropsychiatric Institute, Prince of Wales Hospital, Sydney, New South Wales, Australia

**Jonathan M. Silver, M.D.**
Clinical Professor of Psychiatry, New York University School of Medicine, New York, New York

**Sandeep Vaishnavi, M.D., Ph.D.**
Director, The Neuropsychiatric Clinic at Carolina Partners, Raleigh, North Carolina

**Rodney D. Vanderploeg, Ph.D.**
Clinical Neuropsychologist and Psychology Section Leader, Brain Injury Rehabilitation and Neuropsychology, James A. Haley Veterans Hospital, Tampa, Florida; Associate Professor, Departments of Psychology and Psychiatry and Neurosciences, University of South Florida, Tampa, Florida

**Emma van Reekum, B.S.**
Undergraduate student, Kinesiology B.Sc. program, St. Francis Xavier University, Antigonish, Nova Scotia, Canada

**Robert van Reekum, M.D.**
Assistant Professor, Department of Psychiatry and Institute of Medical Sciences, University of Toronto, Toronto, Ontario, Canada

**Mark F. Walker, M.D.**
Associate Professor of Neurology, Case Western Reserve University; Staff Neurologist, Louis Stokes Cleveland Department of Veterans Affairs Medical Center, Cleveland, Ohio

**William C. Walker, M.D.**
Site Director, Defense and Veterans Brain Injury Center, Hunter Holmes McGuire Veterans Affairs Medical Center, Department of Physical Medicine and Rehabilitation; Ernst and Helga Prosser Professor, Physical Medicine and Rehabilitation, Virginia Commonwealth University School of Medicine, Richmond, Virginia

**John Whyte, M.D., Ph.D.**
Director, Moss Rehabilitation Research Institute, Albert Einstein Healthcare Network, Elkins Park, Pennsylvania

**Stuart C. Yudofsky, M.D.**
D. C. and Irene Ellwood Professor and Chairman, Beth K. and Stuart C. Yu-dofsky Presidential Chair in Neuropsychiatry, Distinguished Service Professor, Menninger Department of Psychiatry and Behavioral Sciences, Baylor College of Medicine; Chairman, Department of Psychiatry, The Methodist Hospital, Houston, Texas

**Nathan D. Zasler, M.D.**
CEO and Medical Director, Concussion Care Centre of Virginia, Ltd., CEO and Medical Director, Tree of Life Services, Inc., and Professor (affiliate), Virginia Commonwealth University Department of Physical Medicine and Rehabilitation, Richmond, Virginia; Associate Professor (adjunct), Department of Physical Medicine and Rehabilitation, University of Virginia, Charlottesville, Virginia; and Chairperson, International Brain Injury Association

## DISCLOSURE OF INTERESTS

*The following contributors to this book have indicated a financial interest in or other affiliation with a commercial supporter, a manufacturer of a commercial product, a provider of a commercial service, a nongovernmental organization, and/or a government agency, as listed below:*

**Erin D. Bigler, Ph.D.**—*Grants and contracts:* At Brigham Young University, the Brain Imaging and Behavior Research Laboratory (Erin D. Bigler, Director), is supported in part by National Institutes of Health grants and contracts, and the University's Neuropsychological Research and Assessment Clinic (E.D. Bigler, Co-director) will offer expert opinion on forensic cases, including those involving traumatic brain injury.

**Jennifer Bogner, Ph.D.**—*Commercial services:* The Ohio Valley Center Substance Abuse Education Series is mentioned in the chapter. The Ohio Valley Center charges for this product to reimburse the cost of production. Dr. Bogner does not personally benefit from such sales.

*The following contributors to this book have indicated they have no competing interests or affiliations to declare:*
Karen E. Anderson, M.D.; David B. Arciniegas, M.D.; Christopher M. Bailey, Ph.D.; Jeffrey T. Barth, Ph.D.; David X. Cifu, M.D.; Douglas B. Cooper, Ph.D.; Jesse R. Fann, M.D., M.P.H.; Kimberly L. Frey, M.S.; Lauren Frey, M.D.; Joseph T. Giacino, Ph.D.; Robert T. Granacher Jr., M.D., M.B.A.; Michael S. Jaffee, M.D.; Matthew Jakupcak, Ph.D.; Ricardo E. Jorge, M.D.; Thomas Kay, Ph.D.; Jan E. Kennedy, Ph.D.; William L. Maxwell, Ph.D., Sc.D.; Kimberly Meyer, M.S.N.; Thomas W. McAllister, M.D.; Una McCann, M.D.; Michael A. McCrea, Ph.D.; Vani Rao, M.D.; Ronald G. Riechers II, M.D.; Robert L. Ruff, M.D., Ph.D.; Suzanne Ruff, Ph.D.; Perminder S. Sachdev, M.B.B.S., M.D., Ph.D.; Jonathan M. Silver, M.D.; Sandeep Vaishnavi, M.D.; Rodney D. Vanderploeg, Ph.D.; Emma van Reekum, B.S.; Robert van Reekum, M.D.; Mark F. Walker, William C. Walker, M.D.; John Whyte, M.D., Ph.D.; Stuart C. Yudofsky, M.D.; Nathan D. Zasler, M.D.

# Preface

**Traumatic brain injury** (TBI) is a worldwide public health problem with a broad range of mental health consequences. In the moments following TBI, neuropsychiatric disturbances are nearly universal. They typically include alterations of consciousness, attention, processing speed, declarative memory, and/or executive function, and frequently are accompanied by emotional and behavioral disturbances as well as sensory and motor problems. In the days to weeks after TBI, neurotrauma-induced neuropsychiatric disturbances are common among persons whose injuries require hospitalization and inpatient rehabilitation; these disturbances often become chronic problems. Recovery following mild TBI usually proceeds rapidly and typically is complete. However, early postinjury neuropsychiatric disturbances at all levels of injury severity often are unrecognized, misunderstood, and inadequately addressed. In such circumstances, these may become chronic disturbances and entail a broad range of secondary psychological health and psychosocial consequences. Preinjury health and psychosocial factors may exacerbate or mitigate the short- and long-term neuropsychiatric consequences of TBI, and a variety of postinjury factors may facilitate or complicate recovery from TBI and its neuropsychiatric sequelae.

Understanding and improving outcomes after TBI therefore requires consideration of not only the effects of external physical forces on the brain but also the person sustaining that injury and the events preceding and following it. The scope of such considerations is necessarily broad and often is quite challenging, especially in the midst of a busy clinical practice. Accordingly, an important objective is to provide physicians, psychologists, nurses, and mental health and rehabilitation specialists with concise and practical guidance on the clinical management of individuals and families affected by TBI.

This book was conceived by Deborah Warden, M.D., to whom it is dedicated, as a clinical manual designed to meet this objective. She facilitated initial communications between the editors of this volume and American Psychiatric Publishing and contributed to early formulations of its contents. She supported the broad view of neuropsychiatry—

inclusive of cognitive, emotional, behavioral, and sensory and motor functions—and encouraged the editors to address the management of neuropsychiatric disturbances commonly experienced by civilians, military service members, and Veterans with TBI. Drawing on the editors' combined backgrounds in psychiatry, neurology, neuropsychology, and physiatry, this volume was developed toward this end.

Internationally known experts in brain injury medicine, rehabilitation psychology, neuropsychology, and the clinical and basic neurosciences contributed chapters on core topics in brain injury medicine. Chapter 1 reviews the epidemiology and pathophysiology of TBI and uses clinical neuroimaging to explain the relationship between brain injury and clinical symptoms. Chapters 2 and 3 offer practical guidance on the medical evaluation and neuropsychological assessment of persons with TBI, respectively. In these chapters, the authors advise applying well-accepted clinical case definitions to history taking and interpretation; recommend thorough consideration of the broad differential diagnosis for early and late postinjury neuropsychiatric disturbances; encourage use of valid and reliable measures to characterize posttraumatic cognitive, emotional, behavioral, sensory, and motor disturbances; and highlight the need to integrate physical, neurological, and mental status examinations, as well as other neurodiagnostic tests, into a comprehensive neuropsychiatric assessment.

The remaining chapters provide concise reviews of the epidemiology, assessment, and treatment of cognitive (Chapters 4 and 5), emotional (Chapters 6–8), behavioral (Chapters 9–12), and other neurological (Chapters 13–16) disturbances among persons with TBI. Chapters focusing more specifically on TBI among older individuals (Chapter 17), athletes (Chapter 18), and military service members and Veterans (Chapter 19) are offered. The diagnostically and therapeutically challenging problem of persistent symptoms after concussion is addressed in detail (Chapter 20), after which the ethical issues and methods of forensic assessment of persons with TBI are considered (Chapter 21). Finally, suggested readings and Web sites relevant to clinicians and to individuals and families affected by TBI are provided in the appendixes.

Because this is a treatment manual rather than an academic monograph, the chapters and reference lists in this volume are brief by design and necessity. Tables and figures are used to organize complex information sets and to make the content more accessible and clinically relevant. Each chapter ends with Key Clinical Points, highlighting concepts, assessment issues, and management approaches useful in everyday clinical practice. Readers are referred to the *Textbook of Traumatic Brain Injury*, 2nd Edition (Silver et al. 2011), for complementary in-depth reviews of the topics addressed in this volume.

This volume was developed over several years, during which the editors balanced the goal of rapid publication against the need to craft a concise, cohesive, and enduring work. We anticipate that this book, thoughtfully considered and carefully completed, will enhance readers' understanding of TBI and inform usefully their care of persons affected by brain injuries.

David B. Arciniegas, M.D.
Nathan D. Zasler, M.D.
Rodney D. Vanderploeg, Ph.D.
Michael S. Jaffee, M.D.

## REFERENCE

Silver JM, McAllister TW, Yudofsky SC: Textbook of Traumatic Brain Injury, 2nd Edition. Washington, DC, American Psychiatric Publishing, 2011

# Acknowledgments

◆

*We are indebted to* Deborah Warden, M.D., for inspiring the creation of this book and facilitating its development, and to Robert E. Hales, M.D., and John McDuffie of American Psychiatric Publishing for their consistent encouragement and unwavering support throughout our work together. We thank our chapter authors for their commitment to improving the care of persons with TBI, excellent contributions to this volume, and patience during the final stages of its production. We appreciate our colleagues, students, friends, family, and advisers who offered insights, feedback, support, encouragement, and forbearance during our development of this volume, especially the following: Laura B. Arciniegas, J.D.; Gabriel Arciniegas; Rafael Arciniegas; Lisa Zasler; Aaron Zasler; Anya Zasler; Maia Zasler; Maytal Zasler; Michelle Koidin Jaffee; Clara Jaffee; Tessa Jaffee; Kimberly L. Frey, M.S.; C. Alan Anderson, M.D.; Hal S. Wortzel, M.D.; Jody Newman, M.A.; Jonathan M. Silver, M.D.; Thomas W. McAllister, M.D.; and Stuart C. Yudofsky, M.D. We also are deeply grateful to our patients, military service members, Veterans, and their families, with whom it is our privilege to work and by whom we are taught every day about living with TBI and its consequences.

This book would not have been possible without T. Angelita Garcia, who served as Managing Editor for this project at the University of Colorado School of Medicine. Ms. Garcia facilitated communications between the editors, authors, and publisher; reviewed the entire manuscript; made suggestions for clarifying and simplifying the text; constructed a master database of all citations used in this work; secured permissions for the use of materials reproduced from other works; and assembled the final manuscript for submission. Her superlative work on this project was essential to its completion, and we deeply appreciate her efforts.

This work was supported in part by the Henry M. Jackson Foundation for the Advancement of Military Medicine. We are grateful for their support and for their commitment to disseminating knowledge about TBI and its management that will benefit members of the armed forces and civilians alike.

# PART I

# INTRODUCTION

# CHAPTER 1

# Overview of Traumatic Brain Injury

*Erin D. Bigler, Ph.D.*
*William L. Maxwell, Ph.D., Sc.D.*

*Traumatic brain injury* (TBI) is a common occurrence and a major public health concern (Lin et al. 2010). According to an epidemiological study based on hospital records in the United States, approximately 51,000 Americans die each year after TBI, with over 1.2 million individuals evaluated in the emergency department (ED) and an additional 290,000 hospitalized (Rutland-Brown et al. 2006). Mild TBI (mTBI) accounts for 80%–90% of ED visits (Zaloshnja et al. 2008). Milder forms of TBI are underdiagnosed in the ED (Powell et al. 2008), and many cases of mTBI are never seen in an ED. As a result, estimates of TBI underrepresent the scope of this problem, which may exceed 2 million cases per year in the United States (Langlois et al. 2006). In a Canadian study that examined not only ED records but also clinic and family practice records within a health care provider system, Ryu et al. (2009) observed the rate of all TBIs to be as high as 653 in 100,000. Hyder et al. (2007) provide a worldwide estimate of 10 million or more people per year affected by TBI. TBI disproportionately occurs in males age 25 years and younger and in patients older than age 65 years (Langlois et al. 2006).

The goal of this chapter is to provide readers with a brief review of the definitions, the neuroanatomy, and the pathophysiology of TBI.

A brief discussion of the relationships between the neuropathology and clinical consequences of TBI is offered as an introduction to the chapters that follow. Given the clinical focus of this volume, neuroimaging is used to illustrate these relationships.

## DEFINITIONS

*Traumatic brain injury* is defined as a traumatically induced physiological disruption of brain function and/or structure resulting from the application of a biomechanical force to the head, rapid acceleration and/or deceleration, or blast-related forces (Kay et al. 1993). TBI is typically classified by the mechanism of injury (e.g., motor vehicle accident, fall, assault, blast), whether the cranium has been breached (penetrating or nonpenetrating), neuroimaging findings, and clinical severity of physical injuries to brain and body (i.e., injury severity score). Although mTBI remains a subject of controversy, the most widely accepted definition of this condition was developed by the American Congress of Rehabilitation Medicine (Box 1–1) (Kay et al. 1993). Injuries whose severity characteristics exceed the limits set in this definition are regarded as moderate to severe and are clarified using other severity metrics (see Chapter 2, "Medical Evaluation"). The most common approach to characterizing TBI severity among persons presenting to the hospital at the time of injury is to use the Glasgow Coma Scale (Teasdale and Jennett 1974), shown in Table 1–1.

The terms *concussion* and *mild TBI* often are used interchangeably in the literature. In the area of sports-related TBI, *concussion* is the more commonly used term. The Zurich consensus statement, developed at the Third International Conference on Concussion in Sport (McCrory et al. 2009), outlines the minimal necessary and sufficient criteria for the presence of a brain injury in this context (Box 1–2). Although sports concussion is a form of mTBI, the majority of mTBIs occur in nonathletes as a consequence of falls, motor vehicle accidents, or assaults. Accordingly, the diagnostic criteria outlined in the Zurich consensus statement do not apply to many other mTBIs.

## ANATOMY OF TRAUMATIC BRAIN INJURY

### Macroscopic Injury

The brain is among the most complex of all biological systems, yet in all mammals its protection from trauma is but a primitive bony casing—

---

**BOX 1–1.   THE AMERICAN CONGRESS OF REHABILITATION MEDICINE DEFINITION OF MILD TRAUMATIC BRAIN INJURY**

---

A traumatically induced physiological disruption of brain function, as manifested by at least one of the following:

1.   Any period of loss of consciousness

2.   Any loss of memory for events immediately before or after the accident

3.   Any alteration in mental state at the time of the accident

4.   Focal neurological deficit(s) that may or may not be transient

The severity of injury also has the following characteristics:

a.   Loss of consciousness of no more than approximately 30 minutes

b.   Glasgow Coma Scale score, when available, of 13–15 at 30 minutes postinjury

c.   Posttraumatic amnesia, if present, lasting not longer than 24 hours

---

*Source.*   Adapted from Kay T, Harrington DE, Adams RE, et al.: "Definition of Mild Traumatic Brain Injury: Report From the Mild Traumatic Brain Injury Committee of the Head Injury Interdisciplinary Special Interest Group of the American Congress of Rehabilitation Medicine." *Journal of Head Trauma Rehabilitation* 8:86–87, 1993.

---

the skull. Bone thickness provides a sturdy barrier between the outside world and the intracranial environment, and for common bumps and blows to the head this barrier protects the intracranial contents exceptionally well and efficiently.

The brain is partly held in place within the three cranial fossae, or cavities, as shown in Figure 1–1 (Blumenfeld 2010). The meninges between the irregular surface of the skull and the brain surface readily support the brain for the kinds of normal movements that humans make, such as jumping, tumbling, and bipedal running. In people below the age of about 40, the brain almost fully fills the cranial vault, being cradled within the three fossae; the two cerebral hemispheres are separated in

**TABLE 1–1.** Glasgow Coma Scale

| Area assessed | Scoring |
| --- | --- |
| Eye opening | 1: None<br>2: To pain<br>3: To speech<br>4: Spontaneous |
| Best verbal response | 1: None<br>2: Incomprehensible speech<br>3: Inappropriate speech<br>4: Confused conversation<br>5: Oriented |
| Best motor response | 1: None<br>2: Extension to painful stimuli (decerebrate posturing)<br>3: Abnormal flexion to painful stimuli (decorticate posturing)<br>4: Flexion/withdrawal to painful stimuli<br>5: Localizing response<br>6: Obeys commands |

*Note.* The Glasgow Coma Scale (GCS) score comprises the values from the three component tests (eye, verbal, and motor scales). Head injuries are classified as severe (GCS 3–8), moderate (GCS 9–12), or mild (GCS 13–15).

*Source.* Teasdale G, Jennett B: Assessment of coma and impaired consciousness: a practical scale. Lancet 2:81–84, 1974.

the midsagittal plane by the falx cerebri, and the tentorium cerebelli provides transverse support between the occipital and temporal cerebral lobes and the cerebellum. Being firmly supported under normal conditions, the brain has little opportunity for any adventitious movement.

Approximately 85–100 cm$^3$ of cerebrospinal fluid (CSF) is within the cranial cavity, and approximately 35 cm$^3$ of CSF is within the ventricular system of the brain. Intraventricular CSF exerts an outward pressure gradient that keeps the brain from collapsing inward, and overall CSF pressure probably exerts a stabilizing effect on the brain and spinal cord under normal conditions. In combination with the overlying sturdy dura mater, the thin layer of CSF on the surface of the brain within the subarachnoid space provides an additional buffer between the inner table of the skull and the brain, where the combination of intraventricular CSF, subarachnoid CSF, and the dura all act somewhat as shock absorbers for anything that jostles the head.

---

**BOX 1–2. DEFINITION AND CHARACTERISTICS OF CONCUSSION IN SPORT ESTABLISHED AT THE THIRD INTERNATIONAL CONFERENCE ON CONCUSSION IN SPORT**

- Concussion is defined as a complex pathophysiological process affecting the brain, induced by traumatic biomechanical forces.

- Concussion may be caused by either a direct blow to the head, face, or neck or a blow elsewhere on the body with an "impulsive" force transmitted to the head.

- Concussion typically results in the rapid onset of short-lived impairment of neurologic function that resolves spontaneously.

- Concussion may result in neuropathological changes, but the acute clinical symptoms largely reflect a functional disturbance rather than a structural injury.

- Concussion results in a graded set of clinical symptoms that may or may not involve loss of consciousness. Resolution of the clinical and cognitive symptoms typically follows a sequential course. In a small percentage of cases, however, postconcussive symptoms may be prolonged.

- No abnormality on standard structural neuroimaging studies is seen in concussion.

*Source.* McCrory et al. 2009.

---

Unfortunately for the modern human, the high-impact forces and rapid acceleration or deceleration of the head experienced in a motor vehicle–pedestrian collision are far different from what the human brain was evolutionarily designed to handle. The very structures that protect the brain under normal conditions now become its foes. The greater wing of the sphenoid, petrous temporal bone, crista galli, sella turcica, tentorium cerebelli, and falx cerebri within the three cranial fossae all become sources of mechanical deformation of the brain. The bony protuberances within the skull result in contusion and are the sites of greatest strain on brain tissues. These anatomical factors most commonly damage the frontotemporal, diencephalic, and cerebellar regions of the brain (Figure 1–1). These anatomical features confer regional vulnerabilities to the brain during TBI, in-

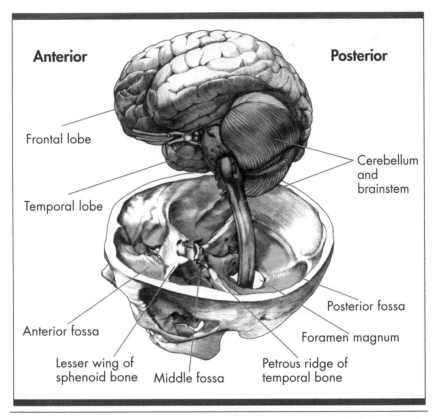

**FIGURE 1–1.** Anterior, middle, and posterior cranial fossae in relation to the base of the brain, highlighting areas vulnerable to compression and contusion when biomechanical forces are applied to the head.

*See Plate 1 to view this figure in color.*

*Source.*    Reprinted from Blumenfeld H: *Neuroanatomy Through Clinical Cases,* 2nd Edition. Sunderland, MA, Sinauer Associates, © 2010. Used with permission.

cluding focal contusions (Figure 1–2) (Ropper and Gorson 2007) and more diffuse injuries, especially to white matter (Bigler et al. 2010). Concussion results from a rotational motion of the cerebral hemispheres in the anterior-posterior plane, around the fulcrum of the fixed-in-place upper brain stem. Neuronal physiology is disrupted at the level of the reticular activating system (situated in the midbrain and diencephalic region), where the maximal rotational forces are induced. The areas most vulnerable to TBI and the neuropsychiatric functions they support are outlined in Table 1–2.

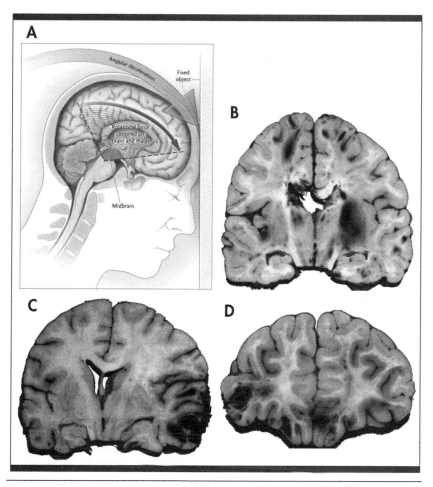

**FIGURE 1–2.** Illustration of traumatic brain injury (TBI) biomechanics and postmortem coronal sections of brain.

*See Plate 2 to view this figure in color.*

*Panel A:* Movement of the brain in response to biomechanical force application. *Panels B, C, and D:* Specimens obtained from patients who sustained TBI in road traffic accidents who died shortly thereafter. Hemorrhagic lesions are seen in the corpus callosum, midline structures, and basal ganglia (*B*), at the lateral aspect of the right temporal lobe (*C*), and on the inferior aspects of the frontal lobes (*D*). The near midline hemorrhagic loci are characteristic of traumatic axonal injury.

*Source.* Panel A reprinted from Ropper AH, Gorson KC: "Clinical Practice: Concussion." *New England Journal of Medicine* 356:166–172, 2007. Used with permission of the Massachusetts Medical Society. Panels B, C, and D reprinted from Graham DI, Nicoll JAR, Bone I: *Introduction to Neuropathology.* London, Hodder Education Publishing, 2006. Used with permission.

**TABLE 1–2.** Brain areas most vulnerable to traumatic brain injury, neuropsychiatric functions in which they are involved, and neuropsychiatric consequences of injury to these areas

| BRAIN AREA | RELEVANT ELEMENTS | EFFECTS OF NEUROTRAUMA |
|---|---|---|
| Frontal lobes | Dorsolateral prefrontal cortices | Executive dysfunction |
| | Ventral (especially lateral orbitofrontal) cortices | Disturbances of comportment and social judgment, including emotional, social, sexual, physical disinhibition |
| | Inferolateral prefrontal cortex | Impaired working memory |
| | Anterior cingulate cortex | Decreased goal-directed cognition, emotion, and behavior (i.e., apathy) |
| Temporal lobes | Temporopolar cortex | Klüver-Bucy–like syndromes, impaired socioemotional processing, loss of empathy, semantic aphasia, visual (object) agnosia, face processing deficits or, rarely, amnesic associative prosopagnosia |
| | Entorhinal-hippocampal complex | Sensory gating deficits, impaired declarative new learning, contributions to attention and working memory impairments |
| | Amygdala | Impaired emotional learning, affective placidity |
| White matter | Upper brain stem, parasagittal white matter, corpus callosum, superficial gray-white matter junctions | Slowed and inefficient information processing; lesions to discrete pathways or tracts that impair information processing in the networks to which the areas contribute |
| | Uncinate fasciculus | Impaired verbal memory; impaired self-awareness, particularly as regards experience of continuous self over time |

**TABLE 1–2.** Brain areas most vulnerable to traumatic brain injury, neuropsychiatric functions in which they are involved, and neuropsychiatric consequences of injury to these areas *(continued)*

| BRAIN AREA | RELEVANT ELEMENTS | EFFECTS OF NEUROTRAUMA |
|---|---|---|
| Thalamus | Motor, sensory, association, limbic, midline, intralaminar, reticular nuclei | Impairment of voluntary motor function, coordination, and motor learning; primary and secondary sensory functions; cognitive, emotional, behavioral, and arousal functions |
| Hypothalamus | Anterior, tuberal, and posterior (including mammillary) nuclei | Autonomic dysfunction, impaired thermoregulation, altered feeding behaviors, endocrine abnormalities, altered sleep-wake and other circadian cycles, pathological laughter or anger |
| Ventral forebrain | Ch1, Ch2, Ch3, Ch4 | Impaired sensory gating, attention, declarative memory, and executive function; hyposmia or anosmia |
| Upper brain stem and brain stem–diencephalic junction | Reticulothalamic system (Ch5, Ch6) | Impaired or absent arousal, including coma |
| | Reticulocortical system, including DA, NE, 5-HT, and Ch5-6 | Diminished arousal, reduced clarity of awareness of the environment, ineffective neural engagement in information processing |

*Note.* 5-HT = serotonin; Ch = cholinergic; DA = dopamine; NE = norepinephrine.

*Source.* Table courtesy of David B. Arciniegas, M.D., University of Colorado School of Medicine. Used with permission.

# Insights From Structural Neuroimaging

Contemporary neuroimaging permits visualization of the major pathologies of TBI from the acute injury period and over months or years thereafter. Computed tomography (CT) of the head is one of the first evaluative procedures typically performed on an individual presenting with a TBI. The advantages of CT include the rapidity with which it can be performed and its sensitivity to significant edema, hemorrhage, contusion, skull fracture, and other critical features of acute brain injury.

Early postinjury CT makes clear that TBI is a heterogeneous condition that injures brain tissues in diverse ways (Figure 1–3) (Saatman et al. 2008). Dramatic focal lesions evident on CT also are generally accompanied by some degree of diffuse injuries to the brain (Bigler et al. 2010). These types of day-of-injury CT scans establish imaging baselines against which subsequent changes and long-term TBI outcomes may be compared.

One of the most common long-term changes, particularly in moderate to severe TBI, is generalized cerebral atrophy. Evidence of such changes may be observed with magnetic resonance imaging (MRI) of the brain as soon as a few weeks postinjury (Bigler et al. 2010). Neuropathological studies also demonstrate postinjury reductions in total brain volume evidence on in vivo neuroimaging. For example, Maxwell et al. (2010) compared brains obtained from healthy subjects who died from non-neurological causes to those of individuals who died after achieving post-TBI outcomes of moderate disability or vegetative state. Brain weight among the healthy subjects was 1,442.7±105.0 g, whereas brain weights were 1,329.6±202.9 g among subjects with moderate post-TBI disability and 1,275±135.5 g among subjects with vegetative states. The observed reductions in brain mass and volume were more severe among subjects with greater severities of injury and worse premortem outcomes.

The volume of individual gray matter structures in regions vulnerable to TBI may be reduced by TBI, which may secondarily result in volume loss in structures that are highly connected to injured brain areas (Bigler et al. 2010; Ross 2011). Loss of thalamic volume is of particular interest in light of this structure's role as a subcortical relay station and integration center between brain areas and for afferent sensory information ascending from the spinal cord to the brain (Fearing et al. 2008; Little et al. 2010; Maxwell et al. 2004). The integrative role of the thalamus within the entire central nervous system confers the potential for changes in this structure, perhaps even subtle ones, to produce multidimensional cognitive, emotional, behavioral, and sensorimotor deficits and functional limitations.

Surface contusions are most common in the frontal polar and inferior orbitofrontal regions, the inferior to medial and temporal po-

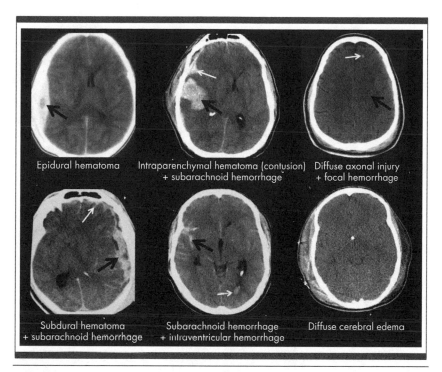

Epidural hematoma

Intraparenchymal hematoma (contusion) + subarachnoid hemorrhage

Diffuse axonal injury + focal hemorrhage

Subdural hematoma + subarachnoid hemorrhage

Subarachnoid hemorrhage + intraventricular hemorrhage

Diffuse cerebral edema

**FIGURE 1–3.** Axial computed tomography scans from patients with Glasgow Coma Scale scores <8, highlighting the heterogeneity of pathologies among persons with similar clinical presentations.

*Black arrows* indicate the first type of pathology listed below each image, and *white arrows* indicate the second type of pathology described.

*Source.* Adapted from Saatman KE, Duhaime AC, Bullock R, et al.: "Classification of Traumatic Brain Injury for Targeted Therapies." *Journal of Neurotrauma* 25:719–738, 2008. The publisher for this copyrighted material is Mary Ann Liebert, Inc. Used with permission.

lar region, and the cerebellum. However, structural damage extends beyond the region of injury identified by conventional neuroimaging (Figures 1–4 and 1–5). The visible effects of TBI on tracts, pathways, and connections demonstrated using diffusion tensor imaging (DTI) in Figures 1–4 and 1–5 are dramatic. However, the best methods of performing and using DTI in clinical practice are not yet fully developed. Tractography is one method of analyzing DTI data, and it is most likely to be revealing among persons with moderate to severe TBI. Although white matter tract discontinuities may be identified among some individuals with persistent symptoms after mild TBI

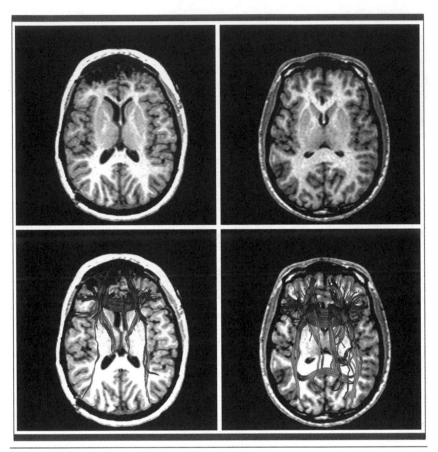

**FIGURE 1–4.** Atrophy of association and commissural tracts of the anterior of the corpus callosum associated with frontal lobe lesion demonstrated by T1-weighted axial magnetic resonance imaging and diffusion tensor imaging in an individual with traumatic brain injury (*left column*) compared to a healthy age-matched individual (*right column*).

*See Plate 3 to view this figure in color.*

*Source.* From Oni MB, Wilde EA, Bigler ED, et al.: "Diffusion Tensor Imaging Analysis of Frontal Lobes in Pediatric Traumatic Brain Injury." *Journal of Child Neurology* 25:976–984, 2010. © 2010 by Sage Publications. Reprinted with permission of Sage Publications.

(Figure 1–6) (Rutgers et al. 2008), visual inspection of DTI tractography images among persons with mTBI often is unrevealing. Quantitative computer-aided examination of the DTI-derived metric fractional anisotropy (FA) provides a method of characterizing white

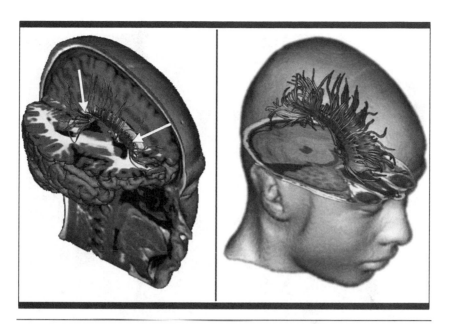

**FIGURE 1–5.** Diffusion tensor imaging (DTI) of the corpus callosum and the consequences of severe traumatic brain injury (TBI)–induced callosal damage on interhemispheric connectivity.

*See Plate 4 to view this figure in color.*

On the *right* is a three-dimensional reconstruction of normal-appearing callosal projection fibers derived from DTI tractography. On the *left* is a three-dimensional reconstruction of a magnetic resonance image from an individual who sustained a severe TBI, showing a partial sagittal view of the medial aspect of the left hemisphere in which the corpus callosum is identified in *white* and TBI-related callosal thinning and loss of projecting fibers are indicated by the *white arrows.*

matter integrity that may facilitate identification of pathological changes produced by TBI. Increased FA in central white matter (where long tracts course), the corpus callosum, thalamus, and upper brainstem in the acute to early postacute stage (within 6 days of injury) may reflect an early postinjury inflammatory reaction (Chu et al. 2010). As that inflammatory reaction subsides and axonal integrity degrades, FA values are reduced (Lipton et al. 2009).

The neuroimaging methods used herein to illustrate the anatomy of TBI offer promise of imminent advances in the clinical characterization of TBI in the early and late postinjury periods. The present technologies permit identification of gross structural abnormalities (e.g., focal contusions, diffuse axonal injury, cerebral edema, intracranial

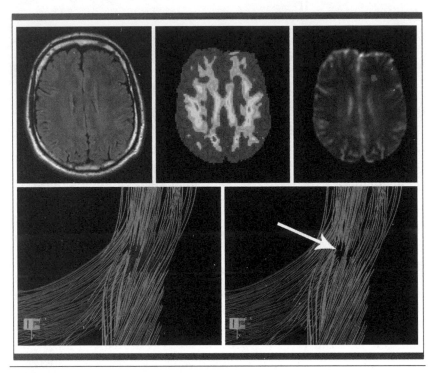

**FIGURE 1–6.** Diffusion tensor imaging (DTI) tractography demonstrating discontinuity of white matter tracts crossing the anterior aspect of the corpus callosum and interfacing with tracts within the region of the frontal forceps.

*See Plate 5 to view this figure in color.*

Fluid-attenuated inversion recovery image in the *top left* shows no abnormalities. Analysis of the fractional anisotropy (FA) map (*top middle*) identifies a region with reduced FA in the white matter of the left frontal lobe, also indicated on the T2-weighted image (*top right*). That region of interest includes fibers within the forceps minor and fronto-temporo-occipital fibers (*bottom left, superior oblique view*), the respective fibers of which are discontinuous (*arrow, bottom right image*).

*Source.* Reprinted from Rutgers DR, Toulgoat F, Cazejust J, et al.: "White Matter Abnormalities in Mild Traumatic Brain Injury: A Diffusion Tensor Imaging Study." *American Journal of Neuroradiology* 29:514–519, 2008. © 2008. Used with permission of American Society of Neuroradiology.

hemorrhages and hematomas), volumetric abnormalities, and altered white matter integrity. Emerging methods of analyzing DTI data, as well as data derived from magnetic resonance spectroscopy, functional MRI, and other advanced imaging techniques, may facilitate identification of more subtle structural abnormalities as well.

# Microscopic Injury

The basis for any level of impairment of neurological function in TBI, regardless of how short lived or chronic the impairment, occurs at the level of the neuron—the fundamental unit of the central nervous system. Neural function is disrupted at the moment of injury by disturbed cell membrane integrity, subsequent ionic changes and disturbed cellular metabolism, altered blood flow within the cerebral microvasculature, and altered transport and abnormal release of neurotransmitters (especially excitatory amino acids such as glutamate), among other processes. Once normal physiological homeostasis has returned, and provided there are no other neuropathophysiological insults, neurons can resume normal function. This disturbance in function, but not structure, may explain the rapid and complete recovery that is commonly observed in the mildest forms of TBI, including sports concussion.

More severe TBI damages neuronal structure and supportive glial cells, leading to dysfunction as well as the potential for neuronal death and subsequent reductions in brain connectivity. Neurotrauma affects axons, dendrites, and cell bodies of neurons. The cell soma may be exposed to transient depolarization, compression due to a related hematoma and development of hypovolemia or ischemia, and excitotoxic insults, among other lesser risks. The axon, located within both subcortical and deep white matter, may be exposed directly to mechanical forces that result in primary axotomy, or to pathophysiological changes that potentiate the incidence of secondary axotomy. Substantial evidence indicates that axonal injury is not the result of neurotrauma-induced "shearing" but rather is the product of a pathological cascade that develops over several hours postinjury and separates axons into fragments (Maxwell et al. 1997). This process is referred to as secondary axotomy, the time course for which differs between axons in different white matter tracts. Primary and secondary axotomy may signal a neuron to enter programmed cell death, which may result in increasing disconnection of cortical and subcortical neuronal circuits during the chronic phase of TBI (Figure 1–7).

Aberrant regulation of ion fluxes across cell membranes is an early and important pathophysiological event. Normal neural transmission is dependent on a rapid exchange of sodium ions regulated in part by voltage-gated sodium channels, of which the Nav1.6 $Na^+$ channel is probably of greatest importance (Caldwell et al. 2000). Transient

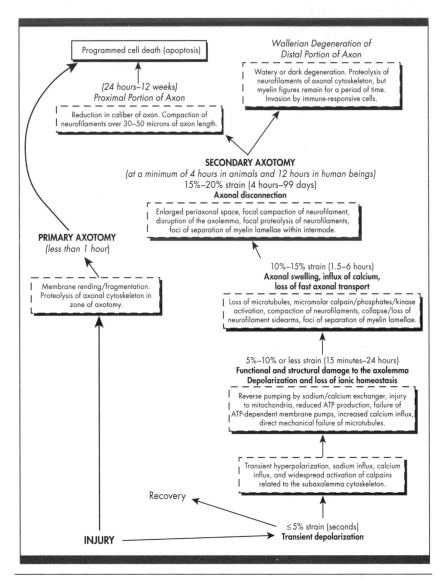

**FIGURE 1–7.** Schematic of the time sequence for primary and secondary axotomy following traumatic brain injury.

mechanical loading at the time of injury mechanically damages Nav1.6 Na$^+$ channels at nodes of Ranvier in adult myelinated central nervous system fibers. Damaged Nav1.6 channels form "pores" that allow an irreversible influx of sodium ions (Stys 2005; Wolf et al. 2001). The resulting ionic redistribution across the axolemma hyperpolarizes the membrane, which compromises $Na^+/Ca^{2+}$ exchange (Wang et al. 2009) and leads to an influx of free calcium ions that impairs or halts neural transmission. Calcium is released from intracellular sources when injury is severe and results in foci of calcium at damaged nodes of Ranvier (Figure 1–8).

Axonal mitochondria attempt to remove excess calcium from the axoplasm but are rapidly saturated by excess free calcium. Sodium influx following TBI also may exacerbate calcium cycling across mitochondrial membranes, due to the energy-dependent reversal of the sodium/calcium exchanger. The subsequent intracellular accumulation further disrupts the metabolic integrity of the neuron (Büki and Povlishock 2006). At the same time, calcium influx results in spontaneous depolymerization of microtubules and results in focal loss of fast axonal transport (Maxwell et al. 1997; Pettus and Povlishock 1996).

Loss of fast axonal transport is probably an early event that does not progress over time. Activated calpains (calcium-dependent cysteine proteases) then act upon structural proteins of the subaxolemma cytoskeleton. This produces protein degradation that disrupts the protein-based organization within the axon. Breakdown of spectrin, the cytoskeletal protein, occurs along the length of axons in the first hours and then again days after the initial injury (Saatman et al. 2003). As this process progresses, axonal swellings and bulbs develop as axons undergo fragmentation and secondary axotomy (Maxwell et al. 2003a) and other neuroinflammatory processes occur (Ziebell and Morganti-Kossmann 2010).

Microtubules (which provide for rapid movement of membrane-limited intracellular components or organelles via fast axonal transport) and neurofilaments (which provide mechanical stability of axons) are also damaged by TBI. A characteristic change in the organization of the axonal cytoskeleton after TBI is *compaction,* a reduction in spacing between neurofilaments (Büki and Povlishock 2006). Sites of compaction of neurofilaments along the length of an axon are landmarks for dissolution or breakage of the axolemma that characterizes secondary axotomy (Maxwell et al. 2003b). A minority of the total number of nerve fibers within an injured tract or area of white matter are affected (i.e., there are small numbers of damaged and degenerating damaged axons among a larger number of intact axons); this is a unique feature of TBI (Jafari et al. 1998; Maxwell et al. 2003b). Some studies suggest that activation of calpains upon post-traumatic intra-axonal influx of $Ca^{2+}$ is a key step in the development

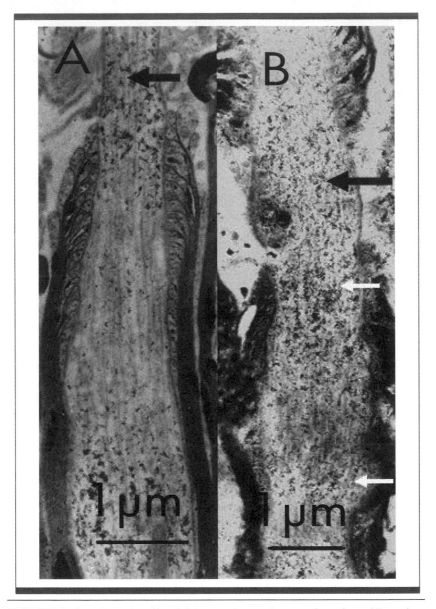

**FIGURE 1–8.**   Longitudinal thin sections of central nodes of Ranvier, processed via the pyroantimonate technique to allow visualization of foci of intracellular free calcium.

In the uninjured animal (*A*), dark scattered deposits are localized to the node of Ranvier (*black arrow*) and the internode (*bottom*). At 15 minutes after traumatic brain injury (*B*), dark scattered deposits are more uniformly distributed throughout the axoplasm, reflecting uncontrolled influx of free calcium ions into the damaged axon.

of compaction of neurofilaments (Büki and Povlishock 2006). Evidence derived from patients in the late postinjury period suggests that loss of white matter volume may continue over at least months following TBI. Very few studies report degenerating or damaged axons during the late postinjury period of TBI (Bramlett and Dietrich 2007; DiLeonardi et al. 2009).

In summary, at the moment of traumatic impact, biomechanical forces induce a series of pathological changes that take minutes to months to stabilize. The variable time course of these neuropathological changes likely relates to the variable clinical course observed in patients with TBI at differing postinjury time intervals. What the clinician may outwardly observe among patients with TBI at any given postinjury time point is the sum total of pathological as well as adaptive and restorative processes that have either occurred or may be occurring. Understanding this pathobiology provides insights for the clinician into what the brain of the patient has experienced and how that may relate to his or her symptoms.

# CLINICAL CONSEQUENCES OF TRAUMATIC BRAIN INJURY

The clinical consequences of TBI depend on a host of preinjury, injury-related, and postinjury factors. Important among these are the type and severity of injury, the presence and extent of focal and/or diffuse pathologies, and the time postinjury at which outcome is assessed. Other important variables that influence clinical outcome are the backdrop of the patient's preinjury ability or capacity and the medical and psychiatric history against which a TBI occurs.

## Cognition

As discussed above in "Anatomy of Traumatic Brain Injury," nonspecific white matter and frontotemporal damage in conjunction with disruption of thalamocortical integrity lead to posttraumatic cognitive problems in the domains of attention, speed of processing, memory, and executive functioning (see Chapter 5, "Cognitive Impairments"). Neuropsychological test results for a person with TBI typically show a reduction in performance in these domains as compared to a control sample or from assumed premorbid ability level (see Chapter 3, "Neuropsychological Assessment").

For example, Figure 1–9 depicts neuropsychological performance assessed longitudinally at approximately 2 months and 1 year postinjury among a group of subjects with Glasgow Coma Scale scores of 6–13 and intracranial abnormalities on day-of-injury CT imaging (Bendlin et al. 2008)—that is, subjects with complicated mild to severe TBI. The most distinct and severe deficits occur proximate to the time of injury. Reduced cognitive processing speed, memory recall, and executive dysfunction are most prominent in the subacute period, and all areas of cognitive function are impaired, when compared to healthy control subjects, in that period as well. Although cognition improves substantially by 1 year postinjury, it does not match that of healthy comparison subjects. This study also investigated pathological changes in the brain using DTI and volumetric MRI analyses, which revealed abnormalities in the corpus callosum and frontotemporal white matter, corresponding to decreased processing speed, as well as frontotemporal atrophy, underlying impaired memory recall and executive function.

A meta-analysis of 16 studies that included a total of 1,380 patients with moderate to severe TBI examined using a broad spectrum of neuropsychological assessments during the first 18 months postinjury and again 4.5 to 11 years postinjury identified "robust, persisting impairments" at both postinjury epochs (Ruttan et al. 2008). Cognition in general was adversely affected by TBI, and attention, processing speed, memory, and executive function were particularly impaired. Thus, in moderate to severe TBI, the level of cognitive deficit at 1 year becomes predictive of persistent chronic deficits.

The cognitive and neuroimaging consequences of mTBI are more challenging to interpret. As noted earlier in this chapter (see "Anatomy of Traumatic Brain Injury"), mTBI is often associated with early cognitive deficits and neurobehavioral symptoms (Levin et al. 1987) (see also Chapter 5, "Cognitive Impairments," and Chapter 18, "Athletes and Sports-Related Concussion"). A subcommittee of the Institute of Medicine's 2007–2008 work group evaluating literature describing the long-term health effects of TBI concluded that there is insufficient evidence of chronic cognitive impairments after a single mild civilian TBI (Dikmen et al. 2009). The authors of this report cautioned that a lack of significant group differences in cognitive functioning among persons with mTBI and appropriately matched comparators does not mean that no individuals in those groups had mTBI-related cognitive impairments. Some individuals may experi-

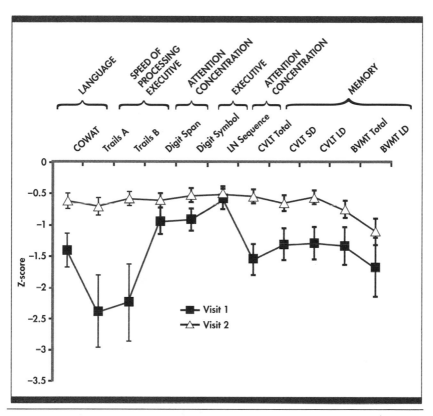

**FIGURE 1–9.** Neuropsychological performance at 2 months (Visit 1) and 1 year (Visit 2) after traumatic brain injury of at least complicated mild severity based on Z-score deviations from performance of a noninjured matched cohort assessed at similar time intervals.

BVMT=Brief Visual Memory Test; COWAT=Controlled Oral Word Association Test; CVLT=California Verbal Learning Test; LD=long delay; LN Sequence=Letter Number Sequencing test; SD=short delay; A=Trail Making Test Part A; Trails B=Trail Making Test Part B.

*Source.* Figure constructed using data presented in Bendlin et al. (2008).

ence late cognitive impairments as a result of the injurious effects of neurotrauma on cognitive-salient brain networks. However, other conditions and factors can mimic or mask such cognitive problems (Carroll et al. 2004; McCrea et al. 2009), and failure to account for them may lead to erroneous conclusions about the relationship between mTBI and long-term cognitive impairments (see Chapter 20, "Persistent Symptoms After a Concussion").

Similarly, conventional neuroimaging (especially CT imaging) is usually unrevealing among persons with mTBI. When abnormalities are present, they tend to be small hemorrhagic lesions or contusions that do not require medical intervention or necessitate hospitalization (Bigler 2004). However, the presence of such abnormalities on day-of-injury CT scans defines complicated mTBI (Williams et al. 1990) and is associated with worse long-term outcomes than uncomplicated mTBI (van der Naalt et al. 1999; Williams et al. 1990). The distinction between complicated and uncomplicated mTBI is blurred by newer imaging techniques, which are better able to detect small hemorrhages as well as metabolic and microstructural abnormalities that previously were opaque to detection by conventional neuroimaging (Morales et al. 2005) (Figure 1–10).

Traditional neuropsychological assessment methods often yield findings of adequate performance in patients with mTBI, even in those experiencing persistent symptoms, yet functional neuroimaging and DTI combined with neurocognitive assessment techniques that measure brain function in milliseconds often show abnormalities (Bigler and Bazarian 2010). It may be that more refined cognitive assessments are essential to reveal the symptoms and problems of patients surviving mTBI.

## Noncognitive Neuropsychiatric Functions

Exacerbation of preinjury psychiatric conditions and the appearance of new-onset neuropsychiatric symptoms are common among persons with TBI (Vaishnavi et al. 2009). Up to about 40% of persons with TBI have two or more psychiatric disorders, and a similar percentage experiences at least one unmet need for cognitive, emotional, or job assistance 1 year after injury. The entire spectrum of TBI severity, from mild to severe, is associated with an increase in psychiatric conditions. For example, in the United Kingdom, of patients admitted to the emergency department after head trauma, 54% experienced behavioral, 39% intellectual, and 29% locomotor disability at 5 years postinjury (Evans et al. 2003). In an Australian study, population levels of clinical depression rose from 17% of patients preinjury to 45% postinjury within the study group, generalized anxiety disorder rose from 13% to 38%, posttraumatic stress disorder increased from 4% to 14%, and panic disorders rose from 1% to 6% (Whelan-Goodinson et al. 2009, 2010).

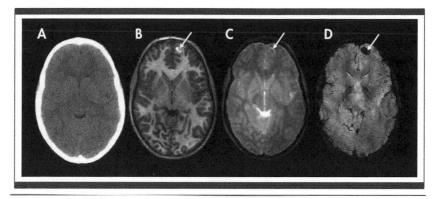

**FIGURE 1–10.** A comparison of neuroimaging methods for identifying day-of-injury intracranial abnormalities.

A normal day-of-injury computed tomography (CT) scan (*A*) is compared with axial T1-weighted magnetic resonance imaging (MRI) (*B*), axial magnetization transfer imaging (MTI) (*C*), and susceptibility-weighted imaging (SWI) (*D*), which were acquired 1 week postinjury. SWI reveals a left frontal hemorrhagic shear injury that is more extensive than the lesion seen on MTI and T1-weighted MRI (indicated by *arrows*) and that is not evident at all on CT.

*Source.* Reprinted from Bigler ED, Maxwell WL: "Neuropathy of Mild Traumatic Brain Injury: Relationship to Neuroimaging Findings." *Brain Imaging and Behavior* 6:108–136, 2012 [PMID: 22434552]. Used with permission of Springer Publishing.

The literature suggests that depression is the most common neuropsychiatric disorder to occur after TBI (Seel et al. 2010). However, and as reviewed extensively in this volume, other disorders of mood and affect, anxiety disorders, posttraumatic stress disorder, aggression, and impaired self-awareness are common neuropsychiatric sequelae of TBI as well. In light of the relationship of frontotemporal and limbic areas to emotion and behavior, as well as the vulnerability of these areas to neurotrauma, the relatively high frequency of emotional and behavioral disturbances common among persons with TBI is not surprising. The connections between frontal and limbic cortices are also vulnerable to disruption by neurotrauma; their disruption may contribute to posttraumatic emotional and behavioral changes by interfering with regulatory interconnections between limbic and other brain structures.

Sleep disturbances are common early and late consequences of TBI at all levels of injury severity (see Chapter 15, "Sleep and Fatigue"). Fatigue is a common posttraumatic symptom and is associated with damage to ventromedial prefrontal cortex (Pardini et al. 2010). A complex interplay between frontotemporolimbic regions is implicated in the neurobiology of motivation and drive (Paus 2001). Accordingly, disorders of diminished motivation (e.g., apathy) are common consequences of TBI (Lane-Brown and Tate 2009) (see Chapter 11, "Apathy"). Endocrine disturbances also may be produced by hypothalamic-pituitary injury (Kokshoorn et al. 2011), a type of injury that also may contribute to diminished drive and motivation after TBI.

Some studies (Ruttan et al. 2008; Till et al. 2008) have questioned the widely held view that cognitive gains made early in recovery are maintained in the long term. In studies of both adults and children, persistent deficits (or dysfunction) in memory, concentration, planning, and language functions have been reported (Anderson and Knight 2010; Hawley 2003), as well as decline in cognitive function in about 30% of survivors of moderate to severe TBI at 4.5–5 years after injury (Kennedy et al. 2009; Ruttan et al. 2008; Till et al. 2008). TBI may also be a risk factor for onset of dementia later in life (Bigler 2009; Omalu et al. 2011).

## Disability

TBI is a leading cause of disability, and an estimated 3.17 million to 3.32 million people in the United States (approximately 1% of the population) are living with long-term disability as a result of TBI (Zaloshnja et al. 2008). Among persons in the United States who received in-hospital treatment after TBI, approximately 43% develop residual disability (Selassie et al. 2008). In the United Kingdom, the annual incidence of posttraumatic disability 1 year after TBI is about 120 per 100,000 patients (Thornhill et al. 2000).

The economic burden of TBI and disability is estimated to be over $60 billion in the United States alone (Maas et al. 2008), with the worldwide impact projected to be in the trillions of dollars (Thurman et al. 2007). The care of and lifestyle changes entailed by TBI, its cognitive and neuropsychiatric sequelae, and the disability they produce represent a major economic, family, and psychosocial burden. Given this rate of disability, the overall physical, neuropsychiatric, and cognitive burden of having sustained a brain injury represents a major challenge in treating patients with TBI.

## CONCLUSION

This chapter reviewed the definitions, neuroanatomy, and pathophysiology of TBI. This review emphasized the vulnerability of frontotemporal, diencephalic, and cerebellar regions of the brain, as well as the white matter within and between these areas, and discussed insights derived from neuroimaging studies regarding focal as well as diffuse brain pathology following TBI. The clinical applications of these insights and neurodiagnostic techniques were also reviewed briefly, including the use of neuroimaging to establish a baseline against which neuroanatomic changes and clinical recoveries are compared. The pathological processes occurring at the neuronal level, including the pathological cascade that results in secondary axotomy, were reviewed, along with the implications of neuronal damage for physical, neurobehavioral, and neurocognitive outcome following TBI. Finally, a brief discussion of the relationships between the neuropathology and clinical consequences of TBI was offered. The subjects discussed briefly in this chapter are reviewed in detail in the remainder of this volume. The overview presented here also illustrates the need to develop more effective measures by which to prevent TBI and to protect against injury when it occurs. Such measures will decrease the substantial personal and economic costs entailed by TBI and improve the lives of individuals and families affected by such injuries.

## *Key Clinical Points*

- Traumatic brain injury is defined as a traumatically induced physiological disruption of brain function and/or structure resulting from the application of a biomechanical force to the head, rapid acceleration and/or deceleration, or blast-related forces.

- At a macroscopic level, TBI most often affects frontotemporal, diencephalic, and cerebellar regions of the brain, as well as the white matter within and between these areas.

- Biomechanical shear/strain forces damage axons and disrupt connections in the brain.

- Axonal damage may be immediately expressed within the first hours of the head injury as a primary axotomy; among those who survive a brain injury, axonal pathology develops over time and largely results in secondary axotomy.

- Neuroimaging is improving the detection of macroscopic pathologies of TBI; diffusion tensor imaging is a particularly interesting technology in light of its sensitivity to white matter pathology.

- TBI produces a wide range of cognitive and other neuropsychiatric problems in the early and late postinjury period; substantial recovery occurs in many persons sustaining such injuries, especially persons with mild TBI, but residual deficits are associated with disability and are costly to persons with TBI, their families, and society.

# REFERENCES

Anderson TM, Knight RG: The long-term effects of traumatic brain injury on the coordinative function of the central executive. J Clin Exp Neuropsychol 32:1074–1082, 2010

Bendlin BB, Ries ML, Lazar M, et al: Longitudinal changes in patients with traumatic brain injury assessed with diffusion-tensor and volumetric imaging. Neuroimage 42:503–514, 2008

Bigler ED: Neuropsychological results and neuropathological findings at autopsy in a case of mild traumatic brain injury. J Int Neuropsychol Soc 10:794–806, 2004

Bigler ED: Traumatic brain injury, in The American Psychiatric Publishing Textbook of Alzheimer Disease and Other Dementias. Edited by Weiner MF, Lipton AM. Washington, DC, American Psychiatric Publishing, 2009, pp 229–246

Bigler ED, Bazarian JJ: Diffusion tensor imaging: a biomarker for mild traumatic brain injury? Neurology 74:626–627, 2010

Bigler ED, Maxwell WL: Neuropathology of mild traumatic brain injury: relationship to neuroimaging findings. Brain Imaging Behav 6:108–136, 2012

Bigler ED, Abildskov TJ, Wilde EA, et al: Diffuse damage in pediatric traumatic brain injury: a comparison of automated versus operator-controlled quantification methods. Neuroimage 50:1017–1026, 2010

Blumenfeld H: Neuroanatomy Through Clinical Cases, 2nd Edition. Sunderland, MA, Sinauer Associates, 2010

Bramlett HM, Dietrich WD: Progressive damage after brain and spinal cord injury: pathomechanisms and treatment strategies. Prog Brain Res 161:125–141, 2007

Büki A, Povlishock JT: All roads lead to disconnection? Traumatic axonal injury revisited. Acta Neurochir (Wien) 148:181–193, discussion 193–194, 2006

Caldwell JH, Schaller KL, Lasher RS, et al: Sodium channel Na(v)1.6 is localized at nodes of Ranvier, dendrites, and synapses. Proc Natl Acad Sci USA 97:5616–5620, 2000

Carroll LJ, Cassidy JD, Peloso PM, et al: Prognosis for mild traumatic brain injury: results of the WHO Collaborating Centre Task Force on Mild Traumatic Brain Injury. J Rehabil Med 43(suppl):84–105, 2004

Chu Z, Wilde EA, Hunter JV, et al: Voxel-based analysis of diffusion tensor imaging in mild traumatic brain injury in adolescents. AJNR Am J Neuroradiol 31:340–346, 2010

Dikmen SS, Corrigan JD, Levin HS, et al: Cognitive outcome following traumatic brain injury. J Head Trauma Rehabil 24:430–438, 2009

DiLeonardi AM, Huh JW, Raghupathi R: Impaired axonal transport and neurofilament compaction occur in separate populations of injured axons following diffuse brain injury in the immature rat. Brain Res 1263:174–182, 2009

Evans SA, Airey MC, Chell SM, et al: Disability in young adults following major trauma: 5 year follow up of survivors. BMC Public Health 3:8, 2003

Fearing MA, Bigler ED, Wilde EA, et al: Morphometric MRI findings in the thalamus and brainstem in children after moderate to severe traumatic brain injury. J Child Neurol 23:729–737, 2008

Hawley CA: Reported problems and their resolution following mild, moderate and severe traumatic brain injury amongst children and adolescents in the UK. Brain Inj 17:105–129, 2003

Hyder AA, Wunderlich CA, Puvanachandra P, et al: The impact of traumatic brain injuries: a global perspective. NeuroRehabilitation 22:341–353, 2007

Jafari SS, Nielson M, Graham DI, et al: Axonal cytoskeletal changes after nondisruptive axonal injury, II: intermediate sized axons. J Neurotrauma 15:955–966, 1998

Kay T, Harrington DE, Adams RE, et al: Definition of mild traumatic brain injury: report from the Mild Traumatic Brain Injury Committee of the Head Injury Interdisciplinary Special Interest Group of the American Congress of Rehabilitation Medicine. J Head Trauma Rehabil 8:86–87, 1993

Kennedy MR, Wozniak JR, Muetzel RL, et al: White matter and neurocognitive changes in adults with chronic traumatic brain injury. J Int Neuropsychol Soc 15:130–136, 2009

Kokshoorn NE, Smit JW, Nieuwlaat WA, et al: Low prevalence of hypopituitarism after traumatic brain injury: a multicenter study. Eur J Endocrinol 165:225–231, 2011

Lane-Brown AT, Tate RL: Apathy after acquired brain impairment: a systematic review of non-pharmacological interventions. Neuropsychol Rehabil 19:481–516, 2009

Langlois JA, Rutland-Brown W, Wald MM: The epidemiology and impact of traumatic brain injury: a brief overview. J Head Trauma Rehabil 21:375–378, 2006

Levin HS, Mattis S, Ruff RM, et al: Neurobehavioral outcome following minor head injury: a three-center study. J Neurosurg 66:234–243, 1987

Lin MR, Chiu WT, Chen YJ, et al: Longitudinal changes in the health-related quality of life during the first year after traumatic brain injury. Arch Phys Med Rehabil 91:474–480, 2010

Lipton ML, Gulko E, Zimmerman ME, et al: Diffusion-tensor imaging implicates prefrontal axonal injury in executive function impairment following very mild traumatic brain injury. Radiology 252:816–824, 2009

Little DM, Kraus MF, Joseph J, et al: Thalamic integrity underlies executive dysfunction in traumatic brain injury. Neurology 74:558–564, 2010

Maas AI, Stocchetti N, Bullock R: Moderate and severe traumatic brain injury in adults. Lancet Neurol 7:728–741, 2008

Maxwell WL, Povlishock JT, Graham DL: A mechanistic analysis of nondisruptive axonal injury: a review. J Neurotrauma 14:419–440, 1997

Maxwell WL, Dhillon K, Harper L, et al: There is differential loss of pyramidal cells from the human hippocampus with survival after blunt head injury. J Neuropathol Exp Neurol 62:272–279, 2003a

Maxwell WL, Domleo A, McColl G, et al: Post-acute alterations in the axonal cytoskeleton after traumatic axonal injury. J Neurotrauma 20:151–168, 2003b

Maxwell WL, Pennington K, MacKinnon MA, et al: Differential responses in three thalamic nuclei in moderately disabled, severely disabled and vegetative patients after blunt head injury. Brain 127:2470–2478, 2004

Maxwell WL, MacKinnon MA, Stewart JE, et al: Stereology of cerebral cortex after traumatic brain injury matched to the Glasgow outcome score. Brain 133:139–160, 2010

McCrea M, Iverson GL, McAllister TW, et al: An integrated review of recovery after mild traumatic brain injury (MTBI): implications for clinical management. Clin Neuropsychol 23:1368–1390, 2009

McCrory P, Meeuwisse W, Johnston K, et al: Consensus statement on concussion in sport: the 3rd International Conference on Concussion in Sport, held in Zurich, November 2008. J Clin Neurosci 16:755–763, 2009

Morales DM, Marklund N, Lebold D, et al: Experimental models of traumatic brain injury: do we really need to build a better mousetrap? Neuroscience 136:971–989, 2005

Omalu B, Bailes J, Hamilton RL, et al: Emerging histomorphologic phenotypes of chronic traumatic encephalopathy in American athletes. Neurosurgery 69:173–183, discussion 183, 2011

Oni MB, Wilde EA, Bigler ED, et al: Diffusion tensor imaging analysis of frontal lobes in pediatric traumatic brain injury. J Child Neurol 25:976–984, 2010

Pardini M, Krueger F, Raymont V, et al: Ventromedial prefrontal cortex modulates fatigue after penetrating traumatic brain injury. Neurology 74:749–754, 2010

Paus T: Primate anterior cingulate cortex: where motor control, drive and cognition interface. Nat Rev Neurosci 2:417–424, 2001

Pettus EH Povlishock JT: Characterization of a distinct set of intra-axonal ultrastructural changes associated with traumatically induced alteration in axolemmal permeability. Brain Res 722(1–2):1–11, 1996

Powell JM, Ferraro JV, Dikmen SS, et al: Accuracy of mild traumatic brain injury diagnosis. Arch Phys Med Rehabil 89:1550–1555, 2008

Ropper AH, Gorson KC: Clinical practice: concussion. N Engl J Med 356:166–172, 2007

Ross DE: Review of longitudinal studies of MRI brain volumetry in patients with traumatic brain injury. Brain Inj 25:1271–1278, 2011

Rutgers DR, Toulgoat F, Cazejust J, et al: White matter abnormalities in mild traumatic brain injury: a diffusion tensor imaging study. AJNR Am J Neuroradiol 29:514–519, 2008

Rutland-Brown W, Langlois JA, Thomas KE, et al: Incidence of traumatic brain injury in the United States, 2003. J Head Trauma Rehabil 21:544–548, 2006

Ruttan L, Martin K, Liu A, et al: Long-term cognitive outcome in moderate to severe traumatic brain injury: a meta-analysis examining timed and untimed tests at 1 and 4.5 or more years after injury. Arch Phys Med Rehabil 89(suppl):S69–S76, 2008

Ryu WH, Feinstein A, Colantonio A, et al: Early identification and incidence of mild TBI in Ontario. Can J Neurol Sci 36:429–435, 2009

Saatman KE, Abai B, Grosvenor A, et al: Traumatic axonal injury results in biphasic calpain activation and retrograde transport impairment in mice. J Cereb Blood Flow Metab 23:34–42, 2003

Saatman KE, Duhaime AC, Bullock R, et al: Classification of traumatic brain injury for targeted therapies. J Neurotrauma 25:719–738, 2008

Seel RT, Macciocchi S, Kreutzer JS: Clinical considerations for the diagnosis of major depression after moderate to severe TBI. J Head Trauma Rehabil 25:99–112, 2010

Selassie AW, Zaloshnja E, Langlois JA, et al: Incidence of long-term disability following traumatic brain injury hospitalization, United States, 2003. J Head Trauma Rehabil 23:123–131, 2008

Stys PK: General mechanisms of axonal damage and its prevention. J Neurol Sci 233:3–13, 2005

Teasdale G, Jennett B: Assessment of coma and impaired consciousness: a practical scale. Lancet 2:81–84, 1974

Thornhill S, Teasdale GM, Murray GD, et al: Disability in young people and adults one year after head injury: prospective cohort study. BMJ 320:1631–1635, 2000

Thurman D, Coronado VG, Selassie AW: The epidemiology of TBI: Implications for public health, in Brain Injury Medicine: Principles and Practice. Edited by Zasler ND, Katz DI, Zafonte RD. New York, Demos, 2007, pp xxviii, 1245–1256, 1275, 1278

Till C, Colella B, Verwegen J, et al: Postrecovery cognitive decline in adults with traumatic brain injury. Arch Phys Med Rehabil 89(suppl):S25–S34, 2008

Vaishnavi S, Rao V, Fann JR: Neuropsychiatric problems after traumatic brain injury: unraveling the silent epidemic. Psychosomatics 50:198–205, 2009

van der Naalt J, Hew JM, van Zomeren AH, et al: Computed tomography and magnetic resonance imaging in mild to moderate head injury: early and late imaging related to outcome. Ann Neurol 46:70–78, 1999

Wang JA, Lin W, Morris T, et al: Membrane trauma and Na+ leak from Nav1.6 channels. Am J Physiol Cell Physiol 297:C823–C834, 2009

Whelan-Goodinson R, Ponsford J, Johnston L, et al: Psychiatric disorders following traumatic brain injury: their nature and frequency. J Head Trauma Rehabil 24:324–332, 2009

Whelan-Goodinson R, Ponsford JL, Schonberger M, et al: Predictors of psychiatric disorders following traumatic brain injury. J Head Trauma Rehabil 25:320–329, 2010

Williams DH, Levin HS, Eisenberg HM: Mild head injury classification. Neurosurgery 27:422–428, 1990

Wolf JA, Stys PK, Lusardi T, et al: Traumatic axonal injury induces calcium influx modulated by tetrodotoxin-sensitive sodium channels. J Neurosci 21:1923–1930, 2001

Zaloshnja E, Miller T, Langlois JA, et al: Prevalence of long-term disability from traumatic brain injury in the civilian population of the United States, 2005. J Head Trauma Rehabil 23:394–400, 2008

Ziebell JM, Morganti-Kossmann MC: Involvement of pro- and anti-inflammatory cytokines and chemokines in the pathophysiology of traumatic brain injury. Neurotherapeutics 7:22–30, 2010

# PART II

# ASSESSMENT

CHAPTER 2

# Medical Evaluation

*David B. Arciniegas, M.D.*

**Comprehensive medical evaluation** is a prerequisite to the treatment of the cognitive, psychiatric, sensorimotor, and functional problems experienced by individuals with traumatic brain injury (TBI). The evaluation necessarily entails characterizing the injury to the brain, other co-occurring injuries, and the care needs attendant on them. However, a thorough evaluation also must address many other issues. As Sir Charles P. Symonds (1937), the acclaimed British neurologist, cautioned in his exposition to the Royal Society of Medicine in 1937, "The later effects of head injury can only be properly understood in light of a full psychiatric study of the individual patient, and in particular, his constitution. In other words, it is not only the kind of injury that matters, but the kind of head" (p. 1092). More recent formulations emphasize the combined influences of preinjury factors, injury factors, and postinjury factors on symptom development and resolution following TBI and encourage consideration of all of these factors when assessing persons with such injuries (Arciniegas and Silver 2013; Silver et al. 2009) (Figure 2–1).

The goal of this chapter is to outline the type of comprehensive medical evaluation performed by physicians in subacute inpatient rehabilitation settings or outpatient clinics. The scope of any specific medical evaluation varies with injury type and severity, the context of

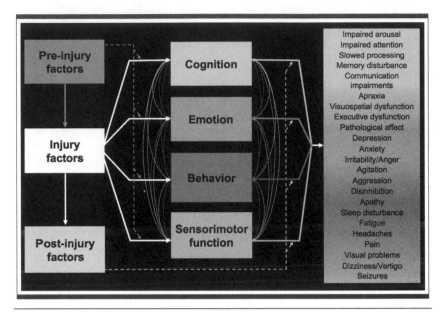

**FIGURE 2–1.** A model of the contributions of pre-injury factors, injury factors, and post-injury factors to posttraumatic neuropsychiatric disturbances.

Injury factors (e.g., inertial and contact forces, cytoxic and metabolic cascade, secondary injury processes) disrupt brain areas supporting cognition, emotion, behavior, and sensorimotor function (*bold solid lines*). Dysfunction in any one of these domains may secondarily affect function in the others (*thin solid lines*). Pre-injury factors (e.g., age, gender, neurogenetics, neurodevelopment, premorbid intellectual function, medical, neurological, psychiatric, and substance use conditions, personality and coping styles, sociocultural background, economic status) may increase vulnerability to or afford resilience from the effects of TBI (*dashed lines*). Post-injury factors (e.g., timely medical and rehabilitative interventions, co-occurring physical injuries and medical complications, medications, education and expectations about TBI and recovery, social supports, post-injury coping styles and psychological issues, disability and role changes, socioeconomic status, medicolegal entanglements) also may modify, for better or worse, the development and resolution of cognitive, emotional, behavioral, and sensorimotor disturbances (*dashed lines*). Collectively, interactions between pre-injury, injury, and post-injury factors produce posttraumatic symptoms, the most common of which are listed in the box on the right side of the figure.

*Source.* Arciniegas DB, Silver JM: "Pharmacotherapy of Neuropsychiatric Disturbances," in *Brain Injury Medicine: Principles and Practice,* edited by Zasler ND, Katz DI, Zafonte RD. © 2013. Reproduced with permission of Demos Medical Publishing LLC.

the evaluation, and the time postinjury at which it is performed. Not all elements of the examination described here will be relevant in all contexts. More specifically, this chapter is not intended to guide the on-scene, emergency department, or neurocritical care assessments of persons with TBI, although elements of the evaluation described in this chapter may be useful in those settings as well.

# HISTORY TAKING

The history-taking portion of the clinical encounter, like any professional interaction, begins with proper introductions. A brief social exchange serves the combined purposes of putting patients and/or caregivers at ease and informing them on the amount of clinician-directed structure likely to be required during the interview. It also provides an opportunity to observe their interpersonal dynamics and identifies the person(s) on whom the examiner's attention will focus (i.e., patient, family, and/or caregiver).

The clinician then states briefly his or her understanding of the ostensible purpose of the encounter (i.e., "I understand that you're here today to talk about *[specific problem or concern]*" or "*[Name of individual making referral]* asked us to meet and discuss/evaluate *[specific problem or concern]*"). Offering such a statement provides an opportunity to ensure that the examiner, the person with TBI, and/or others participating in the clinical encounter are in agreement about the encounter's purpose.

The interview to obtain essential elements of the history (Table 2–1) begins by identifying the patient's and/or the caregiver's chief complaint(s). At the outset, it is essential to put aside any presumption that the presenting problems are consequences of or necessarily related to TBI. A nonspecific open-ended inquiry therefore is used at the outset. An appropriate opening question can be as simple as, "How are you?" "Tell me about yourself." "What's on your mind?" or "What can I do for you today?" Asking the latter question relatively early in the encounter improves the likelihood of identifying issues of greatest concern to the patient and/or caregiver. It is best not to interrupt, direct, or structure spontaneous responses to this question and instead to afford the opportunity for several minutes of uninterrupted response.

A relatively less structured, although entirely clinical, approach is used to elicit the history of present illness from a person with TBI who is able to engage effectively and offer historical information reliably. The clinician guides that individual's anamnesis (i.e., the complete history recalled and recounted by the patient) unobtrusively, and

**TABLE 2–1.**  Essential history-related elements of the evaluation of persons with traumatic brain injury (TBI)

| ELEMENT | COMMENTS |
|---|---|
| History of present illness | Obtain chief complaint(s) and characterize current cognitive, emotional, behavioral, and sensorimotor symptoms as well as their effects on functional status. |
| | Assess onset and duration, quality, intensity, and context in which each problem occurs, as well as precipitating and palliating factors, all prescribed and self-directed treatments, and course over time. |
| | Note the temporal and contextual relationship of the presenting problems to other comorbid conditions. |
| Injury history | Ascertain whether the injury event meets criteria for TBI. |
| | If TBI occurred, estimate duration and course of event-related disturbances of consciousness and/or neurological signs. |
| | Review patient account, witness account(s), and previously recorded descriptions of the injury in medical record(s). |
| | Identify preinjury and peri-injury factors in the differential diagnosis of event-related disturbances of consciousness and/or neurological signs. |
| Preinjury and postinjury medical history | Identify all other medical conditions, neurological disorders, and injuries, as well as their treatment, courses, and outcomes. |
| Preinjury and postinjury mental health history | Identify all psychiatric conditions and substance use disorders, as well as their treatments, courses, and outcomes, regardless of whether they were previously diagnosed and/or treated. |
| Treatments | Identify all prescribed medications, over-the-counter agents, herbal products, nutritional supplements, and rehabilitative interventions, as well as their indications and effects (if any). |
| | Review past medications, surgeries and other procedures, and rehabilitative interventions, as well as their indications and effects. |

**TABLE 2–1.** Essential history-related elements of the evaluation of persons with traumatic brain injury (TBI) *(continued)*

| ELEMENT | COMMENTS |
|---|---|
| Allergies and sensitivities | Identify medication allergies and other environmental allergies. |
| | Identify medication side effects, drug-drug interactions, and idiosyncratic (i.e., rare) medication reactions. |
| Social history | Review intellectual and social development; academic history and highest educational level; occupational history; residence, marital status, and support network; financial status and health care resources; military history; legal history (i.e., past and present civil and criminal matters; assignments of powers of attorney, guardianship, and/or conservatorship); and advance directives. |
| Family history | At a minimum, identify medical, neurological, psychiatric, and substance use disorders in first-degree relatives. |
| Review of systems | Review cognitive function, emotional status (e.g., mood and affect), behavior, self-awareness, sensorimotor function, and general health status, especially issues not addressed by history of present illness. |

identifies clinically important symptoms and signs upon which additional inquiries are focused.

By contrast, unstructured anamnesis can be a countertherapeutic technique when attempted with individuals lacking the ability to communicate effectively, reliably, and/or independently. When opening questions are met with confusion or responses that are unproductive (i.e., tangential, overly inclusive, irrelevant, bizarre), adopting a more structured interview style is appropriate. In such circumstances, the interview focuses on clinically important topics using simple direct questions that are within the patient's abilities to answer.

Interviewing family, caregivers, and other health care professionals knowledgeable about the medical and injury histories is essential to the evaluation of a person with TBI. Knowledgeable and reliable informants are asked to provide the patient's medical history in their own words first (heteroanamnesis). These informants may include spouses, adult children, other family and friends, and others who interact with the person with TBI on a frequent basis. Additionally, collateral data should be obtained through medical record review and communication with other health care professionals involved with the person with TBI.

# HISTORY OF PRESENT ILLNESS

## Symptoms

The history of present illness seeks to clarify the chief complaint(s) and related problems (see Table 2–1). When these are not offered spontaneously, screening for the cognitive, emotional, behavioral, and/or sensorimotor symptoms that are experienced commonly in the immediate and early postinjury periods is appropriate. Self-report symptom inventories administered before or during the clinical interview may facilitate and refine the focus of these inquiries efficiently (Table 2–2).

In some cases, structured clinical interview of the person with TBI and/or a reliable informant may be required to identify clearly pressing clinical concerns. The latter approach is recommended when evaluating persons with TBI whose self-awareness is impaired or who are unable to provide reliable self-report. Because the neuropsychiatric sequelae of TBI are described using medical jargon and may have several possible referents in common parlance, it is important to establish a shared understanding of the terms used during the clinical evaluation. Structured interviews (Table 2–3) provide means of simultaneously assessing for these problems and educating persons with TBI and their families or caregivers about them. Data derived from these measures (as well as self-report scales) also establish baselines against which illness progression and treatment response can be objectively compared.

Each symptom of concern identified during the interview requires clarification with respect to onset, duration, quality, intensity, context of occurrence, precipitating and palliating factors, and course. Symptoms resulting directly from TBI are expected to begin proximate to the time of injury and to improve over time, although the rate and extent of their resolution varies with initial injury severity (Carroll et al. 2004). The relationship between TBI and subsequent symptoms is

---

**TABLE 2–2.** Self-report and/or family report measures used to assess neuropsychiatric symptoms among persons with traumatic brain injury

---

Rivermead Post-Concussion Symptoms Questionnaire

Neurobehavioral Functioning Inventory

Neurobehavioral Symptom Inventory

Cognitive Failures Questionnaire

Multiple Abilities Self-Report Questionnaire

Behavioral Rating Inventory of Executive Function–Adult Version

Beck Depression Inventory–II

Beck Suicide Intent Scale

Beck Anxiety Inventory

State-Trait Anxiety Inventory

PTSD Checklist, including Civilian and Military versions

Center for Neurologic Study–Lability Scale

Apathy Evaluation Scale

Awareness Questionnaire

Epworth Sleepiness Scale

Pittsburgh Sleep Quality Index

---

*Note.* PTSD=posttraumatic stress disorder.

---

most confidently established when this course is followed and when their development and/or persistence are not better accounted for by preinjury conditions or other concurrently sustained injuries. Posttraumatic epilepsy is a noteworthy exception in this regard, with onset occurring weeks, months, or years after injury (see Chapter 14, "Seizures and Epilepsy").

When episodic symptoms (e.g., headaches, seizures) or problems that wax and wane in severity are reported, inquiry into the contexts in which symptoms occur or worsen, precipitating factors in those contexts, palliating factors (if any), and associations with other symptoms (e.g., affective or behavioral disturbances resulting from cognitive failures, cognitive failures resulting from physical symptoms) is essential. The manner in which a person with TBI (and/or family and caregivers) responds to each posttraumatic symptom, including cop-

**TABLE 2–3.** Examples of clinician-administered scales used to characterize neuropsychiatric disturbances among persons with traumatic brain injury

| MEASURE | METHOD(S) |
| --- | --- |
| Neurobehavioral Rating Scale–Revised | Structured patient interview and clinician observation |
| Neuropsychiatric Inventory | Structured informant interview; Clinician version includes clinician observations |
| Mini-International Neuropsychiatric Interview | Structured patient interview |
| Hamilton Depression Rating Scale | Semistructured clinical interview and clinician observation |
| Young Mania Rating Scale | Semistructured clinical interview and clinician observation |
| Pathological Laughing and Crying Scale | Structured clinical interview |
| Hamilton Anxiety Rating Scale | Semistructured clinical interview and clinician observation |
| Agitated Behavior Scale | Clinician observation |
| Overt Behaviour Scale | Semistructured informant interview |
| Overt Aggression Scale | Clinician observation |
| Apathy Evaluation Scale | Semistructured patient interview, clinician observation, and/or informant interview |
| Awareness Questionnaire | Semistructured patient interview, clinician observation, and/or informant interview |

ing strategies used, prescribed and self-directed treatments, and perceived functional consequences, also requires clarification.

Emerging evidence suggests that a minority of persons with moderate to severe TBI may experience modest cognitive decline in the very late postinjury period (i.e., more than 2 years post-TBI) (Till et al. 2008). The factors contributing to such declines are not clear. Over the long term, aging appears to be a contributor to late declines (Himanen et al. 2006). In the early postinjury years, mood, anxiety, and substance use disorders may contribute to apparent cognitive declines (McCrea et al. 2009). There also is evidence that TBI may constitute a risk factor for late neurodegenerative conditions, including chronic traumatic encephalopathy (McKee et al. 2009) and Alzheimer disease (Mauri et al. 2006). At present, the strength of these associations appears to vary with initial injury severity (Mehta et al. 1999), repetitive TBIs (McKee et al. 2009), and/or relevant neurogenetic factors (Jordan 2007; Mauri et al. 2006).

Although late cognitive declines following TBI are possible, cognitive and other symptoms with an initial onset weeks or months after TBI or progressive worsening often are not well explained by TBI alone (Carroll et al. 2004; McCrea et al. 2009). In many cases, these courses are contributed to or explained by comorbid medical, neurological, psychiatric, and/or substance use disorders, adverse medication effects, psychosocial stressors, and medicolegal issues. Screening for such problems is imperative in such circumstances; methods of performing these screenings are discussed in subsequent sections of this chapter.

## Functional Status

Establishing the functional relevance of symptoms reported is a challenging task but an essential element of the comprehensive medical evaluation. In inpatient rehabilitation settings, quantitative assessment is performed routinely with the Functional Independence Measure (FIM; Uniform Data System for Medical Rehabilitation 1997), the Disability Rating Scale (DRS; Rappaport et al. 1982), and other clinician-administered instruments. Qualitative assessments of symptom-related distress and quality of life also are performed commonly in these settings, and are complemented by quantitative assessment using the Satisfaction With Life Scale (Diener et al. 1985), Medical Outcomes Trust Health Survey 36-Item Short Form (SF-36; Findler et al. 2001; Medical Outcomes Trust 1992), or similar measures.

In the outpatient setting, functional disturbances among persons with relatively more severe injuries and impairments are more readily identified by presently available measures than are those associated with mild TBI. An excellent overview measure that may facilitate the identification of functional limitations (i.e., barriers to activity and participation) is provided by the Common Data Elements Traumatic Brain Injury Outcomes Workgroup (Wilde et al. 2010), to which readers are referred for additional consideration of this subject.

## Hypothesis Generation

Using information derived from the history of present illness, the clinician develops hypotheses regarding the patient's symptoms and their causes. Tests of those hypotheses are integrated seamlessly into the clinical interview and, to the greatest extent possible, matched to the patient's needs, abilities, and style. The remainder of the medical evaluation is designed to acquire evidence with which to test those hypotheses, generate alternatives, and inform treatment recommendations.

# INJURY HISTORY

After the clinician has heard the chief complaint(s) and obtained the history of present illness, establishing whether the patient experienced an event that is characterized fairly as a TBI is the next and most critical step in determining whether those symptoms are appropriately regarded as posttraumatic (irrespective of their eventual attribution to neurotrauma and/or other causes). The American Congress of Rehabilitation Medicine's (ACRM's) definition of mild TBI (Kay et al. 1993) and related TBI criteria sets (Department of Veterans Affairs and Department of Defense 2009) provide useful anchors to this step of the evaluation (Table 2–4).

Regardless of the context and time postinjury of the evaluation, the injury history relies on the patient, any witnesses, and medical records to establish the occurrence of an exposure to biomechanical and/or blast-related forces that disrupted brain function and/or structure. However, event-related disturbances of brain function or structure are not specific to TBI, and additional information is required before attributing them unequivocally to TBI.

The injury history seeks to characterize event-related disturbances of consciousness and sensorimotor abnormalities. Distinctions are made between loss of consciousness (LOC), loss of memory (posttraumatic amnesia, or PTA), and alteration of consciousness (AOC). LOC is defined by absence of arousal, with no behavioral response to sensory input and no spontaneous (purposeful or nonpurposeful) behavior. PTA is a dense impairment of declarative memory for peri-injury events. This entails anterograde amnesia, which is the inability to learn and recall new information subsequent to the injury. Retrograde amnesia, a loss of memory for events preceding the injury, also may occur

**TABLE 2–4.** Commonly used clinical case definitions of traumatic brain injury

| ACRM[1] | DoD/DVA[2] |
|---|---|
| Traumatically induced physiological disruption of brain function, as manifested by at least one of the following: | Traumatically induced structural injury and/or physiological disruption of brain function as a result of an external force, indicated by new onset or worsening of at least one of the following clinical signs immediately following the event: |
| Any period of loss of consciousness | Any period of lost or decreased level of consciousness |
| Any loss of memory for events immediately before or after the accident | Any loss of memory for events immediately before or after the injury |
| Any alteration in mental state at the time of the accident (e.g., feeling dazed, disoriented, or confused) | Any alteration in mental state at the time of the injury (e.g., confusion, disorientation, slowed thinking) |
| Focal neurological deficit(s) that may or may not be transient | Neurological deficits (e.g., weakness, loss of balance, change in vision, praxis, paresis/-plegia, sensory loss, aphasia) that may or may not be transient |
| | Intracranial lesion |

[1]Kay T, Harrington DE, Adams RE, et al.: Definition of mild traumatic brain injury: Report from Mild Traumatic Brain Injury Committee of the Head Injury Interdisciplinary Special Interest Group of the American Congress of Rehabilitation Medicine. *The Journal of Head Trauma Rehabilitation* 8(3):86–87, 1993.
[2]Department of Veterans Affairs and Department of Defense: VA/DoD Clinical Practice Guideline for Management of Concussion/Mild Traumatic Brain Injury. *Journal of Rehabilitation Research and Development* 46(6):CP1–68, 2009.

*Source.* Adapted with permission from Arciniegas DB: "Addressing Neuropsychiatric Disturbances During Rehabilitation After Traumatic Brain Injury: Current and Future Methods." *Dialogues in Clinical Neuroscience* 13:325–345, 2011. © Les Laboratoires Servier, Suresnes, France.

and is especially common among persons with relatively more severe TBI. Its scope is usually more limited than that of anterograde amnesia (i.e., loss of memory for moments of preinjury events vs. hours or days of postinjury events). A person with AOC may feel dazed, confused, or disoriented, and may manifest abnormal behavior (e.g., perseveration, disorganization) or severely impaired judgment or self-awareness. Event-related disturbances in sensorimotor function may include focal neurological signs (i.e., signs reflecting focal cortical, subcortical, white matter, cerebellar, or brain stem injury) or seizures.

Broad differential diagnoses are necessary for event-related disturbances of consciousness (Box 2–1) and sensorimotor abnormalities (Box 2–2). Conditions other than TBI may contribute to or account entirely for such problems (Kay et al. 1993; Menon et al. 2010). Their differential diagnoses must be considered before attributing event-related disturbances of consciousness and/or sensorimotor function unequivocally to TBI. This issue is of particular concern among persons whose event-related disturbances of consciousness do not include LOC or PTA, for whom the differential diagnosis of event-related AOC is necessarily broad. Similarly, the differential diagnosis for so-called focal neurological deficits that occur without concurrent disturbance of consciousness and in the absence of penetrating brain injury is extensive and favors injuries to tissues and structures outside the intracranial cavity (i.e., noncerebral tissues) over TBI.

The presence of other conditions in the differential diagnosis for event-related disturbances of consciousness and/or sensorimotor symptoms does not preclude a TBI diagnosis. In some cases, the occurrence of other conditions may explain how a TBI occurred; for example, syncope may result in a fall-related TBI, or alcohol intoxication while driving may result in a traffic accident–related TBI. Co-occurrence of such conditions with TBI also may contribute to persistent postinjury alterations of mental state or neurological function, and their recognition directs treatment efforts productively. Nonetheless, the presence of such conditions necessarily tempers the confidence with which event-related disturbances of consciousness and/or sensorimotor symptoms can be attributed to neurotrauma and used to support a TBI diagnosis.

# CHARACTERIZING TRAUMATIC BRAIN INJURY SEVERITY

When event-related disturbances of consciousness and/or sensorimotor abnormalities can be attributed confidently to neurotrauma-induced disturbances of brain structure and function, the clinician can make a diagnosis of TBI and then needs to characterize its sever-

---

**Box 2–1. Common elements of the differential diagnosis of injury event–related disturbances of consciousness**

- Traumatic brain injury

- Preinjury medical or neurological condition altering consciousness (e.g., delirium)

- Preinjury intoxication or withdrawal from alcohol or other substances

- Peri-injury dehydration and/or hypovolemia

- Peri-injury hypotension

- Peri-injury hyperthermia or hypothermia

- Peri-injury toxin inhalation

- Cerebrovascular events (e.g., transient ischemic attack, stroke)

- Cardiovascular compromise (e.g., cardiac arrest)

- Cerebral hypoxia or hypoxia-ischemia

- Seizure/postictal confusion due to preexisting epilepsy

- Neurotrauma-induced seizures/postictal confusion

- Medication-induced (iatrogenic) confusional state

- Acute stress responses (e.g., severe anxiety reaction, acute stress-induced dissociative state)

---

ity. In general, such characterizations rely on identification of the duration of LOC, PTA, and/or AOC, as well as Glasgow Coma Scale (GCS) scores (Teasdale and Jennett 1974) and neuroimaging findings, when these are available (Table 2–5) (Arciniegas 2011a).

# Prospective Assessment

Performing and interpreting serial assessments of disturbances of consciousness and sensorimotor function in the early postinjury period fa-

---

**BOX 2–2.  COMMON ELEMENTS OF THE DIFFERENTIAL DIAGNOSIS OF EVENT-RELATED SENSORIMOTOR ABNORMALITIES**

---

- Preinjury sensorimotor disorders (e.g., headaches, tinnitus, vertigo)

- Focal cerebral, cerebellar, and/or brain stem injuries

- Cerebrovascular events (e.g., stroke, transient ischemic attack, vasoconstriction)

- Cerebral hypoxia or hypoxia-ischemia

- Subdural or epidural hematomas without overt brain injury

- Simple partial (focal motor or sensory) seizure or postictal paralysis

- Sensory organ injury (e.g., eye, middle or inner ear, nasal or oropharyngeal tissues)

- Cranial nerve injury

- Head and neck injuries

- Spinal cord injury

- Brachial or sacral plexus injury

- Peripheral nerve injury

- Limb or other bodily injury

---

cilitates the characterization of injury severity. Because disturbances of consciousness occur along continua, accurate injury severity characterization depends on serial assessments using measures such as the GCS (Teasdale and Jennett 1974) and/or PTA assessments such as the Galveston Orientation and Amnesia Test (GOAT; Levin et al. 1979) or the Orientation Log (O-Log; Jackson et al. 1998).

For example, the evaluation of an unconscious athlete 30 seconds after injury may yield a GCS score of 3. Taken at face value, this score might suggest a severe TBI. When that same athlete awakens, begins

**TABLE 2–5.** Classification of TBI severity integrating the approaches used by the Department of Veterans Affairs and Department of Defense (2009) and the American Congress of Rehabilitation Medicine (Kay et al. 1993) and extending them to include complicated mild TBI

| | CRITERIA | | | | |
| --- | --- | --- | --- | --- | --- |
| TBI SEVERITY | LOC (HOURS) | PTA (DAYS) | AOC (DAYS) | GCS (AFTER 30 MINUTES) | CT OR MRI |
| Mild | ≤0.5 | ≤1 | ≤1 | 13–15 | Normal |
| Complicated mild | ≤0.5 | ≤1 | ≤1 | 13–15 | Abnormal |
| Moderate | >0.5 to <24 | >1 to <7 | >1 | 9–12 | Normal or abnormal |
| Severe | ≥24 | ≥7 | >1 | 3–8 | Normal or abnormal |

*Note.* AOC=alteration of consciousness (e.g., confusion, disorientation, slowed thinking); CT=computed tomography of the brain; GCS=Glasgow Coma Scale; LOC=loss of consciousness; MRI=magnetic resonance imaging of the brain; PTA=posttraumatic amnesia (densely impaired new learning); TBI=traumatic brain injury.

*Source.* Adapted with permission from Arciniegas DB: "Addressing Neuropsychiatric Disturbances During Rehabilitation After Traumatic Brain Injury: Current and Future Methods." *Dialogues in Clinical Neuroscience* 13:325–345, 2011. © Les Laboratoires Servier, Suresnes, France.

ambulating, and returns to neurological and cognitive baseline 10 minutes later, his GCS score is 15. This clinical course is consistent with the ACRM definition of mild TBI and informs injury severity characterization more usefully than does either GCS score alone. Conversely, if an athlete's on-scene GCS score is 3, his GCS score is 8 in the emergency department 30 minutes later, and he emerges from PTA 2 days later, his TBI severity is most accurately classified as moderate. In both examples, serial assessment using measures of consciousness (i.e., the GCS) and PTA and identifying when they were performed relative to the time of injury is required to characterize TBI severity accurately.

For patients admitted to trauma care or TBI specialty centers, nursing and/or rehabilitation specialists routinely perform injury severity assessments (e.g., GCS, PTA assessment). Unfortunately, such data are often lacking in the medical records of persons whose initial injury care was in the emergency room or other clinical settings (Powell et al. 2008; Ryu et al. 2009). Additionally, few persons with mild TBI present to a hospital for evaluation at the time of injury, and even fewer are hospitalized (Langlois et al. 2006). Accordingly, injury history–taking performed after the peri-injury period often relies on retrospective assessment.

## Retrospective Assessment

Questions about remote event-related disturbances of consciousness (i.e., PTA duration) parallel prospective assessment with the GOAT. The patient is asked to recount both the last memory before the injury and the first memory (or memories) after the injury. With the assistance of the examiner, the patient identifies the point after TBI at which episodic memory becomes relatively continuous (i.e., the point at which the patient can provide a relatively, albeit not entirely, complete first-hand recounting of events). The interval between this point and the last memory prior to TBI is used as an estimate of the duration of PTA. Although external validation of the event recalled by the person with TBI is not possible, this general approach yields reliable estimates of PTA (Bell 2010; McMillan et al. 1996) and may facilitate TBI severity characterization.

Retrospective assessment entails several potential sources of error. Patients often develop personal narratives about their injury experiences that unknowingly conflate first-hand knowledge with information provided by others. If either information source is inaccurate, then the history taken from the person with TBI alone may not be reliable and may not comport fully with accounts offered by others. Accurate self-observation during the peri-injury event also may be compromised or precluded entirely by neurotrauma-induced AOC. It is logically impossible to determine from the first-person perspective (i.e., self-observation) whether a gap in memory for peri-injury events reflects LOC or PTA. Common clinical experience suggests that patients interpret lack of memory for the injury event as "unconsciousness" (i.e., LOC), although it may actually reflect LOC, PTA alone, or some combination of these disturbances of consciousness.

For example, taking at face value a patient's report of 2 hours of LOC leads to classification of TBI severity as moderate (see Table 2–5).

If the patient actually experienced a few minutes of LOC and almost 2 hours of PTA, then his TBI severity is more accurately classified as mild. Because moderate and mild TBI carry different prognoses, and because the TBI severity assigned will influence the etiological interpretation of symptoms and functional problems, careful consideration of these issues is imperative.

In the absence of a witness who can describe the patient's appearance and behavior in the moments following injury and/or a clear on-scene description of the patient in the medical record, clinicians should consider interpreting self-reported absence of memory for the peri-injury period conservatively (i.e., as PTA). Obtaining any and all collateral injury accounts and reviewing medical records are essential to accurate evaluation of TBI severity in such circumstances. If eyewitness accounts or medical records establish that LOC occurred, then the history and TBI severity classification can be modified accordingly.

## Day-of-Injury Neuroimaging

As noted in Chapter 1, "Overview of Traumatic Brain Injury," day-of-injury neuroimaging (usually computed tomography, or CT) also is used to characterize TBI severity. Mild TBI is defined by conventional neuroimaging unrevealing of intracranial abnormalities (see Table 2–5). An individual whose injury severity otherwise meets criteria for mild TBI but whose neuroimaging does demonstrate such abnormalities—usually small hemorrhagic lesions or contusions that do not require medical intervention or necessitate hospitalization—is described as having a complicated mild TBI (Williams et al. 1990). This distinction is important because the outcomes of persons with complicated mild TBI are more like those of persons with moderate TBI than those of persons with uncomplicated mild TBI, and therefore identification of complicated mild TBI may explain atypical (i.e., incomplete) long-term recovery.

## HEALTH AND TREATMENT HISTORY

All of an individual's neurodevelopmental conditions, learning disabilities, medical conditions, neurological disorders, prior injuries, and surgeries, as well as their treatments and outcomes, should be identified in the comprehensive medical evaluation of persons with

TBI. Inquiring about prior TBIs (including recovery course and/or residual symptoms) is particularly important. Such injuries are relatively common and may contribute to atypical recovery following an ostensibly mild TBI (Carroll et al. 2004).

Co-occurring head, neck, sensory organ, and cranial nerve injuries, as well as other physical disorders or injuries, may produce symptoms that overlap with those commonly produced by TBI. Interpreting the history of present illness requires identifying such problems both in relation to the index injury episode and as part of the medical history more generally. These and other conditions constitute preinjury vulnerability factors that may influence the response of the brain to neurotrauma, the development and persistence of posttraumatic symptoms, and the effects of such symptoms on everyday function.

Preinjury psychiatric disorders, including depressive disorders, anxiety disorders, posttraumatic stress disorder, and substance use disorders, are also important concerns in the evaluation of persons with TBI. Preinjury and postinjury psychiatric and substance use disorders adversely affect short- and long-term outcomes following TBI (Carroll et al. 2004; MacMillan et al. 2002) and may contribute substantively to atypical recovery following mild TBI (Carroll et al. 2004; McCrea et al. 2009). These conditions are treatable, and their effective management may reduce the number and perceived severity of other posttraumatic symptoms (Fann et al. 2000, 2001). The identification of preinjury and postinjury psychiatric conditions, preferably using structured diagnostic assessments such as the Mini-International Neuropsychiatric Interview (MINI; Sheehan et al. 1998) or the Schedules for Clinical Assessment in Neuropsychiatry (SCAN; Wing et al. 1990), is an essential element of a comprehensive medical evaluation of persons with TBI.

As part of the comprehensive medical evaluation, the clinician should inquire about prior medical, rehabilitative, and surgical treatments, including their indications, dosages (for medications), durations, and effects. The scope of the assessment encompasses prescribed and self-administered medications (e.g., over-the-counter medications, herbal products, nutritional supplements), as well as those taken before, at the time of, or after TBI. Medication allergies or sensitivities revealed by these treatments are discussed and clarified. Intolerable side effects, drug-drug interactions, and idiosyncratic medication reactions are most appropriately regarded and recorded as medication sensitivities rather than allergies. Among persons with TBI who have received rehabilitative interventions, the treatment target(s), setting (e.g., inpatient, outpatient), time postinjury at which treatment was provided, techniques used, duration, and effects (beneficial or adverse) also require characterization.

# SOCIAL AND FAMILY HISTORY

For the purposes of the comprehensive medical evaluation, the essential elements of social and family histories (i.e., a minimally acceptable data set) are described in Table 2–1, which appears earlier in this chapter. Intellectual and social development may not be characterized easily without the contribution of parents or other people familiar with the patient's history. Intellectual disabilities, learning disorders, lack of friends or childhood playmates, and/or aberrant social behaviors often are identified most easily through the combination of interview of a knowledgeable informant, medical and/or academic record review, and direct interview of the person with TBI. Academic history and educational level include not only the highest grade achieved but also strengths and limitations in subject-specific performance (e.g., math, reading, writing).

Occupational history focuses on the type of work performed, the correspondence between preoccupational training and jobs held, and the stability, longevity, and success achieved in those jobs. Among persons whose employment was terminated, identifying the reasons for that termination may be revealing of cognitive, emotional, behavioral, or sensorimotor problems. Military history requires identification of the military branch in which the individual served, the years and locations of service, role (occupation), whether service included deployment and/or combat, and the terms of discharge from the military. It also is useful to identify the highest rank attained as well as whether the individual "lost rank" during his or her service. As with job terminations, identifying the circumstances for any loss of rank may provide information about TBI or psychological health issues that inform diagnostic and treatment considerations.

The social support network of the person with TBI also is clarified as part of the medical evaluation. This includes not only the people with whom that individual engages, but also the frequency and quality of their interactions. The place and the people with whom the patient resides, if any, are identified, and the stability of residence and financial resources are characterized.

Legal history is a component of the medical evaluation. Soliciting this history requires questions about preinjury and postinjury civil and criminal issues, including current litigation regarding the index injury event. Among persons with severe cognitive impairments, the need for and/or assignment of legally authorized representatives (i.e., proxy medical decision maker, medical power of attorney, guardian, or conservator, as directed by local statutes) should be identified. Finally, for all persons with TBI, it is important to identify whether advance directives have been established. Broaching this subject with the person with TBI and/or the family communicates openness to its discussion, offers permission for its consideration, and facilitates subsequent conversations about this and related matters. These and other forensic issues are discussed at length in Chapter 21, "Forensic Issues and Traumatic Brain Injury."

# REVIEW OF SYSTEMS

In the preceding sections of the evaluation, the clinician is likely to have adequately addressed most or all body systems. Before the clinician begins the examination, however, this section of the evaluation provides an opportunity to review the chief complaint(s) and associated concerns and to summarize information revealed by additional history taking. This review facilitates identification of the most pressing concerns of the person with TBI and others engaged in the clinical encounter and frames the examinations undertaken thereafter.

The review of systems begins with consideration of problems within the neuropsychiatric domains identified in Figure 2–1: cognition, emotion, behavior, and sensorimotor function. Questions are asked about the quality of cognition, including arousal, attention, speed of processing, recognition, declarative memory, language, praxis, visuospatial function, and executive function. Mood (sustained emotional baseline) and affect (moment-to-moment emotional variability), as well as the characteristics of any problems in these domains, should be ascertained. Screening questions are asked regarding behavioral excesses (e.g., disinhibition, agitation, aggression) or deficits (e.g., diminished motivation), as well as concerns about the safety of the person with TBI and of those with whom he or she interacts. Inquiries about typical physical symptoms (e.g., headache, visual disturbances, tinnitus, dizziness, balance and gait abnormalities, sleep disturbances, fatigue) also are made. As noted earlier in this chapter, the self-report, informant report, and clinician-administered measures listed in Tables 2–2 and 2–3 may be very useful guides to this review. A comprehensive medical evaluation also includes a general medical review of systems. In addition to surveying other aspects of nervous system function, the clinician screens for constitutional symptoms, as well as problems of the head, eyes, ears, nose, mouth, and throat, and the cardiovascular, respiratory, gastrointestinal, genitourinary, skin, and musculoskeletal systems.

# EXAMINATION

Thorough general physical, neurological, and mental status examinations are essential components of the medical evaluation of persons with TBI (Table 2–6). Although it is common practice for psychiatrists to defer the general physical and neurological examinations to other physicians, and for some neurologists and physiatrists to defer the elements of the mental status examination (especially emotional and behavioral assessments) to psychiatrists and other mental health clinicians, parsing the examination in this way does not serve persons with TBI well. TBI is associated with a broad range of preinjury and postinjury cognitive, emotional, behavioral, and sensorimotor disturbances, as well as co-occurring physical injuries, the symptoms of which overlap substantially with those that can be produced by TBI. A comprehensive examination that integrates medical, neurological, and mental status examinations is required to clarify the differential diagnoses for such problems.

## Physical Examination

A general physical examination is performed on all patients. Problem-focused examinations are required when evaluating persons with posttraumatic symptoms of types commonly associated with injuries to structures outside the intracranial cavity, including headaches (see Chapter 13, "Headache"), sleep disturbances (see Chapter 15, "Sleep and Fatigue"), and sensory disturbances (see Chapter 16, "Posttraumatic Sensory Impairments"). Surveying for other physical injuries that may mimic, contribute to, or complicate the symptoms of TBI is undertaken as a part of the general physical examination.

**TABLE 2–6.**  Essential elements of the medical examination of persons with traumatic brain injury

| Element | Comments |
|---|---|
| Physical examination | Assess vital signs, height, weight, and body mass index; auscultate the great vessels of the neck; screen cardiac, respiratory, abdominal, musculoskeletal, and other relevant body areas or systems. |
| | Perform problem-focused examinations for headache, sensory complaints, dizziness, and balance problems. |
| Neurological examination | Assess cranial nerves I–XII, reflexes, motor and sensory function, coordination, balance and gait, and subtle neurological signs (e.g., primitive reflexes). |
| Mental status examination | Perform general mental status examination, focusing on appearance and behavior, mood and affect, communication, thought process and content, insight (self-awareness, social cognition), and judgment. |
| | Assess cognition, including arousal, attention, processing speed, working memory, recognition, language and prosody, declarative memory, praxis, visuospatial function, calculation, and executive function. |
| Neurodiagnostic studies | Review prior neuroimaging studies; obtain magnetic resonance imaging of the brain if not done previously. |
| | Perform electrophysiological assessment of persons with suspected posttraumatic epilepsy. |
| | Request laboratory assessments, when clinically indicated (e.g., for suspected endocrinopathy). |
| | Perform neuropsychological evaluation, when clinically indicated. |

# Neurological Examination

In most respects, the neurological examination of persons with TBI (Table 2–7) is similar to that performed in other contexts, with a few noteworthy exceptions. Although assessment of cranial nerve I (i.e., olfaction) is commonly deferred in general neurological practice, it is a required element of the assessment of persons with TBI. Anosmia and hyposmia are relatively common problems after TBI (Swann et al. 2006). In addition to the subjective distress associated with these impairments (and their effects on taste perception), loss of smell presents safety risks to the person with TBI (e.g., inability to detect a fire in one's home early by smelling smoke or to avoid consumption of spoiled food by detecting its odor). Stimuli such as coffee, mint, vanilla, and cinnamon are commonly used to screen for olfactory impairment. Several commercially available smell-testing kits are available to supplement this portion of the examination (see Chapter 16, "Posttraumatic Sensory Impairments").

Eye movement disturbances are relatively common among persons with TBI. These include problems resulting from cranial nerve palsies associated with severe head and face injuries, as well as more subtle disturbances of voluntary control of eye movements due to disturbances in the oculomotor-subcortical circuit, visuospatial attention networks, and their connections to cerebellar and brain stem structures. Impairments of eye movement control associated with TBI, including mild TBI, include disturbances in antisaccades, self-paced saccades, memory-guided sequences, and smooth pursuit (Heitger et al. 2009). Interrupted smooth pursuit eye movements are identifiable on careful examination, and the relevance of visual tracking impairments may be captured by assessments such as the King-Devick test (Galetta et al. 2011) or formal oculomotor examinations (see Chapter 16, "Posttraumatic Sensory Impairments").

Paratonia and primitive reflexes also are included in the examination of persons with TBI. Paratonia may intrude upon the evaluation of resistance to passive manipulation and often is mistaken for intrinsic disturbances of tone (i.e., hypertonicity) such as rigidity or spasticity. *Rigidity* refers to constant hypertonicity that increases resistance to movement by the examiner. *Spasticity* is a velocity-dependent resistance to stretch accompanied by hyperreflexia. By contrast, *paratonia,* which means "beyond tone," describes impairment of volitional motor inhibition during assessment of resistance to passive manipula-

**TABLE 2–7.** Neurological examination

| Section | Elements |
|---|---|
| Cranial nerves | I: Olfaction, using items such as coffee, mint, vanilla, or cinnamon, or using a standardized assessment |
| | II: Visual fields, visual acuity and pupillary responses, and fundus (i.e., retina, disc, macula) |
| | III, IV, VI: Pupillary responses to light and accommodation, extraocular movements and observation for nystagmus |
| | V: Facial sensation and masseter strength |
| | VII: Facial motor function |
| | VIII: Hearing and vestibular function |
| | IX, X: Palatal elevation |
| | XI: Sternocleidomastoid and trapezius strength |
| | XII: Tongue protrusion |
| Motor, Part I | Resistance to passive manipulation, including assessment of intrinsic tone and assessment for paratonia |
| | Observation of bulk and symmetry and observation for involuntary movements |
| Reflexes | Stretch reflexes; responses are graded as 0 (absent), 1+ (diminished, may require evocation maneuvers), 2+ (active), 3+ (brisk, often with spread to other groups), and 4+ (very brisk, with spread and clonus) |
| | When clinically appropriate, brain stem reflexes (e.g., corneal, oculovestibular, gag) |
| | Primitive reflexes, including glabellar, snout, suck, palmomental, and grasp responses |
| Motor, Part II | Assessment for pronator drift |
| | Strength testing of bilateral upper and lower extremities proximally and distally; responses graded as 0 (no muscle movement), 1 (visible or palpable muscle contraction), 2 (full range of motion with gravity eliminated but not against gravity), 3 (movement against gravity but not added resistance), 4 (movement against resistance but subnormal), and 5 (normal strength) |

**TABLE 2–7.** Neurological examination *(continued)*

| SECTION | ELEMENTS |
|---------|----------|
| Sensory | Light touch |
| | Pain (pinprick), temperature |
| | Vibration, proprioception (including finger-to-nose with eyes closed and Romberg tests) |
| Coordination | Finger-nose-finger, fine finger movements, finger-thumb opposition |
| | Rapid repetitive movement, rapid alternating movement |
| | Heel-to-shin movement |
| Gait | Posture, station |
| | Walking, including initiation, stride length, arm swing, turning, toe walking, heel walking, and tandem gait |
| Corticospinal signs | Response to plantar stimulation (assessment for Babinski sign) and assessment for Hoffmann's sign |

tion. Two forms of paratonia occur commonly among persons with TBI: *mitgehen* (from German, "go with"), the inability to inhibit active movement of the extremity despite instructions to the patient to remain passive during the examiner's movement of it, and *gegenhalten* (from German, "hold against" or "go against"), a purposeless resistance by the patient against movement of the extremity by the examiner ("pull-counterpull" phenomenon). *Primitive reflexes* (also known as infantile reflexes or "frontal release signs") are developmentally normal reflexive actions mediated by the central nervous system that emerge among some persons with TBI (see Table 2–7 for examples). The combination of paratonia and primitive reflexes reflects the severity of central nervous system dysfunction (predominantly, but not exclusively, disturbances of frontal-subcortical networks), and predicts cognitive impairments of functional status during the inpatient rehabilitation period after TBI (Wortzel et al. 2009).

Balance disturbances are common after TBI and increase the risk for reinjury (Guskiewicz 2003). Accordingly, balance assessment is an essential component of the examination of persons with TBI. Disturbances of balance may reflect proprioceptive deficits, visual disturbances, vestibular pathology, motor control problems, and/or cerebellar disorders, as well as the effects of medication and other substances. Among the standardized balance assessments developed for use in this context, the Balance Error Scoring System (BESS; Guskiewicz 2001) is among the most easily administered and widely used. Three stances—double leg, single leg, and tandem—are performed on stable and unstable surfaces, and a score is assigned based on the number of errors that occur during the different balance conditions. Normative data are available to guide interpretation of this assessment (Guskiewicz 2001).

The order in which the elements of the neurological examination are assessed varies across clinicians, and this variance is usually inconsequential. An exception to this general rule is the ordering of three elements: resistance to passive manipulation, stretch reflexes, and strength testing (see descriptions in Table 2–7). Special maneuvers are required to elicit primitive reflexes among patients with paratonia, and therefore paratonia must be identified and mitigated (to the greatest extent possible) prior to performing the examination for primitive reflexes. These maneuvers include tilting the head backward and fixing gaze slightly downward in order to place the orbicularis oculi in a neutral position when assessing the glabellar response; placing the jaw and mouth in a partially open and relaxed position prior to assessing snout, suck, and palmomental responses; and placing the hands in a neutral and partially open position to assess palmar grasp. Although performing these maneuvers may not entirely mitigate paratonia-related masking of primitive reflexes, omitting them all but ensures that primitive reflexes will be observed only when they are severe enough to overcome paratonia. Additionally, motor activation associated with strength testing may exaggerate stretch reflexes assessed immediately thereafter; therefore, the assessment of stretch reflexes is performed before strength testing.

## Mental Status Examination

*General mental status examination.* A detailed description of the general mental status examination of persons with TBI (summarized in Table 2–8) is beyond the scope of this chapter; readers are referred to other reviews of this subject for definitions of terms as well as descriptions of specific methods of this portion of the examination (Arciniegas 2013). A few issues especially relevant to performance of this examination among persons with TBI are addressed here.

The use of valid and reliable structured clinical assessments designed specifically for mental status examination is encouraged. The

**TABLE 2–8.** Outline of the mental status examination

| Section | Elements |
|---|---|
| Appearance and behavior | Arousal, apparent age, body habitus and other physical characteristics, position and posture, attire and grooming, personal hygiene, voluntary and involuntary motor activity, eye contact, comportment (demeanor, attitude), motivation, and engagement with examiner |
| Emotion and feeling | Mood (pervasive and sustained emotion and emotional feelings; the emotional "climate") and affect (moment-to-moment emotion and emotional feelings; the emotional "weather") |
| Communication | Voice, speech, language, and paralinguistics (i.e., prosody and kinesics) |
| Thought process | The style and organization of thought (i.e., "how" an individual thinks) |
| Thought content | Perception (e.g., illusions, hallucinations, other perceptual distortions), ideas (e.g., confabulations, delusions, obsessions) and concerns (e.g., intrusive memories, worries, phobias), themes, and thoughts of violence toward self, others, and/or objects (i.e., "what" an individual thinks) |
| Cognition | Arousal, attention, processing speed, working memory, recognition, language and prosody, declarative memory, praxis, visuospatial function, calculation, and executive function |
| Insight | Self-awareness and understanding of the thoughts and actions of others (i.e., social cognition or theory of mind) |
| Judgment | Ability to reason soundly and draw conclusions rationally |

Neurobehavioral Rating Scale–Revised (NBRS-R; McCauley et al. 2001; Vanier et al. 2000) is a brief structured interview that typically requires 15–20 minutes to complete. It includes several cognitive tests as well as questions about mood, affect, and common postconcussive symptoms. It also provides anchors for clinician-based observations of appearance and behavior (including demeanor and attitude), mood and affect, communication, thought process and content, insight, and judgment (e.g., problem solving). Items are rated on a clearly defined 4-point scale, with problems classified as absent, mild, moderate, or severe. In addition to providing a thorough assessment of mental status, the items on the NBRS-R are organized into five factors (executive/cognitive, positive symptoms, negative symptoms, mood/affect, and oral/motor) that contribute usefully to the identification of functionally relevant areas of neuropsychiatric dysfunction.

When persons with TBI are unable to engage effectively in an interview-based mental status examination, observation-based assessment is complemented usefully by informant interviews. The Neuropsychiatric Inventory (NPI; Cummings et al. 1994) is a structured informant-based assessment for neuropsychiatric disturbances commonly observed among persons with neurological disorders, including TBI (Ciurli et al. 2011). The informant is asked screening questions about the occurrence of delusions, agitation/aggression, depression/dysphoria, anxiety, elation/euphoria, apathy/indifference, disinhibition, irritability/lability, aberrant motor behavior, nighttime behavior, and appetite/eating changes in the 4 weeks prior to the interview. Positive responses to screening questions initiate more detailed assessment in each area, yielding ratings of the severity and frequency of neuropsychiatric disturbances. This interview requires 10–20 minutes to complete. Versions of the NPI that incorporate clinician observations (NPI-C; de Medeiros et al. 2010) and that shorten the duration of inquiry to the week preceding interview (NPI-NH; Wood et al. 2000) are particularly useful in inpatient rehabilitation settings or acute long-term care facilities. Use of these (or similar) informant-based interviews also provides a means by which to educate families and caregivers about neuropsychiatric disturbances and the terms used to describe them. After receiving this education, informants may contribute information from a questionnaire version of the NPI (NPI-Q; Kaufer et al. 2000) to subsequent assessments.

Based on data yielded by the NBRS-R or the NPI, the general mental status examination may be enhanced by using one or more symptom-specific scales. Examples of such measures are listed in Tables 2–2 and 2–3 and presented in the report of the Common Data Elements Traumatic Brain Injury Outcomes Workgroup (Wilde et al. 2010).

*Cognitive examination.* The cognitive portion of the mental status examination includes assessments of arousal, attention, processing speed, working memory, recognition, language and prosody, declarative memory, praxis, visuospatial function, calculation, and executive function. These assessments are described in Chapter 3, "Neuropsychological Assessment," and Chapter 5, "Cognitive Impairments," to which readers are referred for detailed reviews.

Consensus is lacking on the best bedside methods of assessing cognition among persons with TBI. The American Neuropsychiatric Association Committee on Research suggests that the Mini-Mental State Examination (MMSE; Folstein et al. 1975) is a useful element of a screening cognitive examination performed by physicians but cautions that such examinations cannot be limited to the MMSE alone (Malloy et al. 1997). The bedside cognitive examination of persons with TBI also requires using specific measures of attention, processing speed, delayed memory, and executive function. The selection of such tests is guided usefully by the stage of posttraumatic encephalopathy of the person being evaluated (Arciniegas 2011a) (see Chapter 5, Table 5–4). Physicians are encouraged to remain mindful of the limitations of presently available bedside cognitive examinations and to develop a repertoire of structured cognitive assessments and individual tests from which to draw when examining persons with TBI.

Regardless of the specific assessment methods used, interpretation of findings on this portion of the mental status examination requires the clinician to estimate preinjury cognitive baseline and thoughtfully compare postinjury performance to estimated preinjury ability. In general, using tests for which there are fully developed, culturally relevant, age- and education-based normative data facilitates this process (Malloy et al. 1997; Strauss et al. 2006). Impairment is commonly defined as performance that falls two or more standard deviations below that of an appropriately matched healthy comparison sample (i.e., $Z$ score $\leq-2$); a more liberal interpretation of mild impairment sometimes sets the threshold at $Z$ score $\leq-1.5$ (Strauss et al. 2006).

When impairments are identified, their functional relevance also must be considered. This is a complex undertaking, especially among persons with mild TBI. Cognitive impairment contributes to functional limitations, but the proportion of variance in functional status accounted for by such impairments is highly variable (Royall et al. 2007). As noted earlier in this chapter, formal assessment often is required to characterize the nature and severity of functional limitations. Even with those data, establishing the cognitive correlates of functional status remains a challenging endeavor and a matter requiring clinical judgment.

# NEURODIAGNOSTIC STUDIES

Neuroimaging, clinical electrophysiology, laboratory assessments, and neuropsychological evaluation may contribute to comprehensive medical evaluation of persons with TBI. The types and uses of such assessments are subjects of controversy, a full discussion of which is beyond the scope of the present work. Instead, a few comments about the uses of these studies in everyday clinical practice are offered.

## Neuroimaging

In the acute setting or when there are concerns about skull fracture or intracranial hemorrhage, CT of the head is appropriate (Department of Veterans Affairs and Department of Defense 2009). The role of structural imaging in the subacute and late postinjury periods is less well established. Among persons with atypical recovery courses, especially those with mild TBI, magnetic resonance imaging (MRI) of the brain may identify abnormalities not appreciated on CT-based assessments (see Chapter 1, "Overview of Traumatic Brain Injury"). Identifying abnormalities located in areas that correspond to cognitive, emotional, behavioral, and sensorimotor symptoms of TBI may contribute to understanding atypical recovery and may inform treatment response expectations. When MRI is performed, it includes T1- and T2-weighted sequences, T2* gradient-recalled echo (T2* GRE) or susceptibility-weighted imaging (SWI), diffusion-weighted imaging (DWI), and apparent diffusion coefficient (ADC) mapping.

Although research using advanced neuroimaging techniques such as diffusion tensor imaging (DTI) and magnetic resonance spectroscopy (MRS) demonstrates differences between groups of subjects with and without TBI, data often do not reliably predict the diagnostic group to which any individual belongs (Wortzel et al. 2011). Additionally, many of the neuroimaging techniques do not yield data that are meaningfully interpretable at the single-subject level because of the unavailability of population-based normative reference data as well as the broad differential diagnosis for the abnormalities they reveal (Wortzel et al. 2011). Similar challenges are encountered when attempting to use functional neuroimaging methods, including single-photon emission computed tomography (SPECT), positron emission tomography (PET), and functional MRI (fMRI), in the evaluation of individual patients (Wortzel et al. 2008). Additional research and refinement is required to establish and define the role of these types of neuroimaging methods in the medical evaluation of persons with TBI.

# Electrophysiological Assessments

Clinical electrophysiology refers to a group of technologies that assess the electrical and magnetic activity of the brain, including conventional electroencephalography (EEG), evoked and event-related potentials (EPs and ERPs, respectively), and quantitative electroencephalography (QEEG). Magnetoencephalography (MEG) is a less commonly available recording method that yields data that complement EEG, QEEG, EP, and ERP data. These assessment methods are of interest for the evaluation of persons with TBI because they measure brain activity at the millisecond level, a temporal resolution that far exceeds that of all presently available neuroimaging methods, and (with high-density recordings) at a spatial resolution similar to that of fMRI, PET, and SPECT.

When clinical history suggests the possibility of seizures, EEG evaluation for interictal epileptiform abnormalities is appropriate (see Chapter 14, "Seizures and Epilepsy"). It is important to remain mindful that interictal EEG is relatively insensitive to epileptiform abnormalities and that the decision to treat patients for posttraumatic seizures rests on the clinical history (i.e., event semiology) rather than the presence or absence of EEG abnormalities.

The use of electrophysiological assessment for detecting nonconvulsive seizures, coma, and brain death among persons with severe TBI, especially in the acute setting, is well developed and widely accepted. The role of electrophysiological assessment among persons with less severe injuries evaluated in the subacute or late postinjury period is less clear (Arciniegas 2011b). QEEG discriminant databases may distinguish between persons with and without TBI. However, these abnormalities are not TBI specific and are indistinguishable from those observed among persons with posttraumatic stress disorder, depression, anxiety disorders, substance use disorders, and sleep deprivation or disorders, as well as some healthy individuals (Arciniegas 2011b; Coutin-Churchman et al. 2003; Nuwer et al. 2005). Accordingly, these assessments are rarely necessary or useful to employ in the clinical evaluation of persons with TBI.

Emerging evidence suggests that QEEG-guided neurofeedback may be of some benefit to persons with TBI (or associated conditions). This treatment seeks to establish patterns of electrophysiological function in the person with TBI that more closely resemble those of healthy individuals (Thornton and Carmody 2009). Performing QEEG is a necessary component of the evaluation of persons with TBI engaging in this treatment. It is important to remain mindful that QEEG findings in this context serve only to establish the electrophysiological baseline that guides treatment and the evaluation of its effects, and that they are not diagnostic of TBI.

## Laboratory Tests

Laboratory tests with the potential to yield results that identify contributors to and/or causes of neuropsychiatric disturbances may be considered. For example, serum chemistries, hepatic and renal function studies, urinalysis and toxicology, and blood levels of prescribed medications (e.g., anticonvulsants, antidepressants, antipsychotics) may identify contributors to posttraumatic encephalopathy and identify other conditions requiring evaluation and treatment. Recent evidence suggests that posttraumatic neuroendocrine disturbances (partial or total hypopituitarism) are problems for a nontrivial minority of persons with moderate to severe traumatic brain injury (Kokshoorn et al. 2011). Optimal methods for assessing and treating other posttraumatic neuroendocrine disturbances are not yet established. In light of these considerations, findings from the medical history and physical examination that raise concerns for specific problems remain the most appropriate guides to the selection and performance of laboratory tests.

## Neuropsychological Evaluation

Neuropsychological evaluation is used to assess for evidence of brain dysfunction as well as the types and severities of cognitive and psychological problems produced by TBI. Although neuropsychological evaluation is not a component of the medical evaluation of persons with TBI, it is often requested by medical providers. Assessments performed by a neuropsychologist may contribute usefully to the development and refinement of the differential diagnosis for neuropsychological difficulties but are not themselves diagnostic of TBI. The types and timings of neuropsychological evaluations relevant to the assessment of persons with TBI are discussed in Chapter 3, "Neuropsychological Assessment."

# CONCLUSION

Comprehensive medical evaluation is a prerequisite to the treatment of the cognitive, psychiatric, sensorimotor, and functional problems experienced by individuals with TBI. The scope of the medical evaluation varies with injury type and severity, the context of the evaluation, and the time postinjury at which it is performed. This chapter focused on the components of a comprehensive medical evaluation of persons with TBI, including approaches to interviewing persons with TBI and their families, essential elements of the medical history, methods by which to clarify the chief complaint(s), history of present illness, injury history, and other essential areas of personal, social, and family history to evaluate. The use of self-report and structured assessments of postconcussive symptoms and related psychiatric disorders was discussed and is encouraged. The examination of persons with TBI was reviewed, and the roles and limitations of other neurodiagnostic assessments were reviewed briefly. This information provides physicians evaluating persons with TBI with a foundation for the evaluation and management of the challenging clinical problems reviewed in the subsequent chapters of this volume.

## *Key Clinical Points*

- Comprehensive medical evaluation of persons with cognitive, emotional, behavioral, and sensorimotor (i.e., neuropsychiatric) disturbances after TBI necessitates consideration of possible preinjury, injury-related, and postinjury contributors.

- Clinical case definitions of TBI require the occurrence of event-related disturbances of consciousness and/or sensorimotor function. A broad differential diagnosis for each type of disturbance must be considered before diagnosing TBI.

- Preinjury and postinjury psychiatric and substance use disorders are common, and assessment for these conditions is a necessary component of the evaluation of persons with posttraumatic symptoms of any kind.

- Self-assessment measures and structured clinical interviews contribute usefully to the evaluation of persons with posttraumatic neuropsychiatric disturbances.

- General physical, neurological, and mental status examinations are essential elements of the evaluation of persons with cognitive, emotional, behavioral, and sensorimotor disturbances after TBI. Integrated performance of these examinations is preferable to their distribution across multiple physicians.

- Although consensus is lacking on the need for structural neuroimaging in evaluations of persons with persistent symptoms in the subacute and late postinjury periods, MRI of the brain can inform usefully on diagnosis and treatment, and its performance is encouraged.

# REFERENCES

Arciniegas DB: Addressing neuropsychiatric disturbances during rehabilitation after traumatic brain injury: current and future methods. Dialogues Clin Neurosci 13:325–345, 2011a

Arciniegas DB: Clinical electrophysiologic assessments and mild traumatic brain injury: state-of-the-science and implications for clinical practice. Int J Psychophysiol 82:41–52, 2011b

Arciniegas DB: Mental status examination, in Behavioral Neurology and Neuropsychiatry. Edited by Arciniegas DB, Anderson CA, Filley CM. Cambridge, UK, Cambridge University Press, 2013, pp 344–393

Arciniegas DB, Silver JM: Pharmacotherapy of neuropsychiatric disturbances, in Brain Injury Medicine: Principles and Practice. Edited by Zasler ND, Katz DI, Zafonte RD. New York, Demos Medical, 2013, pp 1227–1244

Bell K: Is a brief retrospective interview a valid and reliable assessment of duration of post-traumatic amnesia after mild-moderate head injury? Unpublished doctoral dissertation, University of Glasgow, Glasgow, Scotland, 2010

Carroll LJ, Cassidy JD, Peloso PM, et al: Prognosis for mild traumatic brain injury: results of the WHO Collaborating Centre Task Force on Mild Traumatic Brain Injury. J Rehabil Med 43(suppl):84–105, 2004

Ciurli P, Formisano R, Bivona U, et al: Neuropsychiatric disorders in persons with severe traumatic brain injury: prevalence, phenomenology, and relationship with demographic, clinical, and functional features. J Head Trauma Rehabil 26:116–126, 2011

Coutin-Churchman P, Anez Y, Uzcategui M, et al: Quantitative spectral analysis of EEG in psychiatry revisited: drawing signs out of numbers in a clinical setting. Clin Neurophysiol 114:2294–2306, 2003

Cummings JL, Mega M, Gray K, et al: The Neuropsychiatric Inventory: comprehensive assessment of psychopathology in dementia. Neurology 44:2308–2314, 1994

de Medeiros K, Robert P, Gauthier S, et al: The Neuropsychiatric Inventory—Clinician rating scale (NPI-C): reliability and validity of a revised assessment of neuropsychiatric symptoms in dementia. Int Psychogeriatr 22:984–994, 2010

Department of Veterans Affairs, Department of Defense: VA/DoD clinical practice guideline for management of concussion/mild traumatic brain injury. J Rehabil Res Dev 46:CP1–CP68, 2009

Diener E, Emmons RA, Larsen RJ, et al: The Satisfaction With Life Scale. J Pers Assess 49:71–75, 1985

Fann JR, Uomoto JM, Katon WJ: Sertraline in the treatment of major depression following mild traumatic brain injury. J Neuropsychiatry Clin Neurosci 12:226–232, 2000

Fann JR, Uomoto JM, Katon WJ: Cognitive improvement with treatment of depression following mild traumatic brain injury. Psychosomatics 42:48–54, 2001

Findler M, Cantor J, Haddad L, et al: The reliability and validity of the SF-36 health survey questionnaire for use with individuals with traumatic brain injury. Brain Inj 15:715–723, 2001

Folstein MF, Folstein SE, McHugh PR: "Mini-mental state": a practical method for grading the cognitive state of patients for the clinician. J Psychiatr Res 12:189–198, 1975

Galetta KM, Barrett J, Allen M, et al: The King-Devick test as a determinant of head trauma and concussion in boxers and MMA fighters. Neurology 76:1456–1462, 2011

Guskiewicz KM: Postural stability assessment following concussion: one piece of the puzzle. Clin J Sport Med 11:182–189, 2001

Guskiewicz KM: Assessment of postural stability following sport-related concussion. Curr Sports Med Rep 2:24–30, 2003

Heitger MH, Jones RD, Macleod AD, et al: Impaired eye movements in post-concussion syndrome indicate suboptimal brain function beyond the influence of depression, malingering or intellectual ability. Brain 132:2850–2870, 2009

Himanen L, Portin R, Isoniemi H, et al: Longitudinal cognitive changes in traumatic brain injury: a 30-year follow-up study. Neurology 66:187–192, 2006

Jackson WT, Novack TA, Dowler RN: Effective serial measurement of cognitive orientation in rehabilitation: the Orientation Log. Arch Phys Med Rehabil 79:718–720, 1998

Jordan BD: Genetic influences on outcome following traumatic brain injury. Neurochem Res 32:905–915, 2007

Kaufer DI, Cummings JL, Ketchel P, et al: Validation of the NPI-Q, a brief clinical form of the Neuropsychiatric Inventory. J Neuropsychiatry Clin Neurosci 12:233–239, 2000

Kay T, Harrington DE, Adams RE, et al: Definition of mild traumatic brain injury: report from the Mild Traumatic Brain Injury Committee of the Head Injury Interdisciplinary Special Interest Group of the American Congress of Rehabilitation Medicine. J Head Trauma Rehabil 8:86–87, 1993

Kokshoorn NE, Smit JW, Nieuwlaat WA, et al: Low prevalence of hypopituitarism after traumatic brain injury: a multicenter study. Eur J Endocrinol 165:225–231, 2011

Langlois JA, Rutland-Brown W, Wald MM: The epidemiology and impact of traumatic brain injury: a brief overview. J Head Trauma Rehabil 21:375–378, 2006

Levin HS, O'Donnell VM, Grossman RG: The Galveston Orientation and Amnesia Test: a practical scale to assess cognition after head injury. J Nerv Ment Dis 167:675–684, 1979

MacMillan PJ, Hart RP, Martelli MF, et al: Pre-injury status and adaptation following traumatic brain injury. Brain Inj 16:41–49, 2002

Malloy PF, Cummings JL, Coffey CE, et al: Cognitive screening instruments in neuropsychiatry: a report of the Committee on Research of the American Neuropsychiatric Association. J Neuropsychiatry Clin Neurosci 9:189–197, 1997

Mauri M, Sinforiani E, Bono G, et al: Interaction between apolipoprotein epsilon 4 and traumatic brain injury in patients with Alzheimer's disease and mild cognitive impairment. Funct Neurol 21:223–228, 2006

McCauley SR, Levin HS, Vanier M, et al: The Neurobehavioural Rating Scale—Revised: sensitivity and validity in closed head injury assessment. J Neurol Neurosurg Psychiatry 71:643–651, 2001

McCrea M, Iverson GL, McAllister TW, et al: An integrated review of recovery after mild traumatic brain injury (MTBI): implications for clinical management. Clin Neuropsychol 23:1368–1390, 2009

McKee AC, Cantu RC, Nowinski CJ, et al: Chronic traumatic encephalopathy in athletes: progressive tauopathy after repetitive head injury. J Neuropathol Exp Neurol 68:709–735, 2009

McMillan TM, Jongen EL, Greenwood RJ: Assessment of post-traumatic amnesia after severe closed head injury: retrospective or prospective? J Neurol Neurosurg Psychiatry 60:422–427, 1996

Medical Outcomes Trust: SF-36 Health Survey. Boston, MA, Medical Outcomes Trust, 1992

Mehta KM, Ott A, Kalmijn S, et al: Head trauma and risk of dementia and Alzheimer's disease: the Rotterdam Study. Neurology 53:1959–1962, 1999

Menon DK, Schwab K, Wright DW, et al: Position statement: definition of traumatic brain injury. Arch Phys Med Rehabil 91:1637–1640, 2010

Nuwer MR, Hovda DA, Schrader LM, et al: Routine and quantitative EEG in mild traumatic brain injury. Clin Neurophysiol 116:2001–2025, 2005

Powell JM, Ferraro JV, Dikmen SS, et al: Accuracy of mild traumatic brain injury diagnosis. Arch Phys Med Rehabil 89:1550–1555, 2008

Rappaport M, Hall KM, Hopkins K, et al: Disability rating scale for severe head trauma: coma to community. Arch Phys Med Rehabil 63:118–123, 1982

Royall DR, Lauterbach EC, Kaufer D, et al: The cognitive correlates of functional status: a review from the Committee on Research of the American Neuropsychiatric Association. J Neuropsychiatry Clin Neurosci 19:249–265, 2007

Ryu WH, Feinstein A, Colantonio A, et al: Early identification and incidence of mild TBI in Ontario. Can J Neurol Sci 36:429–435, 2009

Sheehan DV, Lecrubier Y, Sheehan KH, et al: The Mini-International Neuropsychiatric Interview (M.I.N.I.): the development and validation of a structured diagnostic psychiatric interview for DSM-IV and ICD-10. J Clin Psychiatry 59(suppl):22–33, quiz 34–57, 1998

Silver JM, McAllister TW, Arciniegas DB: Depression and cognitive complaints following mild traumatic brain injury. Am J Psychiatry 166:653–661, 2009

Spielberger CD, Gorsuch RR, Luchene RE: State-Trait Anxiety Inventory. Palo Alto, CA, Consulting Psychologists Press, 1970

Strauss E, Sherman EMS, Spreen O: A Compendium of Neuropsychological Tests: Administration, Norms, and Commentary, 3rd Edition. New York, Oxford University Press, 2006

Swann IJ, Bauza-Rodriguez B, Currans R, et al: The significance of post-traumatic amnesia as a risk factor in the development of olfactory dysfunction following head injury. Emerg Med J 23:618–621, 2006

Symonds CP: Mental disorder following head injury. Proc R Soc Med 30:1081–1094, 1937

Teasdale G, Jennett B: Assessment of coma and impaired consciousness: a practical scale. Lancet 2:81–84, 1974

Thornton KE, Carmody DP: Traumatic brain injury rehabilitation: QEEG biofeedback treatment protocols. Appl Psychophysiol Biofeedback 34:59–68, 2009

Till C, Colella B, Verwegen J, et al: Postrecovery cognitive decline in adults with traumatic brain injury. Arch Phys Med Rehabil 89(suppl):S25–S34, 2008

Uniform Data System for Medical Rehabilitation: Guide for Uniform Data Set for Medical Rehabilitation (including the Functional Independence Measure instrument), Version 5.1. Buffalo, NY, State University of New York at Buffalo, 1997

Vanier M, Mazaux JM, Lambert J, et al: Assessment of neuropsychologic impairments after head injury: interrater reliability and factorial and criterion validity of the Neurobehavioral Rating Scale—Revised. Arch Phys Med Rehabil 81:796–806, 2000

Wilde EA, Whiteneck GG, Bogner J, et al: Recommendations for the use of common outcome measures in traumatic brain injury research. Arch Phys Med Rehabil 91:1650–1660.e17, 2010

Williams DH, Levin HS, Eisenberg HM: Mild head injury classification. Neurosurgery 27:422–428, 1990

Wing JK, Babor T, Brugha T, et al: SCAN: Schedules for Clinical Assessment in Neuropsychiatry. Arch Gen Psychiatry 47:589–593, 1990

Wood S, Cummings JL, Hsu MA, et al: The use of the Neuropsychiatric Inventory in nursing home residents: characterization and measurement. Am J Geriatr Psychiatry 8:75–83, 2000

Wortzel HS, Filley CM, Anderson CA, et al: Forensic applications of cerebral single photon emission computed tomography in mild traumatic brain injury. J Am Acad Psychiatry Law 36:310–322, 2008

Wortzel HS, Frey KL, Anderson CA, et al: Subtle neurological signs predict the severity of subacute cognitive and functional impairments after traumatic brain injury. J Neuropsychiatry Clin Neurosci 21:463–466, 2009
Wortzel HS, Kraus MF, Filley CM, et al: Diffusion tensor imaging in mild traumatic brain injury litigation. J Am Acad Psychiatry Law 39:511–523, 2011

CHAPTER 3

# Neuropsychological Assessment

*Rodney D. Vanderploeg, Ph.D.*

*Neuropsychology* is the study of brain-behavior relationships and the impact of brain injury or disease on an individual's sensorimotor, cognitive, emotional, and general adaptive capacities. Clinical neuropsychology is an applied science dealing with the cognitive and behavioral manifestation of brain dysfunction. As with all psychological evaluations, neuropsychological assessment involves the patient in a process of answering clinical questions and responding to unique clinical situations that vary somewhat from patient to patient and across practice settings.

Neuropsychological evaluation differs from neurodiagnostic procedures such as computed tomography (CT) or magnetic resonance imaging (MRI) scans that examine the anatomical structure of the brain. With a neuropsychological evaluation, cognitive capabilities are examined, and the findings can be used to make inferences about the brain and its functional status. In this regard, it is similar to neurodiagnostic tests that assess other functional capabilities of the brain. For example, electroencephalography (EEG) and event-related potentials (ERPs) measure the electrical activity of the brain, and positron emission tomography (PET) and single-photon emission computed tomography (SPECT) assess anatomical patterns of cerebral blood flow or metabolic activity. Among these, the neuropsychological evaluation is the only neurodiagnostic procedure that can evaluate how a person cognitively and behaviorally functions in real life. Neuroimaging studies may identify a location of abnormality or dysfunction, but two people with damage in the same brain region may have different behavioral manifestations of that damage. Neuropsychological examinations can identify and quantify those differences.

Neuropsychological tests employ paper-and-pencil, question-and-answer, and sometimes computerized measures designed to assess different aspects of brain-behavior functioning. These measures are designed to meet rigorous psychometric standards, including the establishing of reliability and validity. To interpret findings that reflect underlying brain functioning, the examiner attempts to obtain a patient's optimal performance under standardized and controlled conditions (Lezak et al. 2004). The patient's performance is then compared to normative data from individuals with similar characteristics (e.g., age, gender, and sometimes level of education or ethnic or racial background) both to describe areas of relative strength and to identify areas of cognitive impairment that may reflect underlying brain damage.

Neuropsychologists must be aware of anatomical considerations and behavioral sequelae associated with various etiological conditions in the evaluation and interpretation of data. For example, some cognitive functions depend on well-defined anatomical structures (e.g., lower-level sensorimotor skills and even higher-level perception, such as recognition of familiar faces, depend on functions of the sensorimotor strip and bilateral basal occipital-temporal regions, respectively). Other abilities (e.g., new learning, abstract reasoning, speed of information processing) are diffusely organized or rely on complex, interacting cortical and subcortical networks. Brain injury can result not only in deficits in various cognitive abilities but also in the emergence of new behaviors or symptoms, such as perseverations, confabulations, or unilateral neglect.

# ROLE OF NEUROPSYCHOLOGICAL ASSESSMENT IN TRAUMATIC BRAIN INJURY EVALUATIONS

Neuropsychological evaluation entails assessing psychological and behavioral functions governed by the brain. These evaluations are often used to assess patients for neuropsychological evidence of brain dysfunction when there is uncertainty regarding the occurrence of a clinically significant injury to the brain. When the clinical diagnosis of traumatic brain injury (TBI) is known (e.g., in cases of moderate to severe TBI), neuropsychological testing is used to delineate the cognitive and other psychological sequelae of brain injury. Neuropsychological assessment also can assist with differential diagnosis and help discriminate between alternative explanations for a patient's difficulties. For instance, in TBI, neuropsychological assessment can assist in differentiating between psychological or psychiatric versus brain injury contributions to a patient's difficulties. An example of this would be helping to differentiate between depression and a frontal brain injury in understanding behavioral apathy, abulia, and cognitive difficulties.

In and of itself, neuropsychological assessment cannot definitively diagnose TBI. Its strength is that it provides an objective measure of actual cognitive and behavioral abilities, but testing provides only an indirect measure of brain functioning. Neuropsychological test performance can be affected by factors other than brain integrity, such as fatigue, medications, examiner-patient rapport, patient interest and on-task effort, and so forth. Thus, poor test scores do not necessarily mean that an individual has underlying brain damage. Alternative explanations for poor performance must be excluded. At the same time, it is certainly possible for a person to sustain a TBI with a loss of consciousness of several minutes but to have an excellent recovery such that neuropsychological performance has returned to baseline 1–2 months later. In that case, neuropsychological testing would not identify any prior but subsequently resolved neuropsychological sequelae of a TBI. In fact, this type of recovery is to be expected after mild TBI (Belanger and Vanderploeg 2005; Belanger et al. 2005; Schretlen and Shapiro 2003). In contrast, moderate to severe TBI typically results in some lasting impairments that are detectable on neuropsychological testing even years following injury (Levin 1993; Novack et al. 1995).

Neuropsychologists are typically asked to detail and quantify a given patient's cognitive deficits, as well as to explain how these deficits may affect the patient's daily life. As a result, neuropsychological assessments often serve as the nucleus of rehabilitation and educational intervention plans following TBI and are instrumental in the evaluation of their effectiveness. Neuropsychologists help identify deficits that would be amenable to treatment and identify behavioral capacities that remain relatively intact and potentially useful in a compensatory manner for other impaired cognitive functions. The neuropsychologist often is asked to make treatment recommendations.

These recommendations are typically for immediate treatment purposes (i.e., while the patient is in a rehabilitation treatment facility), as well as to address more long-term issues (e.g., whether the deficits are likely to improve, whether the patient can drive safely, whether the patient can return to work or school). Finally, neuropsychological evaluations can be an important part of monitoring the success of rehabilitation or psychopharmacological interventions.

In educational settings, neuropsychological evaluations can be important in identifying different learning problems following a TBI, help qualify patients with TBI for special educational services, and serve as an important ingredient in setting realistic goals and designing educational plans. Also, neuropsychological evaluations are appearing with increasing frequency in forensic settings, where they are used to help document the presence or absence of cognitive and behavioral impairments secondary to TBI (e.g., in personal injury cases) or in helping to evaluate issues of disability, diminished capacity, or competency.

# COMMON NEUROPSYCHOLOGICAL IMPAIRMENTS FOLLOWING TRAUMATIC BRAIN INJURY

Following a closed (nonpenetrating) TBI, the most common cognitive problems are in the areas of attention/concentration (working memory), new learning and memory, information processing speed, and executive functioning (Levin 1993; Lezak et al. 2004). *Executive abilities* refers to a wide variety of behavioral functions that include anticipation, goal selection, planning, cognitive flexibility, problem solving, abstract reasoning, organization, initiation, self-monitoring, error detection, error correction, control functions, generative behavior, creativity, perseverance, self-awareness, and self-reflection (Vanderploeg 2000). Whether these are distinct or overlapping abilities and their exact neuroanatomical correlates remain uncertain. Despite these uncertainties, executive functions are critical cognitive abilities with far-reaching implications for adaptive functioning during real-life activities.

Although some individual differences are common, the general pattern of impairment in attention, memory, and executive functions is found following all severities of brain injury. Following a mild TBI, these initial difficulties typically resolve within 7–30 days (Belanger and Vanderploeg 2005; Belanger et al. 2005; Schretlen and Shapiro

2003). Following moderate to severe TBI, although impairments improve over time, they typically remain somewhat problematic over the long term (Dikmen et al. 1995; Novack et al. 1995; Ruttan et al. 2008). In all severities of TBI, these core deficits in part reflect either temporary diffuse dysfunction from metabolic/neurotransmitter disruption and brain swelling, or permanent diffuse neurocellular and white matter brain damage. Although information processing speed is not a specific cognitive ability in and of itself, any generalized or diffuse brain dysfunction will impede cognitive efficiency and hence slow motor and cognitive processing speed. With moderate to severe nonpenetrating TBI, dorsolateral and orbitofrontal damage and medial temporal damage are common (Courville 1942; Graham 1996). Hence, the attentional, memory, and executive functions associated with these cortical regions are the most common neuropsychological impairments. With increasing levels of TBI severity, the neuropsychological deficits that remain include problems in most areas of cognitive ability, including global measures such as intellectual performance and on summary neuropsychological measures such as the Halstead Impairment Index (Dikmen et al. 2009).

Unless an individual has a penetrating head injury or focal cortical lesions, specific motor problems (e.g., paresis), language impairment (e.g., aphasias), and visuospatial dysfunction (e.g., neglect) are rare. However, they do occur when specific cortical contusions or hemorrhages affect the cortical regions underlying these cognitive abilities. Penetrating brain injuries are likely to affect focal brain areas, and the resulting cognitive impairments will correspond to the cognitive and behavioral functions of those regions and their interconnecting neural circuits.

Additionally, acute and chronic neurologically based emotional changes are common after moderate to severe TBI, reflecting either overactivation or muting of affective experiences and reactions. Excitable reactions include impulsivity, emotional overreactivity, and irritability. Muted responses include apathy, emotional disinterest, and abulia. Depression and anxiety are not uncommon at various stages of recovery, or in the chronic state. Following mild TBI, the role of neurological injury in the development of acute and chronic post-TBI emotional changes is controversial; chronic neurologically based emotional changes, in my opinion, are highly unusual. However, a subsample will have persistent emotional adjustment difficulties characterized by anxiety, depression, and somatic concerns. The size of this subsample remains controversial, with estimates ranging from less than 5% to 15% (McCrea and American Academy of Clinical Neuropsychology 2008; Vanderploeg et al. 2007). These individuals have been referred to as the "miserable minority" (Ruff et al. 1996).

# Timing of Neuropsychological Assessment After Traumatic Brain Injury

## Mild TBI

As noted above in "Role of Neuropsychological Assessment in Traumatic Brain Injury Evaluations," cognitive recovery is rapid following an uncomplicated mild TBI. A meta-analysis of the mild TBI literature concluded that by 7–10 days after a sports concussion, the neuropsychological ability levels of patients are indistinguishable from those of uninjured controls (Belanger and Vanderploeg 2005). Findings are similar following concussions not related to sports. A meta-analysis by Schretlen and Shapiro (2003) found that individuals who sustained a mild TBI had neuropsychological functioning comparable to that of control subjects by 30 days postinjury.

Based in part on these findings, the Management of Concussion–Mild Traumatic Brain Injury Working Group (2009) states, in the current clinical practice guideline for mild TBI, that "comprehensive neuropsychological/cognitive testing is not recommended during the first 30 days post injury" (p. 42). However, the group also states that following this period, "Patients who have cognitive symptoms that do not resolve or have been refractory to treatment should be considered for referral for neuropsychological assessment. The evaluation may assist in clarifying appropriate treatment options based on individual patient characteristics and conditions" (p. 55).

An exception to these recommendations is in the area of sports concussions, for which player-specific preseason, preinjury baseline neuropsychological test data are available from a brief but sensitive battery. In this context, repeated testing using the same or a similar battery can be important in acute concussion management and in return-to-play decision making. Typically, individuals with concussions are kept from practice and play until their subjective symptoms (e.g., headaches, dizziness, fatigue, irritability, concentration problems) have completely resolved, even under conditions of physical and cognitive demands (i.e., symptom-provocation tests), and repeated neuropsychological testing has shown a return to baseline performance.

## Moderate to Severe TBI

Following emergence from coma, individuals who have sustained a moderate or severe TBI experience a state of confusion and disorientation (i.e., posttraumatic confusional state). During this confusional state, declarative new learning is densely impaired but recovers gradually over time. The period during which this impairment is present—even when it is not the most salient neuropsychological feature of the patient's presentation—is described as the period of posttraumatic amnesia (PTA). This period may last from days to weeks, and sometimes months, post-TBI.

Many neuropsychologists, including me, advocate for delaying formal neuropsychological assessment until individuals emerge from PTA. This is because individuals with PTA tend to perform poorly on virtually all measures and, as a result, neuropsychological assessments performed during this period tend to yield little clinically useful information. However, brief testing performed during the period of PTA may help determine whether specific neurological syndromes are present, such as aphasias, visual field cuts, visual neglect, gross visual perceptual disturbances (e.g., visual agnosia), or focal frontal syndromes such as imitation behavior, utilization behavior, or an environmental dependency syndrome. This type of brief neuropsychological evaluation may be seen as more akin to that completed by behavioral neurologists and neuropsychiatrists.

For example, early detection of a visual field cut or neglect may guide environmental modifications that compensate for such deficits and facilitate the patient's engagement with the environment and others in it (e.g., arranging bed placement within the room such that the patient's intact visual field is oriented toward the door of the room rather than the wall). Similarly, during the period of PTA, a number of patients develop "language of confusion" in which they talk in incomplete sentences, use grammatically incorrect structure, have occasional paraphasic errors, and say things that do not make sense and appear to have little or no relevance to ongoing activities. For those unfamiliar with this phenomenon, the language use (or misuse) of these patients is easily confused with a posttraumatic aphasia.

Early brief bedside cognitive assessment can typically distinguish between these two conditions, resulting in very different treatment or patient handling recommendations.

Brief neuropsychological evaluations during the early portion of the period of PTA can be used to assess and monitor level of arousal, responsiveness, orientation, attention, agitation, and communication abilities. Appropriate measures for these purposes include, among others, the Coma Recovery Scale–Revised (Giacino et al. 2004), Galveston Orientation and Amnesia Test (Levin et al. 1979), Agitated Behavior Scale (Corrigan 1989), and some language/aphasia screening measures. A number of these measures are available at the Center for Outcome Measurement in Brain Injury Web site (www.tbims.org/combi/list.html). Thus, even while patients are in PTA, some abbreviated neuropsychological assessments may prove clinically valuable.

Following a patient's emergence from PTA, a more formal and comprehensive neuropsychological evaluation is indicated. This assessment typically occurs during a patient's acute inpatient rehabilitation treatment stay, but may also occur on an outpatient basis if an inpatient stay is not indicated or possible. The purpose of this evaluation is to identify specific cognitive problems and residual strengths, assist with patient and family education, help establish realistic treatment goals, help develop a rehabilitation treatment plan, and help with prognostication.

Even months and years following a moderate to severe TBI, neuropsychological reevaluations may be indicated to help monitor recovery, assess the effectiveness of treatment, or address new clinical issues and questions as they arise. Questions to consider may include, among others, whether the person with TBI is able to live alone safely, what level of support is required to help the person with TBI function effectively and safely at home, whether the person with TBI is cognitively able and ready to return to work or school, and what level of assistance or support is needed for the person with TBI to return successfully to work or school.

# CONTEXT-SPECIFIC NEUROPSYCHOLOGICAL ASSESSMENT

## Sports Concussions

In high-contact sports, such as football, soccer, and hockey, preseason baseline neuropsychological assessment is becoming a standard at the professional and collegiate levels, and is gaining gradual acceptance at high school and middle school levels. As mentioned above in "Timing of Neuropsychological Assessment After Traumatic Brain Injury," these baseline individual-specific neuropsychological test results can be crucial in acute concussion management and in decisions about returning to play or practice. The standard of care following uncomplicated concussion is rest, both physical and cognitive, with gradual resumption of activities over several days, as long as these activities do not result in emergence of significant acute symptoms (e.g., headaches, dizziness, irritability, concentration problems). In addition to the monitoring of these subjective symptoms, repeated neuropsychological testing with brief, often computerized batteries can be useful for monitoring when cognitive impairments have returned to preinjury levels. Return to play is considered advisable only when both subjective symptoms and objective cognitive performance have returned to normal, even under stress (i.e., following aerobic physical activity and typical cognitive day-to-day demands).

## Military Deployment

With the sports concussion model as a basis, the military has adopted a similar approach to concussion/mild TBI management. Prior to deployment to a combat zone, predeployment baseline assessment is completed using a computerized neuropsychological battery called the Automated Neuropsychological Assessment Metrics (ANAM; Reeves et al. 2001). Medical personnel in the field can readminister the ANAM to an injured service member following a suspected concussion and access that service member's predeployment scores. In the sports concussion management model, personnel should not be assigned to missions until both subjective complaints and objective ANAM performance have returned to baseline, even following aerobic physical activity (Defense and Veterans Brain Injury Center 2008).

## Forensic Contexts

Neuropsychological evaluations are used increasingly in forensic contexts to determine whether a TBI event resulted in continued neuropsychological impairments and to document the nature, extent, severity, and functional implications of such impairments. Among all available neurodiagnostic tests, only neuropsychological evaluations can evaluate and quantify the cognitive and behavioral sequelae of

TBI and their functional implications for everyday life, such as the ability to live independently, drive, shop, work, and manage financial affairs.

Although validity assessment is an important part of any clinical neuropsychological evaluation, it is especially important in forensic evaluations (Larrabee 2005). In personal injury cases, external factors, such as potentially large financial settlements, may influence a patient's motivation during neuropsychological evaluation and may undermine (consciously or unconsciously) a patient's effort to offer his or her best performance during that evaluation. Validity, or effort, testing that addresses this issue is described in greater detail below (see "Neuropsychological Test Interpretation Issues").

# NEUROPSYCHOLOGICAL ASSESSMENT METHODS

## Approaches to Neuropsychological Assessment

There are several neuropsychological schools of thought, which differ with respect to their recommended approaches to neuropsychological assessment. Their differences arise along two continua: 1) fixed versus flexible battery approaches to testing; and 2) quantitative/normative-based versus qualitative/process-based approaches to data interpretation. The Wechsler Adult Intelligence Scale, now in its fourth revision (WAIS-IV; Wechsler 2008), and the Halstead-Reitan Neuropsychological Test Battery (Reitan and Wolfson 2009) are examples of fixed batteries (with respect to the content of the battery) for which the interpretation of results uses primarily quantitative/normative data. On the other end of both continua is a clinically oriented process approach. Such an approach tends to employ a flexible set of tests, rather than a battery whose content is fixed, to address specific clinical populations or issues; the interpretation of performance on these tests relies on qualitative observations and process analyses of a patient's unique performance to help understand the meaning of the results (Milberg et al. 2009). Process observations attempt to address issues such as 1) the type of errors made by the patient; 2) the reason the patient had difficulty with tasks on which errors were made; and 3) the foundational cognitive problem undermining the patient's performance.

Most neuropsychologists vary the tests they select to evaluate patients across different clinical situations. For example, they would not administer motor performance–based visuospatial tasks, such as block design or drawing tasks, to individuals whose arms are paralyzed or otherwise unusable (e.g., in casts because of broken arms or hands). Similarly, neuropsychologists may choose to use somewhat shorter or easier tasks to assess an individual in his or her ninth decade of life than those used to evaluate a 20-year-old adult. In fact, and in appreciation of these varying clinical needs, the latest version of the Wechsler Memory Scale (fourth edition; Wechsler 2009) employs a different set of memory tasks for use with individuals over age 65. Similarly, the California Verbal Learning Test (Delis et al. 2000) has a short form that is often used with older individuals.

Most neuropsychologists use quantitative/normative data to score and interpret test results; at the same time, it is common practice to take qualitative factors that adversely influence performance into account when interpreting test results. Examples of this include recognizing that a similar normative score can be attained following very different behavioral difficulties, such the adverse effects of left-sided neglect versus poor attention to visual detail versus poor organization and planning on drawing or other visuospatial tasks. Not only are the behavioral performance patterns uniquely different but also the rehabilitation implications of those patterns differ. Thus, most neuropsychologists take into account both quantitative and qualitative aspects of performance during test interpretation and discussion of treatment issues.

# Domains Assessed During a Neuropsychological Evaluation

Whether a fixed or a flexible battery approach is used during a comprehensive neuropsychological evaluation, the neuropsychologist typically assesses a full range of brain-behavior abilities. These include attention and concentration; learning and memory; sensory-perceptual abilities; speech and language abilities (sometimes including academic skills such as reading, spelling, and math); visuospatial and visuoconstruction skills; overall intelligence; executive functions (e.g., abstraction, reasoning, problem solving, behavioral self-monitoring, inhibition, self-control, cognitive flexibility); and psychomotor speed, strength, and coordination. Also assessed are underlying foundational functions, such as attention, arousal, and motivation. Although this list of cognitive functions might be organized or labeled differently by various neuropsychologists, these behaviors would generally be evaluated in most comprehensive neuropsychological evaluations. Frequently, assessment of psychological functioning—that is, psychopathology, behavioral adjustment, and interpersonal issues—also is included in a comprehensive neuropsychological evaluation. Table 3–1 identifies cognitive and psychological domains typically assessed and lists tests of each cognitive domain that are commonly used in neuropsychological assessments of adults with TBI. A comprehensive evaluation, including a clinical interview and history, can take anywhere from 4 to 6 hours in many clinical settings, and 8 or more hours in medicolegal and forensic settings; test scoring, interpretation, and report writing require several additional hours.

Rehabilitation neuropsychologists working with patients with TBI also may administer measures to quantify the effects of cognitive impairments on functional day-to-day abilities and on the ability to integrate into the wider community, or to provide a quantification of global functional outcome. Table 3–2 lists some of the more commonly used measures of these types.

## Screening Versus Comprehensive Evaluation

Brief focused evaluations can address important clinical needs when formal comprehensive evaluations are impossible or impractical to complete, such as when assessing individuals during the period of PTA. This type of focused evaluation differs from a screening evaluation, which by its nature is used to attempt to briefly screen most of the important cognitive domains. Generally, in screening evaluations, sensorimotor skills are not included and the cognitive domains that are assessed are not evaluated in depth or detail. Probably the most widely used screening instrument is the Repeatable Battery for the Assessment of Neuropsychological Status (RBANS; Randolph 1998). The RBANS takes less than 30 minutes to administer and has 12 subtests that result in five summary scales: Immediate Memory, Visuospatial/Constructional, Language, Attention, and Delayed Memory. Executive abilities are not assessed in detail, although the Coding subtest does involve executive function and processing speed.

As a rule of thumb, most currently available screening instruments are not as sensitive to brain impairment as is a comprehensive neuropsychological battery, and they are not as sensitive to impairment in various cognitive domains or as effective in evaluating specific subcom-

**TABLE 3–1.** Domains and exemplar tests included in comprehensive neuropsychological evaluations

| DOMAIN OF FUNCTIONING | EXAMPLES OF COMMONLY USED ADULT TESTS |
| --- | --- |
| Preinjury performance estimation | Wechsler Test of Adult Reading (WTAR) |
| | Test of Premorbid Functioning (TOPF) |
| Effort testing (validity assessment) | Word Memory Test (WMT) |
| | Medical Symptom Validity Test (MSVT) |
| | Test of Memory Malingering (TOMM) |
| Overall intelligence | Wechsler Adult Intelligence Scale, 4th Edition (WAIS-IV) |
| Orientation and memory (posttraumatic amnesia) | Galveston Orientation and Amnesia Test (GOAT) |
| Sensory-perceptual abilities | Reitan-Klove Sensory-Perceptual Examination |
| | Visual Field Examination |
| | Finger Agnosia |
| | Finger Tip Number Writing |
| | Bilateral Simultaneous Sensory Stimulation |
| Motor speed and coordination | Halstead-Reitan Battery–Finger Tapping |
| | Grooved Pegboard |
| | WAIS-IV–Digit Symbol-Coding |
| Attention | Stroop Color and Word Test (Stroop CWT) |
| | Halstead-Reitan Battery–Trail Making Test Part A |
| | Brief Test of Attention (BTA) |
| | WAIS-IV Digit Span |
| | WAIS-IV Letter-Number Sequencing |
| | Paced Auditory Serial-Addition Task (PASAT) |
| | Continuous Performance Test II (CPT-II) |

**TABLE 3–1.**  Domains and exemplar tests included in comprehensive
neuropsychological evaluations *(continued)*

| DOMAIN OF FUNCTIONING | EXAMPLES OF COMMONLY USED ADULT TESTS |
| --- | --- |
| Memory | Wechsler Memory Scale, 4th Edition (WMS-4) |
| | Rey Auditory Verbal Learning Test (RAVLT) |
| | California Verbal Learning Test, 2nd Edition (CVLT-II) |
| | Brief Visuospatial Memory Test–Revised (BVMT-R) |
| | Rey Complex Figure Test (RCFT) |
| Language | WAIS-IV Similarities |
| | WAIS-IV Vocabulary |
| | Boston Naming Test (BNT) |
| | Delis-Kaplan Executive Function System (D-KEFS)–Verbal Fluency |
| | Boston Diagnostic Aphasia Examination, 3rd Edition (BDAE-3) |
| Academic abilities | Wide Range Achievement Test, 4th Edition (WRAT-IV) |
| Visual cognitive abilities | WAIS-IV Block Design |
| | WAIS-IV Matrix Reasoning |
| | WAIS-IV Visual Puzzles |
| | WAIS-IV Picture Completion |
| | Rey Complex Figure Test (RCFT) |
| | Visual Form Discrimination |
| | Judgment of Line Orientation |
| | Facial Recognition Test |
| Executive abilities | Halstead-Reitan Battery–Trail Making Test Part B |
| | Halstead-Reitan Battery–Category Test |
| | Wisconsin Card Sorting Test (WCST) |

**TABLE 3–1.** Domains and exemplar tests included in comprehensive neuropsychological evaluations *(continued)*

| DOMAIN OF FUNCTIONING | EXAMPLES OF COMMONLY USED ADULT TESTS |
|---|---|
| Executive abilities *(continued)* | Delis-Kaplan Executive Function System (D-KEFS) |
| | Sorting Test |
| | Trail Making Test |
| | Verbal Fluency Test |
| | Design Fluency Test |
| | Color-Word Interference Test |
| | Tower Test |
| | 20 Questions Test |
| Psychological functioning and adjustment | Minnesota Multiphasic Personality Inventory–2 (MMPI-2) |
| | Personality Assessment Inventory (PAI) |
| | Beck Depression Inventory–II (BDI-II) |
| | Beck Anxiety Inventory (BAI) |

*Source.* For citations for measures, please see the source note to Table 3–2.

ponents of different cognitive abilities (e.g., differentiating between encoding, consolidation, and retrieval memory problems). For these reasons, it is counterintuitive to use a screening battery in the assessment of mild TBI if the goal of the assessment is to determine whether subtle difficulties remain following the typical recovery period (more than 30 days following a mild TBI). On the other hand, it may make clinical sense to use a screening battery in this same context if the patient complains of severe attention and memory problems and if the goal of the evaluation is to determine whether objective evidence can be found to support claims of such cognitive problems.

A neuropsychological screening evaluation also seems counterintuitive in the acute inpatient TBI rehabilitation setting for an individual with a recent moderate to severe TBI. As a rule, these individuals have obvious cognitive problems that are readily apparent to medical and rehabilitation personnel, as well as to many families; in such cases, a screening evaluation simply confirms the obvious. The typical

---

**TABLE 3–2.**   Examples of measures used to assess functional abilities or global outcomes

| Domain | Examples of commonly used adult tests |
|---|---|
| Functional day-to-day abilities | Craig Handicap Assessment and Reporting Technique (CHART) |
| | Community Integration Questionnaire (CIQ) |
| | Mayo-Portland Adaptability Inventory (MPAI) |
| Global functional outcomes | Disability Rating Scale (DRS) |
| | Extended Glasgow Outcome Scale (GOS-E) |

*Source.* Sources for tests not otherwise cited elsewhere in this chapter: TOMM, Tombaugh 1996; Grooved Pegboard, Matthews and Klove 1964; Stroop CWT, Golden 1978; BTA, Schretlan 1997; PASAT, Gronwall 1977; CPT-II, Conners 2000; RAVLT, Schmidt 1996; BVMT-R, Benedict 1997; RCFT, Meyers and Meyers 1995; D-KEFS, Delis et al. 2001; BDAE-3, Goodglass et al. 2001; WRAT-4, Wilkinson et al. 2006; Visual Form Discrimination, Benton 1994; Judgment of Line Orientation, Benton 1994; Facial Recognition Test, Benton 1994; MMPI-2, Butcher et al. 1989; PAI, Morey 2007; BDI-II, Beck et al. 1996; BAI, Beck and Steer 1990; CIQ, Willer et al. 1994; CHART, Whiteneck et al. 1992; MPAI, Malec and Lezak 2003; DRS, Rappaport et al. 1982; GOS-E, Wilson et al. 1998.

goals at this time require a thorough evaluation to 1) identify the specific nature, pattern, and severity of all cognitive problems; 2) help develop a rehabilitation plan; and 3) provide feedback to everyone involved. A screening evaluation would not be a good choice to accomplish these goals. However, use of a screening evaluation such as the RBANS over the ensuing weeks and months may be an efficient and effective way to evaluate progress and determine the effectiveness of the rehabilitation plan.

# Computerized Neuropsychological Assessment

For testing, computers offer the possibility of consistent and standardized administration, increased accuracy of timing of stimulus material presentation and patient response latencies, and error-free scoring and application of norms. As a result, there have been significant developments in the use of computers in neuropsychological assessment, both in computerizing some existing commonly used neuropsychological tests (e.g., Wisconsin Card Sorting Test; Heaton and Psychological Assessment Resources 1993) and in developing entirely new batteries that are relatively quick and efficient (30 minutes' to 2 hours' administration time). However, most of the available batteries have limitations and drawbacks, including generally poor test reliability, questionable or low validity, and significant potential for abuse. Because computerized batteries are standardized, objective, and easy to administer, and because they appear to be easy to clinically interpret (usually because of nice tabular printouts of scores and standardized interpretive statements), it is tempting to take results yielded by these measures at face value. This is particularly problematic with poor scores that are interpreted as indicating impairment or as reflecting brain damage.

Unfortunately, scores can be in the impaired range for many reasons that have nothing to do with an individual's actual neuropsychological abilities or brain dysfunction. Obvious factors include, for example, misunderstanding instructions or unfamiliarity or discomfort with computers. Additional factors are discussed in the next section of this chapter ("Neuropsychological Test Interpretation Issues"). Inadequate clinical neuropsychological expertise and a lack of appreciation of psychometric principles in the interpretation of findings can lead to a very high potential for misuse and the drawing of incorrect conclusions. At the present time, computerized neuropsychological batteries are best suited for the screening of large numbers of individuals or the evaluation of change in populations at risk or in treatment groups. As a result, some computerized batteries are being used in sports concussion or military deployment settings where pretesting and posttesting can be completed (before a sports season or military deployment and following a suspected concussion or other adverse event). Similarly, computerized batteries are being used in pharmacological or other treatment studies. Even in these situations, judicious interpretation of findings by a neuropsychologist is indicated to avoid erroneous conclusions.

# NEUROPSYCHOLOGICAL TEST INTERPRETATION ISSUES

## Premorbid Estimation

In determining whether cognitive abilities are impaired, the neuropsychologist must estimate a patient's innate or premorbid level of cognitive function. Only if current (i.e., postinjury) scores fall below expected preinjury performance levels can neuropsychological test performance be interpreted as indicating impaired cognitive function.

Ideally, actual measures of premorbid cognitive function (e.g., preinjury standardized test scores) would be used to guide interpretation of postinjury neuropsychological test scores. Scores on intelligence tests administered at various points in the educational system, including precollege standardized admissions tests (e.g., Preliminary SAT [PSAT], SAT, ACT), and graduate school standardized admissions tests (e.g., Graduate Record Examination [GRE], Law School Admission Test [LSAT], Medical College Admission Test [MCAT]), might be useful for this purpose. If preinjury standardized testing is not available (as is often the case), past levels of academic achievement (e.g., school grades, high school graduation class rank) can be used to estimate preinjury levels of cognitive functioning. However, it is important to determine whether underperformance or underachievement may have artificially lowered these measures from actual ability, particularly as a result of poor effort, behavioral problems, truancy, psychosocial factors, or medical conditions.

In addition to measures of actual preinjury performance, demographically based prediction models can be used to estimate premorbid levels of cognitive functioning based on educational and vocational background. Table 3–1 offers examples of premorbid cognitive function estimation methods based on reading ability, including ones that take demographic characteristics into account—that is, the Wechsler Test of Adult Reading (WTAR; Wechsler 2001) and the Test of Premorbid Functioning (TOPF; NCS Pearson 2009), which were codeveloped and conormed with the WAIS-III (Wechsler 1997) and WAIS-IV (Wechsler 2008), respectively. When other preinjury data are not available, these methods are commonly used to estimate premorbid cognitive abilities.

## Validity or Effort Assessment

Validity assessment is also a crucial aspect of any neuropsychological evaluation. This assessment attempts to determine whether a patient's test performance is a valid and reliable reflection of his or her actual neuropsychological abilities or whether some other factors account for or contribute to the patient's test performance. Threats to validity include factors such as test-taking anxiety, misunderstanding test instructions, medication side effects, fatigue, comorbid psychological or medical conditions, inadequate effort, low motivation, secondary gain issues, and outright malingering.

A careful history can help determine whether current medications, sleep problems, or comorbid psychological or medical conditions may be contributing to adverse performance. Careful behavioral observation can help in evaluating whether the patient has misunderstood instructions or whether fatigue appears to be a factor over the course of a multiple-hour evaluation. In such circumstances, reiterating test instructions, offering rest breaks, and/or continuing testing at another time can minimize the adverse effects of these factors on neuropsychological test performance.

Inconsistencies in test scores across measures of similar abilities need to be carefully examined, because they often are the result of variable effort and motivation. Similarly, inconsistencies across domains can reflect variable or invalid effort. For example, significantly impaired attention with normal memory functioning is highly unlikely given that good memory performance requires careful and sustained attention to the memory material. A pattern of neuropsychological performance that is inconsistent with the presumed underlying condition is also an indicator of questionable or variable effort. Although memory difficulties are common following moderate to severe TBI, significant decrements in general intelligence are not. Thus, a pattern of low intelligence scores but normal memory performance is an indicator of potential validity concerns.

A variety of test instruments have been developed to assess whether patients are putting forth full and valid effort during neuropsychological testing. Several of these effort testing measures or symptom validity tests are listed in Table 3–1 (e.g., Word Memory Test [WMT; Green 2005b]; Medical Symptom Validity Test [MSVT; Green 2005a]). As a rule, these tests are quite easy even for individuals with low intelligence and neuropsychological problems, although the tests appear, on the surface, to be much more difficult than they actually are. Poor symptom validity test scores suggest poor or variable effort, whereas worse than chance performance on these measures suggests that the patient deliberately attempted to perform poorly and likely is malingering.

## Innate Relative Weakness or Brain Impairment

Everyone has relative strengths and weaknesses in various areas, including the neuropsychological arena. If an individual is administered a large number of cognitive measures, some results will be relatively higher and some will be relatively lower than the average performance. When a person is evaluated after a TBI, a neuropsychologist may be tempted to attribute low scores on one or more tests to that individual's TBI. However, careful consideration must be given to the possibility that current low scores simply reflect innate relatively lower areas of ability.

In determining the presence and severity of injury, the neuropsychologist will find preinjury standardized cognitive testing to be extremely valuable. If preinjury testing showed poorer performance in the areas of attention and memory, then it would be clinically inappropriate to attribute current low scores in these areas to TBI unless current scores were considerably lower than preinjury levels of performance. Unfortunately, such preinjury standardized testing is rarely available, and when it is available, it typically does not cover the domains that are most likely to be impaired following TBI—that is, attention, memory, processing speed, and executive functioning. Although no good solution to this problem exists, a careful history can be helpful in identifying areas of neuropsychological functioning that were relative strengths and weaknesses. Asking the patient to describe his or her academic performance and to identify courses that he or she experienced as particularly difficult or easy may be especially useful toward that end. Asking about any difficulties with paying attention in class and about memorization abilities in classes also can be informative, and asking about interests and hobbies can provide clues to areas of relative strength. One should not assume that an individual's areas of relative cognitive strength are reflective of his or her overall neuropsychological abilities, and one should avoid concluding, perhaps incorrectly, that relatively lower scores on tests of other cognitive abilities reflect the effects of TBI.

## Comorbidities

Just as individuals have areas of innate cognitive strengths and weaknesses, some individuals have pre-TBI conditions or postinjury comorbidities that overlap with and confound interpretation of TBI-related cognitive impairments. Individuals with attention deficit disorder, learning disabilities, conduct disorder, alcohol or substance abuse, and even depression are more likely to sustain a subsequent TBI (Vassallo et al. 2007). All of these conditions, as well as other comorbidities such as anxiety and psychosis, have neuropsychological correlates. It is extremely important not to attribute current post-TBI problems to TBI when they are actually secondary to such preexisting or comorbid conditions.

# CONCLUSION

Neuropsychological evaluation contributes usefully to the evaluation of adults with TBI. This type of clinical evaluation is used to assess patients for neuropsychological evidence of brain dysfunction when there is uncertainty about whether a clinically significant TBI has occurred, to assess the types and severities of cognitive and psychological sequelae of TBI, and to help develop a differential diagnosis for a patient's neuropsychological difficulties. Importantly, neuropsychological assessment cannot provide a definitive diagnosis of TBI. It offers an objective measure of actual cognitive and behavioral abilities, but interpretation of performance on neuropsychological testing requires consideration of a broad range of factors other than brain integrity.

## *Key Clinical Points*

- Neuropsychological evaluation is the only neurodiagnostic procedure that can evaluate how a person is cognitively and behaviorally functioning in everyday life. This evaluation can delineate the cognitive and behavioral sequelae of brain injury and assist with differential diagnosis and treatment planning.

- Following a closed (nonpenetrating) TBI, the most common neuropsychological problems are in the areas of attention/concentration (working memory), new learning and memory, information processing speed, and executive functioning.

- Because cognitive recovery is typically rapid following a mild TBI, comprehensive neuropsychological testing is not recommended during the first 30 days postinjury. The exception to this is in the area of sports concussions, because preinjury baseline data are often available and postinjury reassessments can be important in acute concussion management.

- Although comprehensive formal neuropsychological testing is not indicated during the period of posttraumatic amnesia following a moderate to severe TBI, short assessments can be helpful in determining whether specific neurological syndromes are present, such as aphasia, visual field cut, visual neglect, visual agnosia, or focal frontal syndromes.

- Validity assessment is a crucial aspect of any neuropsychological evaluation, particularly in the forensic arena.

- To avoid erroneous conclusions, computerized neuropsychological assessment should be completed only by neuropsychologists with psychometric and TBI expertise.

- Interpretation of neuropsychological test findings is complicated by validity and effort concerns, uncertain levels of a patient's premorbid functioning, and preinjury or comorbid conditions that could affect performance.

# REFERENCES

Beck AT, Steer RA: Beck Anxiety Inventory: Manual. San Antonio, TX, Psychological Corporation, 1990

Beck AT, Steer RA, Brown GK: Beck Depression Inventory: Manual, 2nd Edition. San Antonio, TX, Psychological Corporation, 1996

Belanger HG, Vanderploeg RD: The neuropsychological impact of sports-related concussion: a meta-analysis. J Int Neuropsychol Soc 11:345–357, 2005

Belanger HG, Curtiss G, Demery JA, et al: Factors moderating neuropsychological outcomes following mild traumatic brain injury: a meta-analysis. J Int Neuropsychol Soc 11:215–227, 2005

Benedict RHB: Brief Visuospatial Memory Test–Revised (BVMT-R): Professional Manual. Lutz, FL, Psychological Assessment Resources, 1997

Benton AL: Contributions to Neuropsychological Assessment: A Clinical Manual, 2nd Edition. New York, Oxford University Press, 1994

Butcher JN, Dahlstrom WG, Graham JR, et al: MMPI-2: Minnesota Multiphasic Personality Inventory–2: Manual for Administration, Scoring and Interpretation. Minneapolis, University of Minnesota Press, 1989

Conners CK: Continuous Performance Test II. Toronto, ON, Canada, Multi-Health Systems, 2000

Corrigan JD: Development of a scale for assessment of agitation following traumatic brain injury. J Clin Exp Neuropsychol 11:261–277, 1989

Courville CB: Coup-contrecoup mechanism of craniocerebral injuries: some observations. Arch Surg 45:19–43, 1942

Defense and Veterans Brain Injury Center: Consensus Conference on the Acute Management of Concussion/Mild Traumatic Brain Injury (mTBI) in the Deployed Setting. Washington, DC, Defense and Veterans Brain Injury Center, 2008

Delis DC, Kramer JH, Kaplan E, et al: California Verbal Learning Test (CVLT-II)–Adult Version, 2nd Edition. San Antonio, TX, NCS Pearson, 2000

Delis DC, Kaplan E, Kramer JH: Delis-Kaplan Executive Function System (D-KEFS). San Antonio, TX, NCS Pearson, 2001

Dikmen S, Machamer JE, Winn HR, et al: Neuropsychological outcome at 1-year post head injury. Neuropsychology 9:80–90, 1995

Dikmen S, Machamer J, Temkin N: Neurobehavioral consequences of traumatic brain injury, in Neuropsychological Assessment of Neuropsychiatric and Neuromedical Disorders, 3rd Edition. Edited by Grant I, Adams KM. New York, Oxford University Press, 2009, pp 597–617

Giacino JT, Kalmar K, Whyte J: The JFK Coma Recovery Scale—Revised: measurement characteristics and diagnostic utility. Arch Phys Med Rehabil 85:2020–2029, 2004

Golden CJ: Stroop Color and Word Test. Chicago, IL, Stoelting, 1978

Goodglass H, Kaplan E, Barresi B: Boston Diagnostic Aphasia Examination (BDAE), 3rd Edition. Philadelphia, PA, Lippincott Williams & Wilkins, 2001

Graham DI: Neuropathology of head injury, in Neurotrauma. Edited by Narayan RK, Povlishock J, Wilberger J. New York, McGraw-Hill Professional, 1996, pp 43–60

Green P: Medical Symptom Validity Test (WSVT) for Windows: User's Manual and Program, Revised. Edmonton, AB, Canada, Green's Publishing, 2005a

Green P: Word Memory Test (WMT) for Windows: User's Manual and Programs, Revised. Edmonton, AB, Canada, Green's Publishing, 2005b

Gronwall DM: Paced Auditory Serial Addition Task: a measure of recovery from concussion. Percept Mot Skills 44:367–373, 1977

Heaton RK, Psychological Assessment Resources: Wisconsin Card Sorting Test Manual, Revised and Expanded. Odessa, FL, Psychological Assessment Resources, 1993

Kaplan E, Goodglass H, Weintraub S: Boston Naming Test, 2nd Edition. Philadelphia, PA, Lippincott Williams & Wilkins, 2001

Larrabee GJ: Assessment of malingering, in Forensic Neuropsychology: A Scientific Approach. Edited by Larrabee GJ. New York, Oxford University Press, 2005, pp 115–158

Levin H: Neurobehavioral sequelae of closed head injuries, in Head Injury, 3rd Edition. Edited by Cooper PR. Baltimore, MD, Williams & Wilkins, 1993, pp 525–551

Levin HS, O'Donnell VM, Grossman RG: The Galveston Orientation and Amnesia Test: a practical scale to assess cognition after head injury. J Nerv Ment Dis 167:675–684, 1979

Lezak MD, Howieson DB, Loring DW: Neuropsychological Assessment, 4th Edition. New York, Oxford University Press, 2004

Malec J, Lezak MD: Manual for the Mayo-Portland Adaptability Inventory (MPAI-4) for Adults, Children and Adolescents. Rochester, MN, Mayo Clinic and Medical School, 2003

Management of Concussion–Mild Traumatic Brain Injury Working Group: VA/DoD Clinical Practice Guideline for Management of Concussion/ Mild Traumatic Brain Injury (mTBI). Department of Veterans Affairs and Department of Defense. Washington, DC, Department of Veterans Affairs, Department of Defense, 2009. Available at: http://www.healthquality. va.gov/management_of_concussion_mtbi.asp. Accessed June 23, 2012.

Matthews CG, Klove K: Instruction Manual for the Adult Neuropsychological Test Battery. Madison, University of Wisconsin Medical School, 1964

McCrea M, American Academy of Clinical Neuropsychology: Mild Traumatic Brain Injury and Postconcussion Syndrome: The New Evidence Base for Diagnosis and Treatment. New York, Oxford University Press, 2008

Meyers JE, Meyers KR: Rey Complex Figure Test and Recognition Trial. Lutz, FL, Psychological Assessment Resources, 1995

Milberg WP, Hebben N, Kaplan E: The Boston process approach to neuropsychological assessment, in Neuropsychological Assessment of Neuropsychiatric and Neuromedical Disorders, 3rd Edition. Edited by Grant I, Adams KM. New York, Oxford University Press, 2009, pp 42–65

Morey LC: Personality Assessment Inventory (PAI): Professional Manual, 2nd Edition. Lutz, FL, Psychological Assessment Resources, 2007

NCS Pearson: Test of Premorbid Functioning. San Antonio, TX, NCS Pearson, 2009

Novack TA, Kofoed BA, Crossno B: Sequential performance on the California Verbal Learning Test following traumatic brain injury. Clin Neuropsychol 9:38–43, 1995

Randolph C: Repeatable Battery for the Assessment of Neuropsychological Status (RBANS). San Antonio, TX, NCS Pearson, 1998

Rappaport M, Hall KM, Hopkins K, et al: Disability rating scale for severe head trauma: coma to community. Arch Phys Med Rehabil 63:118–123, 1982

Reeves D, Winter K, Culligan K, et al: Automated Neuropsychological Assessment Metrics (ANAM). Pensacola, FL, Space and Naval Warfare Systems Command, 2001

Reitan RM, Wolfson D: The Halstead-Reitan Neuropsychological Test Battery for Adults: theoretical, methodological, and validation bases, in Neuropsychological Assessment of Neuropsychiatric and Neuromedical Disorders, 3rd Edition. Edited by Grant I, Adams KM. New York, Oxford University Press, 2009, pp 3–24

Ruff RM, Camenzuli L, Mueller J: Miserable minority: emotional risk factors that influence the outcome of a mild traumatic brain injury. Brain Inj 10:551–565, 1996

Ruttan L, Martin K, Liu A, et al: Long-term cognitive outcome in moderate to severe traumatic brain injury: a meta-analysis examining timed and untimed tests at 1 and 4.5 or more years after injury. Arch Phys Med Rehabil 89(suppl):S69–S76, 2008

Schmidt M: Rey Auditory Verbal Learning Test: A Handbook. Los Angeles, CA, Western Psychological Services, 1996

Schretlen D: Brief Test of Attention Professional Manual. Lutz, FL, Psychological Assessment Resources, 1997

Schretlen DJ, Shapiro AM: A quantitative review of the effects of traumatic brain injury on cognitive functioning. Int Rev Psychiatry 15:341–349, 2003

Tombaugh TN: Test of Memory Malingering. New York, Multi-Health Systems, 1996

Vanderploeg RD: The interpretation process, in Clinician's Guide to Neuro-psychological Assessment, 2nd Edition. Edited by Vanderploeg RD. Mahwah, NJ, Erlbaum, 2000, pp 103–143

Vanderploeg RD, Curtiss G, Luis CA, et al: Long-term morbidities following self-reported mild traumatic brain injury. J Clin Exp Neuropsychol 29:585–598, 2007

Vassallo JL, Proctor-Weber Z, Lebowitz BK, et al: Psychiatric risk factors for traumatic brain injury. Brain Inj 21:567–573, 2007

Wechsler D: Wechsler Adult Intelligence Scale, 3rd Edition. San Antonio, TX, NCS Pearson, 1997

Wechsler D: Wechsler Test of Adult Reading. San Antonio, TX, NCS Pearson, 2001

Wechsler D: Wechsler Adult Intelligence Scale, 4th Edition. San Antonio, TX, NCS Pearson, 2008

Wechsler D: Wechsler Memory Scale, 4th Edition. San Antonio, TX, NCS Pearson, 2009

Whiteneck GG, Charlifue SW, Gerhart KA, et al: Quantifying handicap: a new measure of long-term rehabilitation outcomes. Arch Phys Med Rehabil 73:519–526, 1992

Wilkinson GS, Robertson GJ, Psychological Assessment Resources: WRAT4: Wide Range Achievement Test, Professional Manual, 4th Edition. Lutz, FL, Psychological Assessment Resources, 2006

Willer B, Ottenbacher KJ, Coad ML: The Community Integration Questionnaire: a comparative examination. Am J Phys Med Rehabil 73:103–111, 1994

Wilson JT, Pettigrew LE, Teasdale GM: Structured interviews for the Glasgow Outcome Scale and the extended Glasgow Outcome Scale: guidelines for their use. J Neurotrauma 15:573–585, 1998

# PART III

# MANAGEMENT

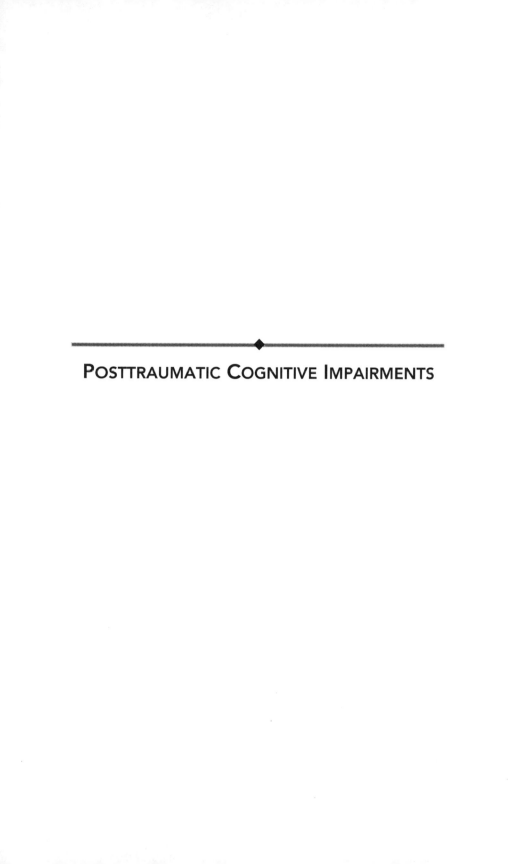

# POSTTRAUMATIC COGNITIVE IMPAIRMENTS

CHAPTER 4

# Disorders of Consciousness

*John Whyte, M.D., Ph.D.*
*Joseph T. Giacino, Ph.D.*

***Traumatic brain injury*** (TBI) is a leading cause of disorders of consciousness (DOC), including coma, vegetative state (VS), and the minimally conscious state (MCS). The scientific landscape in DOC has changed dramatically over the last decade, with new conceptual developments, greater understanding of natural history and underlying mechanisms, improved assessment techniques, and emerging treatments. Refining the diagnostic criteria for DOC has advanced clinical management and long-term care planning for patients with these conditions. Notwithstanding these advances, error rates as high as 41% continue to be seen in distinguishing among these conditions, with the majority of errors involving misdiagnosing patients in MCS as being in VS (Schnakers et al. 2009). Recovery of consciousness generally reflects increasing restoration of neurocognitive function, but progression from coma to full consciousness does not always proceed in a linear manner. Although the conditions captured by the term *disorders of consciousness* often have overlapping features, distinctions among them can be made using specialized assessment procedures. In this chapter, we describe the clinical diagnostic criteria for coma, VS, and MCS. We also describe the posttraumatic confusional state (PTCS) and distinguish all of these conditions from the locked-in syndrome (LIS).

# Definitions and Differential Diagnosis

## Coma

*Coma* is defined pathophysiologically as failure of the reticular system, which is primarily responsible for mediating tonic arousal functions (Plum and Posner 1982). On bedside examination, the patient has no voluntary movement, and behavioral responses are limited to reflex activity. The eyes remain continuously closed; when manually opened, they do not fixate or follow visual stimuli. The continuous absence of spontaneous or stimulus-induced eye opening is characteristic of coma, and the electroencephalogram (although not required for diagnosis) reveals absence of sleep-wake cycles. Coma generally resolves within 2–4 weeks and, in most cases of continued unconsciousness, evolves into VS or MCS.

## Vegetative State

The term *vegetative state* was coined by Jennett and Plum in 1972 to denote a clinical condition in which the vegetative functions (e.g., cardiovascular, respiratory, and thermoregulation functions) remain preserved in the setting of complete loss of higher cortical function. VS is distinguished from coma by the reemergence of the sleep-wake cycle, signaled clinically by periods of spontaneous eye opening (Jennett and Plum 1972). As when a patient is in coma, bedside examination yields no observable response to command, no intelligible speech (although moaning may occur), and no other evidence of purposeful or voluntary behavior (Multi-Society Task Force on PVS 1994a, 1994b). Infrequently, behaviors such as inappropriate smiling, crying, or grimacing, and even randomly produced single words (Schiff et al. 1999), may be observed, but these behaviors are not tied to specific environmental precipitants. For example, the patient may cry when spoken to by a family member but also in response to the sound of a door closing. When VS lasts 1 month or more, this condition is referred to as *persistent vegetative state* (PVS). For persons with TBI, VS is considered permanent after 12 months (Multi-Society Task Force on PVS 1994a, 1994b).

# Minimally Conscious State

The *minimally conscious state* is characterized by the presence of inconsistent but clearly discernible behavioral signs of consciousness (Giacino et al. 2002). Signs of consciousness must be reproducible, and care must be taken to differentiate these events from random or spontaneous occurrences of the same behavior, by demonstrating their contingent relationship to relevant environmental events. Serial reassessment may help confirm the diagnosis when initial examination findings are ambiguous or variable as a result of behavioral variability. Visual pursuit is often the first sign of the transition from VS to MCS because it frequently presages other signs of conscious awareness (Giacino and Whyte 2005). Akinetic mutism (Cairns et al. 1941), characterized by severely diminished drive or intention (Giacino and Kalmar 1997), represents a distinct subcategory of MCS. In akinetic mutism, unlike other forms of MCS, arousal and vigilance are often well preserved and do not account for the marked behavioral aspontaneity and anergia that define this condition. In addition, the lesion profile in akinetic mutism typically localizes to the posterior diencephalon or basal and mesial frontal regions, rather than the more common neurotrauma-induced pattern of diffuse axonal injury and multifocal contusions.

Emergence from MCS occurs when the patient clearly demonstrates reliable communication through verbal or gestural yes-no responses, or recovery of functional object use (Giacino et al. 2002), both of which require preservation of large-scale distributed cortical processing networks and enable meaningful environmental interaction.

# Posttraumatic Confusional State

Although emergence from MCS is marked by recovery of basic communication and/or practic functions (i.e., praxis), severe cognitive, behavioral, and affective disturbances persist. Patients commonly exhibit temporal and spatial disorientation, distractibility, anterograde amnesia, impaired judgment, perceptual disturbance, restlessness, sleep disorder, and emotional lability. This symptom constellation has been termed *posttraumatic confusional state* (Stuss et al. 1999). During PTCS, 24-hour supervision and assistance are required to ensure the patient's safety and completion of routine self-care activities. Sherer et al. (2005) found that 70% of patients with TBI admitted to an inpatient rehabilitation facility met operational criteria for PTCS.

Among patients emerging from MCS, the percentage meeting the criteria for PTCS is likely substantially higher.

## Locked-In Syndrome

LIS is not a disorder of consciousness; however, it is characterized by severely reduced behavioral responsiveness and therefore must be differentiated from coma, VS, and MCS to ensure proper clinical management. LIS is marked by tetraplegia and anarthria in the setting of well-preserved cognitive function (Plum and Posner 1966). Arousal and alertness may be compromised during the acute stage, but these impairments generally resolve within a period of days (Smart et al. 2008). The average time to diagnosis has been estimated to be 2.5 months, and family members usually detect signs of consciousness (in 55% of cases) before medical staff (in 23% of cases) are able to do so (Laureys et al. 2005). In classic LIS, patients have complete paralysis of the orobuccal musculature and all four extremities. Vertical eye movements are generally spared and allow nonverbal communication through directional gaze, although ocular bobbing may interfere with eye movement control during the acute stage. Perceptual functions are also spared, because ascending afferent axons remain intact.

## EPIDEMIOLOGY

Estimates of the incidence and prevalence of posttraumatic VS and MCS are crude for a number of reasons. Diagnostic classification systems, such as the ICD-10 (World Health Organization 1992/2010), do not recognize MCS, and no population-based surveillance systems are available to capture cases across settings. Some individuals who are in VS at the time of hospital discharge escape notice during emergence while residing in nonspecialized custodial care facilities. Additionally, few incidence and prevalence studies distinguish among the diagnoses that led to the disorder of consciousness, so the estimates provided here combine those of traumatic and nontraumatic etiologies. The annual incidence of VS at 1 month postinjury in the United States is estimated to be 46 cases per million, after excluding congenital and neurodegenerative causes (Jennett 2002).

Prevalence figures are even more elusive because they are influenced not only by obstacles to surveillance but also by adequacy of care and decisions to withdraw artificial nutrition and hydration. Prevalence estimates for VS in the United States range from 25,000 (Multi-Society Task Force on PVS 1994a, 1994b) to 420,000 (Spudis 1991). Prevalence rates are also influenced by survival time, an index that is not always considered in published estimates. Mean survival after 1 month in VS is reported to be 2–5 years; mean survival increased to 10 years for those alive at 1 year postinjury and increased to more than 20 years for those alive at 4 years postinjury (Beaumont and Kenealy 2005).

Fins et al. (2007) used a severity model to project an annual incidence of 8,844–25,088 MCS cases per year in the United States. Strauss et al. (2000) concluded that the prevalence of MCS in the United States is between 112,000 and 280,000. However, the reliability of these estimates is questionable because they are calculated indirectly. Prospective collection of epidemiological data is required to more precisely characterize the demography of MCS.

# PATHOPHYSIOLOGY

The pathophysiology of coma, VS, and MCS has been investigated in postmortem analyses and through structural and functional neuroimaging studies. Lesion profiles are largely determined by the primary mechanism of injury. In traumatic coma, centripetal acceleration-deceleration forces cause diffuse axonal injury, producing immediate loss of consciousness. Focal mesodiencephalic lesions may also be sufficient to cause coma. Positron emission tomography studies demonstrate that resting brain metabolism is reduced by 40%–50% during coma, reflecting global brain dysfunction (Laureys and Boly 2007).

The prototypical lesion profile in traumatic VS involves extensive bihemispheric white matter injury, occurring in up to 71% of cases. More severe diffuse axonal injury is manifested by punctate lesions distributed throughout the corpus callosum (grade 2) or the corpus callosum and rostral brain stem (grade 3) (Adams et al. 2000). Associated ischemic injury is evident in the thalamus (80%) and watershed areas (43%). Functional neuroimaging studies suggest that traumatic VS is best construed as a disconnection syndrome. Functional magnetic resonance imaging (fMRI) studies employing auditory, visual, or noxious stimulation show activation of primary auditory, visual, and somatosensory cortices, with severely reduced brain metabolism in secondary frontotemporoparietal association cortices. The so-called default mode network, a set of functionally interconnected brain regions that activate when the brain is not engaged in externally driven tasks, is also markedly downregulated in VS. Recent investigations indicate that the extent of default network connectivity is proportionally related to level of consciousness, with systematically increasing connectivity evident in the progression from coma, through VS and MCS, and on to LIS and finally healthy controls (Vanhaudenhuyse et al. 2010). These findings suggest that retention of default network activity may be a necessary condition for conscious awareness.

Pathophysiological studies of traumatic MCS also show a preponderance of thalamic lesions and grade 2 and 3 diffuse axonal injury. One postmortem study found greater sparing of corticocortical and corticothalamic connections in MCS (Jennett et al. 2001). Functional neuroimaging studies show that in MCS, in contrast to VS, connectivity between primary and associative cortices is intact, suggesting greater preservation of the distributed neural systems that are necessary to support cognitive processing.

In LIS, the persistent inability to speak or move the extremities is due to disruption of the corticospinal and corticobulbar tracts at the level of the ventral pons. Basilar thrombosis accounts for approximately 60% of cases. Functional neuroimaging studies typically show complete preservation of cortical regions, including the default network (Vanhaudenhuyse et al. 2010). The cerebellum is hypometabolic, likely giving rise to the ubiquitous motor incoordination deficits.

# PROGNOSIS

Prognostic research on DOC has been limited by several factors. The differential diagnosis among these disorders is challenging, and the evidence needed to establish a specific diagnosis confidently is documented inconsistently in medical records. MCS is more recently defined than VS (Giacino et al. 2002) and, along with confusional states, is not documented in a standard fashion. Thus, it is difficult to conduct prognostic studies using administrative databases. Prospective studies of prognosis are challenged by the fact that most patients with DOC are discharged to private homes and nursing facilities within weeks or months of injury, so far more is known about the patterns of early evolution of DOC than about the fate of those who continue to suffer from a disorder of consciousness at a later time (Multi-Society

Task Force on PVS 1994a, 1994b). Moreover, most prognostic studies have concentrated on dichotomous outcomes, such as return versus nonreturn of consciousness or death versus survival, so little is known about the degree of functional improvement that can be anticipated if consciousness does return.

Despite these limitations, the prognosis for recovery of consciousness from VS is related to the time since injury, depth of unconsciousness, and rate of functional change (Whyte et al. 2005). Recovering from VS to MCS early after injury is a positive prognostic sign for further recovery (Giacino and Kalmar 1997). Neuropathological variables that predict variations in recovery among those with DOC have not been conclusively identified (Giacino and Whyte 2005). Some evidence suggests that patients with callosal and dorsolateral brain stem lesions who remain in VS for at least 2 months have a much lower probability of recovery of consciousness by 1 year than those without lesions in these locations (Kampfl et al. 1998). Among adults who remain vegetative 1 month after TBI, about half will regain consciousness by 1 year postinjury (Multi-Society Task Force on PVS 1994a, 1994b). Although recovery is most likely in the early months, some patients continue to regain consciousness up to and even beyond 1 year postinjury, in contrast to the much lower proportion of patients with nontraumatic injuries who demonstrate late recoveries (Multi-Society Task Force on PVS 1994a, 1994b). In view of the small but important number of well-documented late recoveries in the literature and the implications of an incorrect diagnosis of "permanent vegetative state," the American Congress of Rehabilitation Medicine (1995) recommended abandoning the term *permanent vegetative state* in favor of referencing the cause of the injury (e.g., trauma, stroke) and the length of time postonset, because both of these factors carry prognostic information.

Much less is known about the prognosis for further recovery from MCS or confusional states at later time points. One study of patients in MCS at least 1 month postinjury found considerable recovery in 16 of 18 patients over several years' time, with duration of MCS not strongly correlated with the ultimate outcome (Lammi et al. 2005). Prediction of the time course of recovery from confusion is less well studied.

Life expectancy in DOC is reduced, and various factors contribute to this shortening. The death rate in the first year is high (one-third to one-half), likely owing, in part, to the complications associated with brain injuries severe enough to induce VS (Multi-Society Task

Force on PVS 1994a, 1994b). However, beyond the first year, extended survival is possible, although it remains shortened in comparison to the general population (Strauss et al. 1999). Increased mortality is likely due to factors that affect TBI survivors more generally, such as cardiovascular disease related to immobility, pneumonia and sepsis, and seizures (Shavelle et al. 2001; Strauss et al. 2004). Little is known about how caregivers' views of aggressive medical care evolve over time, so decisions not to treat late complications may contribute to reduced survival.

# CLINICAL ASSESSMENT

## Behavioral Assessment

Consciousness—an internal subjective state—cannot be assessed directly and therefore must be inferred from other sources of information. Behavioral assessment remains the gold standard for detecting signs of consciousness in patients with severe speech and motor impairments. Perhaps surprisingly, no practice standards have been established to govern the methodology, frequency, or duration of behavioral assessment. This seems a particularly glaring omission in view of the inherent challenges posed by reliance on indirect measures of consciousness. Ultimately, the examiner's task is to systematically elicit and distinguish voluntary, automatic, and reflexive behaviors.

The high rate of misdiagnosis reported in the literature likely reflects cumulative "error" contributed by the examiner, patient, and environment. The risk of examiner error increases when the scope of the assessment is too narrow or when interpretation of responses rests on subjective judgment alone. Patient variability due to fluctuations in arousal, subclinical seizure activity, occult illness, or pain may interfere with assessment, and sensory, motor, or cognitive deficits may confound assessment as well. Environmental factors, such as sedating medications, restrictions in range of movement caused by restraints and immobilization techniques, poor positioning, or distracting ambient noise, heat, or light, may also interfere with assessment. These sources of error are of particular concern when major decisions, such as end-of-life planning, rest on the results.

To maximize accuracy, two different but complementary methods of assessment have been devised. In the first of these, assessment and scoring procedures are standardized with the aim of generating a global profile of cerebral function that is reproducible across examiners. Primary indications for standardized assessment include differential diagnosis, outcome prediction, and evaluation of treatment effectiveness. The second approach employs quantitative assessment procedures that are individually tailored to address very specific questions (e.g., Can the individual see? Is a particular movement occurring in response to command?) (DiPasquale and Whyte 1996).

**Standardized assessment.** Many different behavioral rating scales have been constructed to assess patients with diminished levels of responsiveness, but with varying degrees of supporting research (Majerus et al. 2005). Table 4–1 presents a partial listing of scales. At a minimum (Giacino and Smart 2007), standardized behavioral rating scales should do the following:

- Capture a broad range of behavior across a continuum of complexity
- Have sufficient reliability to produce reasonably stable findings across raters
- Have acceptable validity to assure that the scale is measuring the construct under investigation
- Have adequate sensitivity to detect subtle signs of consciousness and sufficient specificity to avoid false-positive errors
- Guide appropriate diagnostic, prognostic, and treatment formulations

In a systematic review of 13 behavioral assessment scales for DOC, Seel et al. (2010) found insufficient evidence to support use of these measures for differential diagnosis or outcome prediction because most studies were not conducted in a masked manner, raising the risk of bias. Following review of the available evidence concerning standardization, content validity, reliability, criterion and/or construct validity, diagnostic validity, and prognostic validity, the authors recommended the Coma Recovery Scale—Revised (CRS-R) for assessment of DOC, with minor reservations. The CRS-R was also selected as the measure of choice for assessment of recovery of consciousness by the Moderate/Severe Traumatic Brain Injury: Rehabilitation Subgroup of the National Institute of Neurological Disorders and Stroke (NINDS) Common Data Element Working Group (www.commondataelements.ninds.nih.gov/TBI.aspx) based on its psychometric characteristics and availability in 10 languages.

**TABLE 4–1.** Neurobehavioral assessment scales designed for patients with disorders of consciousness

| Scale | Target setting | Target populations |
|---|---|---|
| Disorders of Consciousness Scale | Inpatient rehabilitation unit | Coma, VS, MCS |
| Sensory Modality Assessment and Rehabilitation Technique | Inpatient rehabilitation unit | VS, MCS |
| Wessex Head Injury Matrix | ICU/Inpatient rehabilitation unit | Coma, VS, MCS |
| Western Neuro Sensory Stimulation Profile | Inpatient rehabilitation unit | VS, MCS |

*Note.* ICU=intensive care unit; MCS=minimally conscious state; VS=vegetative state.

The CRS-R is intended for use by medical and allied health professionals and comprises six subscales addressing auditory, visual, motor, oromotor/verbal, communication, and arousal functions. Subscale items are hierarchically arranged, corresponding to brain stem, subcortical, and cortically mediated functions. Administration and scoring guidelines are manualized. The scale is well represented in the scientific literature and has been used to investigate diagnostic accuracy (Giacino et al. 2004; Schnakers et al. 2008), the relationship between behavioral and neurophysiological markers of consciousness (Coleman et al. 2009; Newcombe et al. 2010; Smart et al. 2008), outcome prediction (Giacino and Kalmar 1997; Vanhaudenhuyse et al. 2008), and treatment effectiveness (Schiff et al. 2007).

Other behavioral assessment scales recommended by the American Congress of Rehabilitation Medicine DOC Task Force (Seel et al. 2010), with moderate reservations, are listed in Table 4–1.

*Quantitative individualized behavioral assessment.* Although standardized assessment has many advantages, by its nature it cannot always clarify questions of interest regarding individual patients. For example, a patient may be reported by caregivers to smile or laugh in response to television comedy shows, an observation that, if accurate, would indicate interaction with the environment. In other cases, a specific confounding sensory or motor deficit may interfere with the clear interpretation of a score from a standardized scale, such as when a patient may not follow a command because of impaired hearing and vision. Finally, standardized scales may not be able to address clinical questions more specific than state of consciousness. For example, an examiner may be aware that the patient demonstrates visual tracking on a scale item, but may still be interested in the state of the individual visual fields or the presence of hemi-inattention.

Quantitative individualized behavioral assessment (QIBA) makes use of the principles of single-subject experimental design to answer questions like this (Whyte and DiPasquale 1995; Whyte et al. 1999) and can be a useful adjunct to standardized assessment. In brief, a question of clinical interest is identified, and an individualized assessment protocol is designed that operationalizes the examiner's stimuli and the patient's behaviors that constitute a response. To confirm a patient's reactions to comedy shows, for example, one might identify a set of video vignettes from comedy shows and a similar set from news programs, and show these to the patient in random order. Smiling and laughing would be defined in very specific terms, and then the presence or absence of these behaviors would be examined for its association with the type of video vignette.

In Table 4–2, we show the application of the QIBA method to the assessment of command following. The patient was given a standard set of verbal commands, in random order, across many assessment sessions. After the command was given (or after the silent interval was started, in the case of silent observation), a defined degree of elbow flexion occurring within 10 seconds was defined as a response. Note that if an examiner had simply given the verbal command "Bend your elbow," he or she would have seen a fairly high frequency of response. However, this type of response occurred with similar frequency in response to "Hold still" but more often following either verbal command than during silent observation. These observations suggested either that the patient had a profound language comprehension problem, with some preservation of consciousness, or that despite being unconscious, she increased her frequency of spontaneous movement in response to noise of any kind. A subsequent protocol demonstrated that this patient was vegetative but responsive to noise.

# Electrophysiological Assessment

Routine assessment using electroencephalography (EEG) or more prolonged recording may reveal frequent occult seizure activity that

**TABLE 4–2.**  Responses of a patient to commands using a quantitative individualized behavioral assessment approach

| | PATIENT RESPONSE | |
|---|---|---|
| EXAMINER INSTRUCTION | FLEXES ELBOW | NO RESPONSE |
| Bend your arm | 34 (40% of time) | 50 |
| Hold still | 36 (43% of time) | 48 |
| [Silent observation] | 24 (29% of time) | 60 |

*Note.*  Results indicate the patient's responses across multiple sessions.

could be suppressing consciousness. Short-latency evoked potentials may help clarify the integrity of visual and auditory pathways and, thereby, help identify potential confounds in the assessment of consciousness (e.g., when a patient fails to follow a command to "look at the cup" for reasons of visual or auditory impairments). The resting EEG spectrum is also associated with prognosis (Kotchoubey et al. 2005).

Some researchers have used cognitive event-related potentials (i.e., relatively late evoked waves associated with various steps in cognitive processing) and similar techniques to explore the contents of consciousness independent of motor responses. Many of these techniques make use of the general tendency for rare or unexpected events to evoke larger electrical responses than repetitive familiar events. Thus, one can assess whether the nervous system "discriminates" between a rare high tone and more common low tones, a rare word and more common nonwords, or even a rare anomalous end of a sentence and common sentences that end in expected ways. Although such differences clearly signify discrimination at some level of the nervous system, surprisingly complex processing is possible in sleep or under anesthesia. More compelling evidence for consciousness in the absence of behavioral responses is electrophysiological evidence of command following. In one study, for example, 22% of patients who were assessed as vegetative using behavioral assessment demonstrated larger evoked responses to words from one of five equally probable semantic categories (e.g., furniture) when they were instructed to attend to that category (Kotchoubey et al. 2005). Commands to engage in mental imagery, similarly, may activate motor areas (Kranczioch et al. 2009). Such electrophysiological techniques have already been shown, in principle, to be able to detect some evidence of consciousness that is not behaviorally observable. However, none of these techniques has been sufficiently studied in terms of sensitivity, specificity, or prognostic power to be routinely applied clinically.

# Neuroimaging

*Structural imaging.* To date, structural imaging has played only a minor role in assessing patients with DOC. In the early period of DOC, computed tomography (CT) or magnetic resonance imaging (MRI) may be used to screen for treatable complications such as chronic fluid collections or communicating hydrocephalus, which may impede recovery. Use of structural imaging for prognostic prediction, however, has been of limited value (Whyte et al. 2005). This is likely due to a combination of factors, including the fact that diffuse axonal injury, often implicated in prolonged DOC, is poorly imaged, and the fact that the brain systems that are necessary and sufficient for supporting consciousness are not fully defined. Recent advances in high-resolution MRI and image analysis allow sensitive detection of atrophy in relatively small deep structures such as the thalamus (Kim et al. 2008). Diffusion tensor imaging and tractography show promise in quantifying the degree of damage to specific white matter pathways. Together, these may become useful additions to the prognostic armamentarium, but they are not sufficiently validated at present to serve this role.

*Functional imaging.* Functional neuroimaging technologies are gradually moving closer to clinical application. These procedures are likely to eventually be viewed as complementary to behavioral assessment methods. Neuroimaging paradigms designed to detect active cognitive processing in patients without behavioral evidence of consciousness are now in investigational use. These procedures are expected to play an important role in diagnostic and prognostic decision making (Giacino et al. 2006). In active fMRI paradigms, the subject is instructed to perform a mental task while imaging data are acquired. The activation profile triggered by the instructional set can then be compared to profiles obtained at rest, or during a second instructional set known to activate a non-overlapping cortical network. In effect, active imaging paradigms, like some of the electrophysiological assessment methods, are designed to detect covert command-following.

In the first study of this type, Owen et al. (2006) instructed a patient with a behavioral diagnosis of traumatic VS undergoing fMRI to imagine either playing tennis or walking around the rooms of her home. In healthy volunteers, these two mental imagery tasks produce distinct regions of activation: in the supplementary motor area for tennis playing and the parahippocampal place area for home navigation. When the patient was instructed to imagine playing tennis, activation was observed in the supplementary motor area, but when she was instructed to imagine walking through her house, activation shifted to the premotor cortex, parahippocampal gyrus, and posterior parietal cortex. These contingent shifts in task-specific activity were interpreted as voluntary responses reflecting the intention of the patient. Based on these findings, the authors concluded that the patient was not in VS. Preserved command-following capacity has also been demonstrated in a series of patients with minimal or no behavioral signs of awareness by asking them to silently name objects (Rodriguez Moreno et al. 2010). Complete activation of the object-naming network was observed in two of five MCS patients and one of three VS patients, none of whom were able to name or identify objects on bedside examination.

The covert command-following paradigm has been reconfigured for assessment of communication ability (Monti et al. 2010). In one of 31 patients diagnosed with MCS on the CRS-R, it was possible to convert directed imagery tasks into a yes-no communication system by instructing the patient to imagine playing tennis as a proxy for "yes" and walking around the house for "no." Using this procedure, the patient accurately and reliably answered five of six questions concerning the name of a family member. These compelling results hold promise for augmented communication in patients unable to harness compensatory devices due to accompanying sensory and motor impairments.

## Clinical Assessment Summary

Specialized behavioral rating scales, electrophysiological measures, and functional neuroimaging may add additional data to diagnostic decision making. However, these measures are also susceptible to patient variability and technical limitations. Little is known, at present, about the rate of misdiagnosis from each modality or about the number of assessments required to accurately detect intermittent signs of consciousness. In the absence of a true gold standard, the optimal approach to assessment is one that incorporates multimodal measures that can be repeated over time.

# TREATMENT

## Health Maintenance

Recovery of function occurs to varying degrees for a significant proportion of patients with DOC, but no treatments have yet been rigorously proven to enhance that recovery. Thus, much of the early care of patients with DOC focuses on minimizing presumed adverse influences on recovery, preserving bodily health in support of eventual cognitive recovery, and reducing the burden of care while patients remain in these states.

Several neurological complications of TBI may suppress recovery. Frequent occult seizures may result in a patient being frequently or chronically in a postictal state, although evidence-based guidelines regarding the appropriate nature and timing of screening for seizures in this population are lacking. Communicating hydrocephalus may limit recovery; occasionally, abrupt improvements occur after shunting. However, the differentiation of communicating hydrocephalus from hydrocephalus *ex vacuo* is challenging in a population in which diffuse cerebral atrophy is common. Moreover, even an accurate diagnosis of communicating hydrocephalus does not ensure clinical response to shunting because this condition often coexists with other catastrophic forms of brain damage that also limit recovery.

Recent research suggests a high prevalence of endocrine dysfunction related to damage to the hypothalamic-pituitary axis in TBI, particularly in the context of severe injury (Lieberman et al. 2001). Evidence indicates that deficiencies in growth hormone and other hormones may depress cognitive function in patients without brain damage, but the magnitude of this effect in patients with very marginal neural function and, hence, the likely effect of treatment are unknown. As with epilepsy, no evidence-based guidelines are available for timing or content of endocrine screening.

Cognitive function may be depressed for iatrogenic reasons, as when sedating drugs are used to treat co-occurring symptoms. Understandably, few clinical trials have directly addressed this issue. However, a randomized controlled trial of seizure prophylaxis with phenytoin found significantly worse cognitive function in the treatment group than the placebo group early after injury but not later (Dikmen et al. 1991). One might expect even more negative effects of phenytoin on patients with DOC. Thus, any unnecessary medications with potential sedating effects should be withdrawn and less sedating alternatives should be substituted when ongoing treatment is required. One may choose, for example, local nerve or botulinum toxin blocks to control hypertonia rather than centrally acting medications.

Patients with DOC may have a wide range of medical complications typical of the wider population of individuals with severe brain injury and/or multiple trauma. Dysautonomia, in which patients present with some combination of hypertonia, hypertension, tachycardia, sweating, and fever, is characteristic of this patient population in the early weeks after injury, particularly in those with brain stem involvement (Baguley et al. 1999). Episodes may vary in frequency and severity. They may occur without apparent provocation, but may also be triggered by noxious influences, thus limiting the aggressiveness of physical care. Rigorous treatment research is lacking, but treatment ranges from managing individual symptoms (e.g., β-blockers for tachycardia and hypertension, glycopyrrolate for sweating) to use of centrally acting agents such as morphine or gabapentin, which appear promising from case reports (Baguley et al. 2007), but which may involve a trade-off between physical symptoms and alertness.

Patients with DOC universally require some form of feeding tube and incontinence management. Although most patients can be managed with a gastrostomy tube, some with gastric transit deficits or gastroesophageal reflux require jejunal or combination tubes. Urinary incontinence is generally due simply to unconsciousness or is of the uninhibited detrusor type; however, detrusor-sphincter dyssynergia, a risk factor for infection, can occur, so screening of postvoid residuals is warranted. Incontinence is generally best managed with adult diapers and a regular bowel program rather than a catheter, unless skin breakdown is a problem.

Whether caused by the dysautonomic syndrome or by more typical upper motor neuron syndromes, hypertonia is common among those with DOC and may lead to progressive joint contracture and skin breakdown. There is reason to be aggressive in treatment of hypertonia early after injury, because severe deformity may limit functional progress once consciousness returns. However, as with dysautonomia, centrally acting treatments, including intrathecal baclofen, may control tone at the cost of risk to cognitive function. Phenol nerve and motor point blocks and botulinum toxin blocks are ideal alternatives for patients with focal hypertonia, but it is more difficult to manage widespread hypertonia with these methods. Even without significant hypertonia, such patients require regular passive range-of-motion exercises and/or resting splints to maintain joint mobility. Immobility also predisposes to skin breakdown, such that regular turning is required, and patients may need special beds for pressure relief. Thrombophlebitis is another potential concern of immobility, but evidence-based screening recommendations have not been developed for the DOC population, and the optimal duration of prophylactic treatment, if any, is unknown.

Patients who remain unconscious for prolonged periods may be difficult to place in nursing homes and difficult to care for at home. Thus, efforts should be made to simplify the care regimen as much as possible. This may involve attempts at decannulation, and at reducing the frequency of required turning at night (often in conjunction with special bedding), as well as the consolidation of medication and feeding times.

# Enhancing Recovery

Although no treatment to accelerate or improve recovery from DOC is currently supported by peer-reviewed Class I evidence, this is a very active area of research, and there are some promising leads with regard to such interventions (discussed below). However, this entire enterprise is limited by the lack of mechanistically relevant clinical subgrouping. VS, in particular, is defined by the "absence" of behavioral evidence of consciousness. That absence can, in principle, be caused by near total destruction of the neural structures that support cognition and consciousness, or by less profound but key areas of damage such as the supplementary motor area and mesial frontal areas that mediate drive functions and may have greater recovery potential. With this in mind, no single treatment is likely to be of benefit to all patients in VS.

# Environmental Treatments

Sensory stimulation and physical management interventions can be categorized as environmental treatments. Sensory stimulation involves the controlled application of specific types and intensities of sensory stimuli for the purpose of provoking coordinated behavioral activity and enhancing neuroplasticity. The effectiveness of sensory stimulation has been reviewed in five studies over the last 20 years, most recently in 2007. Overall, these reviews agree that the evidence for the efficacy of sensory stimulation programs is weak, but the evidence *against* this effect is similarly weak (Lombardi et al. 2002; Martin and Whyte 2007). Thus, sensory stimulation, combined with physical management to maintain and enhance health, is a typical standard of care, at least during the acute phase of DOC.

With respect to the use of integrated systems of rehabilitation care, there is Class IV evidence (i.e., case series, retrospective reviews) that patients with severe TBI who receive early "formalized" multidisciplinary rehabilitation obtain significantly higher scores on physical, cognitive, and functional outcome measures; have shorter inpatient lengths of stay; and have less residual functional disability during the postacute period (Tanhehco and Kaplan 1982; Timmons et al. 1987). Similarly, "slow to recover" patients (mean initial Glasgow Coma Scale score=5.9) admitted to a long-term rehabilitation unit (mean time to admission>12 months) evidenced significant improvements from admission to discharge (mean length of stay=359 days), with 85% able to be discharged to community-based settings (Gray and Burnham 2000).

## Neuromodulation Treatments

Numerous pharmacological agents as well as hyperbaric oxygen have been advocated for the treatment of DOC. Many of the agents tried have noradrenergic, dopaminergic, or mixed catecholaminergic profiles, with the intent to enhance arousal, drive, and potentially neuroplasticity. These treatments have been directed toward enhancing the course of recovery in the relatively acute period or, less commonly, toward symptomatic improvement in the more chronic phase. Consequently, only Class III evidence exists to support the use of most of these treatments. A meta-analysis of single-subject methylphenidate assessments, which used the drug's short duration of action and multiple crossovers to control for variations in natural recovery, found no evidence that the drug enhanced the following of commands by patients in VS or MCS (Martin and Whyte 2007).

Caregivers and clinicians therefore often find themselves in a position of selecting treatments for patients with DOC that are insufficiently supported by evidence. When making such selections, one must recognize that treatments such as drugs and other physiologically active treatments, intended to substantially alter the function of the nervous system, are capable of powerful adverse effects as well.

Interestingly, some of the most convincing evidence for the ability to modulate consciousness in the chronic period comes not from stimulant or catecholaminergic drugs but instead from the hypnotic agent zolpidem. Although the initial reports that zolpidem could restore consciousness were case reports (Clauss and Nel 2006), the facts that this effect was seen after a single 10-mg dose in several patients after years of unconsciousness, that the patients returned to VS several hours later, and that the effect could be replicated with repeated dosing, made the concern about natural recovery less relevant. Subsequent placebo-controlled single-subject research has verified this phenomenon but shown it to occur for only a small minority of patients with DOC (Whyte and Myers 2009). Zolpidem is an omega-1 $\gamma$-aminobutyric acid type A (GABA$_A$) agonist, which would be expected to have primarily inhibitory neural effects. The neural substrate by which it exerts this effect on consciousness is unknown.

Because neural transmission is modulated through brain electrical activity, it is possible to influence cognition and behavior by titrating the frequency, intensity, and spread of electrical impulses delivered to key structures. Deep brain stimulation (DBS) involves implantation of an electrical pulse generator in the chest wall and of a targeted stimulator lead in the brain, and delivery of electrical pulses through that lead to relevant brain structures. DBS studies conducted in the late 1980s and early 1990s in patients reportedly diagnosed with persistent VS provided reasonably good evidence of increased arousal following introduction of DBS (Kanno et al. 1987; Tsubokawa et al. 1990). However, convincing evidence of meaningful improvement in behavioral output was lacking in these studies.

More recently, Schiff et al. (2007) employed a novel DBS protocol targeting the anterior intralaminar thalamic nuclei in a patient who had remained in posttraumatic MCS for 6.5 years prior to enrollment in the study. Using a single-subject, double-blind, alternating crossover design, significant improvements were noted in level of arousal, upper extremity motor control, and oral feeding during the DBS-On condition. These effects were maintained over time.

## Family Support and Care Planning

Most patients with DOC were, at some point in their post-TBI course, on the verge of death as a result of injury. Hence, their mere survival is initially a source of optimism for relatives and friends. However, the fact that return of consciousness does not automatically follow can be enormously traumatic and may trigger a wide range of individual re-sponses, including denial (seeing evidence of consciousness where it does not exist), anger (feeling that inadequate clinical care is respon-sible), or avoidance (resisting participation in care), as well as more active and adaptive coping strategies that involve information seeking and problem solving. The situation may also have profound effects on the family system, leading to closer collaboration or greater con-flict among family members. In most cases, neither the uncertainty of the prognosis nor the emotional state of caregivers invites early dis-cussions of end-of-life care. However, discussion of do not resuscitate (DNR) status may be appropriate even in the context of continued hope, given the likelihood of further brain damage from an arrest. However, as time passes, the prognosis becomes progressively more predictable, and caregivers may also be able to deliberate more easily and/or clearly on future treatment decisions.

For these reasons, we favor a psychoeducational model of family support and decision making that includes regular updating. This ap-proach involves providing education about DOC, prognosis, and treatment options so that caregivers can operate in an informed state. It also involves responding to the very real emotional trauma they ex-perience from having a loved one who is largely lost to them but who still requires care. For example, presenting a line graph of weekly CRS-R scores provides a visual representation of the rate and degree of change over time and may help families appreciate the likelihood of further improvement. As time passes, if recovery is occurring, its pace is roughly predictive of future outcome (Whyte et al. 2005). If no recovery is apparent, the odds of return of consciousness are pre-dictably reduced, and the level of function that might be achieved even if consciousness returns is diminished. Thus, caregivers who wanted the most aggressive care early after injury may shift toward an interest in more palliative care at a later point, and sometimes to the withdrawal of food and hydration.

In most jurisdictions in the United States, a patient judged to be permanently unconscious may have supportive care withdrawn, whereas patients with severely impaired consciousness (e.g., MCS or confusional state) typically need a very specific advance directive to that effect—something very few individuals have—for supportive care to be withdrawn. This background of changing prognosis and caregiver emotional status requires an ongoing counseling process; however, beyond the first few weeks or months postinjury, most such patients are cared for by nonspecialist physicians, so there is little opportunity for ongoing expert consultation.

## Future of Treatments for Disorders of Consciousness

There is greater optimism than ever before that effective rehabilitation treatments may be found at least for some patients with DOC. The rapidly evolving imaging and electrophysiological measures of brain structure and function may provide greater ability to identify mechanistically relevant patient subgroups who will respond to specific treatments. However, enormous structural and policy obstacles stand in the way of realizing this potential. Many patients with DOC never have contact with neurorehabilitation practitioners with expertise in their condition, and those able to receive such services early often lose contact with those expert systems within months of injury. This issue, driven by funding restrictions on clinical care, limits ongoing counseling about changing prognosis, enrollment in longitudinal research and clinical trials, and expert management of patients' clinical condition.

In 2006, a group of clinical and research experts in DOC issued a Report to Congress that recommended an alternative model to enhance both clinical care and research (Berube et al. 2006). In brief, this model recommended early admission to expert rehabilitation centers, focusing on treatment of medical comorbidities and complications, accurate assessment, care simplification, and initial family education. Patients who failed to demonstrate recovery during this early process would then be discharged to a lower level of care but would retain contact with the specialty center for periodic follow-up and expert consultation, and research enrollment. The cost-effectiveness of this proposed model is unknown, however. At the present time, clinicians must rely primarily on minimizing complications and supporting caregivers in decision making.

## CONCLUSION

Substantial challenges face individuals with posttraumatic DOC and their families, as well as the clinicians caring for them. Recent conceptual refinements and improvements as well as new insights into the pathophysiology of DOC have yielded improved assessment techniques and diagnostic confidence. Treatment continues to focus largely on health maintenance, environmental interventions, and family support and care planning. Pharmacotherapy and neuromodulation treatments are emerging as well, but remain variable in the benefits they afford for persons with DOC. Nonetheless, there is increasing optimism among researchers and clinicians working in this area for the development of effective rehabilitation strategies for patients with disorders of consciousness.

# *Key Clinical Points*

- Patients with severe TBI typically evolve through the stages of coma, vegetative state, minimally conscious state, and posttraumatic confusion prior to developing more coherent behavioral function. The duration of this progression through disorders of consciousness (DOC) depends on the underlying injury severity, and progress may stall at any point beyond coma.

- Traumatic cases of DOC are characterized by bihemispheric white matter pathology, prominent damage to the thalamus, or both, suggesting that DOC are more related to neural connectivity than to a specific critical site.

- Accurate diagnosis is important for accurate prognostication, optimal rehabilitation treatment planning, and informed and ethical decision making. Structured and repeated behavioral assessment using a standardized instrument such as the Coma Recovery Scale–Revised, supplemented by quantitative individualized behavioral assessment, is the mainstay of clinical evaluation, but the emergence of promising electrophysiological and imaging methods will likely lead to more multimodal assessment strategies.

- Although many treatments have been advocated to enhance recovery from DOC, no treatment is associated with definitive evidence of efficacy in large numbers of patients. The predominant clinical priority is to optimize overall health and ease of management while waiting for natural recovery to proceed.

- Because of the neuropathological variability associated with DOC, it is unlikely that any single treatment can benefit all patients with these disorders. Thus, future research is needed to identify pathophysiologically defined subgroups with the potential to respond to specific treatments.

# REFERENCES

Adams JH, Graham DI, Jennett B: The neuropathology of the vegetative state after an acute brain insult. Brain 123:1327–1338, 2000

American Congress of Rehabilitation Medicine: Recommendations for use of uniform nomenclature pertinent to patients with severe alterations in consciousness. Arch Phys Med Rehabil 76:205–209, 1995

Ansell BJ, Keenan JE: The Western Neuro Sensory Stimulation Profile: a tool for assessing slow-to-recover head-injured patients. Arch Phys Med Rehabil 70:104–108, 1989

Baguley IJ, Nicholls JL, Felmingham KL, et al: Dysautonomia after traumatic brain injury: a forgotten syndrome? J Neurol Neurosurg Psychiatry 67:39–43, 1999

Baguley IJ, Heriseanu RE, Gurka JA, et al: Gabapentin in the management of dysautonomia following severe traumatic brain injury: a case series. J Neurol Neurosurg Psychiatry 78:539–541, 2007

Beaumont JG, Kenealy PM: Incidence and prevalence of the vegetative and minimally conscious states. Neuropsychol Rehabil 15:184–189, 2005

Berube J, Fins J, Giacino J, et al: The Mohonk Report: A Report to Congress. Disorders of Consciousness: Assessment, Treatment and Research Needs, 2006. Available at: http://www.northeastcenter.com/the-mohonk-report-disorders-of-consciousness-assessment-treatment research-needs.pdf. Accessed November 15, 2010.

Cairns H, Oldfield RC, Pennybacker JB, et al: Akinetic mutism with an epidermoid cyst of the 3rd ventricle. Brain 64:273–290, 1941

Clauss R, Nel W: Drug induced arousal from the permanent vegetative state. NeuroRehabilitation 21:23–28, 2006

Coleman MR, Davis MH, Rodd JM, et al: Towards the routine use of brain imaging to aid the clinical diagnosis of disorders of consciousness. Brain 132:2541–2552, 2009

Dikmen SS, Temkin NR, Miller B, et al: Neurobehavioral effects of phenytoin prophylaxis of posttraumatic seizures. JAMA 265:1271–1277, 1991

DiPasquale MC, Whyte J: The use of quantitative data in treatment planning for minimally conscious patients. J Head Trauma Rehabil 11:9–17, 1996

Fins JJ, Master MG, Gerber LM, et al: The minimally conscious state: a diagnosis in search of an epidemiology. Arch Neurol 64:1400–1405, 2007

Giacino JT, Kalmar K: The vegetative and minimally conscious states: a comparison of clinical features and functional outcome. J Head Trauma Rehabil 12:36–51, 1997

Giacino JT, Smart CM: Recent advances in behavioral assessment of individuals with disorders of consciousness. Curr Opin Neurol 20:614–619, 2007

Giacino J, Whyte J: The vegetative and minimally conscious states: current knowledge and remaining questions. J Head Trauma Rehabil 20:30–50, 2005

Giacino JT, Ashwal S, Childs N, et al: The minimally conscious state: definition and diagnostic criteria. Neurology 58:349–353, 2002

Giacino JT, Kalmar K, Whyte J: The JFK Coma Recovery Scale–Revised: measurement characteristics and diagnostic utility. Arch Phys Med Rehabil 85:2020–2029, 2004

Giacino JT, Hirsch J, Schiff N, et al: Functional neuroimaging applications for assessment and rehabilitation planning in patients with disorders of consciousness. Arch Phys Med Rehabil 87(suppl):S67–S76, 2006

Gill-Thwaites H: The Sensory Modality Assessment Rehabilitation Technique: a tool for assessment and treatment of patients with severe brain injury in a vegetative state. Brain Inj 11:723–734, 1997

Gill-Thwaites H, Munday R: The Sensory Modality Assessment and Rehabilitation Technique (SMART): a valid and reliable assessment for vegetative state and minimally conscious state patients. Brain Inj 18:1255–1269, 2004

Gray DS, Burnham RS: Preliminary outcome analysis of a long-term rehabilitation program for severe acquired brain injury. Arch Phys Med Rehabil 81:1447–1456, 2000

Jennett B: The vegetative state. J Neurol Neurosurg Psychiatry 73:355–357, 2002

Jennett B, Plum F: Persistent vegetative state after brain damage: a syndrome in search of a name. Lancet 1:734–737, 1972

Jennett B, Adams JH, Murray LS, et al: Neuropathology in vegetative and severely disabled patients after head injury. Neurology 56:486–490, 2001

Kampfl A, Schmutzhard E, Franz G, et al: Prediction of recovery from posttraumatic vegetative state with cerebral magnetic-resonance imaging. Lancet 351:1763–1767, 1998

Kanno T, Kamei Y, Yokoyama T, et al: Neurostimulation for patients in vegetative status. Pacing Clin Electrophysiol 10:207–208, 1987

Kim J, Avants B, Patel S, et al: Structural consequences of diffuse traumatic brain injury: a large deformation tensor-based morphometry study. Neuroimage 39:1014–1026, 2008

Kotchoubey B, Lang S, Mezger G, et al: Information processing in severe disorders of consciousness: vegetative state and minimally conscious state. Clin Neurophysiol 116:2441–2453, 2005

Kranczioch C, Mathews S, Dean PJ, et al: On the equivalence of executed and imagined movements: evidence from lateralized motor and nonmotor potentials. Hum Brain Mapp 30:3275–3286, 2009

Lammi MH, Smith VH, Tate RL, et al: The minimally conscious state and recovery potential: a follow-up study 2 to 5 years after traumatic brain injury. Arch Phys Med Rehabil 86:746–754, 2005

Laureys S, Boly M: What is it like to be vegetative or minimally conscious? Curr Opin Neurol 20:609–613, 2007

Laureys S, Pellas F, Van Eeckhout P, et al: The locked-in syndrome: what is it like to be conscious but paralyzed and voiceless? Prog Brain Res 150:495–511, 2005

Lieberman SA, Oberoi AL, Gilkison CR, et al: Prevalence of neuroendocrine dysfunction in patients recovering from traumatic brain injury. J Clin Endocrinol Metab 86:2752–2756, 2001

Lombardi FL, Taricco M, De Tanti A, et al: Sensory stimulation for brain injured individuals in coma or vegetative state. Cochrane Database Syst Rev (2):CD001427, 2002

Majerus S, Gill-Thwaites H, Andrews K, et al: Behavioral evaluation of consciousness in severe brain damage, in The Boundaries of Consciousness: Neurobiology and Neuropathology (Progress in Brain Research, Vol 150). Boston, MA, Elsevier, 2005, pp 397–413

Martin RT, Whyte J: The effects of methylphenidate on command following and yes/no communication in persons with severe disorders of consciousness: a meta-analysis of n-of-1 studies. Am J Phys Med Rehabil 86:613–620, 2007

Monti MM, Vanhaudenhuyse A, Coleman MR, et al: Willful modulation of brain activity in disorders of consciousness. N Engl J Med 362:579–589, 2010

Multi-Society Task Force on PVS: Medical aspects of the persistent vegetative state (1). N Engl J Med 330:1499–1508, 1994a

Multi-Society Task Force on PVS: Medical aspects of the persistent vegetative state (2). N Engl J Med 330:1572–1579, 1994b

Newcombe VF, Williams GB, Scoffings D, et al: Aetiological differences in neuroanatomy of the vegetative state: insights from diffusion tensor imaging and functional implications. J Neurol Neurosurg Psychiatry 81:552–561, 2010

Owen AM, Coleman MR, Boly M, et al: Detecting awareness in the vegetative state. Science 313:1402, 2006

Pape TL, Heinemann AW, Kelly JP, et al: A measure of neurobehavioral functioning after coma, part I: theory, reliability, and validity of Disorders of Consciousness Scale. J Rehabil Res Dev 42:1–17, 2005

Plum F, Posner J: The Diagnosis of Stupor and Coma. Philadelphia, PA, FA Davis, 1966

Plum F, Posner J: The Diagnosis of Stupor and Coma (Contemporary Neurology), 3rd Edition. New York, Oxford University Press, 1982

Rodriguez Moreno D, Schiff ND, Giacino J, et al: A network approach to assessing cognition in disorders of consciousness. Neurology 75:1871–1878, 2010

Schiff N, Ribary U, Plum F, et al: Words without mind. J Cogn Neurosci 11:650–656, 1999

Schiff ND, Giacino JT, Kalmar K, et al: Behavioural improvements with thalamic stimulation after severe traumatic brain injury. Nature 448:600–603, 2007

Schnakers C, Hustinx R, Vandewalle G, et al: Measuring the effect of amantadine in chronic anoxic minimally conscious state. J Neurol Neurosurg Psychiatry 79:225–227, 2008

Schnakers C, Vanhaudenhuyse A, Giacino J, et al: Diagnostic accuracy of the vegetative and minimally conscious state: clinical consensus versus standardized neurobehavioral assessment. BMC Neurol 9:35, 2009

Seel RT, Sherer M, Whyte J, et al: Assessment scales for disorders of consciousness: evidence-based recommendations for clinical practice and research. Arch Phys Med Rehabil 91:1795–1813, 2010

Shavelle RM, Strauss D, Whyte J, et al: Long-term causes of death after traumatic brain injury. Am J Phys Med Rehabil 80:510–516, quiz 517–519, 2001

Sherer M, Nakase-Thompson R, Yablon SA, et al: Multidimensional assessment of acute confusion after traumatic brain injury. Arch Phys Med Rehabil 86:896–904, 2005

Shiel A, Horn SA, Wilson BA, et al: The Wessex Head Injury Matrix (WHIM) main scale: a preliminary report on a scale to assess and monitor patient recovery after severe head injury. Clin Rehabil 14:408–416, 2000

Smart CM, Giacino JT, Cullen T, et al: A case of locked-in syndrome complicated by central deafness. Nat Clin Pract Neurol 4:448–453, 2008

Spudis EV: The persistent vegetative state, 1990. J Neurol Sci 102:128–136, 1991

Strauss D, Shavelle RM, Ashwal S: Life expectancy and median survival time in the permanent vegetative state. Pediatr Neurol 21:626–631, 1999

Strauss D, Ashwal S, Day SM, et al: Life expectancy of children in vegetative and minimally conscious states. Pediatr Neurol 23:312–319, 2000

Strauss D, Shavelle RM, DeVivo MJ, et al: Life expectancy after traumatic brain injury. NeuroRehabilitation 19:257–258, 2004

Stuss DT, Binns MA, Carruth FG, et al: The acute period of recovery from traumatic brain injury: posttraumatic amnesia or posttraumatic confusional state? J Neurosurg 90:635–643, 1999

Tanhehco J, Kaplan PE: Physical and surgical rehabilitation of patient after 6-year coma. Arch Phys Med Rehabil 63:36–38, 1982

Timmons M, Gasquoine L, Scibak JW: Functional changes with rehabilitation of very severe traumatic brain injury survivors. J Head Trauma Rehabil 2:64–73, 1987

Tsubokawa T, Yamamoto T, Katayama Y, et al: Deep-brain stimulation in a persistent vegetative state: follow-up results and criteria for selection of candidates. Brain Inj 4:315–327, 1990

Vanhaudenhuyse A, Schnakers C, Brédart S, et al: Assessment of visual pursuit in post-comatose states: use a mirror (letter). J Neurol Neurosurg Psychiatry 79:223, 2008

Vanhaudenhuyse A, Noirhomme Q, Tshibanda LJ, et al: Default network connectivity reflects the level of consciousness in non-communicative brain-damaged patients. Brain 133:161–171, 2010

Whyte J, DiPasquale MC: Assessment of vision and visual attention in minimally responsive brain injured patients. Arch Phys Med Rehabil 76:804–810, 1995

Whyte J, Myers R: Incidence of clinically significant responses to zolpidem among patients with disorders of consciousness: a preliminary placebo controlled trial. Am J Phys Med Rehabil 88:410–418, 2009

Whyte J, DiPasquale MC, Vaccaro M: Assessment of command-following in minimally conscious brain injured patients. Arch Phys Med Rehabil 80:653–660, 1999

Whyte J, Katz D, Long D, et al: Predictors of outcome in prolonged posttraumatic disorders of consciousness and assessment of medication effects: a multicenter study. Arch Phys Med Rehabil 86:453–462, 2005

World Health Organization: The ICD-10 Classification of Mental and Behavioural Disorders: Clinical Descriptions and Diagnostic Guidelines. Geneva, World Health Organization, 1992/2010

CHAPTER 5

# Cognitive Impairments

*David B. Arciniegas, M.D.*
*Kimberly L. Frey, M.S.*
*Thomas W. McAllister, M.D.*

**Cognitive impairments** are common consequences of traumatic brain injury (TBI) in both the early and late postinjury periods (Dikmen et al. 2009). Posttraumatic cognitive impairments contribute to early and late postinjury disability among persons with TBI (Sigurdardottir et al. 2009) and are sources of distress for persons with TBI and their families (Ponsford et al. 2003). The high frequency and important functional consequences of posttraumatic cognitive impairments requires health care providers working with persons with TBI to be familiar with the evaluation and management of these problems.

Toward that end, we review in this chapter the evaluation and treatment of posttraumatic cognitive impairments. We begin by defining the major domains of cognition and describing acute posttraumatic encephalopathy. The latter is used as a conceptual framework for understanding the common types and typical courses of cognitive impairments experienced by persons with TBI. We then offer a practical overview of the evaluation and treatment of persons with posttraumatic cognitive impairments.

# DEFINITIONS

In the broadest philosophical sense, *cognition* is the mental process of knowing (from the Latin *cognoscere*, meaning "to come to know"). The term's use in general psychology captures a broad array of mental processes, including sensation, perception, information processing, learning and remembering, experience, imagining, reasoning, and judging. In clinical parlance, *cognition* refers to a constellation of mental functions involved in the acquisition, processing, and use of information. These processes include, but are not limited to, arousal, attention and processing speed, working memory, recognition, declarative memory, communication, praxis, visuospatial function, executive function, and self-awareness (insight).

Cognition is distinguished, and often discussed separately, from the other major categories of neuropsychiatric function—that is, emotion, behavior, and sensorimotor function. However, distinctions among these categories of neuropsychiatric function and the mental processes they comprise cannot be taken too absolutely: cognition is inexorably intertwined with emotion, behavior, and somatic processes such that disturbances in noncognitive domains affect cognition, and vice versa (Barsalou et al. 2007). As discussed in later sections of this chapter, the evaluation and treatment of problems in any category of neuropsychiatric function therefore require consideration of their potential cross-category contributors.

A common practice in clinical and research settings is to discuss specific cognitive processes as if they are entirely separable. Factor analyses of the neuropsychological tests used to assess cognitive domain–specific performance offer some assurances that conclusions drawn from their use are tenable and of heuristic value. However, performance on tests usually associated with one cognitive domain (e.g., declarative memory) is influenced by abilities and/or impairments in other domains (e.g., arousal, attention, working memory, language, executive function). It therefore is prudent to remain circumspect about the causes of and contributors to any particular cognitive impairment revealed by such tests, especially among persons in whom cognitive impairments are multiple and/or severe.

Having acknowledged these issues, we begin our discussion of posttraumatic cognitive impairments by defining each of the major cognitive domains. In this context, we comment on the frequency and manner in which each domain is affected by TBI (Table 5–1) (Dikmen et al. 2009).

**TABLE 5–1.** Summary of conclusions drawn by the Institute of Medicine (IOM) regarding the evidence of long-term cognitive outcomes following penetrating, severe, moderate, and mild traumatic brain injury (TBI)

| TBI TYPE | IOM CONCLUSIONS | COGNITIVE DOMAINS AFFECTED |
|---|---|---|
| Penetrating | Sufficient evidence | Varies with the affected brain region and volume of tissue lost |
| Severe | Sufficient evidence | Common<br>　Attention<br>　Processing speed<br>　Declarative memory<br>　Executive function<br>Less common<br>　Language<br>　Praxis<br>　Visuospatial function |
| Moderate | Limited/suggestive evidence | Processing speed<br>Declarative memory<br>Executive function |
| Mild | Inadequate/insufficient evidence | |

# Cognitive Function and Dysfunction

*Arousal.* *Arousal* refers to a state of wakefulness that establishes the capacity to respond appropriately to internal or external stimuli. Arousal occurs along a continuum, with coma and manic excitement representing the extremes of hypoarousal and hyperarousal, respectively.

Early impairments of arousal (i.e., loss of consciousness) are common features of TBI at all severity levels. For the vast majority of persons with TBI, loss of consciousness is a transient and relatively brief consequence of TBI (Arciniegas 2011a). However, a nontrivial minority of persons, usually those with very severe TBI, experience very slow and sometimes incomplete recovery of arousal and/or awareness (Katz et al. 2009). The conditions that have disturbances of arousal and awareness as the central feature are described as disorders of consciousness, and include coma, vegetative states, and the minimally conscious state (Giacino et al. 2002); these problems are discussed at length in Chapter 4, "Disorders of Consciousness."

**Attention.** *Attention* refers to a collection of processes that permit selection of an internal or external stimulus for cognitive processing, maintaining focus on a stimulus over time (sustained attention), and alternating between two or more attentional targets (alternating, or divided, attention; also described as executive control of attention). *Inattention* may be used to denote impairment in any of these functions, although the term most accurately refers to impaired selective attention. Disturbances of the ability to sustain attention are described as impaired vigilance, difficulty concentrating, or distractibility.

Impairments of selective and sustained attention are common in the early period after TBI and tend to resolve before disturbances in higher-level cognition and memory (Stuss et al. 1999). Impairments of higher-level attention, including alternating or divided attention, may persist despite improvements in selective and simple sustained attention, especially among persons with moderate or severe TBI (Dikmen et al. 2009). Although referred to simply as attention problems, these higher-level disturbances appear to reflect impairments in executive control of attention and cohere with other disturbances of executive function (Ciaramelli et al. 2006; Serino et al. 2006).

**Processing speed.** The speed of information processing is described clinically as reaction time or response latency (i.e., the interval between stimulus presentation and behavioral response). Processing speed is among the most common impairments following TBI (Dikmen et al. 2009). The severity of processing speed impairments tends to parallel initial injury severity, with the most severe and persistent deficits (i.e., bradyphrenia) following severe TBI. These impairments are also seen following mild TBI, and are most prominent during the early postinjury period (Mathias et al. 2004). Processing speed impairments may contribute to difficulty using other cognitive abilities efficiently and may produce performance impairments on neuropsychological tests of other cognitive functions (Ciaramelli et al. 2006).

**Working memory.** Also described as *immediate memory* or *registration*), *working memory* refers to the ability to maintain attention to a stimulus for a brief period after its presentation; that is, working memory is the cognitive function that permits a stimulus to which attention is directed and sustained to be held "in mind" or "online" when the stimulus is no longer physically present. This concept of working memory is sometimes extended to the manipulation of information held "in mind"; performing such information manipulations also is described as executive control of working memory.

Working memory impairments are common in the early period following TBI at all injury severity levels (Ciaramelli et al. 2006; McAllister et al. 2006). Although working memory impairments tend to improve over time even after severe TBI (Sanchez-Carrion et al. 2008), their persistence may contribute substantially to attention, memory, and executive dysfunction in the late postinjury period (Ciaramelli et al. 2006).

**Recognition.** *Recognition* refers to the ability to integrate sensory information at a cortical level (i.e., cortically based perception) in a manner that permits the association of the information with similar prior percepts. Recognition occurs within a single sensory modality (i.e., vision, hearing, somatosensation, smell, taste), and impairments of recognition are described as agnosias.

Agnosias are relatively uncommon consequences of TBI. When they arise, they are most commonly associated with focal contusion or traumatic ablation to sensory association cortices required for recognition or with damage to the white matter connecting sensory association cortices to other brain areas.

**Memory.** Memory, like attention, is not a unitary cognitive function. Instead, *memory* is a term used to describe a diverse set of processes involved in learning and recalling information. These processes are generally categorized into declarative (explicit) and procedural (implicit) types.

*Declarative memory* refers to the encoding, storage, and retrieval of semantic (factual), episodic (event), and personal (autobiographical) information, and often is subdivided into verbal, visual, and spatial types. *Encoding* refers to the construction of a neural representation of a stimulus (a percept) that may be maintained briefly and/or stored for later recall; this process is described clinically as *immediate memory* or *registration,* and overlaps conceptually with simple working memory. *Consolidation* is a gradual process by which stable neural representations of encoded information are developed. *Retrieval* refers to the recall of information that has been encoded and consolidated, whether spontaneously (free recall) or in response to semantic or recognition cues.

Clinicians commonly distinguish between registration (immediate, or working, memory), short-term memory (i.e., recall after a relatively brief delay), and long-term memory (i.e., recall after a relatively long delay) and describe impairment in memory as *amnesia.* It is important to be aware that the correspondence between the terms used to describe memory in clinical practice does not match precisely their use in nonclinical literatures (Cowan 2008). It therefore is useful to describe memory-related clinical phenomena in narrative (in lieu of or in addition to terms of art) and not to presume that there is consensus on the intended referents of memory-related terms.

*Posttraumatic amnesia* (PTA) refers to a dense impairment in new learning and recall produced by neurotrauma. Difficulty learning information subsequent to the moment of injury is described as *anterograde amnesia,* whereas inability to retrieve previously learned (i.e., encoded, although not necessarily consolidated) information is referred to as *retrograde amnesia. Orientation* refers to memory for temporal information (e.g., current day, date, month, season, year), location (e.g., building, floor/level, city, county, state), circumstances, and personal identity. Impaired orientation (literally *disorientation*) is a prominent feature of PTA. Although disorientation is associated with other memory impairments, it is contributed to by inattention as well (Tittle and Burgess 2011).

*Procedural memory* denotes the process by which skills are learned and recalled. In contrast to declarative memory, which describes memory for "who," "what," "when," and "where," procedural memory describes memory for "how" to do things. Procedural memory is largely, although not entirely, dissociable from declarative memory (Beaunieux et al. 2006). It also overlaps conceptually and clinically with praxis: the acquisition of new skills is procedural learning, their use at a later date reflects procedural recall, and their demonstration on demand or request defines praxis. Among adults with TBI, procedural memory often is less affected than declarative memory, and its preservation is capitalized on in the early postinjury rehabilitation of persons in PTA (Ehlhardt et al. 2008).

**Communication.** Communication comprises language, paralinguistic functions (prosody and kinesics), speech, and voice. *Language* is a systematic means of communicating using conventionalized and meaningful symbols, including sounds, gestures, signs, and marks. Its elements include naming, fluency, repetition, and comprehension. *Naming* is the ability to attach linguistic labels to objects and actions; *fluency* describes the production of syntactically correct phrases comprised, on average, of six or more words without undue word-finding pauses; *repetition* describes the ability to reproduce phrases one hears or reads; and *comprehension* describes the ability to recognize and attach meaning to linguistic symbols. Disturbances of language are termed *aphasias*.

*Prosody* refers to the affective import introduced into communication, and *kinesics* describes its gestural accompaniment. Like language, prosody entails motor (fluency), repetition, and sensory (comprehension) elements. Disturbances of these paralinguistic functions are *aprosodias*.

Although language is commonly conveyed verbally, it is not equivalent to speech or voice. *Speech* narrowly refers to the use of the tongue, lips, jaw, and other orophangeal muscles to articulate words. Impairment of their use for this purpose is described as *dysarthria*. *Voice* is a product of the laryngeal function of phonation (i.e., the production of sounds by the vocal folds through quasi-periodic vibration), impairment of which is described as *dysphonia*.

Aphasia and aprosodia are relatively uncommon consequences of TBI (Dikmen et al. 2009) and tend to be associated with focal lesions of the dominant and nondominant hemisphere language-related structures, respectively. Functional communication impairments, which include mild or subtle disturbances of language, prosody, speech, and voice and of the effective use of language in social contexts, are relatively common consequences of TBI and, therefore, important targets of treatment (Cicerone et al. 2005).

**Praxis.** *Praxis* refers to the ability to execute skilled purposeful movements on demand given normal comprehension of the request and the elementary motor abilities to execute it. Impairments of this ability are described as apraxias, and are classified into three types: limb-kinetic, ideomotor, and ideational. *Limb-kinetic apraxia* describes the inability to make finely graded, precise, individual finger movements on demand. *Ideomotor apraxia* refers to the inability to perform a single previously learned skilled movement on demand. *Ideational apraxia* refers to the inability to carry out a specific sequence of tasks on demand; this sequential form of praxis overlaps conceptually with executive control of motor programming.

Apraxia is a less common consequence of TBI than attention, memory, or executive function impairments (Dikmen et al. 2009). When it occurs, however, it is a potentially disabling problem and an important target of rehabilitative treatments (Cicerone et al. 2011).

**Visuospatial function.** *Visuospatial function* refers to the ability to assess spatial relationships between objects in the environment and also between the environment and oneself. The most dramatic disturbance of visuospatial function is hemispatial neglect (a disorder of spatial attention), which is a relatively uncommon consequence of nonpenetrating TBI (Dikmen et al. 2009). Among persons with working memory and declarative memory impairments after TBI, disturbances in their visuospatial components (i.e., the visuospatial "sketchpad" or working memory, spatial components of declarative memory) are not uncommon and tend to be associated with right hemisphere injuries (Cicerone et al. 2011).

**Executive function.** *Executive function* refers to cognitive processes that manage and control "basic" aspects of cognition (i.e., executive control functions) as well as intrinsically complex cognitive skills such as information retrieval and generation, set shifting, inhibitory control, environmental autonomy, planning and organization, pattern recognition, problem solving, and abstraction. Other terms used to describe the components of this cognitive domain include *volition,* or conscious decision making and action; *purposive action,* the initiation and maintenance of behaviors that increase the likelihood of a desired end; *monitoring,* the ongoing assessment of the goal-directed success of a previously decided behavior sequence; *mental flexibility,* which may entail set shifting as well as the ability to integrate feedback, including self-monitoring, and to consider alternative actions; and *judgment,* the capacity to assess one's current situation and potential future action options, assign outcome probabilities to those options, and pursue the one that best fits the short- and long-term goals.

Executive dysfunction is a common early and late posttraumatic cognitive impairment among persons with moderate and severe TBI (Dikmen et al. 2009). Among persons with mild TBI, executive dysfunction is a common problem in the early postinjury period (Erez et al. 2009; Hartikainen et al. 2010) and may be contributed to by TBI and/or other neuropsychiatric disturbances in the late postinjury period (McCrea et al. 2009). Across injury types and postinjury periods, executive dysfunction contributes to functional disability (Erez et al. 2009; Ponsford et al. 2008).

**Insight.** *Insight* refers to the capacity for understanding one's own mental processes, problems, and circumstances (i.e., self-awareness), as well as the ability to understand the mental processes of others and the significance of events or actions. The capacity for self-awareness and insight into the minds and actions of others are related but psychologically distinct functions that are characterized by substantial interindividual differences even among healthy individuals (Gardner 1983).

*Anosognosia,* or lack of recognition of illness in oneself, is the prototypical impairment of insight. It is associated historically with left hemiparesis due to right hemisphere (especially parietal) stroke. Analyses of neuroanatomical and cognitive correlates of impaired self-awareness suggest that it is a multifaceted problem that occurs along a continuum of severity (Sherer et al. 2005). Its occurrence may follow injury to one or more elements of a broad network of cerebral structures, including at least prefrontal and parietal areas, as well as cortical, subcortical, and white matter structures comprising the spatial attention network. Impaired self-awareness after TBI is associated strongly with deficits in executive function (Ciurli et al. 2010; Ownsworth et al. 2002). The relationship between impaired insight into the minds and acts of others (e.g., social awareness, theory of mind) and executive dysfunction is less well established but remains a subject of active investigation (Muller et al. 2010; Ownsworth et al. 2002).

# Acute Posttraumatic Encephalopathy

Cognitive impairments, which are the defining feature of TBI for many individuals, usually include loss of consciousness, PTA, and/or other disturbances of cognition (Kay et al. 1993; Menon et al. 2010). Impairments of arousal, attention and processing speed, working memory, declarative memory, and executive function are common in the early postinjury period, and their severity varies with initial TBI severity (Nakase-Thompson et al. 2004; Stuss et al. 1999). Resolution of these problems typically follows a relatively predictable course: arousal returns before selective and simple sustained attention, and recovery of these functions tends to precede recovery of new learning and recall, which, in turn, precedes recovery of higher cognitive functions, including executive function and executive control of basic cognitive functions (Erez et al. 2009; Stuss et al. 1999).

The complex constellation of co-occurring cognitive problems as well as their evolution over the early postinjury period renders their succinct description quite challenging. The prominence of neurotrauma-induced declarative memory impairments during the early postinjury period, the prognostic value of their duration (Frey et al.

2007), and the common practice of identifying their termination have fostered the common practice of thinking about patients as being either "in PTA" or "out of PTA." The cognitive presentation of persons in the very early period after TBI is predominated by impairments of attention rather than amnesia (Corrigan et al. 1992; Kean et al. 2010; Stuss et al. 1999). Describing such presentations as "PTA" risks misunderstanding the phenomenology and neurobiology of the early postinjury period and, hence, may misdirect clinical efforts toward a less salient or relevant cognitive target (i.e., memory, rather than attention). Emergence from PTA also does not indicate cognitive or functional recovery and does not obviate the need for cognitively focused interventions: functionally important disturbances of executive function persist at least transiently after PTA resolves (Erez et al. 2009; Hagen et al. 1972; Hartikainen et al. 2010). Additionally, the focus on cognitive disturbances alone in the early postinjury period minimizes the functional importance and clinical challenges presented by concurrent noncognitive neuropsychiatric disturbances (Arciniegas and McAllister 2008; Ciurli et al. 2011).

We suggest describing the cognitive and noncognitive neuropsychiatric manifestation of neurotrauma-induced disturbances of brain function and structure as an acute posttraumatic encephalopathy (Arciniegas 2011a). The term *encephalopathy* (i.e., disorder or disease of the brain) captures the broad-ranging clinical manifestations of neurotrauma-induced alterations of brain function, and the modifier *acute posttraumatic* anchors the onset of encephalopathy to the immediate postinjury period and identifies TBI as its principal cause. This condition comprises five stages through which patients tend to pass sequentially: posttraumatic coma, posttraumatic confusional state (or delirium), posttraumatic amnesia, posttraumatic dysexecutive syndrome, and recovery (Figure 5–1). Each stage of acute posttraumatic encephalopathy is named according to its most salient (but not sole) cognitive feature and is described with its noncognitive neuropsychiatric features (Table 5–2).

It may be conceptually correct to describe patients who fail to recover cognitively as remaining persistently encephalopathic. However, the clinical conditions of such patients are generally described using a more specific diagnostic term that captures their phenomenological and temporal characteristics (e.g., persistent vegetative state, chronic minimally conscious state, dementia due to TBI, chronic mild neurocognitive disorder). The practice of describing

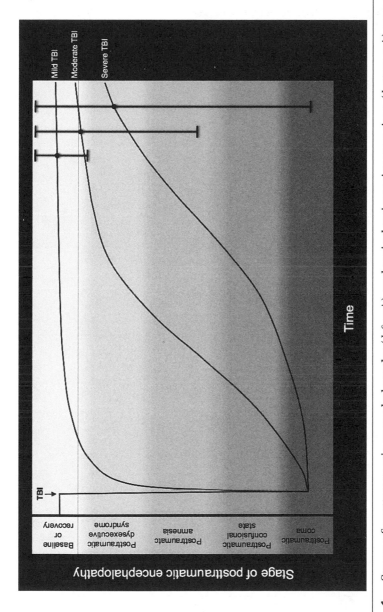

**FIGURE 5–1.** Stages of posttraumatic encephalopathy (*left axis*) and typical trajectories over time (*bottom axis*) associated with mild, moderate, or severe traumatic brain injury (TBI), with typical ranges of outcomes (*whisker bars*). ***Shown in color as Plate 6.***

**TABLE 5–2.**  The stages of posttraumatic encephalopathy

| STAGE | DESCRIPTION | ADDITIONAL FEATURES |
|---|---|---|
| Posttraumatic coma | Absence of arousal | Preserved brainstem reflexes, but no behavioral response to sensory input and no spontaneous behavior (purposeful or non-purposeful) |
| Posttraumatic confusional state | Reduced clarity of awareness of the environment, as evidenced by a reduced ability to focus, sustain, or shift attention | Alterations of arousal, disturbances of sleep-wake cycle, motor restlessness, perceptual disturbances; impaired processing speed, working memory, episodic memory, language/communication, and executive function; emotional lability, disinhibition, agitation, and/or aggression; fluctuating features, fluctuating severity |
| Posttraumatic amnesia | Impaired declarative new learning, including orientation as well as autobiographical information, for the peri-injury and immediate postinjury period | Impaired processing speed as well as higher-level attention, working memory, and executive function impairments are often present but are less severe than during the preceding confusional state; impaired new learning is not attributable to lower-level cognitive impairments; emotional and behavioral disturbances |
| Posttraumatic dysexecutive syndrome | Impaired intrinsic executive function and impaired executive control functions | Emotional and behavioral disturbances |
| Recovery | Return to baseline cognitive function | Injury-related disturbances of cognition are no longer present or, if present, are better accounted for by another neuropsychiatric condition; noncognitive neuropsychiatric symptoms may be present |

the late cognitive sequelae of TBI in this manner reduces this risk of confusing incomplete resolution of acute posttraumatic encephalopathy with chronic traumatic encephalopathy (Omalu et al. 2005), a delayed-onset TBI-induced neurodegenerative disorder associated with repetitive concussions (mild TBI). At the same time, adopting a common semantic convention for the description of acute- and delayed-onset neurotrauma-induced encephalopathies facilitates the development of common clinical and research approaches to these problems. We hope that this approach to describing the complex constellations of cognitive and other neuropsychiatric problems occurring in the early postinjury period reduces the nosological challenges that presently complicate the study and treatment of persons with such problems.

# EVALUATION

Comprehensive neuropsychiatric evaluation is a prerequisite to the treatment of any problem presented by a patient with TBI. At a minimum, this evaluation includes detailed history taking; characterization of preinjury and postinjury developmental, medical, neurological, psychiatric, substance, and psychosocial issues; physical and neurological examinations; mental status examination; and relevant laboratory and neurodiagnostic assessments (see Chapter 2, "Medical Evaluation").

## Cognitive Assessment

There are numerous measures that may be used to characterize post-traumatic cognitive complaints and impairments. Among patients able to offer reliable self-report, a variety of symptom inventories may inform the clinical evaluation of posttraumatic cognitive impairments (Table 5–3). When bedside cognitive assessments are performed, the clinician should select measures that capture the cognitive and noncognitive neuropsychiatric disturbances characteristic of the stage of acute posttraumatic encephalopathy of the patient to whom they are administered (Table 5–4) (Arciniegas 2011a).

As patients transition between stages of acute posttraumatic encephalopathy, using combinations of assessments that capture those transitions may guide treatment usefully. When the combination of clinical interview and bedside examination does not adequately inform clinical diagnosis or treatment planning, then formal neuropsychological assessment is warranted (see Chapter 3, "Neuropsychological Assessment"). Regardless of the method used to characterize cognitive im-

**TABLE 5–3.** Examples of self-report and clinician-administered instruments used to assess cognitive complaints and impairments among persons with traumatic brain injury

| MEASURE | METHOD(S) |
| --- | --- |
| Cognitive Failures Questionnaire | Self-report |
| Multiple Abilities Self-Report Questionnaire | Self-report |
| Behavioral Rating Inventory of Executive Function–Adult Version | Self-report, informant report |
| Neurobehavioral Functioning Inventory | Self-report and/or family report |
| Neurobehavioral Rating Scale–Revised | Structured clinical interview and clinician observation |
| Awareness Questionnaire | Semistructured clinical interview, clinician observation, informant interview, and/or self-report |

**TABLE 5–4.** Assessments of the cognitive and noncognitive features of the prerecovery stages of posttraumatic encephalopathy

| POSTTRAUMATIC ENCEPHALOPATHY STAGE | RECOMMENDED ASSESSMENTS |
| --- | --- |
| Posttraumatic coma | Coma Recovery Scale–Revised (CRS-R) |
| Posttraumatic confusional state | Delirium Rating Scale–Revised-98 (DRS-R-98) <br> Confusion Assessment Protocol (CAP) |
| Posttraumatic amnesia | Orientation Log (O-Log) <br> Galveston Orientation and Amnesia Test (GOAT) |
| Posttraumatic dysexecutive syndrome | Mini-Mental State Examination (raw and Z-score) <br> Clock Drawing Test (standardized scoring) <br> Frontal Assessment Battery (raw and Z-score) <br> Neurobehavioral Rating Scale–Revised (NBRS-R) <br> Hanks' Brief Inpatient Neuropsychological Battery |

pairments, pretreatment assessment is required to identify the targets of treatment and to establish the baseline against which the effects of treatment will be compared.

# Neuroimaging

Structural magnetic resonance imaging (MRI) of the brain may be useful in the development of a treatment plan for posttraumatic cognitive impairments. When performed, clinical studies should include T1- and T2-weighted sequences, T2* gradient recalled echo (T2* GRE) or susceptibility-weighted imaging (SWI), diffusion-weighted imaging (DWI), and apparent diffusion coefficient (ADC) mapping. Diffusion tensor imaging (DTI) and/or magnetic resonance spectroscopy (MRS) are research techniques that may become useful adjuncts to the neuroimaging examination as well. Severe damage (including traumatic ablation) of areas required for specific cognitive functions suggests a relative lack of anatomical target for rehabilitative or pharmacotherapeutic interventions. Such findings guide treatment toward education, support, and compensatory strategy development for patients and caregivers and may allow realistic expectations to be set regarding cognitive recovery and treatment response. By contrast, relatively normal findings from neuroimaging suggest preserved targets for rehabilitative and pharmacotherapeutic interventions and may increase optimism regarding their effectiveness.

# Differential Diagnosis

The differential diagnosis for cognitive impairments in both the early and late postinjury periods is quite broad. Its elements require consideration and, where appropriate, management before rehabilitative interventions or pharmacotherapies for posttraumatic cognitive impairments are prescribed. The elements of this differential diagnosis include, but are not limited to, preinjury cognitive impairments, learning disorders, and intellectual disabilities; preinjury medical, neurological, psychiatric, and substance use disorders; co-occurring vascular and/or hypoxic-ischemic brain injuries, central nervous system infections, neurosurgically induced lesions (e.g., decompressive lobectomy with craniectomy resulting in the "syndrome of the trephined" or "sinking skin flap syndrome"); postinjury medical, neurological, or psychiatric conditions (e.g., depression, anxiety, headache, pain, fatigue, sleep disturbances, seizures, sensory problems) and substance use disorders; medications, including prescribed medications, over-the-counter agents, and psychoactive herbal products and supplements; and symptom elaboration or malingering.

Adverse cognitive side effects of prescribed medications (e.g., sedative-hypnotics, antidepressants with anticholinergic properties, first- or second-generation antipsychotics, anticonvulsants) and over-the-counter medications (e.g., antihistamines, anticholinergics, psychoactive herbal remedies), as well as intoxication or withdrawal from alcohol or illicit substances, also merit specific attention during consideration of the differential diagnosis of posttraumatic cognitive impairments. Administration of prophylactic anticonvulsants after the first postinjury week is of particular concern; consistent with established practice guidelines for TBI (Marion 2006), this treatment approach is not recommended, and its discontinuation reduces the cognitive burden of these agents. Individual clinical circumstances may necessitate the use of these or other medications that impair cognition, and a proscriptive approach to pharmacotherapy in patients with TBI therefore is not reasonable. However, avoiding, eliminating, or using the minimum necessary dose of such medications and discontinuing them as soon as is feasible is recommended. The clinician should complete changes in medication management before drawing conclusions about severity, prognosis, and the need to initiate cognition-specific rehabilitative or pharmacological treatments.

Another important consideration is the extent to which a patient's cognitive complaints and/or impairments comport with those usually associated with the type and severity of injury that the patient experienced. Cognitive impairments and related functional limitations are worst in the immediate postinjury period and gradually (although sometimes incompletely) improve thereafter (Carroll et al. 2004; Dikmen et al. 2009). The presence of cognitive impairments that are unusual in type or severity, recovery trajectories that deviate from the expected course (e.g., decline rather than improvement), or functional limitations that are not well explained by the types and severities of cognitive impairments necessitates consideration of noncognitive contributors to the clinical presentation.

## Functional Status

Cognition plays an important role in many daily activities, but the proportion of variance in functional status accounted for by most cognitive tests is relatively modest (Royall et al. 2007). Similarly, cognitive impairments—especially those in the mild to moderate range—do not themselves diminish decisional capacity or establish de facto incompetence. Assessments of functional status and decisional capacity are distinct undertakings from cognitive examination.

Such assessments are required to establish the relevance of cognitive complaints and/or impairments identified during other portions of the evaluation. Clinical interview of the patient and, when possible and relevant, of his or her family, caregivers, and employers may identify functional limitations requiring intervention and their most likely cognitive contributors. Noncognitive contributors to functional limitations, including cognitive, emotional, behavioral, physical, and psychosocial factors, also must be considered. When questions about everyday functional abilities remain, consultation with and/or evaluation by a rehabilitation specialist with expertise in standardized evaluations of functional status (e.g., rehabilitation psychologist, occupational therapist) may be necessary. Formal assessment of the patient's function in his or her usual environments (e.g., home, work) by a rehabilitation therapist sometimes is needed to identify the functional limitations, their cognitive contributors, and the methods of intervention that are most likely to be helpful.

## TREATMENT

The treatment of posttraumatic cognitive impairments is a complex subject, and one about which much has been written but with remarkably little agreement. Some clinicians approach the posttraumatic cognitive complaints as high-priority treatment issues for every patient, whereas others maintain a therapeutic nihilism that precludes their prescription of any treatment for posttraumatic cognitive impairments. We suggest that neither of these is a reasonable clinical approach. The treatment needs of each patient, as well as the potential benefits of rehabilitative and medication interventions, vary with his or her personal characteristics, the severity of TBI, the time since injury, the types and severities of cognitive impairments, the presence of noncognitive TBI sequelae, and the functional relevance of the patient's cognitive complaints and/or impairments (Arciniegas 2011a).

For example, treatment is directed principally at problems other than cognition in the immediate postinjury period and during the initial stages of acute posttraumatic encephalopathy following moderate or severe TBI. Initial interventions are directed at secondary injury processes, management of other physical injuries, oxygenation, hydration, metabolic support, reinjury risk reduction, and family education and support (Marion 2006). In this context, cognition is an important treatment target to the extent that addressing it reduces the risk of reinjury, facilitates engagement in and/or adherence to medical or rehabilitative interventions, promotes more rapid progression through acute posttraumatic encephalopathy, and limits the duration and/or extent of postinjury disability. As time since injury elapses and recovery is made from other bodily injuries, posttraumatic cognitive impairments are often made more apparent, their functional consequences are better appreciated, and the need to address them effectively becomes a pressing clinical concern. In the acute and postacute injury periods, treatment of posttraumatic cognitive impairments is one of the principal tasks of physicians, psychologists, and rehabilitation specialists.

Among persons with mild TBI, initial interventions include rest, education, and realistic expectation setting (Bell et al. 2008) (see Chapter 18, "Athletes and Sports-Related Concussion"). Time-limited symptom-focused management of somatic symptoms (e.g., headache, dizziness, sleep disturbances) and management of co-occurring noncerebral injuries (including pain control) also may be appropriate. Because mild TBI, by definition, entails a loss of consciousness lasting no more than 30 minutes and confusional or amnestic states lasting no more than 24 hours, posttraumatic cognitive impairments following mild TBI are predominantly dysexecutive (Erez et al. 2009; Halterman et al. 2006; Hartikainen et al. 2010; Nolin 2006). Typical recovery following mild TBI is characterized by relatively rapid resolution of these problems without specific intervention (Carroll et al. 2004; McCrea et al. 2009), obviating cognition as a treatment target in many cases. Among patients demonstrating atypical recovery from mild TBI (i.e., persistence of cognitive and noncognitive symptoms beyond the first several months postinjury), careful consideration of the differential diagnosis of such problems is essential before initiating cognition-specific interventions (see Chapter 20, "Persistent Symptoms After a Concussion").

The various examples presented highlight the challenges of adopting a single approach (i.e., "treat everyone" or "treat no one") to the management of posttraumatic cognitive impairments. In the following sections, we provide a brief overview of common treatments provided to persons with posttraumatic cognitive impairments and their families.

# Education

Providing education about TBI, cognition, functional status, and the expected recovery course is an essential component of the treatment of persons with posttraumatic cognitive impairments and their families or caregivers (Bell et al. 2005, 2008). At the same time, the clinician should become educated by those individuals and their families about their circumstances and beliefs about recovery after TBI, as a prerequisite to establishing shared realistic treatment expectations and goals. Education about treatment usefully includes discussion of the importance of supporting or improving real-world function and quality of life through time-limited (rather than chronic) cognitive rehabilitation interventions.

Spontaneous recovery often contributes to cognitive improvement following TBI. Education on this point may help patients and caregivers anticipate a time after which recovery of cognitive impairment plateaus and continued impairment-focused cognitive rehabilitation may not be appropriate. When education about spontaneous recovery is coupled with education on the distinction between cognitive recovery (i.e., improvement in cognitive abilities) and functional recovery (i.e., compensation and other adaptation), individuals experiencing persistent cognitive impairments may transition more easily from a remediation-focused treatment approach to one emphasizing improvement in everyday function. The latter approach focuses on compensatory strategy development, modification of the environment or tasks to reduce performance barriers, and setting realistic performance expectations. Successful implementation of this treatment approach requires ongoing education about its merits and goals.

Patients and caregivers often expect brain injury medicine subspecialists to prescribe medications for cognitive impairments. This expectation is often coupled with unrealistic expectations about the benefits or the adverse effects of pharmacotherapy. Unambiguously framing pharmacotherapy as adjunctive to all other interventions and educating patients and families about realistic (i.e., modest) treatment expectations are required before and during the use of pharmacological treatments. Education about spontaneous recovery also improves patient and family acceptance of the treatment discontinuation trials required to determine whether pharmacotherapy is effective and its continuation necessary.

## Supportive Therapy

Supportive therapy focuses on the personal, social, occupational, and functional challenges presented by posttraumatic cognitive impairments. It is an important component of the treatment plan for persons with these impairments, as well as their caregivers and families. Supportive therapy begins by acknowledging the patient's experience of cognitive problems and their everyday consequences. The clinician and patient collaboratively identify solutions to those issues. Among patients for whom posttraumatic cognitive impairments become persistent problems, support is coupled with education to foster functional compensation and adaptation. Providing supportive therapy helps to establish a therapeutic alliance and creates a context for discussing and promoting adherence to prescribed rehabilitative and pharmacological treatments.

## Environmental and Behavioral Interventions

Understanding the context in which a patient's cognitive impairments result in functional problems permits modifying it in a manner that capitalizes on remaining cognitive strengths, reduces performance failures, mitigates cognitive impairment–related disability, and alleviates patient and caregiver distress. Eliminating external or internal sources of distraction and overstimulation may allow a patient to focus more effectively despite attentional impairments. Developing a predictable schedule for performing tasks (including personal care, meals, work, social activities, and sleep), using structured procedures to perform them, and reducing opportunities for environmental disruptions may improve the consistency and success of task performance. Organizing the daily scheduling to coincide with periods when the individual is well rested, providing breaks during the day, and teaching the patient and others to monitor for signs of physical and/or cognitive fatigue may reduce actual or perceived performance failures. Resetting patient and family expectations about the speed and depth of verbal exchanges, encouraging others to allow sufficient time for the person with TBI to respond or accomplish tasks, and teaching others not to interrupt adaptive schedules and routines also may facilitate performance successes.

For patients with impairments in working memory and/or declarative memory, setting up task routines that do not exceed memory span (the amount of information that can be held "in mind") and that are free from interference (i.e., interposed irrelevant tasks) may improve the likelihood of successful task completion. When necessary, encouraging the use of personal "cognitive prosthetics" (e.g., memory notebooks, personal digital assistants, timers, alarms) and appropriate placement of cues (e.g., signs, lights, alarms, verbal cues from others) in the environment may facilitate task initiation, maintenance, and completion. Similarly, reinforcing spontaneous adaptive behaviors and providing no reinforcement for maladaptive behaviors also may promote effective task performance.

The treatment of posttraumatic cognitive impairments therefore focuses not only on the person with those impairments but also on his or her environment, the manner in which the individual functions therein, and the people with whom the person interacts. Individually tailored environmental modification and behavioral interventions— irrespective of the setting in which treatment occurs—are essential elements of any treatment plan designed to improve the functional performance of persons with posttraumatic cognitive impairments.

## Cognitive Rehabilitation

The range of rehabilitative interventions for posttraumatic cognitive impairments is broad, and a detailed review of these treatments is beyond the scope of this volume. Clinicians providing care to persons with posttraumatic cognitive impairments are encouraged to familiarize themselves with cognitive rehabilitative treatments used commonly in inpatient and outpatient settings and with the evidence supporting them. The evidence-based reviews of cognitive rehabilitation performed by the Brain Injury Interdisciplinary Special Interest Group of the American Congress of Rehabilitation Medicine (Cicerone et al. 2000, 2005, 2011) and the Task Force on Cognitive Rehabilitation of the European Federation of Neurological Societies (Cappa et al. 2003, 2005) are summarized in Tables 5–5 and 5–6.

These reports evaluated rehabilitation interventions for cognitive impairments following TBI and stroke. Although substantial dissimilarities between TBI and stroke limit the translation of stroke rehabilitation approaches to the care of persons with TBI, the focal cognitive disorders of traumatic contusions and missile injuries are often quite stroke-like and may respond to cognitive rehabilitation interventions developed for stroke survivors. For this reason, these interventions also are included in Tables 5–5 and 5–6.

Matching treatments to the patients for whom they are most likely to be useful and providing them at a time postinjury when they are likely to facilitate improvements greater than those conferred by spontaneous re-

**TABLE 5–5.**   General cognitive rehabilitation interventions for persons with traumatic brain injury (TBI)

| Intervention | Comment |
| --- | --- |
| Comprehensive-holistic neuropsychological rehabilitation | Reduces cognitive and functional disability among persons with moderate to severe TBI when offered during postacute rehabilitation. Integrated treatment of individual and group psychotherapies emphasizing emotional, behavioral, and interpersonal function may facilitate success of cognition-specific interventions. |
| Compensatory strategy training | Most useful after emergence from posttraumatic amnesia or in the late postinjury period. Most useful when applied to functionally important and personally relevant activities. |
| Self-regulation and self-monitoring instruction | Most useful for persons with executive dysfunction, impaired attention (including neglect states) or memory, and/or emotional dysregulation. |
| Computer-based tasks without therapist involvement | Not effective and strongly discouraged. |

covery remain uncertain and controversial endeavors (Committee on Cognitive Rehabilitation Therapy for Traumatic Brain Injury 2011). As suggested in Tables 5–5 and 5–6, some cognitive rehabilitation interventions appear to be useful during the acute rehabilitation period (i.e., aphasia therapies, treatments of visual perceptual deficits, errorless learning), some may be useful in the acute rehabilitation period following emergence from PTA (e.g., compensatory strategy training), and others appear more useful in the postacute rehabilitation period (e.g., comprehensive-holistic neuropsychological rehabilitation, individual and group-based interventions for executive dysfunction, higher-level attention training). However, the optimal timing and best practices for most of these interventions are not well established.

Fortunately, little risk of harm is associated with the provision of cognitive rehabilitation. However, these treatments are not inexpen-

**TABLE 5–6.** Domain-specific rehabilitation interventions for posttraumatic cognitive impairments

| COGNITIVE DOMAIN | COMMENT |
| --- | --- |
| Attention | Attention training during the acute recovery and early rehabilitation periods confers benefits no greater than spontaneous recovery. |
| | Attention training is recommended during the postacute rehabilitation period, including direct attention and metacognitive strategy training targeting improved real-world function. |
| | Clinician-guided computer-based attention training may be used as an adjunct to other cognitive rehabilitation interventions when it includes more than repeated task exposure alone. |
| | Computer-based attention training without clinician involvement is not recommended. |
| Memory | Memory strategy training, including internalized strategies and external compensations, may be useful for mild memory impairments. |
| | Functionally relevant external memory compensations (e.g., notebooks) and/or errorless learning may facilitate learning specific skills or knowledge among persons with severe memory impairments. |
| | Group-based interventions may be useful. |
| Communication | Individual and group interventions during acute and postacute rehabilitation may improve language deficits, communication, and pragmatic conversational skills. |
| | Nonrepetitive, clinician-guided computer-based interventions may be a useful adjunct treatment for cognitive-linguistic deficits. |
| Praxis | Specific gestural or strategy training during acute rehabilitation may improve apraxia. |

**TABLE 5–6.** Domain-specific rehabilitation interventions for posttraumatic cognitive impairments *(continued)*

| COGNITIVE DOMAIN | COMMENT |
|---|---|
| Vision and visuospatial function | Visual scanning, visuo-spatio-motor training, alertness and sustained attention training, caloric or galvanic vestibular stimulations, transcutaneous electrical stimulation of neck muscles, or limb activation technologies may improve hemispatial neglect; strategies based on reading, copying and figure description, video feedback, trunk orientation, forced use of the left eye, and prism goggles may be helpful for some patients as well. |
| | Visual perceptual deficits may improve with systematic training of visuospatial deficits and visual organization skills. |
| | Computer-based interventions to extend visual fields (but not to improve hemispatial neglect) may be useful when combined with other standard visual and/or visuospatial rehabilitation interventions. |
| Executive function | Metacognitive strategy training (i.e., self-monitoring and self-regulation, including emotional self-regulation) may improve executive function. |
| | Individual and group-based interventions for executive dysfunction, and particularly problem-solving difficulties, directed at personally relevant everyday situations and functional activities may be useful during the postacute rehabilitation period. |

sive, their costs are often not covered by third-party payers, and the treatment-related expenses may be prohibitive for many patients and families. For these reasons, we are supportive of problem-focused cognitive rehabilitation directed at improving real-world function and quality of life when it is provided in a time-limited and fiscally responsible manner. When undertaken during the period of spontaneous recovery, interventions directed at mitigating functional disability and facilitating adaptive engagement in other treatment and in community life may be appropriate; however, clinicians, patients, and families are encouraged to remain circumspect about the need for, benefits of, and costs associated with rehabilitation interventions undertaken during this period.

As recovery proceeds, cognitive impairments that interfere with daily function are important and useful targets of treatment. For individuals for whom cognitive impairments become chronic problems, we encourage employing time-limited treatments that emphasize functional problem-focused compensatory strategy development and/or adaptation over the remediation of cognitive impairments, and we discourage engaging patients in chronic cognitive rehabilitation.

# Pharmacotherapy

Medications are best regarded as adjuncts to educational, supportive, environmental, behavioral, and rehabilitative interventions. Their administration may alter the cerebral neurochemical milieu in a manner that enhances the effectiveness of rehabilitative interventions. Some medications also may promote neural and cognitive recovery, although evidence in support of this suggestion is limited (Liepert 2008).

Authors of several extensive literature reviews have synthesized and summarized the available pharmacotherapies for posttraumatic cognitive impairments (Arciniegas and Silver 2006; Chew and Zafonte 2009; Warden et al. 2006; Wheaton et al. 2011; Writer and Schillerström 2009). Medications described in these reports and their common uses in this population are summarized in Table 5–7. Clinicians working in this area are encouraged to familiarize themselves with these reports on the cognitive rehabilitation and pharmacotherapy of posttraumatic cognitive impairments. Additionally, before prescribing these or any other medications, clinicians are encouraged to refer to each medication's product information sheet as well as other reference materials for complete reviews of dosing, side effects, drug-drug interactions, treatment risks, and treatment contraindications. It is important to remain mindful that many third-party payers often do not provide support for these treatments, and the U.S. Food and Drug Administration has not approved any medication for use as a treatment of posttraumatic cognitive impairment. Accordingly, the use of medications to treat individuals with these impairments is a matter of empirical trial and one whose relative benefits and costs must be considered carefully.

**TABLE 5–7.** Medications used to treat posttraumatic cognitive impairments

| MEDICATION | CLASS | DAILY DOSE RANGE | COGNITIVE TARGETS |
|---|---|---|---|
| Methylphenidate | MRRI | 5–60 mg (target dose: 0.3 mg/kg twice daily) | Arousal, attention, processing speed, working memory, declarative memory, general cognition |
| Dextroamphetamine | MRRI | 5–60 mg (target dose: 0.3 mg/kg twice daily) | Attention, processing speed, secondary improvements in other cognitive domains |
| Amantadine | Uncompetitive NMDA-R antagonist | 50–200 mg | Arousal, attention, executive function, general cognition |
| Modafinil | Mixed pro-monoaminergic effects | 100–400 mg | Arousal; may improve other cognitive domains in a manner similar to methylphenidate but evidence of such effects is lacking |
| Bromocriptine | Dopamine agonist | 2.5–90 mg | Arousal, working memory, executive function (including executive control of attention and working memory) |
| Carbidopa-levodopa | Dopamine agonist | One to two 25/100-mg tablets three to four times daily | Arousal |

**TABLE 5–7.** Medications used to treat posttraumatic cognitive impairments *(continued)*

| Medication | Class | Daily dose range | Cognitive targets |
|---|---|---|---|
| Donepezil | AChEI | 5–10 mg | Attention, processing speed, working memory, declarative memory; may secondarily benefit executive function |
| Rivastigmine | AChEI | 1.5–12 mg | Declarative memory; may secondarily benefit attention, processing speed and executive function |
| Citicoline | Stimulant/ nootropic with multiple neurochemical effects | 1 g | Declarative memory |

*Note.* AChEI=acetylcholinesterase inhibitor; MRRI=monoamine releaser and reuptake inhibitor; NMDA-R=*N*-methyl-D-aspartate receptor.

The pharmacotherapy of cognitive impairments in the immediate postinjury period or prior to emergence from the posttraumatic confusional state is underdeveloped (see Chapter 4, "Disorders of Consciousness"). Some evidence suggests that treatment with amantadine during the immediate postinjury period may hasten recovery of arousal (Wheaton et al. 2009); whether this effect reflects this agent's stabilization of glutamate signaling via uncompetitive antagonism of *N*-methyl-D-aspartate (NMDA) receptors, indirect facilitation of dopaminergic function via antagonism of NMDA receptors on ventral tegmental area neurons, or both these and other actions remains uncertain. There are reports describing the use of acetylcholinesterase inhibitors (e.g., physostigmine) to facilitate emergence from the posttraumatic confusional state (i.e., delirium) and/or posttraumatic amnesia (Arciniegas 2011b). However, acute neurotrauma produces functionally disruptive elevations of cerebral catecholamines, acetyl-choline, and most, if not all, other cerebral neurotransmitters (Arciniegas 2011b; Shaw 2002). The duration of these neurotransmitter excesses varies with initial injury severity, the presence of focal lesions, and other individual patient characteristics; this variability complicates medication selection and prediction of treatment effects attendant on early postinjury pharmacological interventions. Therefore, the treatment of the cognitive components of the early stages of acute posttraumatic encephalopathy in the first days to weeks following the postinjury period is primarily nonpharmacological. Pharmacotherapy is reserved for the treatment of functionally important non-cognitive features of the posttraumatic confusional state (e.g., hallucinations, delusions, severe emotional disturbances, restlessness, agitation, aggression).

In the subacute period after more severe injuries (i.e., during or after emergence from PTA) or in the late period after TBI of any severity, there are two general approaches to the pharmacotherapy of posttraumatic cognitive impairments: catecholaminergic (i.e., dopaminergic, noradrenergic) augmentation and cholinergic augmentation (Arciniegas and Silver 2006; Chew and Zafonte 2009; Warden et al. 2006). Medications that augment the cerebral dopaminergic and/or noradrenergic function are used most often to improve processing speed or to support arousal, and they may improve sustained attention, working memory, declarative memory, and executive function. Methylphenidate is the most extensively studied and commonly used medication for these types of posttraumatic cognitive impairments, and appears most effective as a treatment for processing speed impairments. The acetylcholinesterase inhibitors (e.g., donepezil, rivastigmine) increase cerebral cholinergic function and are most useful for the treatment of posttraumatic attention and declarative memory impairments (Kim et al. 2009; Silver et al. 2006; Tenovuo et al. 2009; Zhang et al. 2004). Treatment responders may experience secondary benefits in other cognitive functions, including executive function (Silver et al. 2009). It has been suggested that citicoline (also known as cytidine diphosphate choline, or CDP-choline), which augments both cerebral catecholaminergic and cholinergic function, may improve subacute posttraumatic cognitive impairments and related postconcussive symptoms (Zafonte et al. 2009); however, a multicenter double-blind placebo-controlled trial failed to find such an effect (Zafonte et al. 2012).

When medications are used to treat cognitive impairments, beginning with relatively low dosages and slowly advancing to maximally tolerated and effective levels is encouraged (i.e., start low, go slow, but go). Heightened vigilance for side effects and drug-drug interactions needs to be maintained, and performing relatively frequent and assiduous assessments for such problems is prudent. Treatment also should be discontinued periodically to determine whether it remains necessary (especially during the period of spontaneous recovery). When a single medication does not provide adequate relief of symptoms or cannot be tolerated at therapeutic doses, augmentation using a second low-dose agent with a different mechanism of action may be useful.

# CONCLUSION

Cognitive complaints and/or impairments are common among persons with TBI in the early and late postinjury periods. Comprehensive neuropsychiatric assessment is required prior to undertaking cognition-specific treatments, and may direct treatment toward noncognitive contributors to cognitive complaints and/or impairments. The evaluation and management of posttraumatic cognitive impairments require consideration of initial TBI severity, time since injury, stage of posttraumatic encephalopathy, and the functional relevance of the cognitive and noncognitive disturbances. Treatment entails the provision of educational, supportive, environmental, and behavioral interventions to patients, as well as their families and caregivers. Cognitive rehabilitation, especially compensatory strategies and adaptive approaches, may be useful, particularly among persons with persistent posttraumatic cognitive impairments. Pharmacotherapy may be a useful adjunct to other interventions by altering the cerebral neurochemical milieu in a manner that facilitates engagement in and response to nonpharmacological interventions. Regardless of the specific modes of treatment employed, treatment of posttraumatic cognitive impairments is most useful when it addresses real-world functional challenges experienced by patients and caregivers, incorporates realistic treatment-response expectations, and ensures that patients and families are provided the support and resources needed to cope effectively with cognitive impairments and their consequences.

## *Key Clinical Points*

- Biomechanically induced cognitive impairments are defining features of TBI; these impairments include loss of consciousness, posttraumatic amnesia, and other alterations of consciousness.

- Among persons with moderate to severe TBI, residual disturbances of attention, processing speed, declarative memory, and executive function are relatively common.

- Most persons sustaining mild TBI experience complete and relatively rapid cognitive recovery; atypical recovery often involves, but may not be fully explained by, noncognitive conditions.

- Evaluation of posttraumatic cognitive impairments requires comprehensive neuropsychiatric assessment using stage-specific cognitive and functional assessments.

- Treatment of posttraumatic cognitive impairments is directed at functionally important cognitive impairments and provided to patients and their families and caregivers.

- Education, supportive therapy, and environmental and behavioral interventions are essential components of the treatment of posttraumatic cognitive impairments; treatment also may include problem-focused and time-limited cognitive rehabilitation and, when necessary, combined rehabilitative and pharmacotherapeutic interventions.

# REFERENCES

Arciniegas DB: Addressing neuropsychiatric disturbances during rehabilitation after traumatic brain injury: current and future methods. Dialogues Clin Neurosci 13:325–345, 2011a

Arciniegas DB: Cholinergic dysfunction and cognitive impairment after traumatic brain injury, part 2: evidence from basic and clinical investigations. J Head Trauma Rehabil 26:319–323, 2011b

Arciniegas DB, McAllister TW: Neurobehavioral management of traumatic brain injury in the critical care setting. Crit Care Clin 24:737–765, viii, 2008

Arciniegas DB, Silver JM: Pharmacotherapy of posttraumatic cognitive impairments. Behav Neurol 17:25–42, 2006

Barsalou LW, Breazeal C, Smith LB: Cognition as coordinated non-cognition. Cogn Process 8:79–91, 2007

Beaunieux H, Hubert V, Witkowski T, et al: Which processes are involved in cognitive procedural learning? Memory 14:521–539, 2006

Bell KR, Temkin NR, Esselman PC, et al: The effect of a scheduled telephone intervention on outcome after moderate to severe traumatic brain injury: a randomized trial. Arch Phys Med Rehabil 86:851–856, 2005

Bell KR, Hoffman JM, Temkin NR, et al: The effect of telephone counselling on reducing post-traumatic symptoms after mild traumatic brain injury: a randomised trial. J Neurol Neurosurg Psychiatry 79:1275–1281, 2008

Cappa SF, Benke T, Clarke S, et al: EFNS guidelines on cognitive rehabilitation: report of an EFNS task force. Eur J Neurol 10:11–23, 2003

Cappa SF, Benke T, Clarke S, et al: EFNS guidelines on cognitive rehabilitation: report of an EFNS task force. Eur J Neurol 12:665–680, 2005

Carroll LJ, Cassidy JD, Peloso PM, et al: Prognosis for mild traumatic brain injury: results of the WHO Collaborating Centre Task Force on Mild Traumatic Brain Injury. J Rehabil Med 43(suppl):84–105, 2004

Chew E, Zafonte RD: Pharmacological management of neurobehavioral disorders following traumatic brain injury: a state-of-the-art review. J Rehabil Res Dev 46:851–879, 2009

Ciaramelli E, Serino A, Di Santantonio A, et al: Central executive system impairment in traumatic brain injury. Brain Cogn 60:198–199, 2006

Cicerone KD, Dahlberg C, Kalmar K, et al: Evidence-based cognitive rehabilitation: recommendations for clinical practice. Arch Phys Med Rehabil 81:1596–1615, 2000

Cicerone KD, Dahlberg C, Malec JF, et al: Evidence-based cognitive rehabilitation: updated review of the literature from 1998 through 2002. Arch Phys Med Rehabil 86:1681–1692, 2005

Cicerone KD, Langenbahn DM, Braden C, et al: Evidence-based cognitive rehabilitation: updated review of the literature from 2003 through 2008. Arch Phys Med Rehabil 92:519–530, 2011

Ciurli P, Bivona U, Barba C, et al: Metacognitive unawareness correlates with executive function impairment after severe traumatic brain injury. J Int Neuropsychol Soc 16:360–368, 2010

Ciurli P, Formisano R, Bivona U, et al: Neuropsychiatric disorders in persons with severe traumatic brain injury: prevalence, phenomenology, and relationship with demographic, clinical, and functional features. J Head Trauma Rehabil 26:116–126, 2011

Committee on Cognitive Rehabilitation Therapy for Traumatic Brain Injury: Cognitive Rehabilitation Therapy for Traumatic Brain Injury: Evaluating the Evidence. Washington, DC, Institute of Medicine, 2011

Corrigan JD, Mysiw WJ, Gribble MW, et al: Agitation, cognition and attention during post-traumatic amnesia. Brain Inj 6:155–160, 1992

Cowan N: What are the differences between long-term, short-term, and working memory? Prog Brain Res 169:323–338, 2008

Dikmen SS, Corrigan JD, Levin HS, et al: Cognitive outcome following traumatic brain injury. J Head Trauma Rehabil 24:430–438, 2009

Ehlhardt LA, Sohlberg MM, Kennedy M, et al: Evidence-based practice guidelines for instructing individuals with neurogenic memory impairments: what have we learned in the past 20 years? Neuropsychol Rehabil 18:300–342, 2008

Erez AB, Rothschild E, Katz N, et al: Executive functioning, awareness, and participation in daily life after mild traumatic brain injury: a preliminary study. Am J Occup Ther 63:634–640, 2009

Folstein MF, Folstein SE, McHugh PR: "Mini-mental state": a practical method for grading the cognitive state of patients for the clinician. J Psychiatr Res 12:189–198, 1975

Frey KL, Rojas DC, Anderson CA, et al: Comparison of the O-Log and GOAT as measures of posttraumatic amnesia. Brain Inj 21:513–520, 2007

Gardner H: Frames of Mind: The Theory of Multiple Intelligences. New York, Basic Books, 1983

Giacino JT, Ashwal S, Childs N, et al: The minimally conscious state: definition and diagnostic criteria. Neurology 58:349–353, 2002

Giacino JT, Kalmar K, Whyte J: The JFK Coma Recovery Scale—Revised: measurement characteristics and diagnostic utility. Arch Phys Med Rehabil 85:2020–2029, 2004

Hagen C, Malkmus D, Durham P: Rancho Los Amigos Scale. Downey, CA, Communication Disorders Service, 1972

Halterman CI, Langan J, Drew A, et al: Tracking the recovery of visuospatial attention deficits in mild traumatic brain injury. Brain 129:747–753, 2006

Hartikainen KM, Waljas M, Isoviita T, et al: Persistent symptoms in mild to moderate traumatic brain injury associated with executive dysfunction. J Clin Exp Neuropsychol 32:767–774, 2010

Katz DI, Polyak M, Coughlan D, et al: Natural history of recovery from brain injury after prolonged disorders of consciousness: outcome of patients admitted to inpatient rehabilitation with 1–4 year follow-up. Prog Brain Res 177:73–88, 2009

Kay T, Harrington DE, Adams RE, et al: Definition of mild traumatic brain injury: report from the Mild Traumatic Brain Injury Committee of the Head Injury Interdisciplinary Special Interest Group of the American Congress of Rehabilitation Medicine. J Head Trauma Rehabil 8:86–87, 1993

Kean J, Trzepacz PT, Murray LL, et al: Initial validation of a brief provisional diagnostic scale for delirium. Brain Inj 24:1222–1230, 2010

Kim YW, Kim DY, Shin JC, et al: The changes of cortical metabolism associated with the clinical response to donepezil therapy in traumatic brain injury. Clin Neuropharmacol 32:63–68, 2009

Levin HS, O'Donnell VM, Grossman RG: The Galveston Orientation and Amnesia Test: a practical scale to assess cognition after head injury. J Nerv Ment Dis 167:675–684, 1979

Liepert J: Pharmacotherapy in restorative neurology. Curr Opin Neurol 21:639–643, 2008

Marion DW: Evidenced-based guidelines for traumatic brain injuries. Prog Neurol Surg 19:171–196, 2006

Mathias JL, Beall JA, Bigler ED: Neuropsychological and information processing deficits following mild traumatic brain injury. J Int Neuropsychol Soc 10:286–297, 2004

McAllister TW, Flashman LA, McDonald BC, et al: Mechanisms of working memory dysfunction after mild and moderate TBI: evidence from functional MRI and neurogenetics. J Neurotrauma 23:1450–1467, 2006

McCauley SR, Levin HS, Vanier M, et al: The Neurobehavioural Rating Scale–Revised: sensitivity and validity in closed head injury assessment. J Neurol Neurosurg Psychiatry 71:643–651, 2001

McCrea M, Iverson GL, McAllister TW, et al: An integrated review of recovery after mild traumatic brain injury (MTBI): implications for clinical management. Clin Neuropsychol 23:1368–1390, 2009

Menon DK, Schwab K, Wright DW, et al: Position statement: definition of traumatic brain injury. Arch Phys Med Rehabil 91:1637–1640, 2010

Muller F, Simion A, Reviriego E, et al: Exploring theory of mind after severe traumatic brain injury. Cortex 46:1088–1099, 2010

Nakase-Thompson R, Sherer M, Yablon SA, et al: Acute confusion following traumatic brain injury. Brain Inj 18:131–142, 2004

Nolin P: Executive memory dysfunctions following mild traumatic brain injury. J Head Trauma Rehabil 21:68–75, 2006

Omalu BI, DeKosky ST, Minster RL, et al: Chronic traumatic encephalopathy in a National Football League player. Neurosurgery 57:128–134, discussion 128–134, 2005

Ownsworth TL, McFarland K, Young RM: The investigation of factors underlying deficits in self-awareness and self-regulation. Brain Inj 16:291–309, 2002

Ponsford J, Olver J, Ponsford M, et al: Long-term adjustment of families following traumatic brain injury where comprehensive rehabilitation has been provided. Brain Inj 17:453–468, 2003

Ponsford J, Draper K, Schonberger M: Functional outcome 10 years after traumatic brain injury: its relationship with demographic, injury severity, and cognitive and emotional status. J Int Neuropsychol Soc 14:233–242, 2008

Royall DR, Lauterbach EC, Kaufer D, et al: The cognitive correlates of functional status: a review from the Committee on Research of the American Neuropsychiatric Association. J Neuropsychiatry Clin Neurosci 19:249–265, 2007

Sanchez-Carrion R, Fernandez-Espejo D, Junque C, et al: A longitudinal fMRI study of working memory in severe TBI patients with diffuse axonal injury. Neuroimage 43:421–429, 2008

Serino A, Ciaramelli E, Di Santantonio A, et al: Central executive system impairment in traumatic brain injury. Brain Inj 20:23–32, 2006

Shaw NA: The neurophysiology of concussion. Prog Neurobiol 67:281–344, 2002

Sherer M, Hart T, Whyte J, et al: Neuroanatomic basis of impaired self-awareness after traumatic brain injury: findings from early computed tomography. J Head Trauma Rehabil 20:287–300, 2005

Sigurdardottir S, Andelic N, Roe C, et al: Cognitive recovery and predictors of functional outcome 1 year after traumatic brain injury. J Int Neuropsychol Soc 15:740–750, 2009

Silver JM, Koumaras B, Chen M, et al: Effects of rivastigmine on cognitive function in patients with traumatic brain injury. Neurology 67:748–755, 2006

Silver JM, Koumaras B, Meng X, et al: Long-term effects of rivastigmine capsules in patients with traumatic brain injury. Brain Inj 23:123–132, 2009

Stuss DT, Binns MA, Carruth FG, et al: The acute period of recovery from traumatic brain injury: posttraumatic amnesia or posttraumatic confusional state? J Neurosurg 90:635–643, 1999

Tenovuo O, Alin J, Helenius H: A randomized controlled trial of rivastigmine for chronic sequels of traumatic brain injury: what it showed and taught? Brain Inj 23:548–558, 2009

Tittle A, Burgess GH: Relative contribution of attention and memory toward disorientation or post-traumatic amnesia in an acute brain injury sample. Brain Inj 25:933–942, 2011

Trzepacz PT, Baker RW, Greenhouse J: A symptom rating scale for delirium. Psychiatry Res 23:89–97, 1988

Vanier M, Mazaux JM, Lambert J, et al: Assessment of neuropsychologic impairments after head injury: interrater reliability and factorial and criterion validity of the Neurobehavioral Rating Scale–Revised. Arch Phys Med Rehabil 81:796–806, 2000

Warden DL, Gordon B, McAllister TW, et al: Guidelines for the pharmacologic treatment of neurobehavioral sequelae of traumatic brain injury. J Neurotrauma 23:1468–1501, 2006

Wheaton P, Mathias JL, Vink R: Impact of early pharmacological treatment on cognitive and behavioral outcome after traumatic brain injury in adults: a meta-analysis. J Clin Psychopharmacol 29:468–477, 2009

Wheaton P, Mathias JL, Vink R: Impact of pharmacological treatments on cognitive and behavioral outcome in the postacute stages of adult traumatic brain injury: a meta-analysis. J Clin Psychopharmacol 31:745–757, 2011

Writer BW, Schillerstrom JE: Psychopharmacological treatment for cognitive impairment in survivors of traumatic brain injury: a critical review. J Neuropsychiatry Clin Neurosci 21:362–370, 2009

Zafonte R, Friedewald WT, Lee SM, et al: The Citicoline Brain Injury Treatment (COBRIT) trial: design and methods. J Neurotrauma 26:2207–2216, 2009

Zafonte RD, Bagiella E, Ansel BM, et al: Effect of citicoline on functional and cognitive status among patients with traumatic brain injury: Citicoline Brain Injury Treatment Trial (COBRIT). JAMA 308:1993–2000, 2012

Zhang L, Plotkin RC, Wang G, et al: Cholinergic augmentation with donepezil enhances recovery in short-term memory and sustained attention after traumatic brain injury. Arch Phys Med Rehabil 85:1050–1055, 2004

# POSTTRAUMATIC EMOTIONAL AND BEHAVIORAL DISTURBANCES

CHAPTER 6

# Disorders of Mood and Affect

*Ricardo E. Jorge, M.D.*
*David B. Arciniegas, M.D.*

**Disorders of mood and affect** are common consequences of traumatic brain injury (TBI). The pathogenesis of these
disorders following TBI is complex and, in all likelihood, variable with
respect to etiology. In some cases, especially in the early period following TBI, the development of these disorders may reflect the effects of
neurotrauma on the several distributed neural networks that generate and regulate emotion (Jorge et al. 1993a). For some patients, particularly those in whom depressive disorders develop in the late
postinjury period, psychological and social factors appear to be etiologically important (Jorge et al. 1993a; Whelan-Goodinson et al.
2010).

Regardless of whether the development of these conditions reflects the effects of neurotrauma on cognitive and emotional processing, preinjury psychiatric and psychological factors, postinjury
psychological or social problems, the influence of environment and
family, or some combination of these factors, TBI disorders of mood
and affect negatively influence the recovery process and constitute a
major determinant of functional and psychosocial outcome (Bombardier et al. 2010; Seel et al. 2010).

The high frequency and functional importance of disorders of
mood and affect among persons with TBI make these disorders an es-

sential subject for practicing clinicians to understand. Therefore, in this chapter, we describe the evaluation and management of the most common of these disorders among persons with TBI: depressive disorders, manic and mixed mood states (bipolar spectrum disorders), and pathological laughing and crying.

# DEPRESSIVE DISORDERS

## Epidemiology

Depressive disorders develop commonly among persons with TBI, with estimated frequencies ranging from 6% to 77% (Seel et al. 2010). Most experts on this subject accept an estimated first-year post-TBI depression frequency in the range of 25%–50% (Kim et al. 2007; Seel et al. 2010) and lifetime rates of 26%–64% (Hibbard et al. 1998; Koponen et al. 2002). Although the risk of developing depression is generally regarded as being highest in the first post-TBI year, the risk of this condition remains increased even decades after injury.

## Risk Factors

The list of identified risk factors for depressive disorders after TBI is extensive. At a minimum, such risk factors include neurogenetics, preinjury personal and psychosocial factors, injury-related neurobiological factors, and postinjury psychosocial factors, as well as the interactions of these various factors.

*Neurogenetics.* The role of genetics in the development of post-TBI neuropsychiatric disorders, including depression, is an active area of investigation. The apolipoprotein E4 (APOE4) genotype may be relevant to some TBI outcomes but does not appear to influence the rate of depressive disorders following either mild TBI (Chamelian et al. 2004) or more severe TBI (Koponen et al. 2004). Polymorphisms in genes whose products are involved in the regulation of ascending neurotransmitter systems also are of interest. For instance, polymorphisms of the serotonin transporter gene 5HTT do not appear to influence the occurrence or severity of depression after TBI (Chan et al. 2008) but may modify response to treatment. For example, response to citalopram in this population is influenced by genotype, with adverse treatment effects occurring more frequently among persons with specific 5HTT polymorphisms (including rs25531) and favorable treatment response predicted by the C-677(T) polymorphism of the methylene tetrahydrofolate reductase (MTHFR) gene and the val66met polymorphism of the brain-derived neurotrophic factor (BDNF) gene (Lanctôt et al. 2010). Further investigations are required to clarify the relevance of this class of preinjury risk factor on the development and resolution of depressive disorders among persons with TBI.

*Preinjury personal and psychosocial factors.* The development and persistence of depression after TBI is also influenced by psychosocial factors. These include, among others, poor preinjury occupational status, poor premorbid social functioning and/or poverty, previous history of psychiatric diagnosis (including depression) or brain injury, alcohol abuse, fewer years of formal education, female gender, and a tendency to experience high levels of stress. With time after injury, persons with TBI may experience substantial changes in autonomy, self-image, and close relationships; these changes, particularly in the face of maladaptive coping styles, lack of social supports, or other external stressors, may also contribute to the development of depressive disorders, especially those with new onset in the late postinjury period.

*Injury-related neurobiological factors.* Among the neurobiological mechanisms involved in the development of posttraumatic depression, especially those occurring in the early postinjury period, are damage to left dorsolateral and ventrolateral prefrontal cortices, frontoparietal white matter integrity, left basal ganglia, and proximity to the left frontal pole (Jorge et al. 1993b; Koponen et al. 2006; Lipsey et al. 1983; Matthews et al. 2011). Depression phenotype also may be influenced by the anatomy of injury, with major depression alone correlating most strongly with left anterior lesions and anxious depression correlating with right hemisphere lesions (Jorge et al. 2004). Rao et al. (2010) observed relationships between persons with depression following TBI and impaired performance on tests of frontotemporal functioning, lower choline/creatine and $N$-acetylaspartate/creatine ratios in the right basal ganglia, and lower regional brain volumes in the right frontal and left occipital and temporal lobes.

Irrespective of issues related to injury laterality, these findings suggest that damage to anterior cerebral and dorsolateral prefrontal structures is associated with an increased risk for depression following TBI. It is possible that injury to these areas compromises the top-down regulation of emotion and/or results in disinhibition of ventral limbic/paralimbic structures involved in emotional generation, thereby increasing the risk for depression after TBI.

The neurochemical bases of post-TBI depression remain uncertain, although serotonergic disturbances have been suggested to play a role in this problem (Mobayed and Dinan 1990). As noted earlier in "Neurogenetics," response to treatment with citalopram may be modified by polymorphisms in the genes coding for 5-HTT, MTHFR, and BDNF, although there is no evidence presently that these or other genes modifying neurotransmission or repair alter the risk for developing depression after TBI. These remain understudied issues and ones in need of further investigation.

*Postinjury psychosocial factors.* Preinjury and postinjury psychosocial factors influence the development of depression following TBI (Seel et al. 2010). Early- and late-onset post-TBI depressions are influenced by patients' perceived lack of social support or close confiding relationships. In particular, lack of an intimate partner, lack of a close friend, and/or discordant close relationships are associated with depression following TBI. Unemployment issues, including postinjury job loss, lower income levels, and financial problems, also are risk factors for depression after TBI.

## Clinical Assessment

*Differential diagnosis.* The first step toward effectively treating depression after TBI is accurate clinical diagnosis. Considering the differential diagnosis of mood disturbances among persons with TBI therefore is a prerequisite to other evaluations as well as treatment. The differential diagnosis of post-TBI depressive disorders includes delirium-associated mood disturbances, substance-related mood disturbances (including those related to substance intoxications or withdrawals), medication-induced depressive symptoms, dysthymia, bipolar spectrum disorders, adjustment disorder with depressed mood, pathological laughing and crying (PLC), posttraumatic stress disorder (PTSD), posttraumatic apathy, personality change due to a general medical condition (especially labile type), and pre-TBI depressive and/or personality disorders, among other neuropsychiatric conditions.

Pre-TBI mood (especially depressive) disorders are common among persons with TBI (Hibbard et al. 1998; Whelan-Goodinson et al. 2009) and must be included in the differential diagnosis of any post-TBI depressive disorder. When such disorders are part of the pre-TBI history, it may not be possible to assert with certainty the role of TBI in the development and maintenance of postinjury depressive disorders. Similarly, preinjury personality disorders and substance use disorders may contribute to the development of depressive symptoms following TBI. These conditions also merit consideration as contributing or alternative explanations for post-TBI depressive symptoms.

Depressive symptoms may develop during the posttraumatic confusional state (i.e., posttraumatic delirium) or during a post-TBI substance withdrawal syndrome. These symptoms are usually evident as such rather than as a frank depression by virtue of the co-occurrence of other symptoms of delirium or substance withdrawal. They tend to be labile in character and resolve in concert with the conditions underlying them. Medication-induced depressive symptoms are often more challenging to identify as such; when suspected, tapering and/or discontinuing potentially causative medication is appropriate.

Apathy is frequently observed among TBI patients, particularly those with more severe injuries, and may be mistaken for or comorbid with depression (Kant et al. 1998a; Seel et al. 2010). Apathy is a syndrome of diminished goal-directed behavior (as manifested by lack of effort, initiative, and productivity), cognition (as manifested by decreased interests, lack of plans and goals, and lack of concern about one's own health or functional status), and emotion (as manifested by flat affect, emotional indifference, and restricted responses to important life events) (Marin et al. 1995). Apathy is distinguished from depression by virtue of the absence of the core psychological symptoms of depression: persistent and excessive sadness as well as negative valence and distorted appraisal of the self, the world, and one's future. In general, patients and their families are more likely to endorse the description of a patient with apathy as "lacking emotion" or "emotionally absent" and to reject characterization of such a patient as "persistently and excessively sad."

PTSD also is in the differential diagnosis for depression after TBI, and often PTSD and depression are comorbid conditions. The presence of PTSD is suggested by reexperiences of the trauma through flashbacks or vivid nightmares, avoidance of circumstances related to the trauma, and emotional withdrawal or blunting. Because the treatment for comorbid PTSD and depression differs from the treatment of depression alone, identification of this comorbidity is essential (see Chapter 8, "Posttraumatic Stress Disorder").

*Diagnostic assessment.* Standard diagnostic criteria for depression are appropriately applied to the diagnosis of depression among persons with TBI (Jorge et al. 1993a). Structured or semistructured psychiatric interviews are useful when attempting to establish a diagnosis of depression (and other psychiatric disorders) after TBI (Fann et al. 2005; Starkstein and Lischinsky 2002) (see Chapter 3, "Neuropsychological Assessment").

Although physical postconcussive and depressive symptoms may overlap, the number and perceived severity of postconcussive symptoms as well as neuropsychological impairments remit substantively in response to treatment of post-TBI depression (Fann et al. 2000, 2001). Accordingly, it is not appropriate to parse physical from psychological symptoms when diagnosing depression after TBI. Instead, all potentially relevant symptoms should be counted toward this diagnosis.

Assigning a diagnosis of mood disorder due to a general medical condition (TBI) with major depressive-like episode/depressive features, or of major depressive disorder, or of depressive disorder not otherwise specified (NOS) rests on an individual clinician's confidence as regards the causal relationship between a TBI and the depressive episode. Among patients without a pre-TBI mood disorder who develop depression in the early postinjury period, and for which there are no significant medical or medication contributors, it may be reasonable to attribute that episode to the neurobiological effects of TBI on the brain and, hence, to offer a mood disorder "due to TBI" diagnosis. Among patients with a pre-TBI mood disorder or whose depression develops in the late postinjury period, it may be more difficult to establish confidently that the depressive episode is a direct physiological consequence of TBI. In such circumstances, a conservative approach is to offer a diagnosis of major depressive disorder (or, as appropriate, dysthymic disorder or depressive disorder NOS) and to regard TBI as important and a possible treatment-informing comorbidity rather than as the cause of the patient's depressive disorder.

After establishing a categorical diagnosis of depression, assessing symptom severity using scales that are valid and reliable in this population is encouraged (see Chapter 3). Particularly useful scales include the Beck Depression Inventory (BDI; Green et al. 2001), Hamilton Rating Scale for Depression (HAM-D; Fedoroff et al. 1992), the Depression Scale of the Neurobehavioral Functioning Inventory (Seel and

Kreutzer 2003), and the Center for Epidemiologic Studies Depression Scale (Starkstein and Lischinsky 2002). Clinician-administered scales augment and, among persons with limited insight due to TBI, sometimes offer advantages over self-report measures. Regardless of whether clinician-administered, self-report, or both types of symptom severity measures are used, administration at baseline (initial assessment) and serially during treatment is encouraged. Such assessments provide information regarding the effects (or lack of effect) of treatments and may serve usefully as a psychoeducational tool during the counseling and psychotherapeutic portions of depression treatment.

*Laboratory and neurodiagnostic studies.* Physical examination, including vital signs, as well as height and weight (to calculate body mass index), is a requisite element of the pretreatment evaluation (see Chapter 2, "Medical Evaluation"). Neuroimaging is enhancing the understanding of the neurobiological bases of mood disorders among persons with TBI, and is a useful component of the evaluation of persons with TBI generally. If neuroimaging has not been performed previously, it may contribute usefully to the evaluation of persons with posttraumatic depressive disorders. Quantitative electroencephalographic (EEG) and more complex electrophysiological responses may be relevant to the study of depression among persons with TBI (Larson et al. 2009; Reza et al. 2007). However, electrophysiological studies are not presently regarded as useful elements of the clinical evaluation of patients with mood disorders following TBI. If the history or examination suggests endocrine or diagnostically relevant physical conditions, then performing problem-focused laboratory studies is appropriate (American Psychiatric Association 2010). In light of the relatively high frequency of neuroendocrine abnormalities in this population (Rothman et al. 2007), screening for thyroid dysfunction is encouraged as part of the pretreatment depression evaluation. The American Psychiatric Association (2010) also suggests that physicians consider screening persons with depression for human immunodeficiency virus (HIV) infections, and encourages pretreatment urine and/or serum toxicology screening for alcohol and other substances of abuse.

# Treatment

*Psychotherapy.* Regardless of the relative contributions of neurotrauma, psychological, social, and other factors to depressive disorders after TBI, education regarding TBI and recovery expectations, reassurance, and frequent support are recommended as part of all treatment plans for persons with these disorders (Bell et al. 2008; Snell et al. 2009). Cognitive-behavioral therapy (CBT) may decrease depressive, anxious, and anger symptoms as well as improve problem-solving skills, self-esteem, and psychosocial functioning following TBI (Anson and Ponsford 2006a, 2006b). Even when depression itself does not respond to this psychotherapeutic intervention, CBT may help develop skills needed to cope more effectively with persistent postconcussive, including mood, symptoms.

Peer support programs for persons with TBI and their families increase knowledge about TBI, improve general outlook, enhance coping with depression, and improve quality of life (Hibbard et al. 2002). Attending to the psychological needs of spouses, families, and caregivers of persons with TBI is also important because post-TBI depression is strongly associated with significant family dysfunction (Groom et al. 1998) and because depression is common among caregivers of persons with TBI (Harris et al. 2001). Helping family members develop problem-solving and behavioral coping strategies also appears to decrease the severity of depression in the family member with TBI (Leach et al. 1994). Engaging both the patient and his or her family members therefore is essential in the treatment of depression following TBI.

**Pharmacotherapy.** The Selective serotonin reuptake inhibitors (SSRIs) and tricyclic antidepressants (TCAs) may improve depression following TBI (Warden et al. 2006). Effective treatment of post-TBI depression with SSRIs also reduces comorbid irritability and aggression (Kant et al. 1998b) as well as the number and perceived severity of co-occurring postconcussive and cognitive symptoms (Fann et al. 2000, 2001), although the beneficial effect of antidepressant treatment on posttraumatic cognitive impairments is not reported invariably (Lee et al. 2005).

Table 6–1 describes the starting dosages and typical total daily dosages of medications used to treat depression among persons with TBI. Before prescribing these or any other medications, clinicians are encouraged to refer to each medication's product information sheet as well as other reference materials for complete reviews of dosing, side effects, drug-drug interactions, treatment risks, and treatment contraindications. Concerns about both the tolerability and effectiveness of TCAs in this population have led most experts to regard TCAs

**TABLE 6–1.** Medications used to treat depression

| Medication | Starting dosage | Target total daily dosage |
| --- | --- | --- |
| Citalopram | 5–10 mg/day | 10–40 mg |
| Escitalopram | 5–10 mg/day | 5–30 mg |
| Sertraline | 25 mg/day | 25–200 mg |
| Fluoxetine | 10 mg/day | 10–60 mg |
| Paroxetine | 5–10 mg/day | 10–50 mg |
| Mcthylphenidate | 5 mg twice daily | 5–60 mg |
| Dextroamphetamine | 5 mg twice daily | 5–60 mg |
| Nortriptyline | 25 mg/day | 25–150 mg |
| Desipramine | 50 mg/day | 50–200 mg |
| Mirtazapine | 15 mg/day | 15–45 mg |
| Bupropion XL | 150 mg/day | 150–450 mg |
| Venlafaxine XR | 37.5 mg/day | 37.5–225 mg |

as second-line pharmacotherapies for depression after TBI and to recommend SSRIs as the first-line agents for this purpose. Among the SSRIs, sertraline and citalopram are favored in light of their beneficial effects, relatively limited side effects, and short half-lives.

The use of other SSRIs, especially fluoxetine and paroxetine, is limited by their relatively greater potential for adverse effects and drug-drug interactions. For example, fluoxetine is a robust inhibitor of the cytochrome P450 (CYP450) enzymes 2D6, 2C19, and 3A and is associated with problematic drug-drug interactions when coadministered with a substrate, inhibitor, or inducer of these enzymes. Fluoxetine also is metabolized to norfluoxetine, an active metabolite that has a half-life (with long-term use) of approximately 16 days and that also inhibits these CYP450 isoenzymes. If patients develop problematic side effects or drug-drug interactions during treatment with fluoxetine, the slow elimination of fluoxetine and norfluoxetine places patients at risk for a longer duration of such problems than would be likely with other SSRIs. Paroxetine also is a potent inhibitor of 2D6 and 2C19, and its significant antimuscarinic effects increase the risk of treatment-related cognitive dysfunction even among healthy adults (Schmitt et al. 2001). These issues limit enthusiasm for the use of fluoxetine or paroxetine to treat depression among persons with TBI.

Methylphenidate also has been compared to sertraline and placebo in a double-blind, parallel-group study (Lee et al. 2005). Both agents improved depression, and methylphenidate, but not sertraline, also improved neuropsychological performance. Gualtieri and Evans (1988) observed similar methylphenidate-induced benefits on depression after TBI. Although methylphenidate would be an uncommon first-line intervention for depression after TBI in an outpatient setting, it may be useful for this purpose in an inpatient (including acute rehabilitation) setting or when rapidity of treatment response is essential. Early positive responses to methylphenidate in such circumstances are generally followed by a transition to maintenance therapy with an SSRI. Methylphenidate and other stimulants, including dextroamphetamine, are also used commonly to augment partial responses to SSRIs, especially when cognitive impairments and/or fatigue are residual symptoms during treatment with conventional antidepressants.

The efficacy and tolerability of other antidepressants, including the serotonin-norepinephrine reuptake inhibitors (SNRIs), bupropion, and the monoamine oxidase inhibitors (MAOIs), for the treatment of depression among persons with TBI are not well established. Many of these agents are used commonly in clinical practice and, in general, they appear to be similar to the SSRIs with respect to their benefits and adverse effects. The MAOIs are a noteworthy exception to this generality, and their use is discouraged among persons with cognitive or other neurobehavioral impairments because of the possibility of reduced adherence to the dietary restrictions required when taking MAOIs. Bupropion also is of concern in light of its propensity for lowering seizure threshold. This risk is greatest with the immediate-release form of bupropion (Alper et al. 2007); accordingly, using the sustained-release form of bupropion is prudent in this population, and maintaining heightened vigilance for treatment-related seizures during treatment initiation and dose escalation is essential.

*Electroconvulsive therapy.* Electroconvulsive therapy (ECT) may be used for treatment of depression among persons with TBI who fail to respond to other interventions. When ECT is used for the treatment of posttraumatic depression, we recommend treatment with the lowest possible energy levels that will generate a seizure of adequate duration (>20 seconds), use of pulsatile currents, increased spacing of treatments (2–5 days between treatments), and fewer treatments in an entire course (i.e., four to six). If the patient also has significant cognitive (especially memory) impairments due to TBI, nondominant unilateral ECT is the preferred technique.

# Mania, Mixed Mood Episodes, and Bipolar Disorder

## Epidemiology

Mania and mixed mood episodes are relatively uncommon consequences of TBI (Silver et al. 2001). Estimated frequencies of secondary mania among persons with TBI range from 1.7% to 9% (Silver et al. 2001; van Reekum et al. 2000), and clinical experience among neurorehabilitation specialists working in nonpsychiatric settings suggests that this condition occurs at a low frequency. When secondary mania occurs, it tends to do so soon (i.e., within several months) after injury (Jorge et al. 1993b). The average duration of fully symptomatic episodes of secondary mania is approximately 2 months, but mood symptoms may persist for as long as 6 months despite resolution of other manic symptoms. Recurrence of secondary mania and the development of subsequent bipolarity are not typical and strongly suggest the presence (or "unmasking") of an underlying bipolar disorder.

The estimated lifetime relative risk for bipolar disorder after TBI ranges from 1.1 (Silver et al. 2001)—a level of risk not statistically different from that of the general population—to 5 (van Reekum et al. 2000). These estimates are influenced strongly by small sample sizes, selection biases, and diagnostic ascertainment issues. In the largest and most compelling of these studies (Silver et al. 2001), the observed frequency of bipolar disorder (defined as the occurrence of at least one hypomanic or manic episode) was not elevated relative to that of the general population and was further attenuated by controlling for the effects of comorbid alcohol abuse.

## Risk Factors

The limited evidence on and variable methods used to define and study mania and mixed mood episodes among persons with TBI preclude drawing definitive conclusions about risk factors for these conditions. Jorge et al. (1993b), in a study of early post-TBI mania, observed no clear relationship between mania and TBI severity, posttraumatic epilepsy, post-TBI physical or cognitive impairments, level of social functioning, or the presence of family or personal history of psychiatric disorders. Shukla et al. (1987) also observed no relationship between posttraumatic mania and family history of bipolar disorder, but did note associations between post-TBI mania and injury severity (as estimated by duration of posttraumatic amnesia) as well as posttraumatic epilepsy. Complicating matters, the frequency of TBI may be elevated among unaffected family members of persons with bipolar disorder (Malaspina et al. 2001), suggesting the possibility that some heritable element of the bipolar phenotype (e.g., increased novelty seeking, reduced harm avoidance, cognitive deficits) may increase the risk for TBI. Comorbid alcohol use disorders also affect the apparent, but not actual, risk for bipolar disorder among persons with TBI.

Injuries involving the right hemisphere, particularly the right basoventral, anterior temporal, orbitofrontal, caudate, and thalamic areas, are associated with the development of mania due to TBI (Jorge et al. 1993b; Oster et al. 2007). Although the association with right hemisphere injuries is a common observation across many studies and is often cited in the neurobehavioral literature, the cerebral injuries with which secondary manic states are most commonly associated are usually bilateral.

## Clinical Assessment

*Differential diagnosis.* The differential diagnosis of mood disorders with manic or mixed features among persons with TBI is broad, encompasses preinjury and postinjury psychiatric disorders, and overlaps substantially with that of post-TBI depressive disorders (see preceding section, "Depressive Disorders," for review of that differential diagnosis). Several additional conditions merit consideration in this context, including emotional disturbances associated with delirium; mood disorders due to the effect of drugs, including intoxication and/or withdrawal states; posttraumatic epilepsy; and personality change due to TBI.

Transient euphoric and irritable symptoms may develop during the posttraumatic confusional state (i.e., posttraumatic delirium), during a post-TBI substance intoxication or withdrawal syndrome, or as a result of some medications, all of which preclude diagnosis of post-TBI mood disorder with manic or mixed features. These symptoms rarely take on the appearance of true mania, given their transience, lability, and co-occurrence with other symptoms of an acute confusional state. Such symptoms generally resolve in concert with the conditions in which they arise. When medication-induced manic-like symptoms or mixed mood symptoms are suspected, medication taper or discontinuation is appropriate.

Posttraumatic epilepsy and its treatments are associated with the development of emotional disturbances, including manic-like symptoms and/or mixed mood states. Similarly, psychosis associated with epilepsy also may entail the concurrent development of emotional disturbances. Manic or mixed mood episodes that develop in this context may be temporally linked to seizures (or postictal psychosis) or may have a more prolonged course.

Finally, personality change due to TBI may include mood instability, disinhibited or impulsive behavior, and hyperactivity. Patients with such personality changes, however, lack the pervasive and sustained alteration of mood that characterizes manic or mixed syndromes.

*Diagnostic assessment.* The diagnosis of post-TBI manic episodes, mixed mood episodes, or bipolar disorders requires the unequivocal presence of the cardinal feature of such episodes: a distinct period of abnormally and persistently elevated, expansive, or irritable mood lasting at least 4 days for hypomanic episodes or 1 week for manic episodes. Any other cognitive, vegetative, or behavioral disturbance counted toward that diagnosis must be either clear attendants of the sustained and pervasive mood disturbance(s) or, if otherwise present, clearly exacerbated in severity and frequency during the mood disturbance(s).

Overdiagnosis of mania and bipolar disorder in this population is common in many communities and clinical practices. This problem appears to derive most often from misattribution of TBI-related disturbances in affect regulation (i.e., frequent brief episodes of irritability or laughing), impulsive or disinhibited behaviors, alterations in sleep and appetitive behaviors, and cognitive disturbances, to bipolar spectrum disorders despite the absence of the cardinal (mood) disturbance that the diagnosis of mania, mixed mood episode, or bipolar disorder requires. This distinction is not a matter of semantics: the treatment of paroxysmal disturbances of affect and disinhibited behaviors differs from treatments offered to persons with mania or bipolar disorder. In particular, unopposed SSRIs are prescribed routinely and appropriately for the treatment of posttraumatic disturbances of affect and behavioral dyscontrol syndromes, a practice that is generally inadvisable among persons with secondary mania or bipolar disorders (Dealberto et al. 2008).

The methods used to diagnose manic episodes, mixed mood episodes, and bipolar disorder among persons with TBI are the same as those used to make primary (idiopathic) diagnoses of these types (Jorge and Robinson 2003). Using structured or semistructured psychiatric interviews to diagnose these conditions is encouraged, and the Young Mania Rating Scale (Young et al. 1978) is useful as a measure of symptom severity and treatment response in this population (Daniels and Felde 2008; Oster et al. 2007).

*Laboratory and neurodiagnostic studies.* The evaluation of persons with TBI and suspected bipolar spectrum disorders follows the general principles and components of a complete psychiatric evaluation as outlined in the American Psychiatric Association's (1995) "Practice Guideline for Psychiatric Evaluation of Adults." Physical examination, including vital signs with height and weight (to calculate body mass index), is a requisite element of the pretreatment evaluation.

Structural neuroimaging is a useful component of the evaluation of persons with TBI generally. If it has not been performed previously, it may contribute usefully to the evaluation of persons with TBI and mania, mixed mood episodes, or bipolar disorders. Video-EEG monitoring and 24-hour ambulatory recordings may be useful in the differential diagnosis of patients presenting with paroxysmal behavioral disturbances that have unclear etiology or that are associated with intraepisode or postepisode alterations of consciousness. This is particularly relevant to the evaluation of persons with TBI and bipolar spectrum disorders, in light of the possible associations between such disorders and posttraumatic epilepsy. Otherwise, electrophysiological studies are not presently regarded as useful elements of the clinical evaluation in the context of bipolar spectrum disorders.

If the clinical history or examination suggests that the patient has other endocrine or concurrent physical conditions, then performing problem-focused laboratory studies is appropriate (American Psychiatric Association 2010; Hirschfeld 2002). In light of the relatively high frequency of neuroendocrine abnormalities in persons with TBI (Rothman et al. 2007), screening for thyroid dysfunction is encouraged as part of the pretreatment evaluation. As with the evaluation of persons with depression, screening for HIV infection as well as performing urine and/or serum toxicology screening for alcohol and other substances of abuse is encouraged.

# Treatment

*Pharmacotherapy.* The literature describing pharmacotherapy for mania among persons with TBI is insufficient to permit the development of formal treatment standards, guidelines, or options (Warden et al. 2006). A broad range of agents used to treat idiopathic manic and mixed mood states are used to treat secondary mania and bipolar spectrum disorders among persons with TBI (Table 6–2). Before prescribing these or any other medications, clinicians are encouraged to refer to each medication's product information sheet as well as other reference materials for complete reviews of dosing, side effects, drug-drug interactions, treatment risks, and treatment contraindications. The literature and common clinical experience suggest that most of these medications effectively treat TBI-related manic and/or mixed mood states. Their use in clinical practice therefore is informed by their tolerability.

Valproate may exacerbate cognitive impairments in some persons with TBI, especially during the acute titration period, but it appears less likely to do so than either carbamazepine or lithium (Dikmen et al. 2000; Hornstein and Seliger 1989; Massagli 1991). Nonetheless, use of any of these agents necessitates careful and continuous assessment for the development of treatment-related motor impairments (e.g., tremor, incoordination, ataxia, gait disturbances) and cognitive impairments, as well as other adverse somatic side effects (e.g., weight gain, gastrointestinal problems/diarrhea, hematological abnormalities, hepatotoxicity, alopecia). Additionally, the risk of polycystic ovary syndrome requires consideration of alternative treatments in females.

Given that lithium carbonate is often used as a first-line treatment for persons with idiopathic bipolar disorder, it merits special comment as a treatment of mania among persons with TBI. Intolerance of dosages necessary to effect mood stabilization appears to be more common among persons with TBI than among those with primary mania or mixed mood states. This intolerance is often attributable to the adverse cognitive and motor effects of lithium carbonate, which appears more likely to produce nausea, tremor, ataxia, and lethargy in persons

**TABLE 6–2.** Medications used to treat mania and/or mixed mood episodes among persons with traumatic brain injury

| MEDICATION | STARTING DOSAGE | TARGET TOTAL DAILY DOSAGE |
|---|---|---|
| Valproate | 250 mg three times daily | 1,500–4,500 mg (maximum 60 mg/ kg/day; usual serum concentration: 50–125 µg/mL) |
| Quetiapine | 25–50 mg/day | 300–800 mg |
| Carbamazepine | 100 mg/day | 200–1,600 mg (usual serum concentration: 4–12 µg/mL) |
| Lithium | 150 mg at bedtime | 300–1,500 mg (with serum level 0.5– 1.2 mEq/L) |

with neurological disorders than in the general psychiatric population. Additionally, lithium carbonate lowers seizure threshold; in light of the lingering risk for posttraumatic epilepsy (see Chapter 14, "Seizures and Epilepsy"), as well as the potential comorbidity between posttraumatic epilepsy and mania, this effect is concerning with respect to lithium's use in patients with TBI. As such, common limitations of the use of this agent in this population include partial response, relapse of symptoms, or need for a second mood-stabilizing medication. When lithium is used in persons with TBI, vigilance for adverse effects (even at ostensibly "therapeutic" dosages and serum levels) is essential.

Several of the newer anticonvulsants (e.g., lamotrigine, oxcarbazepine) and the atypical antipsychotics (e.g., risperidone, olanzapine, ziprasidone, aripiprazole) may be useful in the treatment of posttraumatic mania, but few reports have been published of their use among persons with posttraumatic mania. Clinicians interested in using these agents for these patients are advised to undertake such treatments cautiously and with careful monitoring for adverse cognitive, motor, cardiac, and metabolic side effects.

In the absence of evidence demonstrating the clear superiority of one of these agents over the others, we generally recommend either valproate or quetiapine as a first-line treatment given their effectiveness for acute mania, rapid-cycling bipolar disorder, and antimanic prophylaxis, as well as their reasonable tolerability in persons with TBI. When these agents, alone or in combination, prove ineffective, then the use of one or more of the other agents listed in Table 6–2 may be required.

*Psychotherapy.* The TBI literature provides no clear guidance regarding the psychotherapeutic approach to persons with mania or mixed mood states after TBI. Education and supportive interventions regarding both TBI and the mood disturbance with which the patient presents are reasonable and commonsense interventions. Additional psychoeducational and psychotherapeutic interventions are modeled after those used in the management of persons with idiopathic bipolar disorders, as described in the American Psychiatric Association's "Practice Guideline for the Treatment of Patients With Bipolar Disorder" (American Psychiatric Association 2002; Hirschfeld 2002).

*Electroconvulsive therapy.* ECT appears to be effective for treatment-resistant or life-threatening manic or mixed mood episodes among persons with TBI. When ECT is used for the treatment of posttraumatic depression, we recommend treatment with the lowest possible energy levels that will generate a seizure of adequate duration (>20 seconds), using pulsatile currents, increased spacing of treatments (2–5 days between treatments), and fewer treatments in an entire course (i.e., four to six). If the patient also has significant cognitive (especially memory) impairments due to TBI, unilateral ECT is the preferred technique.

# PATHOLOGICAL LAUGHING AND CRYING

Pathological laughing and crying (also known as emotional lability, pseudobulbar affect, emotional incontinence, and involuntary emotional expression disorder, among other names) is the prototypical disorder of affect (Wortzel et al. 2008). The clinical features of this condition are presented in Table 6–3. Recognizing PLC is important not only for diagnostic accuracy but also because the treatment implications, both pharmacological and psychotherapeutic, of this diagnosis are different from treatments recommended for some of the mood disorders with which it is confused, especially bipolar spectrum disorders.

## Epidemiology

During the first year post-TBI, the frequency of PLC ranges from 5% to 11% (Tateno et al. 2004; Zeilig et al. 1996). The prevalence of PLC in the late period following TBI is not well established, but common clinical experience suggests that it may become a long-term problem in persons with TBI, especially among persons with relatively more severe injuries.

**TABLE 6–3.** Diagnostic criteria for pathological laughing and crying due to traumatic brain injury

| | |
|---|---|
| Required features | Frequent, brief episodes of uncontrollable laughing and/or crying. |
| | The intensity of each episode of laughing and/or crying is excessive in relation to its inciting stimulus. |
| | The laughing and crying is stereotyped (i.e., phenomenologically identical) across episodes. |
| | The episodes neither reflect nor produce a persistent change in the prevailing mood. |
| | The episodes of laughing and/or crying reflect a change in the patient's customary affect. |
| | The episodes are subjectively distressing (e.g., are embarrassing) and/or impair social, occupational, or other important aspects of function. |
| | The episodes are a direct result of traumatic brain injury. |
| Variable features | The episodes may occur spontaneously (i.e., with no apparent inciting stimulus). |
| | The displays of affect may be of a valence contradictory to that expected given the context in which they occur (i.e., laughing when crying would be expected, or vice versa). |
| | Feelings experienced while laughing or crying may be congruent or incongruent with the apparent valence of the display of affect (i.e., feeling mirth while crying, feeling sad while laughing). |
| | Feelings may be entirely absent during the episodes (i.e., feeling nothing while crying or laughing). |
| Exclusory features | The laughing and/or crying is not an ictal display of affect (i.e., dacrystic or gelastic epilepsy). |

# Risk Factors

The principal risk factors for PLC appear to be the location and extent of anatomical injury (Rabins and Arciniegas 2007; Wortzel et al. 2008). The dorsal (dorsolateral and anterior prefrontal) cortical, internal capsular, and pontocerebellar elements of the cortico-limbic-subcortico-thalamic-ponto-cerebellar (CLSTPC) network facilitate voluntary regulation of emotional expression and mediate associated subjective experiences (i.e., feelings). Injury to and/or dysfunction of these elements of the CLSTPC network are most commonly implicated as critical to the development of PLC (Olney et al. 2011; Wortzel et al. 2008). Some evidence (Sackeim et al. 1982) indicates that crying-predominant PLC is more strongly associated with left hemisphere injuries than is laughing-predominant PLC, which is more strongly associated with right hemisphere injuries. However, both forms of PLC are most common among persons with bilateral injuries.

Evidence in other conditions (especially stroke) indicates that anatomical disruption of the brain stem serotonergic (median and dorsal raphe) nuclei and/or their ascending serotonergic efferents to targets within the CLSTPC network is associated with PLC (Rabins and Arciniegas 2007). Deficits in dopaminergic or noradrenergic function, and/or excessive glutamatergic function, within the CLSTPC network also are sometimes suggested as contributing to the development of PLC; however, these suggestions are based entirely on the effects of pharmacotherapies that directly or indirectly affect serotonergic function as well.

At the present time, there is no evidence suggesting that neurogenetics, development, age, gender, pre-TBI psychiatric or substance use history, pre-TBI or post-TBI psychosocial factors, or other factors influence the risk of developing PLC after TBI.

# Clinical Assessment

*Differential diagnosis.* Mood disorders and ictal displays of affect are included in the differential diagnosis of PLC. Recognizing the disturbance of emotional regulation as paroxysmal—not clearly linked to or influencing the patient's prevailing mood, and not associated with or producing cognitive, vegetative, and behavioral disturbances entailed by disorders of mood—facilitates distinguishing PLC from depressive and bipolar spectrum disorders. Ictal laughing (gelastic seizure) and ictal crying (dacrystic or quiritarian seizure) are manifestations of complex partial epilepsy in which the seizure itself (i.e., the ictus) is characterized by laughing or crying. As complex partial seizures, by definition, they entail ictal alteration of consciousness and are followed by at least a brief period of postictal confusion. They are frequently associated with ictal epileptiform discharges on electroencephalography, and sometimes associated with interictal epileptiform abnormalities. The occurrence of alterations in consciousness during episodes of crying and laughing is inconsistent with a diagnosis of PLC. When such alterations are present, a diagnosis of PLC is unlikely. Treatment of PLC is not the same as that of gelastic or dacrystic seizures, highlighting the importance of distinguishing between these conditions.

Also in the differential diagnosis is essential crying, an uncommon, lifelong, and (probably) hereditary propensity for crying in response to stimuli of modest or greater sentimental value (Green et al. 1987). This condition lies at the borderline between normal affective variability and a medical disorder. Unlike PLC, essential crying does not produce significant subjective distress or functional impairment and therefore does not require treatment. Personality disorders in which disturbances of affect regulation feature prominently (e.g., borderline personality disorder, histrionic personality disorder) also are in the differential diagnosis of PLC. Unlike pathological laughing and crying, the disturbances of affect in personality disorders are not stereotyped or discretely paroxysmal and tend to be linked more clearly to personally relevant sentimental (and usually relational or interpersonal) stimuli.

*Diagnostic assessment.* Interview and observation of the patient as well as interview of a knowledgeable informant are generally sufficient to establish a diagnosis of PLC. Clinicians unfamiliar with this interview may find the Pathological Laughter and Crying Scale (PLACS; Robinson et al. 1993) useful for diagnosing this condition, characterizing its severity, and monitoring response to treatment. In light of the need to distinguish PLC from depression and bipolar spectrum disorders, concurrent assessment for these conditions using the methods described earlier in this chapter (see "Depressive Disorders") is recommended. Depression and PLC may co-occur following TBI, and the presence of depression does not exclude a diagnosis of PLC if criteria for both are met. It is possible, although not yet reported, that the same may be true for PLC and manic or mixed mood episodes.

*Laboratory and neurodiagnostic assessments.* No specific laboratory or neurodiagnostic assessments are recommended for diagnosing PLC. Neuroimaging is frequently obtained as part of the evaluation for TBI and may inform on the anatomical underpinnings of PLC in this context. When the history does not provide information needed to determine whether the displays of affect represent seizures, PLC, or both, video-EEG monitoring may be required to clarify the diagnosis.

# Treatment

The management of PLC consists of pharmacotherapy with education and counseling of patients and their family members. The PLC literature overwhelmingly demonstrates the effectiveness of relatively low dosages of serotonergically and noradrenergically active antidepressants for PLC, regardless of whether this condition manifests predominantly as crying, laughing, or both (Wortzel et al. 2008). This treatment approach is especially noteworthy in light of the potential for misdiagnosis of PLC as one or another form of bipolar disorder: the latter diagnosis generally leads clinicians to avoid prescription of an unopposed SSRI and tends to drive prescription of "mood stabilizers" (especially anticonvulsants and/or lithium). In fact, unopposed SSRIs are the treatment of choice for persons with bipolar disorder, and most but not all "mood stabilizers" are ineffective as treatments for PLC. Accordingly, the importance of diagnostic accuracy and the potential for misdiagnosis to drive pharmacological mismanagement cannot in this context be overstated.

SSRIs are the first-line treatments of PLC, and often reduce the frequency and severity of this condition within a few days of treatment initiation. These and other treatments for PLC are presented in Table 6–4. Before prescribing these or any other medications, clinicians are encouraged to refer to each medication's product information sheet as well as other reference materials for complete reviews of dosing, side effects, drug-drug interactions, treatment risks, and treatment contraindications. Using SSRIs with relatively short half-lives, limited drug-drug and CYP450 interactions, and favorable side-effect profiles is recommended. TCAs may also be effective for PLC, with nortriptyline being the most commonly used agent in this class. Medications that enhance dopamine and/or norepinephrine neurotransmission, including methylphenidate, also may improve PLC.

**TABLE 6–4.** Medications used to treat pathological laughing and crying due to traumatic brain injury

| Medication | Starting dosage | Target total daily dosage |
|---|---|---|
| Citalopram | 5–10 mg/day | 10–40 mg |
| Escitalopram | 5–10 mg/day | 5–30 mg |
| Sertraline | 25 mg/day | 25–200 mg |
| Fluoxetine | 10 mg/day | 10–60 mg |
| Paroxetine | 5–10 mg/day | 10–50 mg |
| Nortriptyline | 10 mg/day | 25–150 mg |
| Methylphenidate | 5 mg twice daily | 5–60 mg |
| Carbidopa-levodopa | 25/100-mg tablet three times daily | 25/100-mg tablet, up to two tablets four times daily |
| Mirtazapine | 15 mg/day | 15–45 mg |
| Venlafaxine XR | 37.5 mg/day | 37.5–225 mg |
| Lamotrigine | 25 mg/day | 100 mg |
| Amantadine | 50 mg/day | 50–200 mg |
| Dextromethorphan-quinidine | 20/10-mg capsule once daily | 20/10-mg capsule once or twice daily |

There is a limited literature describing lamotrigine as a possible treatment for PLC in the context of TBI and epilepsy (Chahine and Chemali 2006). Among patients whose PLC is accompanied by irritability/anger, aggressive behaviors, and/or self-destructive behaviors, treatment with anticonvulsants adjunctively to SSRIs also may confer benefit across these symptoms. Finally, dextromethorphan-quinidine or amantadine—both of which are uncompetitive N-methyl-D-aspartate receptor antagonists—also may improve PLC due to TBI (Wortzel et al. 2008). The latency between treatment initiation and improvement in PLC is similar for amantadine and the SSRIs (2–5 days), whereas the latency between treatment initiation and response with dextromethorphan-quinidine in PLC is often longer (4–5 weeks) than with SSRIs. Although both dextromethorphan-quinidine and amantadine may be effective treatments for PLC, tolerability and the potential for drug-drug interactions attendant on their use are concerning; they are therefore best reserved for use in the treatment of PLC when other agents have proved ineffective or intolerable.

# CONCLUSION

Disorders of mood and affect are common consequences of TBI. The pathogenesis of mood disorders following TBI is complex and reflects the combined effects of neurotrauma on cognitive and emotional processing, preinjury psychiatric and psychological factors, postinjury psychological or social problems, the influence of environment and family, or some combination of these factors. Disorders of mood and affect can negatively influence the recovery process during the early period following TBI and constitute a major determinant of long-term functional and psychosocial outcomes.

In this chapter, we reviewed the characteristics, epidemiology, risk factors, evaluation, and treatment of the most common disorders of mood and affect experienced by persons with TBI. Although these presentations, by design, were brief, our intent was to provide readers with practical recommendations regarding the evaluation and management of adults with these conditions. Additional research in this area is both needed and under way, so clinicians are advised to complement the views and suggestions offered here with updates informed by emerging research findings.

## *Key Clinical Points*

- Depression is among the most common neuropsychiatric sequelae of TBI. The evaluation and management of this condition are similar to those of primary (idiopathic) major depressive disorder.

- Depression that develops in the early postinjury period may be related more strongly to the neurobiological effects of TBI on emotion than is later-onset depression. Depression that develops in the late postinjury period is more strongly associated with psychological and social stressors and dysfunction.

- Mania, mixed mood states, and bipolar spectrum disorders are uncommon but serious consequences of TBI. In most respects, the evaluation and management of these conditions are similar to those of idiopathic bipolar spectrum disorders.

- Pathological laughing and crying is an infrequent consequence of TBI, but one whose treatments are distinct from those of the bipolar spectrum disorders for which it is frequently mistaken. Selective serotonin reuptake inhibitors are first-line treatments for this condition.

# REFERENCES

Alper K, Schwartz KA, Kolts RL, et al: Seizure incidence in psychopharmacological clinical trials: an analysis of Food and Drug Administration (FDA) summary basis of approval reports. Biol Psychiatry 62:345–354, 2007

American Psychiatric Association: Practice guideline for psychiatric evaluation of adults. Am J Psychiatry 152(11 suppl):63–80, 1995

American Psychiatric Association: Practice guideline for the treatment of patients with bipolar disorder (revision). Am J Psychiatry 159(suppl):1–50, 2002

American Psychiatric Association: Treatment of Patients With Major Depressive Disorder. Washington, DC, American Psychiatric Association, 2010

Anson K, Ponsford J: Evaluation of a coping skills group following traumatic brain injury. Brain Inj 20:167–178, 2006a

Anson K, Ponsford J: Who benefits? Outcome following a coping skills group intervention for traumatically brain injured individuals. Brain Inj 20:1–13, 2006b

Bell KR, Hoffman JM, Temkin NR, et al: The effect of telephone counselling on reducing post-traumatic symptoms after mild traumatic brain injury: a randomised trial. J Neurol Neurosurg Psychiatry 79:1275–1281, 2008

Bombardier CH, Fann JR, Temkin NR, et al: Rates of major depressive disorder and clinical outcomes following traumatic brain injury. JAMA 303:1938–1945, 2010

Chahine LM, Chemali Z: Du rire aux larmes: pathological laughing and crying in patients with traumatic brain injury and treatment with lamotrigine. Epilepsy Behav 8:610–615, 2006

Chamelian L, Reis M, Feinstein A: Six-month recovery from mild to moderate traumatic brain injury: the role of APOE-epsilon4 allele. Brain 127:2621–2628, 2004

Chan F, Lanctôt KL, Feinstein A, et al: The serotonin transporter polymorphisms and major depression following traumatic brain injury. Brain Inj 22:471–479, 2008

Daniels JP, Felde A: Quetiapine treatment for mania secondary to brain injury in 2 patients. J Clin Psychiatry 69:497–498, 2008

Dealberto MJ, Marino J, Bourgon L: Homicidal ideation with intent during a manic episode triggered by antidepressant medication in a man with brain injury. Bipolar Disord 10:111–113, 2008

Dikmen SS, Machamer JE, Winn HR, et al: Neuropsychological effects of valproate in traumatic brain injury: a randomized trial. Neurology 54:895–902, 2000

Fann JR, Uomoto JM, Katon WJ: Sertraline in the treatment of major depression following mild traumatic brain injury. J Neuropsychiatry Clin Neurosci 12:226–232, 2000

Fann JR, Uomoto JM, Katon WJ: Cognitive improvement with treatment of depression following mild traumatic brain injury. Psychosomatics 42:48–54, 2001

Fann JR, Bombardier CH, Dikmen S, et al: Validity of the Patient Health Questionnaire–9 in assessing depression following traumatic brain injury. J Head Trauma Rehabil 20:501–511, 2005

Fedoroff JP, Starkstein SE, Forrester AW, et al: Depression in patients with acute traumatic brain injury. Am J Psychiatry 149:918–923, 1992

Green A, Felmingham K, Baguley IJ, et al: The clinical utility of the Beck Depression Inventory after traumatic brain injury. Brain Inj 15:1021–1028, 2001

Green RL, McAllister TW, Bernat JL: A study of crying in medically and surgically hospitalized patients. Am J Psychiatry 144:442–447, 1987

Groom KN, Shaw TG, O'Connor ME, et al: Neurobehavioral symptoms and family functioning in traumatically brain-injured adults. Arch Clin Neuropsychol 13:695–711, 1998

Gualtieri CT, Evans RW: Stimulant treatment for the neurobehavioural sequelae of traumatic brain injury. Brain Inj 2:273–290, 1988

Harris JK, Godfrey HP, Partridge FM, et al: Caregiver depression following traumatic brain injury (TBI): a consequence of adverse effects on family members? Brain Inj 15:223–238, 2001

Hibbard MR, Uysal S, Kepler K, et al: Axis I psychopathology in individuals with traumatic brain injury. J Head Trauma Rehabil 13:24–39, 1998

Hibbard MR, Cantor J, Charatz H, et al: Peer support in the community: initial findings of a mentoring program for individuals with traumatic brain injury and their families. J Head Trauma Rehabil 17:112–131, 2002

Hirschfeld RMA: Guideline Watch: Practice Guideline for the Treatment of Patients With Bipolar Disorder, 2nd Edition. Washington, DC, American Psychiatric Association, 2002. Available at: http://psychiatryonline.org/content.aspx?bookid=28&sectionid=1682557. Accessed December 7, 2012.

Hornstein A, Seliger G: Cognitive side effects of lithium in closed head injury. J Neuropsychiatry Clin Neurosci 1:446–447, 1989

Jorge R, Robinson RG: Mood disorders following traumatic brain injury. Int Rev Psychiatry 15:317–327, 2003

Jorge RE, Robinson RG, Arndt SV, et al: Comparison between acute- and delayed-onset depression following traumatic brain injury. J Neuropsychiatry Clin Neurosci 5:43–49, 1993a

Jorge RE, Robinson RG, Starkstein SE, et al: Secondary mania following traumatic brain injury. Am J Psychiatry 150:916–921, 1993b

Jorge RE, Robinson RG, Moser D, et al: Major depression following traumatic brain injury. Arch Gen Psychiatry 61:42–50, 2004

Kant R, Duffy JD, Pivovarnik A: Prevalence of apathy following head injury. Brain Inj 12:87–92, 1998a

Kant R, Smith-Seemiller L, Zeiler D: Treatment of aggression and irritability after head injury. Brain Inj 12:661–666, 1998b

Kim E, Lauterbach EC, Reeve A, et al: Neuropsychiatric complications of traumatic brain injury: a critical review of the literature (a report by the ANPA Committee on Research). J Neuropsychiatry Clin Neurosci 19:106–127, 2007

Koponen S, Taiminen T, Portin R, et al: Axis I and II psychiatric disorders after traumatic brain injury: a 30-year follow-up study. Am J Psychiatry 159:1315–1321, 2002

Koponen S, Taiminen T, Kairisto V, et al: APOE-epsilon4 predicts dementia but not other psychiatric disorders after traumatic brain injury. Neurology 63:749–750, 2004

Koponen S, Taiminen T, Kurki T, et al: MRI findings and Axis I and II psychiatric disorders after traumatic brain injury: a 30-year retrospective follow-up study. Psychiatry Res 146:263–270, 2006

Lanctôt KL, Rapoport MJ, Chan F, et al: Genetic predictors of response to treatment with citalopram in depression secondary to traumatic brain injury. Brain Inj 24:959–969, 2010

Larson MJ, Kaufman DA, Kellison IL, et al: Double jeopardy! The additive consequences of negative affect on performance-monitoring decrements following traumatic brain injury. Neuropsychology 23:433–444, 2009

Leach LR, Frank RG, Bouman DE, et al: Family functioning, social support and depression after traumatic brain injury. Brain Inj 8:599–606, 1994

Lee H, Kim SW, Kim JM, et al: Comparing effects of methylphenidate, sertraline and placebo on neuropsychiatric sequelae in patients with traumatic brain injury. Hum Psychopharmacol 20:97–104, 2005

Lipsey JR, Robinson RG, Pearlson GD, et al: Mood change following bilateral hemisphere brain injury. Br J Psychiatry 143:266–273, 1983

Malaspina D, Goetz RR, Friedman JH, et al: Traumatic brain injury and schizophrenia in members of schizophrenia and bipolar disorder pedigrees. Am J Psychiatry 158:440–446, 2001

Marin RS, Fogel BS, Hawkins J, et al: Apathy: a treatable syndrome. J Neuropsychiatry Clin Neurosci 7:23–30, 1995

Massagli TL: Neurobehavioral effects of phenytoin, carbamazepine, and valproic acid: implications for use in traumatic brain injury. Arch Phys Med Rehabil 72:219–226, 1991

Matthews SC, Strigo IA, Simmons AN, et al: A multimodal imaging study in U.S. veterans of Operations Iraqi and Enduring Freedom with and without major depression after blast-related concussion. Neuroimage 54(suppl):S69–S75, 2011

Mobayed M, Dinan TG: Buspirone/prolactin response in post head injury depression. J Affect Disord 19:237–241, 1990

Olney NT, Goodkind MS, Lomen-Hoerth C, et al: Behaviour, physiology and experience of pathological laughing and crying in amyotrophic lateral sclerosis. Brain 134:3458–3469, 2011

Oster TJ, Anderson CA, Filley CM, et al: Quetiapine for mania due to traumatic brain injury. CNS Spectr 12:764–769, 2007

Rabins PV, Arciniegas DB: Pathophysiology of involuntary emotional expression disorder. CNS Spectr 12(suppl):17–22, 2007

Rao V, Munro CA, Rosenberg P, et al: Neuroanatomical correlates of depression in post traumatic brain injury: preliminary results of a pilot study. J Neuropsychiatry Clin Neurosci 22:231–235, 2010

Reza MF, Ikoma K, Ito T, et al: N200 latency and P300 amplitude in depressed mood post-traumatic brain injury patients. Neuropsychol Rehabil 17:723–734, 2007

Robinson RG, Parikh RM, Lipsey JR, et al: Pathological laughing and crying following stroke: validation of a measurement scale and a double-blind treatment study. Am J Psychiatry 150:286–293, 1993

Rothman MS, Arciniegas DB, Filley CM, et al: The neuroendocrine effects of traumatic brain injury. J Neuropsychiatry Clin Neurosci 19:363–372, 2007

Sackeim HA, Greenberg MS, Weiman AL, et al: Hemispheric asymmetry in the expression of positive and negative emotions: neurologic evidence. Arch Neurol 39:210–218, 1982

Schmitt JA, Kruizinga MJ, Riedel WJ: Non-serotonergic pharmacological profiles and associated cognitive effects of serotonin reuptake inhibitors. J Psychopharmacol 15:173–179, 2001

Seel RT, Kreutzer JS: Depression assessment after traumatic brain injury: an empirically based classification method. Arch Phys Med Rehabil 84:1621–1628, 2003

Seel RT, Macciocchi S, Kreutzer JS: Clinical considerations for the diagnosis of major depression after moderate to severe TBI. J Head Trauma Rehabil 25:99–112, 2010

Shukla S, Cook BL, Mukherjee S, et al: Mania following head trauma. Am J Psychiatry 144:93–96, 1987

Silver JM, Kramer R, Greenwald S, et al: The association between head injuries and psychiatric disorders: findings from the New Haven NIMH Epidemiologic Catchment Area study. Brain Inj 15:935–945, 2001

Snell DL, Surgenor LJ, Hay-Smith EJ, et al: A systematic review of psychological treatments for mild traumatic brain injury: an update on the evidence. J Clin Exp Neuropsychol 31:20–38, 2009

Starkstein SE, Lischinsky A: The phenomenology of depression after brain injury. NeuroRehabilitation 17:105–113, 2002

Tateno A, Jorge RE, Robinson RG: Pathological laughing and crying following traumatic brain injury. J Neuropsychiatry Clin Neurosci 16:426–434, 2004

van Reekum R, Cohen T, Wong J: Can traumatic brain injury cause psychiatric disorders? J Neuropsychiatry Clin Neurosci 12:316–327, 2000

Warden DL, Gordon B, McAllister TW, et al: Guidelines for the pharmacologic treatment of neurobehavioral sequelae of traumatic brain injury. J Neurotrauma 23:1468–1501, 2006

Whelan-Goodinson R, Ponsford J, Johnston L, et al: Psychiatric disorders following traumatic brain injury: their nature and frequency. J Head Trauma Rehabil 24:324–332, 2009

Whelan-Goodinson R, Ponsford JL, Schonberger M, et al: Predictors of psychiatric disorders following traumatic brain injury. J Head Trauma Rehabil 25:320–329, 2010

Wortzel HS, Oster TJ, Anderson CA, et al: Pathological laughing and crying: epidemiology, pathophysiology and treatment. CNS Drugs 22:531–545, 2008

Young RC, Biggs JT, Ziegler VE, et al: A rating scale for mania: reliability, validity and sensitivity. Br J Psychiatry 133:429–435, 1978

Zeilig G, Drubach DA, Katz-Zeilig M, et al: Pathological laughter and crying in patients with closed traumatic brain injury. Brain Inj 10:591–597, 1996

CHAPTER 7

# Anxiety Disorders

*Jesse R. Fann, M.D., M.P.H.*
*Matthew Jakupcak, Ph.D.*

**The spectrum** of traumatic brain injury (TBI) severity, from mild to severe, is associated with an increased risk for anxiety symptoms. Anxiety problems can occur at any time after injury and vary from subtle changes in mood and behavior to severe panic and agoraphobia, significant agitation, or profound avoidance. Although rigorous, prospective epidemiological studies of anxiety after TBI are lacking, anxiety is often most profound shortly following injury, when the patient is dealing with acute postconcussive symptoms, adjustment to physical injury and neurocognitive deficits, and grief. Anxiety may also be temporarily increased due to the withdrawal or tapering of medications, such as sedatives or opioids, used in the acute post-TBI period. Moreover, a history of psychiatric conditions such as anxiety is more common in persons with TBI than in those without TBI, suggesting that anxiety and anxiolytics may be risk factors for sustaining a TBI (Fann et al. 2002). In addition to well-defined syndromes, symptoms such as fatigue, insomnia, perseveration, or apathy can occur in combination with anxiety. Therefore, the development of anxiety symptoms following TBI can be due to a combination of biological factors resulting from disruption of neurotransmitter and neuroendocrine systems caused by the TBI; psychological factors associated with a traumatic injury; and behavioral, interpersonal, and social consequences of the TBI.

The somatic symptoms of anxiety disorders can be difficult to differentiate from postconcussive symptoms, such as headache, nausea, dizziness, and paresthesias. Also, the cognitive sequelae of TBI, such as decreased attention and concentration, can be exacerbated by the presence of comorbid anxiety. The picture can be further complicated by comorbid substance use, which can be an attempt to self-treat anxiety symptoms.

Severe anxiety rarely requires psychiatric hospitalization. More commonly, anxiety problems are identified in the context of other complaints, such as cognitive problems, somatic complaints, depression, impulsivity, social withdrawal, and agitation (Draper and Ponsford 2009). Often first noted by caregivers or acquaintances, anxiety symptoms can interfere with rehabilitation and are a common cause of caregiver burden. Symptoms that are commonly comorbid with anxiety, such as agitation, anger, and aggression, can cause the family considerable distress and can remain a chronic problem. Additionally, personality changes after TBI can be characterized predominantly by apprehension, aggression, disinhibition, or lability (Kim 2002), although a wide array of personality changes, including amplification of premorbid traits, may occur (Hibbard et al. 2000).

Anxiety levels can also increase at other critical junctures, such as at hospital discharge, follow-up assessments, vocational reentry, and injury anniversaries. Even in the absence of overt posttraumatic stress disorder (PTSD), reminders of the injury or other cues, such as those that increase feelings of grief or guilt, can exacerbate anxiety symptoms. Anxiety levels may decline over time as adaptation occurs through the course of recovery. Brief and less impairing distress during care onset and critical points during follow-up may suggest a disorder of adjustment (adjustment disorder, with depression, anxiety, or both).

Diagnostically, more severe and ongoing anxiety may present in the form of persistent worry, fatigue, muscle tension, restlessness, and impaired sleep over time, suggesting a generalized anxiety disorder. Such a picture may develop insidiously and may be fueled by persisting physical and cognitive deficits (e.g., in multitasking) that make performing usual roles more difficult and frustrating. In contrast, very rapid-onset increases in anxiety with marked autonomic response, including agitation, heart palpitations, sweating, gastric upset, or shortness of breath, may indicate panic attacks or, if recurrent, panic disorder. Obsessions may be difficult to differentiate from perseverative thoughts, which are common following TBI. Both may be associated with repetitive behaviors, but the latter are usually associated with more profound feelings of anxiety and worry. Persisting anxiety that impairs function and impedes medical treatment indicates a need for intervention.

# EPIDEMIOLOGY

The prevalence of depression and PTSD has most often been the focus of research into the psychiatric sequelae of TBI. However, other anxiety disorders are also common, including generalized anxiety disorder (GAD), panic with or without agoraphobia, social and simple phobias, and obsessive-compulsive disorder (OCD). These disorders may be comorbid with PTSD and depression or they may develop as stand-alone psychiatric disorders. In a study by Jorge et al. (2004), 23 of 30 patients (76.7%) with major depression also met criteria for comorbid anxiety disorder, compared with 9 of 44 patients (20.4%) without a mood disorder. Bombardier et al. (2010) reported that patients with TBI were nine times more likely to have a panic or other anxiety disorder if they were depressed than were those who were not depressed. Bryant et al. (2010) found that 91% of patients with PTSD experienced a comorbid psychiatric disorder, whereas non-PTSD anxiety disorders occurred in the absence of PTSD or depression in 23.3% of severely injured patients.

The reported prevalence of specific anxiety disorders in patients with TBI varies considerably across research studies, likely due to differences in sample characteristics (e.g., clinical setting, TBI severity, sample size, time since injury) and assessment procedures (e.g., retrospective vs. prospective assessments). Table 7–1 reports observed rates of specific anxiety disorders across various studies (Bryant et al. 2010; Deb et al. 1999; Fann et al. 1995; Hibbard et al. 1998; Whelan-Goodinson et al. 2010). Preexisting psychiatric conditions may inform the risk for developing anxiety disorders following TBI (Ashman et al. 2004; Deb et al. 1999). Among patients with TBI, women may be more likely than men to develop an anxiety disorder (Ashman et al. 2004), and patients who are younger and have lower levels of education may be at increased risk for anxiety following injury (Deb et al. 1999). Although preexisting psychiatric symptoms may increase risk for anxiety disorders following TBI, a significant number of persons without a history of psychiatric disorders will experience new-onset anxiety within the months or years following TBI.

**TABLE 7–1.**  Observed prevalence of specific anxiety disorders following traumatic brain injury across studies

| | | | ANXIETY DISORDERS | | | | | |
| STUDY | SAMPLE SIZE | MEAN TIME POST-TBI | GAD | PTSD | OCD | PANIC | PHOBIAS |
| --- | --- | --- | --- | --- | --- | --- | --- |
| Fann et al. (1995) | 50 | 2.7 years | 24% | NA | NA | 4% | 2% |
| Hibbard et al. (1998) | 100 | 7.6 years | 8% | 17% | 14% | 11% | 7% |
| Deb et al. (1999) | 100 | 1 year | 3% | 3% | 2% | 9% | 1% |
| Bryant et al. (2010) | 817 | 1 year | 13.4% | 13% | 4% | 7.5% | 9%–12.8% |
| Whelan-Goodinson et al. (2010) | 100 | 0.5–5.5 years | 17% | 14% | 1% | 6% | 1%–7% |

*Note.*   GAD=general anxiety disorder; NA=not assessed; OCD=obsessive-compulsive disorder; PTSD=posttraumatic stress disorder; TBI=traumatic brain injury.

The Bryant et al. (2010) study results provide a clearer estimate of the prevalence of specific anxiety disorders and the incidence of new-onset anxiety disorders in persons with mild TBI. Investigators examined prevalence rates of mood and anxiety disorders measured prospectively in a sample of 817 civilian patients hospitalized for traumatic injury, 40% of whom had experienced a mild TBI. At 1 year postinjury, 22% of patients had a new-onset psychiatric disorder, with higher rates observed in patients who had sustained a mild TBI (24.8%) relative to patients without TBI (20.5%). Compared to patients without TBI, patients with mild TBI were more likely to develop PTSD, agoraphobia and panic, or social phobia in the year following injury. At 1-year postinjury, the percentages with new-onset anxiety disorders were as follows: GAD 10%, PTSD 7.8%, agoraphobia 7.2%, social phobia 4.9%, panic 3.7%, and OCD 1.8%. The overall 1-year prevalence rates for each anxiety disorder were higher among persons with preinjury psychiatric disorders, although their relative frequencies were similar to those among persons with new-onset post-TBI anxiety disorders (see Table 7–1). The results reported by Bryant et al. (2010) and in several other studies suggest that non-PTSD anxiety disorders such as GAD are nearly as common as or more common than PTSD in patients with mild TBI. In this study, anxiety disorders also occurred in the absence of PTSD or depression.

Rates of PTSD and non-PTSD anxiety disorders vary according to specific populations. Among Iraq and Afghanistan War Veterans who screen positive for TBI, PTSD is more common (64%) than depression (43.6%) or non-PTSD anxiety disorders (35.6%) (Carlson et al. 2010). The predominance of PTSD in these Veterans is not surprising given the context of deployment and the nature of events (e.g., blasts from explosive devices) that typically cause concussions during combat. However, the rates of PTSD and non-PTSD anxiety disorders observed in these populations are not appropriately extrapolated to civilian populations.

# CLINICAL ASSESSMENT

Knowledge of a patient's specific physical and cognitive impairments is required to design an appropriate and effective treatment plan for anxiety disorders after TBI. A detailed understanding of the patient's physical and psychological stage in rehabilitation and functional goals aids in choosing the most appropriate psychopharmacological or psychotherapeutic treatment modality. Knowledge of the patient's current functional, social, and vocational status is required to tailor the psychiatric treatment to specific practical needs and limitations. For example, initial treatment with a potentially sedating medication in a fatigued, cognitively impaired, anxious patient with TBI who is not participating optimally in physical therapy may not be appropriate.

Once the clinician has developed rapport with a patient, it is helpful to discuss the events that led up to the patient's impairment (e.g., the circumstances of the car crash that led to the TBI) to explore the psychodynamic significance of these events. Such an understanding provides valuable context when exploring goals and potential roadblocks during the course of treatment.

Interviewing the patient's family, friends, and caregivers can provide critical information about the patient's past and present mental state. Patients may report different symptoms from those observed by people close to them. Close communication with family and other caregivers and acquaintances can provide critical longitudinal information about the progress of psychiatric treatment.

The phenomenological presentation of psychiatric symptoms in patients with brain injury may differ from symptoms that arise de novo or in other medical settings. Although psychopathology based on the DSM-IV-TR criteria (American Psychiatric Association 2000) should be thoroughly explored, psychiatric symptoms that do not meet these criteria but still lead to significant functional impairment are common in the rehabilitation setting. These syndromes, or symptom clusters, still may warrant close monitoring and treatment to maximize functioning. Therefore, in addition to monitoring and documenting psychiatric signs and symptoms, clinicians should closely monitor functional status (e.g., activities of daily living, progress in physical and occupational therapy, role functioning) as an indicator of overall progress.

Anxiety intervention should begin with defining treatment end points according to measurable outcomes. Examples of useful measures for anxiety include the Brief Symptom Inventory Anxiety subscale (Meachen et al. 2008) and the GAD-7 (Spitzer et al. 2006), although the latter has not yet been validated in TBI populations. Improved participation in rehabilitation therapies, which may be the outcome of most concern to the referring physician, can be monitored easily with the Pittsburgh Rehabilitation Participation Scale (Lenze et al. 2004).

Realistic expectations, including the possibility of incomplete remission of symptoms, must be conveyed at the outset so that the patient, who is already frustrated with the often slow and arduous rehabilitation process, does not become even more hopeless or overwhelmed if some symptoms persist. Because patients may have strong preexisting beliefs and preferences for specific treatment approaches, adequate time must be spent on providing education about the natural course of recovery, potentially disabling consequences, and available evidence-based treatment approaches for anxiety. Collaboration with rehabilitation psychologists and counselors can provide significant depth of assessment and breadth of intervention. Often, appropriately applied treatments may not have been given ample time to work. This problem may be exacerbated by imposed pressures on rehabilitation centers to work within predetermined payment structures and lengths of stay on the basis of medical diagnoses (Carter et al. 2000).

# TREATMENT

## Overview and General Principles

Despite the high prevalence of anxiety after TBI, the evidence for the treatment of post-TBI anxiety disorders is limited. However, there are some principles for the treatment of TBI neuropsychiatric symptoms that are based on the limited evidence-based and expert opinion. We suggest that both pharmacological and nonpharmacological approaches are often required to optimally treat anxiety disorder among persons with TBI.

## Nonpharmacological Interventions

Nonpharmacological treatments are often well received by patients and their families, partly because they return some semblance of control back to the patient. Practices such as exercise and meditation are often attractive because they empower the patient and reinforce his or her sense of self-efficacy. Psychotherapy for the patient and family should be encouraged. One goal of therapy is to treat loss of self-esteem or overt anxiety and depression associated with loss of cognitive functioning. Specific goals include providing a realistic new baseline for the patient, as well as providing emotional support and education for both the patient and his or her family. Cognitive and behavioral approaches, such as those that address avoidance behaviors, can be very helpful in this patient population. Behavioral approaches taught to the family may be more helpful for the more severely injured patients. In patients with the necessary cognitive skills, approaches such as cognitive restructuring and teaching new skills are beneficial. Mindfulness training, in particular, has been popular and may be helpful for some patients. The learning of such skills can allow the patient to actually experience personal growth after the emotional trauma of brain injury, and is often appreciated.

Behavioral interventions for moderate to severe TBI typically include behavior modification and cognitive-behavioral therapy (CBT) delivered as components of comprehensive, multidisciplinary rehabilitation treatment. Behavior modification applies principles of reinforcement and shaping (e.g., token economies or extinction procedures) to reduce behavioral and emotional disturbances, and CBT is used for education and skills training to promote patients' awareness of deficits and to increase positive coping following injury (Cattelani et al. 2010). Although anxiety symptoms are often present in patients undergoing rehabilitation for TBI, few studies to date have examined the efficacy of behavioral therapies for treating specific anxiety disorders that are comorbid with TBI.

In general, strong evidence supports the efficacy of CBT for treating GAD, panic and agoraphobia, social phobia, and OCD (Arch and Craske 2009). CBT for anxiety disorders typically introduces the patient to 1) education regarding the anxiety disorder, 2) cognitive restructuring techniques used to challenge maladaptive beliefs, and 3) exposure exercises used to promote mastery and habituation to anxiety cues. The emphasis on education and skill building in CBT is congruent with global rehabilitation goals, although most of the support for CBT to treat anxiety in TBI relies on case reports (Hiott and Labbate 2002; Soo and Tate 2007). Preliminary clinical trials of individual and group CBT suggest that CBT may increase awareness of skill deficits and improve coping in persons with TBI and anxiety, although anxiety symptoms may not fully resolve during brief courses of therapy (Hodgson et al. 2005). Thus, CBT may need to be adapted for persons with TBI (e.g., shorter sessions and longer treatment course, use of complementary written materials, involvement of a support person) or augmented by alternative therapies.

Mindfulness or meditation training is an alternative treatment that is beneficial for a number of physical and mental health disorders

(Grossman et al. 2004). Meditation has been shown to improve cognitive functioning (Zeidan et al. 2010), and preliminary evidence suggests that mindfulness meditation may improve quality of life in persons with TBI (Bedard et al. 2003). Furthermore, several studies have found that mindfulness- and acceptance-based behavioral therapies are efficacious treatments for anxiety disorders (Evans et al. 2008; Miller et al. 1995; Roemer et al. 2008). The development of cognitive therapy followed early forms of behavioral therapy, and acceptance-based behavioral therapies are sometimes referred to as a "third wave" form of CBT. Acceptance-based behavioral therapies differ from traditional CBT approaches in that they do not directly seek to challenge or restructure patients' thoughts but rather they encourage patients to practice nonjudgmental, nondirective awareness of their thoughts and somatic sensations to circumvent fear-related avoidant behaviors.

Biofeedback is an alternative treatment that provides physiological monitoring and feedback to patients while they practice relaxation and concentration exercises. Biofeedback applies operant learning principles to promote and reinforce patients' normative brain and autonomic functioning. Biofeedback has been associated with improvements in memory recall in patients with TBI (Thornton and Carmody 2008) and decreased headache frequency in people with recurring headaches (Nestoriuc et al. 2008). Preliminary evidence suggests that biofeedback may also be beneficial for treating anxiety disorders such as GAD (Rice et al. 1993), specific phobias (Telch et al. 2000), and panic (Meuret et al. 2004). Preliminary studies of biofeedback with electroencephalographic recording and photic feedback (Schoenberger et al. 2001) and with music therapy (Guétin et al. 2009) for improving mood after TBI have been reported, but further study is required.

Acupuncture is an alternative form of medicine that stimulates specific points on the body through the introduction of small needles into the skin and muscle tissues. Traditional Chinese medicine applies acupuncture needles with the understanding that stimulating specific body points can redirect the body's energy pathways, whereas contemporary or medical forms of acupuncture pinpoint nerve bundles or motor points specifically associated with injury (Pilkington 2010). Although limited research is available on the benefits of acupuncture for TBI, acupuncture may be beneficial for treating chronic pain associated with traumatic injury (Nayak et al. 2001) and may decrease pain levels in individuals with recurring headaches (Sun and Gan 2008). Some evidence suggests that acupuncture is beneficial for short-term anxiety states, although additional research is required to determine whether acupuncture benefits individuals with chronic anxiety disorders (Pilkington 2010). In a case report involving classical Chinese acupuncture, a patient with severe TBI, multiple injuries, and severe pain reported subjective but not objective improvement on the Hospital Anxiety and Depression Scale (Donnellan 2006).

## Pharmacotherapy

Medications, when used in the treatment of patients with mild TBI or their family members, are most usefully regarded as adjuncts to other interventions, including all of the nonpharmacological interventions described in the preceding section of this chapter. For patients with TBI, medications can help reduce the reluctance or inability to begin the recovery process. In a sense, medications "grease the wheel" and allow the patient to begin moving through the recovery process more easily.

For persons with relatively more severe TBI, medications may be the primary treatment. The basic principle of "start low, go slow, but go" is especially relevant for the treatment of anxiety, due to the potentially sedating nature of many anxiolytics. Clinicians also need to continually reassess each patient's clinical condition (preferably using instruments that have been validated in patients with TBI), monitor drug-drug interactions, and augment partial treatment responses.

Because few randomized placebo-controlled studies have evaluated pharmacotherapies for anxiety disorders among persons with TBI, many of the following recommendations are based on case series and expert consensus (Warden et al. 2006) or are extrapolated from other neurological populations. Heterogeneous study populations, including those varying in time elapsed since injury, confound the interpretation of study results.

When TBI occurs in the context of preexisting anxiety problems, continuing a previously effective medication regimen is logical. However, the occurrence of TBI may facilitate the emergence of side effects that were not previously experienced. In many cases, these side effects can be managed successfully by reducing the dose of the medication used. When this does not afford relief from adverse side effects, a change in pharmacotherapy may be required.

Selective serotonin reuptake inhibitors (SSRIs), in general, as well as tricyclic antidepressants, may improve anxiety among persons with TBI. Antidepressants appear to be particularly useful for anxiety that co-occurs with depression (Ashman et al. 2009). For example, in an 8-week placebo run-in study of sertraline 25–150 mg/day for major depression in patients within 2 years of mild TBI, patients had a significant reduction in anxiety on the Symptom Checklist–90 (SCL-90) (Fann et al. 2000). However, in a case series of fluoxetine treatment for major depressive disorder with melancholia after moderate to severe TBI, three of eight patients complained of anxiety (Cassidy 1989). Because the initial activating effects of serotonergic agents may be particularly problematic for anxious individuals, and may then lead to nonadherence or early discontinuation, these medications should be started at 50% or 25% of the usual starting dosage. As in treating depression, the higher range of dosages may need to be reached to eventually achieve maximum therapeutic effect. Potential side effects that may be more pronounced after TBI, such as sedation, apathy, agitation, and sexual dysfunction, should be monitored closely. Antidepressants also may be useful for the management of obsessive-compulsive symptoms after TBI, as they are for primary OCD. In a case report, venlafaxine 150 mg/day successfully treated new-onset compulsions after TBI, with a Yale-Brown Obsessive Compulsive Scale (Y-BOCS) score decreasing from 35 to 3 over 10 weeks and remaining stable over 4 months (Khouzam and Donnelly 1998).

Valproic acid, gabapentin, and pregabalin may be of benefit for anxiety, especially in patients with concomitant mood lability or seizures (Pande et al. 2000). Buspirone is another option for generalized anxiety symptoms; however, it has been associated, albeit rarely, with seizures and movement disorders (LeWitt et al. 1993). These agents may also be helpful for patients with anger and aggression. Due to potential neurotoxic side effects, slow titration is indicated.

There is good evidence for the use of β-blockers for agitation and aggression after TBI (Fleminger et al. 2006), but β-blockers have also been used for anticipatory anxiety in non-TBI populations. Caution should be exercised when using β-blockers in patients with ongoing dizziness or light-headedness. Bradycardia and hypotension are potential side effects; contraindications include asthma, chronic obstructive pulmonary disease, type 1 diabetes mellitus, congestive heart failure, persistent angina, significant peripheral vascular disease, and hyperthyroidism. Pindolol is less likely to cause bradycardia.

Antipsychotics should not be used as first-line treatments for anxiety after TBI and should be reserved for patients with psychotic symptoms. Among the newer-generation antipsychotics, which have fewer extrapyramidal side effects than typical neuroleptics, quetiapine and olanzapine may be the most useful for sleep and anxiety. Sedation, weight gain, and QTc prolongation should be monitored closely.

Benzodiazepines and/or sedative-hypnotics are occasionally necessary for short-term treatment for acute anxiety, particularly in the first few weeks after injury and when insomnia is prominent and functionally impairing. Benzodiazepines (e.g., lorazepam, clonazepam, alprazolam) should be used initially at lower dosages because of their propensity to exacerbate or cause cognitive impairment and sedation (Table 7–2). However, benzodiazepines are not recommended for long-term use because patients with TBI may be more susceptible to their potential adverse reactions and because benzodiazepines may actually cause a paradoxical agitation in these patients (Lee et al. 2003). The high prevalence of substance abuse in patients with TBI also adds to the risk of treatment complications during long-term benzodiazepine use; among patients with alcohol, sedative-hypnotic, or other pre-TBI or post-TBI substance use disorders, it is prudent to avoid prescribing benzodiazepines for the treatment of post-TBI anxiety disorders. If a benzodiazepine is required, using a scheduled (rather than as-needed) dose of a short-acting agent (e.g., lorazepam) is encouraged. If an as-needed approach is used initially, then dosing should be promptly transitioned to a regular schedule as soon as the effective daily total dose is determined. Enlisting the assistance of a family member or caregiver, if available, may reduce the risk of benzodiazepine overuse and improve monitoring for medication-induced side effects or paradoxical disinhibition or agitation.

# CONCLUSION

Anxiety disorders are common problems among persons with TBI. When these problems occur, they may interfere with cognition, exacerbate other neuropsychiatric disturbances, and compromise everyday function. Behavioral modification and CBT are common components of comprehensive rehabilitation interventions for persons with TBI. Strong evidence supports the use of CBT for treating specific anxiety disorders, although fewer studies have examined the efficacy of CBT for anxiety in persons with TBI. Adaptations for individuals with cog-

**TABLE 7–2.** Pharmacological agents commonly used for combined anxiety and insomnia after traumatic brain injury

| MEDICATION | SUGGESTED DOSAGE RANGE | COMMON SIDE EFFECTS/ CAUTIONS |
|---|---|---|
| **Anxiolytics for anxiety (short-term, 2–12 weeks)** | | |
| Lorazepam | 0.5–6 mg divided daily | Sedation, confusion, orthostasis, tolerance/abuse, respiratory depression |
| Clonazepam | 0.5–4 mg divided daily | Sedation, confusion, orthostasis, tolerance/abuse, respiratory depression |
| Alprazolam | 0.25–3 mg divided daily | Sedation, confusion, orthostasis, tolerance/abuse, respiratory depression |
| **Sedative-hypnotics for anxiety-related insomnia** | | |
| Zolpidem | 2.5–10 mg at bedtime | Sedation, mild confusion risk |
| Zaleplon | 2.5–10 mg at bedtime | Sedation, mild confusion risk |
| Eszopiclone | 0.5–3 mg at bedtime | Sedation, mild confusion risk |
| Ramelteon | 4–12 mg at bedtime | Nausea, gastrointestinal upset |
| Trazodone | 12.5–150 mg at bedtime | Sedation, orthostasis, dry mouth, priapism (uncommon) |
| Temazepam | 7.5–30 mg hs | Sedation, confusion risk |

nitive impairments are likely helpful but require further study. In patients with nonresponsive or persistent anxiety symptoms, alternative approaches such as mindfulness meditation and acceptance-based behavioral strategies, biofeedback, or acupuncture may be beneficial. Medications may serve as useful adjuncts to nonpharmacological interventions, particularly among persons with relatively more severe TBI and/or those who are unable to engage effectively in psychotherapies. Antidepressants are the most commonly used agents for post-TBI anxiety, but the range of pharmacotherapies that may be useful is broad. In general, the use of benzodiazepines is discouraged, especially among persons requiring long-term pharmacotherapies for anxiety and those with comorbid substance use disorders.

## *Key Clinical Points*

- Non-PTSD anxiety disorders such as generalized anxiety disorder, panic, obsessive-compulsive disorder, and social phobia are more common in patients following TBI than in the general population.

- Depression and substance abuse commonly co-occur with anxiety after TBI.

- Nonpharmacological treatments that incorporate both behavioral and cognitive components hold promise for patients with TBI and anxiety, particularly if these treatments address avoidance behaviors.

- Selective serotonin reuptake inhibitors appear to be effective for longer-term treatment of anxiety following TBI.

- Benzodiazepines can be used for short-term anxiolysis, but their use entails significant risks of sedation, cognitive dysfunction, possible disinhibition, and the development of benzodiazepine abuse and/or dependence.

# REFERENCES

American Psychiatric Association: Diagnostic and Statistical Manual of Mental Disorders, 4th Edition, Text Revision. Washington, DC, American Psychiatric Association, 2000

Arch JJ, Craske MG: First-line treatment: a critical appraisal of cognitive behavioral therapy developments and alternatives. Psychiatr Clin North Am 32:525–547, 2009

Ashman TA, Spielman LA, Hibbard MR, et al: Psychiatric challenges in the first 6 years after traumatic brain injury: cross-sequential analyses of Axis I disorders. Arch Phys Med Rehabil 85(suppl):S36–S42, 2004

Ashman TA, Cantor JB, Gordon WA, et al: A randomized controlled trial of sertraline for the treatment of depression in persons with traumatic brain injury. Arch Phys Med Rehabil 90:733–740, 2009

Bedard M, Felteau M, Mazmanian D, et al: Pilot evaluation of a mindfulness-based intervention to improve quality of life among individuals who sustained traumatic brain injuries. Disabil Rehabil 25:722–731, 2003

Bombardier CH, Fann JR, Temkin NR, et al: Rates of major depressive disorder and clinical outcomes following traumatic brain injury. JAMA 303:1938–1945, 2010

Bryant RA, O'Donnell ML, Creamer M, et al: The psychiatric sequelae of traumatic injury. Am J Psychiatry 167:312–320, 2010

Carlson KF, Nelson D, Orazem RJ, et al: Psychiatric diagnoses among Iraq and Afghanistan war veterans screened for deployment-related traumatic brain injury. J Trauma Stress 23:17–24, 2010

Carter GM, Relles DA, Wynn BO, et al: Interim Report on an Inpatient Rehabilitation Facility Prospective Payment System. Santa Monica, CA, RAND, 2000

Cassidy JW: Fluoxetine: a new serotonergically active antidepressant. J Head Trauma Rehabil 4(2):67–69, 1989

Cattelani R, Zettin M, Zoccolotti P: Rehabilitation treatments for adults with behavioral and psychosocial disorders following acquired brain injury: a systematic review. Neuropsychol Rev 20:52–85, 2010

Deb S, Lyons I, Koutzoukis C, et al: Rate of psychiatric illness 1 year after traumatic brain injury. Am J Psychiatry 156:374–378, 1999

Donnellan CP: Acupuncture for central pain affecting the ribcage following traumatic brain injury and rib fractures: a case report. Acupunct Med 24:129–133, 2006

Draper K, Ponsford J: Long-term outcome following traumatic brain injury: a comparison of subjective reports by those injured and their relatives. Neuropsychol Rehabil 19:645–661, 2009

Evans S, Ferrando S, Findler M, et al: Mindfulness-based cognitive therapy for generalized anxiety disorder. J Anxiety Disord 22:716–721, 2008

Fann JR, Katon WJ, Uomoto JM, et al: Psychiatric disorders and functional disability in outpatients with traumatic brain injuries. Am J Psychiatry 152:1493–1499, 1995

Fann JR, Uomoto JM, Katon WJ: Sertraline in the treatment of major depression following mild traumatic brain injury. J Neuropsychiatry Clin Neurosci 12:226–232, 2000

Fann JR, Leonetti A, Jaffe K, et al: Psychiatric illness and subsequent traumatic brain injury: a case control study. J Neurol Neurosurg Psychiatry 72:615–620, 2002

Fleminger S, Greenwood RRJ, Oliver DL: Pharmacological management for agitation and aggression in people with acquired brain injury. Cochrane Database Syst Rev (4):CD003299, 2006

Grossman P, Niemann L, Schmidt S, et al: Mindfulness-based stress reduction and health benefits: a meta-analysis. J Psychosom Res 57:35–43, 2004

Guétin S, Soua B, Voiriot G, et al: The effect of music therapy on mood and anxiety-depression: an observational study in institutionalised patients with traumatic brain injury. Ann Phys Rehabil Med 52:30–40, 2009

Hibbard MR, Uysal S, Kepler K, et al: Axis I psychopathology in individuals with traumatic brain injury. J Head Trauma Rehabil 13:24–39, 1998

Hibbard MR, Bogdany J, Uysal S, et al: Axis II psychopathology in individuals with traumatic brain injury. Brain Inj 14:45–61, 2000

Hiott DW, Labbate L: Anxiety disorders associated with traumatic brain injuries. NeuroRehabilitation 17:345–355, 2002

Hodgson J, McDonald S, Tate R, et al: A randomised controlled trial of a cognitive-behavioural therapy program for managing social anxiety after acquired brain injury. Brain Impair 6:169–180, 2005

Jorge RE, Robinson RG, Moser D, et al: Major depression following traumatic brain injury. Arch Gen Psychiatry 61:42–50, 2004

Khouzam HR, Donnelly NJ: Remission of traumatic brain injury–induced compulsions during venlafaxine treatment. Gen Hosp Psychiatry 20:62–63, 1998

Kim E: Agitation, aggression, and disinhibition syndromes after traumatic brain injury. NeuroRehabilitation 17:297–310, 2002

Lee HB, Lyketsos CG, Rao V: Pharmacological management of the psychiatric aspects of traumatic brain injury. Int Rev Psychiatry 15:359–370, 2003

Lenze EJ, Munin MC, Quear T, et al: The Pittsburgh Rehabilitation Participation Scale: reliability and validity of a clinician-rated measure of participation in acute rehabilitation. Arch Phys Med Rehabil 85:380–384, 2004

LeWitt PA, Walters A, Hening W, et al: Persistent movement disorders induced by buspirone. Mov Disord 8:331–334, 1993

Meachen SJ, Hanks RA, Millis SR, et al: The reliability and validity of the Brief Symptom Inventory–18 in persons with traumatic brain injury. Arch Phys Med Rehabil 89:958–965, 2008

Meuret AE, Wilhelm FH, Roth WT: Respiratory feedback for treating panic disorder. J Clin Psychol 60:197–207, 2004

Miller JJ, Fletcher K, Kabat-Zinn J: Three-year follow-up and clinical implications of a mindfulness meditation-based stress reduction intervention in the treatment of anxiety disorders. Gen Hosp Psychiatry 17:192–200, 1995

Nayak S, Shiflett SC, Schoenberger NE, et al: Is acupuncture effective in treating chronic pain after spinal cord injury? Arch Phys Med Rehabil 82:1578–1586, 2001

Nestoriuc Y, Martin A, Rief W, et al: Biofeedback treatment for headache disorders: a comprehensive efficacy review. Appl Psychophysiol Biofeedback 33:125–140, 2008

Pande AC, Pollack MH, Crockatt J, et al: Placebo-controlled study of gabapentin treatment of panic disorder. J Clin Psychopharmacol 20:467–471, 2000

Pilkington K: Anxiety, depression and acupuncture: a review of the clinical research. Auton Neurosci 157:91–95, 2010

Rice KM, Blanchard EB, Purcell M: Biofeedback treatments of generalized anxiety disorder: preliminary results. Biofeedback Self Regul 18:93–105, 1993

Roemer L, Orsillo SM, Salters-Pedneault K: Efficacy of an acceptance-based behavior therapy for generalized anxiety disorder: evaluation in a randomized controlled trial. J Consult Clin Psychol 76:1083–1089, 2008

Schoenberger NE, Shif SC, Esty ML, et al: Flexyx Neurotherapy System in the treatment of traumatic brain injury: an initial evaluation. J Head Trauma Rehabil 16:260–274, 2001

Soo C, Tate RL: Psychological treatment for anxiety in people with traumatic brain injury. Cochrane Database Syst Rev (3):CD005239, 2007

Spitzer RL, Kroenke K, Williams JB, et al: A brief measure for assessing generalized anxiety disorder: the GAD-7. Arch Intern Med 166:1092–1097, 2006

Sun Y, Gan TJ: Acupuncture for the management of chronic headache: a systematic review. Anesth Analg 107:2038–2047, 2008

Telch MJ, Valentiner DP, Ilai D, et al: The facilitative effects of heart-rate feedback in the emotional processing of claustrophobic fear. Behav Res Ther 38:373–387, 2000

Thornton KE, Carmody DP: Efficacy of traumatic brain injury rehabilitation: interventions of QEEG-guided biofeedback, computers, strategies, and medications. Appl Psychophysiol Biofeedback 33:101–124, 2008

Warden DL, Gordon B, McAllister TW, et al: Guidelines for the pharmacologic treatment of neurobehavioral sequelae of traumatic brain injury. J Neurotrauma 23:1468–1501, 2006

Whelan-Goodinson R, Ponsford JL, Schonberger M, et al: Predictors of psychiatric disorders following traumatic brain injury. J Head Trauma Rehabil 25:320–329, 2010

Zeidan F, Johnson SK, Diamond BJ, et al: Mindfulness meditation improves cognition: evidence of brief mental training. Conscious Cogn 19:597–605, 2010

# CHAPTER 8

# Posttraumatic Stress Disorder

*Jan E. Kennedy, Ph.D.*
*Michael S. Jaffee, M.D.*
*Douglas B. Cooper, Ph.D.*

**We discuss** briefly in this chapter the definition, epidemiology, and clinical assessment of posttraumatic stress disorder (PTSD), as well as overlapping neurochemical and neuroanatomical changes associated with PTSD and traumatic brain injury (TBI). We also summarize the major treatments for PTSD, including pharmacological, psychological, and other treatments. Each section, where relevant, incorporates the unique characteristics of PTSD in the context of TBI, including mild TBI (mTBI).

## DEFINITIONS

Acute emotional responses following exposure to trauma are common, expected, and temporary. In contrast, PTSD represents a continuation and magnification of anxiety-related symptoms. According to DSM-IV-TR criteria (American Psychiatric Association 2000), three characteristic symptom clusters—reexperiencing, avoidance, and hyperarousal—must be present for at least 1 month and cause impairments in functioning to meet diagnostic criteria for PTSD (Table 8–1). The reexperiencing symptoms of PTSD, such as nightmares, flashbacks, and

214 Management of Adults With Traumatic Brain Injury

**TABLE 8–1.** Diagnostic criteria for posttraumatic stress disorder according to DSM-IV-TR

| CRITERION | SYMPTOMS |
|---|---|
| A. Experienced, witnessed, or was confronted with event(s) involving actual or threatened death, serious injury, or compromised physical integrity of self or others | Intense fear<br>Helplessness<br>Horror |
| B. Reexperiencing of traumatic event | Recurrent or intrusive memories<br>Recurrent distressing dreams<br>Sense of reliving the trauma<br>Psychological or physiological distress when reminded of the trauma |
| C. Avoidance | Efforts to avoid trauma-associated thoughts, feelings, or conversations<br>Efforts to avoid activities, places, or people that revive memories of trauma<br>Inability to recall parts of the trauma<br>Withdrawal from activities or people<br>Emotional numbing |
| D. Increased autonomic arousal | Sleep disturbance<br>Irritability<br>Difficulty concentrating<br>Hypervigilance<br>Exaggerated startle response |

*Note.* Adapted from American Psychiatric Association: *Diagnostic and Statistical Manual of Mental Disorders,* 4th Edition, Text Revision. Washington, DC, American Psychiatric Association, 2000. Used with permission.

intrusive memories, are unique to this disorder, distinguishing it from other anxiety disorders. Avoidance symptoms and autonomic hyperarousal are common to both PTSD and other anxiety disorders.

The symptoms must cause marked impairment in social, occupational, or other important areas of function and persist for at least 1 month after the traumatic experience. If the duration of symptoms is less than 3 months, PTSD is considered acute; if symptoms last 3 months or more, PTSD is classified as chronic. Delayed onset of PTSD refers to the development of symptoms meeting criteria for this disorder 6 or more months after the traumatic event to which they are related; in some cases, delayed onset may occur years after traumatic exposure.

# CO-OCCURRENCE WITH TRAUMATIC BRAIN INJURY

Of the many emotional disorders commonly exhibited after TBI, PTSD is one of the most prevalent. The emotional trauma associated with high-speed motor vehicle collisions, assaults, falls, and military combat can be sufficient to meet Criterion A of the DSM-IV-TR diagnostic criteria for PTSD. This criterion requires not only that "the person experienced, witnessed, or was confronted with an event or events that involved actual or threatened death or serious injury, or a threat to the physical integrity of self or others," but also that the person's response to that event or events involved intense fear, helplessness, or horror (American Psychiatric Association 2000, p. 467).

Other symptoms of PTSD overlap with persistent postconcussive symptoms (Figure 8–1) (Stein and McAllister 2009). These include cognitive symptoms such as poor attention and memory, behavioral disturbances such as impulsivity and disinhibition, and emotional disorders such as depression and affective lability. Secondary effects of both disorders can include social isolation, interpersonal difficulties, and functional impairments in work and home environments.

Debate is ongoing in both clinical and academic circles about whether PTSD can develop in individuals who sustained TBIs with loss of consciousness (Rattok et al. 1996). One argument is that PTSD cannot develop in the context of an injury that produces dense amnesia for the traumatic event—for example, severe TBI involving posttraumatic amnesia (PTA) of days to weeks. Harvey et al. (2005), however, lay out a cogent argument for the coexistence of these conditions by systematically addressing each of the primary issues in this debate and providing a rationale for mitigating factors or resolutions for each issue. Briefly summarized, the authors argue that symptoms of PTSD are plausible given that persons with TBI often experience preserved "islands" of memory for peri-injury events. These islands of memory may be sufficiently traumatic to constitute the cardinal symp-

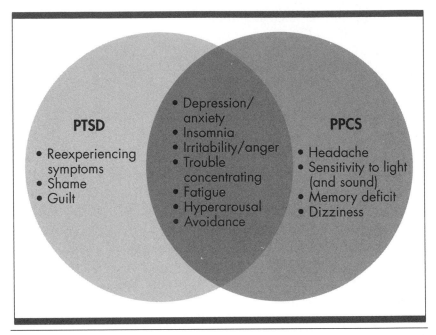

**FIGURE 8–1.**   Overlap between posttraumatic stress disorder (PTSD) and persistent postconcussive symptoms (PPCS).

*Source.*   Reprinted from Stein MB, McAllister TW: "Exploring the Convergence of Posttraumatic Stress Disorder and Mild Traumatic Brain Injury." *American Journal of Psychiatry* 166:768–776, 2009. © American Psychiatric Association. Used with permission.

toms of PTSD and serve as the focus for subsequent PTSD symptoms. They also argue that persons experiencing PTA have a tendency to fill in the gaps of peri-injury memory with information derived from secondary sources (e.g., pictures of accident scene, stories from accident observers). These "reconstructed" memories (i.e., personal narratives), the authors suggest, also can be psychologically traumatic and serve as the foundation for PTSD. These arguments suggest that PTSD and TBI are not mutually exclusive conditions.

# NEUROCHEMICAL AND NEUROANATOMICAL CONSIDERATIONS

The neurochemical and structural changes associated with TBI and PTSD overlap in some respects. This overlap provides a potential link between these conditions at a physiological level.

# Neurochemical Abnormalities

Alterations in the noradrenergic and serotonergic transmitter systems as well as the hypothalamic-pituitary-adrenal axis are common among individuals with PTSD (see Southwick et al. 2005 for review). Excessive neurotransmitter releases and dysfunction after TBI (sometimes described as a "neurotransmitter storm") include acute elevations of norepinephrine and serotonin, among other neurotransmitters. Chronic stress responses leading to endocrine changes contribute to both postconcussive and PTSD-type symptoms. Corticosteroids and corticotropin-releasing hormone (CRH) involved in stress responses decrease brain metabolism in prefrontal and temporal areas and impair metabolic neuronal response to physiological insult or structural injury. Chronic exposure to increased corticosteroids and CRH may result in reductions of dendritic arborization and, consequently, cognitive impairments, as well as reduced neurogenesis and neural recovery (Hoffman and Harrison 2009).

# Structural Changes

Several structural commonalities link TBI and PTSD (Hoffman and Harrison 2009; Stein and McAllister 2009). Symptoms of PTSD arise from alterations in the functioning of the frontal and anterior temporal areas of the brain and the regions and neuronal networks linking these areas. Prefrontal cortex hypoactivity and amygdala hyperactivity are the primary functional changes linked to PTSD. Similarly, the areas of greatest vulnerability to damage from TBI are the prefrontal cortex, the ventral portions of the frontal lobe, and the anterior temporal lobe due to the shearing forces of these brain areas against the skull.

The overlap between regional brain abnormalities associated with PTSD and TBI is illustrated in Figure 8–2 (Stein and McAllister 2009). This neuroanatomical overlap is particularly interesting as a potential explanation for the co-occurrence of TBI and PTSD among persons with blast-related injuries. Energy from blast explosions that is focused by the orbital sockets and nasal sinuses produces cortical damage in the orbitofrontal area. Destruction of the neuronal myelin, as seen on diffusion tensor imaging (DTI), impairs connections from this area to subcortical structures such as the amygdala that are involved in the pathogenesis of PTSD. Prefrontal damage leads to behavioral disinhibition, characteristic of TBI and PTSD; this damage is also associated with deficits in attention and working memory and

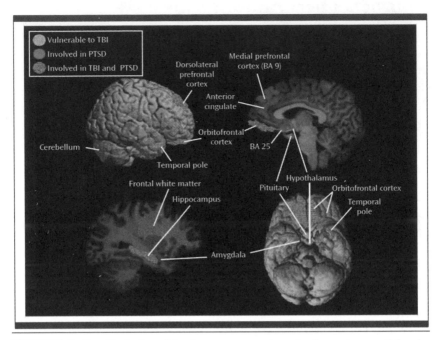

**FIGURE 8–2.** Relationship between regional alterations of brain structure associated with posttraumatic stress disorder (PTSD) and traumatic brain injury (TBI).

Several brain regions have been consistently implicated in PTSD, including the amygdala, the hippocampus, the orbitofrontal cortex, and the dorsolateral and dorsomedial prefrontal cortex. Several brain regions are vulnerable to the typical biomechanical forces associated with TBI, including the orbitofrontal cortex, the dorsolateral prefrontal cortex, the temporal pole, and the hippocampus. Overlap areas include the orbitofrontal cortex, the dorsolateral prefrontal cortex, and the hippocampus. In addition, tracts connecting the amygdala and the medial prefrontal cortex course through the subfrontal white matter and are thus vulnerable to disruption by TBI. BA=Brodmann area.

*See Plate 7 to view this figure in color.*

*Source.*   Reprinted from Stein MB, McAllister TW: "Exploring the Convergence of Posttraumatic Stress Disorder and Mild Traumatic Brain Injury." *American Journal of Psychiatry* 166:768–776, 2009. © American Psychiatric Association. Used with permission.

with decreased inhibition of the limbic areas, including the amygdala. The amygdala is involved in the processing of fear. As such, the autonomic hyperarousal symptoms of PTSD can be related to functional alterations in this area of the anterior temporal lobe.

Damage to the prefrontal cortex and cortical-subcortical tracks from TBI may contribute to the development and symptom severity of

PTSD. Conflicting evidence exists regarding whether persistent post-concussive symptoms contribute to the development of PTSD symptoms or whether PTSD symptoms cause postconcussive symptoms to persist. Efforts to differentiate TBI- and PTSD-related symptoms through neuroimaging or through neurological or neuropsychological assessment have been generally disappointing, due to the degree of overlap and nonspecificity of symptoms and the similarity in neurobiological substrates underlying these conditions (Brenner et al. 2009; Cooper et al. 2011).

Emerging research has been elucidating the pathophysiology and effects of blast-related TBI. Findings suggest a more diffuse injury pattern of the affected neural structures in blast injury, as well as associated brain inflammation and dysfunction of the extracellular matrix (Ling et al. 2009). Researchers are beginning to better understand potential long-term consequences of exposure to repetitive mTBIs. A chronic traumatic encephalopathy due to accumulation of tau proteins with associated cognitive dysfunction has been described (Cantu 2007; Casson et al. 2006; McCrory 2002; McKee et al. 2009; Omalu et al. 2006, 2011). This and other post-TBI dementing illnesses require further study as potential late complications that may affect the remission and/or treatment response of post-TBI PTSD.

# EPIDEMIOLOGY

## Posttraumatic Stress Disorder

PTSD was first defined as a mental disorder in DSM-III (American Psychiatric Association 1980) in response to the increased recognition of this condition among Vietnam War Veterans. In general, the severity of the psychological trauma relates in a direct fashion to the development of PTSD. This relationship is consistently found for sexual assault, combat exposure, natural disaster, and terrorist attack (Kessler et al. 1995). Mortality risk and acute stress reactions also mediate the development of later PTSD. The presence of traumatic and stressful experiences throughout life increases the incidence, severity, and chronicity of PTSD (Solomon and Mikulincer 2006). The prevalence of PTSD is higher in those populations at risk for repeated exposure to traumatic experiences, such as paramedics and first responders. Studies have shown that the incidence of PTSD among American firefighters is 22.2% and among Canadian firefighters is

17.3% (Corneil et al. 1999). In comparison, the estimated lifetime prevalence of PTSD is approximately 7%–9% among community samples in the United States (Kessler 2000; Yehuda 2004). The lifetime prevalence of PTSD is twice as high among females as among males (Breslau 2001). Although females are exposed to fewer traumatic events overall, they are at greater risk for rape and sexual assault trauma.

PTSD frequently runs a chronic course, with symptoms waxing and waning over many years (Solomon and Mikulincer 2006). Comorbid conditions are frequently present, including depression, other anxiety disorders, and substance use disorders (Brady et al. 2000). PTSD is often associated with physical health problems (Hidalgo and Davidson 2000; Hoge et al. 2007). Psychosocial support, however, may be an ameliorating factor in the subsequent expression of PTSD (Brailey et al. 2007).

## Posttraumatic Stress Disorder and Traumatic Brain Injury

Carlson et al. (2011) performed a systematic review of the incidence and prevalence studies of mTBI and PTSD in both civilian and military populations published between 1980 and 2009. This article is an excellent resource for additional information about the topic.

*Military and Veteran populations.* The process by which PTSD can develop following TBI is illustrated in the military context. Psychological stress inherent in the combat environment affects recovery from combat-related TBI (Vasterling et al. 2006). Both the circumstances at the specific time of the injury as well as general environmental factors in the deployed setting are potentially influential in the recovery process. This interaction is particularly pronounced following mTBI. Although PTSD can occur after TBI of any severity, complaints and distress are more frequent following mTBI. It has become increasingly apparent that the combination of post-deployment PTSD and a history of deployment-related mTBI is a common and important but poorly understood phenomenon associated with current military conflict.

A recent Veterans Affairs (VA) study reported that nearly half of 13,000 Veterans from Operation Iraqi Freedom (OIF)/Operation Enduring Freedom (OEF) who were screened for TBI had at least one psychiatric diagnosis (Carlson et al. 2010). PTSD and depression were the most common diagnoses in this group. Veterans who screened positive for TBI had significantly (three times) greater rates of PTSD than those who screened negative. Another study reported that service members who received an mTBI during deployment to OIF were more likely to meet PTSD criteria than OIF Veterans with other injuries (Hoge et al. 2008). The concurrent presence of TBI and other physical injuries and/or the overall level of severity of injuries may modulate this relationship.

A recent study in a large group of OIF males who were Navy seamen and Marines (MacGregor et al. 2010) found that among individuals with moderate to severe physical injuries (Injury Severity Scale [ISS] score>3), PTSD was less common among those with TBI (of any severity) than among those without TBI. Results for those with mTBI and for those with more severe TBI were not reported separately in this study. However, among those with mild overall injuries (ISS<4), a greater number of those with mTBI had PTSD than did those without TBI. In addition, recent findings in an OIF sample with mTBI indicated that those with other physical injuries reported fewer PTSD symptoms than did those with no other associated injuries (Kennedy et al. 2010).

Exposure to combat and being injured in combat increase the risk of developing PTSD (Hoge et al. 2007). With regard to the specific effects of blast injury, research illustrates a similar clinical pattern between service members injured in a combat zone and civilians injured in the Oklahoma City federal building blast. In both settings, those injured by blast had a risk of developing PTSD that was significantly greater in those who had an mTBI as part of their injury pattern than in those whose injuries did not include an mTBI (Hoge et al. 2008; Walilko et al. 2009).

The specific nature and amount of traumatic exposure vary for U.S. Veterans of different war eras, yielding different rates of PTSD for each conflict (Kennedy et al. 2007). Approximately 30% of Vietnam Veterans and 10% of Gulf War Veterans have experienced clinically significant PTSD symptoms. Approximately 12%–13% of combat personnel deployed to Iraq and Afghanistan have PTSD symptoms following combat deployments with heavy enemy engagement, with numbers increasing to 17%–25% at 3–6 months after their return (Milliken et al. 2007). Compared with other types of trauma, combat trauma is particularly distressing. In a national sample of 1,703 men reporting a traumatic event in the National Comorbidity

Survey, those reporting combat trauma as the worst trauma were more likely to have lifetime PTSD, delayed PTSD symptom onset, and unresolved PTSD symptoms. The negative influence of PTSD symptoms on life in general was revealed by higher rates of unemployment and divorce, as well as increased likelihood of having been fired from a job and of engaging in physical spouse abuse (Prigerson et al. 2001).

The "burden of adversity" hypothesis provides a model for understanding the dynamics involved in the development and course of cumulative negative conditions experienced by service members exposed to OIF/OEF combat deployments (Brenner et al. 2009). This model is based on the idea of cumulative disadvantage in which the collective presence of genetic and environmental risk factors over time leads to a trajectory of physical and psychiatric risk that becomes more and more divergent from the normal course of recovery and resilience. As applied to military service members previously deployed to OIF/OEF, the model proposes that after a TBI, postconcussive symptoms lead to stressors across a range of areas, including physical, emotional, cognitive, psychosocial, vocational, financial, and recreational functioning. Increased chronic disability results from the interaction between these stressors and premorbid factors. Treatment emphasizes early symptom identification and management to alter the negative life course trajectory.

*Civilian populations.* The increased rate of PTSD following mTBI is not limited to the active-duty deployed population. In a study of civilian trauma center patients, those with mTBI were more likely to develop PTSD (11.8%) than were those with no TBI (7.5%). Longer duration of PTA was associated with less severe intrusive memories, suggesting a protective effect of amnesia on reexperiencing in this mTBI group (Bryant et al. 2009).

Several studies have also investigated the incidence and prevalence of PTSD across the more severe end of the brain injury spectrum. At a large civilian medical center, Bombardier et al. (2006) conducted a prospective cohort study of 124 patients with complicated mild, moderate, and severe TBI followed across the first 6 months postinjury (Figure 8–3). The investigators tracked the rate and phenomenology of PTSD symptoms every 30 days. Cumulative incidence of PTSD at 6 months post-TBI was 11.3%. The majority of these individuals (86%) also met criteria for an additional psychiatric disorder. Arousal symptoms (DSM-IV-TR Criterion D) and reexperiencing phenomena (Criterion B) were more common than avoidance behaviors (Crite-

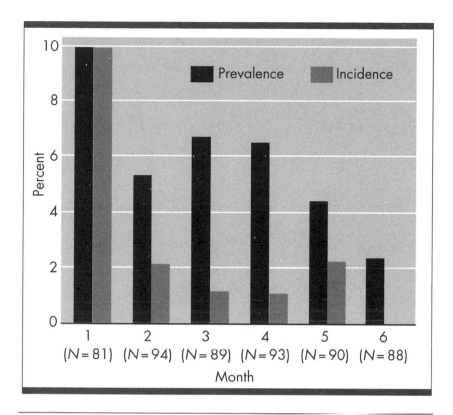

**FIGURE 8–3.** Incidence and prevalence of subjects who met posttraumatic stress disorder symptom criteria each month.

*Source.* Reprinted from Bombardier CH, Fann JR, Temkin N, et al.: "Posttraumatic Stress Disorder Symptoms During the First Six Months After Traumatic Brain Injury." *Journal of Neuropsychiatry and Clinical Neurosciences* 18:501–508, 2006. © American Psychiatric Association. Used with permission.

rion C) in this sample (Figure 8–4). In a selected sample of patients with severe TBI, Bryant et al. (2000) found a higher incidence (27%) of PTSD than that reported by Bombardier et al. (2006) but a similar picture of symptom presentation, dominated by emotional reactivity and hyperarousal.

## CLINICAL ASSESSMENT

The gold standard for diagnosis of PTSD is the use of a structured or semistructured clinical interview, although research studies often use self-report symptom ratings to indicate the presence of the disorder.

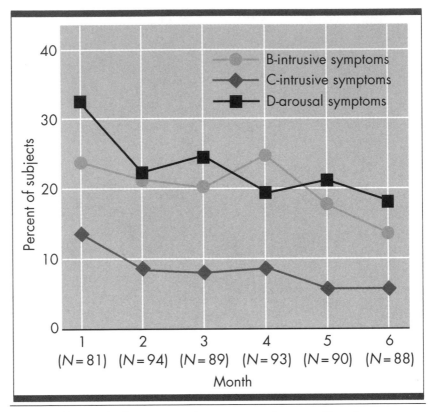

**FIGURE 8–4.**   Endorsement of posttraumatic stress disorder symptom clusters by month.

*B, C,* and *D* refer to the corresponding lettered criteria for posttraumatic stress disorder in DSM-IV-TR.

*Source.*   Reprinted from Bombardier CH, Fann JR, Temkin N, et al.: "Posttraumatic Stress Disorder Symptoms During the First Six Months After Traumatic Brain Injury." *Journal of Neuropsychiatry and Clinical Neurosciences* 18:501–508, 2006. © American Psychiatric Association. Used with permission.

Several of the most commonly used instruments are the PTSD Checklist (PCL; Blanchard et al. 1996), the four-question Primary Care PTSD Screen (PC-PTSD; Prins et al. 2003), and the Trauma Symptom Inventory (TSI; Briere et al. 1995). Estimates of the correspondence of these ratings to clinically verified diagnoses range in value, and the use of these instruments requires familiarity with their specific characteristics and clinical yields (Golding et al. 2009).

Diagnosing PTSD in an individual with a history of TBI and persistent postconcussive symptoms is not a straightforward endeavor. Because the symptoms of PTSD and the late consequences of TBI may overlap, the clinician can have difficulty determining whether an individual's presentation is best described as reflecting PTSD, the late effects of TBI, or both. This challenge is even greater among persons with mTBI, among whom persistent postconcussive symptoms reflect atypical, and often polyetiological, recovery (Carroll et al. 2004; McCrea et al. 2009).

Different paradigms exist for understanding the relationship between PTSD and mTBI symptoms. One currently popular way to conceptualize this relationship is to recognize that these conditions may mutually affect one another. For example, cognitive models propose that PTSD is maintained when trauma survivors have inadequate cognitive resources to manage their traumatic memories and to use adaptive cognitive strategies (Ehlers and Clark 2000). Symptoms from TBI likely compromise the ability to cope with the stress of PTSD (e.g., through disinhibition of executive control processes), and PTSD likewise compromises the ability to navigate the cognitive and other manifestations of TBI (Jackson et al. 2008; Moore et al. 2006). Other examples of interaction include mutual effects on symptom severity and temporal effects in which causality of symptoms is a function of time after the injury. The time-dependent nature of the relationship between TBI and PTSD is characterized by initial postconcussive symptoms, closely tied to acute neurochemical changes from the TBI, and persistent symptoms that become increasingly related to other factors such as the presence of comorbid PTSD. An excellent review of this issue, offered from a cognitive neuroscience perspective, is provided by Vasterling et al. (2009).

# TREATMENT

Rehabilitation and outcome after TBI are hindered by the presence of PTSD. Patients with PTSD following severe TBI report poorer health, lower functional capacity, less life satisfaction, and more symptoms of depression than a similar TBI group without PTSD (Bryant et al. 2001; Johansen et al. 2007). Similarly, outcomes 3–4 months after mTBI also relate to the presence of PTSD (Hoge et al. 2008). Based on these findings, the Defense and Veterans Brain Injury Center (DVBIC), a collaboration between military treatment facilities and VA hospitals, has consistently recommended that patients identified with TBI be screened and evaluated for PTSD and that positive findings be incorporated into a multidisciplinary integrated treatment approach to achieve adequate recovery in patients exhibiting PTSD following TBI. PTSD treatments may need to be adapted when applied to the patient with TBI. Treatment plans are developed to encompass evaluation and management of all potential TBI symptoms, including those in the physical, cognitive, and emotional areas.

The importance of early identification and treatment of symptoms of PTSD among individuals with TBI is well acknowledged. For example, in a sequential model for the treatment of postconcussive symptoms (Terrio et al. 2009), the first step involves providing positive expectations for recovery and treatment of ongoing psychiatric symptoms such as those related to PTSD or depression. Somatic symptoms are addressed second, including treatments for headaches and sleep. Cognitive symptoms are treated as needed once the other steps have been completed and associated symptoms adequately managed. This model is similar to the current joint Department of Veterans Affairs/Department of Defense mTBI clinical practice guidelines (www.dvbic.org/sites/default/files/Co-occurring-Conditions-Toolkit.pdf).

Research addressing treatment of the patient with TBI and PTSD is now appearing in the literature, although the scope of that literature remains relatively limited. An examination of the VA systems of care and provider perspectives across the country (Sayer et al. 2009) identified administrative, assessment, and treatment challenges related to patients with TBI and PTSD symptoms. For example, the integration of TBI and PTSD treatments has been hampered by separate administrative structures within medical/neurological and behavioral health lines. Assessment of these patients is lengthy and complex, particularly for OIF/OEF Veterans compared to civilians, due to the added effects of deployment stress. No clear guidance is available for modifying evidence-based treatment for PTSD to accommodate patients with TBI. Providers perceived that these patients require more time, attention, repetition, and flexibility to achieve benefit from PTSD treatment. Some PTSD providers felt that prolonged exposure therapy was a better choice than cognitive processing therapy for patients with mTBI and PTSD; this preference appeared to be based on the relatively less memory-demanding nature of exposure therapy. Medications contraindicated for either TBI or PTSD were regarded as best to avoid, and an emphasis was placed on treating concurrent conditions such as sleep problems and pain. Additionally, ancillary services such as vocational or employment counseling, family interventions, and education about the co-occurrence of TBI and PTSD are important but potentially overlooked aspects of care in these cases.

One of the primary concerns in the treatment of PTSD in individuals with co-occurring TBI surrounds memory dysfunction and its potential effect on participation and follow-through in psychotherapy for PTSD. A well-designed randomized controlled trial by Bryant et al. (2003) examined the efficacy of cognitive-behavioral therapy (CBT) for individuals with acute stress disorder and a history of mTBI. Although the sample sizes were small (12 per treatment arm), the study demonstrated a dramatic reduction in the subsequent development of PTSD in those subjects who participated in CBT (8%) versus those who received supportive counseling (58%), despite sustaining an mTBI within 2 weeks of the initiation of treatment. This study did not examine cognition as a variable of interest.

By contrast, Wild and Gur (2008) looked specifically at the effect of verbal memory on CBT for PTSD. Their findings indicated that verbal memory difficulties diminished the effectiveness of CBT and response to treatment, even when the authors controlled for other potential mediating variables (i.e., IQ, attention, PTSD severity, depression, substance use). Although this study did not include subjects with co-occurring mTBI, the findings suggest that the degree of memory dysfunction may be more predictive of poor treatment outcome than diagnostic categories (e.g., mTBI).

In short, few empirically validated therapies exist to treat comorbid PTSD and postconcussion symptoms in civilian, Veteran, or military populations, despite the critical need for such therapies, as discussed by Lew et al. (2008) with regard to the military and Veteran health care delivery systems. Rigorous research by DVBIC and the Defense Centers of Excellence produced a manual of management recommendations for patients with TBI and PTSD, as well as other comorbidities such as pain or substance abuse (www.dvbic.org/strategies-symptom-management).

# Pharmacotherapy

Definitive empirical evidence for the efficacy of specific pharmacological treatment for combined TBI and PTSD is lacking. However, case studies, limited controlled trials, and consensus-based guidelines help inform clinicians treating these individuals. Several classes of medication have been found effective for the treatment of both post-concussive and posttraumatic stress-related symptoms (Table 8–2); readers are encouraged to consider the extended review of this subject by McAllister (2009). Among persons with TBI, the use of benzodiazepines and other sedating antianxiety medications to treat PTSD is discouraged; these agents may interfere with cognition, motor function, and neural recovery and therefore are not the best first choices for the management of PTSD symptoms in this population (Hoffman and Harrison 2009).

## Psychological and Behavioral Therapies

Several forms of psychological and behavioral therapy are effective for PTSD (Table 8–3). One major class focuses on controlled exposure and extinguishing the intrusive reexperiencing symptoms. Examples include eye movement desensitization and reprocessing (EMDR) and prolonged exposure therapy. Another major type of therapy concentrates on correcting dysfunctional thoughts and the associated emotional and behavioral disturbances involved in PTSD. Both trauma-focused and more general non-trauma-focused CBT and cognitive processing therapy are included in this type of approach. Although they are not targeted treatments for PTSD, stress management techniques such as relaxation training and biofeedback are often helpful in managing associated anxiety symptoms.

Early provision of CBT after concurrent mTBI and psychological trauma (i.e., within 2 weeks of the trauma event) to persons with acute stress disorder appears to be more effective at preventing the development of PTSD than supportive counseling (Bryant et al. 2003). In light of the benefits of CBT afforded during the early period after mTBI (when cognitive symptoms would be expected to be at their worst), the common supposition that posttraumatic cognitive impairments preclude participation in CBT appears less tenable. As noted earlier in the "Treatment" section, Sayer et al. (2009) suggested that persons with more severe posttraumatic cognitive impairments may require a longer treatment period, greater attention, more repetition, and some flexibility in treatment in order to benefit from psychotherapies for PTSD. However, recent evidence suggests that programs comprising psychoeducational groups, cognitive skill building, and a modified form of cognitive processing therapy can be helpful to patients with comorbid TBI and PTSD (Chard et al. 2011).

**TABLE 8–2.** Medications used commonly to treat the neuropsychiatric consequences of TBI, PTSD, or both

| MEDICATION CLASS | SUBTYPES | COMMON USES IN TBI | COMMON USES IN PTSD | POTENTIAL ISSUES IN COMORBID TBI AND PTSD |
|---|---|---|---|---|
| Antidepressants | SSRIs, SNRIs, TCAs, HCAs, MAOIs | Depression, anxiety, affective lability, disinhibition, aggression | PTSD symptoms, comorbid depressive and anxiety symptoms | Limited evidence. Anticholinergic effects adversely affect cognition. Some agents may lower seizure threshold. |
| Anxiolytics | SSRIs, buspirone, benzodiazepines | Anxiety, agitation | PTSD symptoms, other comorbid anxiety disorders | Limited evidence. Benzodiazepines may impair cognition and motor function, produce paradoxical agitation/disinhibition; also carry risk for abuse or dependence. |
| Anticonvulsants | Valproate, carbamazepine, lamotrigine | Early seizure prophylaxis, treatment of PTE, secondary mania, disinhibition, aggression | PTSD symptoms, comorbid bipolar disorder or epilepsy | Limited evidence. May adversely affect cognition, motor function. Multiple systemic side effects, including hepatic, hematological, dermatological, and reproductive consequences. |
| Catecholaminergic modulators | Dopaminergic and/or noradrenergic agonists, reuptake inhibitors, or antagonists | Augmentation of catecholaminergic function for arousal, speed of processing, attention problems | Antagonists of β-adrenergic receptors (β-blockers) for hyperarousal | Limited evidence. Agents that augment cerebral catecholaminergic function may exacerbate PTSD-related hyperarousal. β-Blockers may exacerbate TBI-related cognitive impairments. Central nervous stimulants carry risk for abuse or dependence. |

**TABLE 8–2.** Medications used commonly to treat the neuropsychiatric consequences of TBI, PTSD, or both (continued)

| MEDICATION CLASS | SUBTYPES | COMMON USES IN TBI | COMMON USES IN PTSD | POTENTIAL ISSUES IN COMORBID TBI AND PTSD |
|---|---|---|---|---|
| Cholinergic modulators | Cholinesterase inhibitors | Memory and other cognitive impairments | Not commonly used | Limited evidence. Augmentation of central nervous system cholinergic tone may exacerbate sleep disturbances (nightmares) and reexperiencing symptoms (intrusive memories) of PTSD. |
| Antipsychotics | Typical antipsychotics, atypical antipsychotics | Psychosis, severe acute or chronic aggression | Augmentation of antidepressants, mood stabilization, and treatment of severe acute or chronic aggression | Limited evidence. May exacerbate cognitive impairments and produce motor disturbances (acute or tardive extrapyramidal effects, acute or chronic dykinesias or dystonias). Metabolic syndrome. |

*Note.* HCA=heterocyclic antidepressant; MAOI=monoamine oxidase inhibitor; PTE=posttraumatic epilepsy; PTSD=posttraumatic stress disorder; SNRI=serotonin-norepinephrine reuptake inhibitor; SSRI=selective serotonin reuptake inhibitor; TBI=traumatic brain injury; TCA=tricyclic antidepressant.

*Source.* Adapted from McAllister TW: "Psychopharmacological Issues in the Treatment of TBI and PTSD." *Clinical Neuropsychologist* 23:1338–1367, 2009. Copyright 2012 by Taylor and Francis Informa UK LTD—Journals. Used with permission.

**TABLE 8–3.** Effective forms of psychological and behavioral therapy for posttraumatic stress disorder

Trauma-focused individual or group cognitive-behavioral therapy

Individual or group cognitive-behavioral therapy not focused on trauma

Individual stress management treatment focused on relaxation and stress reduction techniques

Individual therapy focused on controlled prolonged exposure to trauma elements

Cognitive processing therapy

Eye movement desensitization and reprocessing

Additional research will better define the types of psychotherapies that are beneficial to persons with comorbid PTSD and TBI. Until such studies are performed and inform on the modifications of psychotherapeutic interventions required by comorbid TBI, the available evidence suggests that many persons with these comorbid conditions will benefit from the psychotherapies that are part of the standard repertoire of treatments for PTSD (American Psychiatric Association 2006).

## Other Treatments

Environmental enrichment is a treatment for PTSD among persons with TBI that is predicated on the shared structural, functional, and neurochemical characteristics of these conditions (Hoffman and Harrison 2009). This approach originates from extensive research in animal models in which environments that encourage mental activation through exploration lead to enhanced recovery from brain damage. Environmental enrichment can reverse the negative effects of chronic stress by lowering stress hormones such as adrenocorticotropic hormone and corticosterone. This treatment has been shown to increase neuronal density, dendritic branching, synapses, and growth factor expressions, leading to increased total brain and cortical weight. The positive effect of this treatment on stress reduction is assumed to relate to the patient's greater sense of control over the environment.

A related concept linked to improved recovery is resilience (Karatsoreos and McEwen 2011). Resilience is predicated on a complex constellation of neurological and organismal factors, including growth factors, chaperone molecules, and circadian rhythms that permit an individual to respond adaptively to stressors in the environment. The concept of resilience (or, conversely, vulnerability) is relevant to understanding the development of PTSD and, possibly, the adverse effects of TBI on the neural systems that are usually engaged when responding to stress. Therapies designed to enhance resilience prior to trauma or to encourage its restoration after trauma may become important elements of the treatment of PTSD.

Modern technological innovations have been applied to the treatment of TBI and PTSD. For example, the imaginal and/or in vivo exposure component of PTSD treatment has been adapted to a virtual reality environment. This alternative methodology minimizes avoidance and facilitates emotional processing. Currently, virtual reality systems have the disadvantages of being costly and limited in number; however, with technological advances, they have the potential to provide powerful and efficient tools for rehabilitation after trauma. Mobile technology has been applied to care, in the form of assistive devices to implement reminders, schedules, and a link to information. Telehealth initiatives provide service delivery and education to rural and underserved populations.

## CONCLUSION

The events that produce TBI may be psychologically traumatizing and place individuals experiencing them at risk for PTSD. This syndrome begins with a psychologically traumatic event that produces intense fear, helplessness, and/or horror, after which reexperiencing, avoidance, and hyperarousal symptoms develop. Many, but not all, of these symptoms are similar to the persistent postconcussive symptoms experienced by some TBI survivors. The neuroanatomical and neurobiological bases of PTSD and TBI (and, presumably, persistent postconcussive symptoms) overlap, which may in part explain some of the similarities in the clinical presentations of persons with these conditions. The course of PTSD is variable, but it may become a chronic problem for some persons with TBI. The pharmacotherapies, psychotherapies, and other interventions for PTSD offered to persons with TBI are similar to those offered to persons without TBI. When medications are used, agents that are least likely to exacerbate cognitive, motor, or other neurological problems are preferred. The range of psychotherapies for PTSD is broad, and preliminary evidence suggests that they can be provided to many persons with TBI—especially persons with mTBI—with no or only modest modifications. The psychotherapy of PTSD provided to persons with more severe cognitive impairments remains underdeveloped. In such circumstances, prolonged exposure therapies involving greater attention, more repetition, and some flexibility in treatment approach may be useful for the treatment of PTSD.

## *Key Clinical Points*

- TBI and posttraumatic stress disorder (PTSD) can co-occur, especially among persons with histories of mild TBI.

- The neuroanatomical and neurobiological bases of PTSD and TBI overlap, as do some of their symptoms.

- Reexperiencing, shame, and guilt are not typical postconcussive symptoms; their presence suggests that the patient has PTSD.

- Pharmacotherapies used to treat PTSD among persons with TBI are similar to those offered to people without TBI. Agents less likely to exacerbate neurological problems are preferred.

- Psychotherapies are important in the treatment of PTSD among persons with TBI. Early studies suggest that such therapies can be offered with little or no modification, especially to persons with mild TBI.

- Psychotherapy for PTSD provided to persons with more severe cognitive impairments needs further study. Prolonged, more flexible exposure therapies for PTSD may prove useful.

# REFERENCES

American Psychiatric Association: Diagnostic and Statistical Manual of Mental Disorders, 3rd Edition. Washington, DC, American Psychiatric Association, 1980

American Psychiatric Association: Diagnostic and Statistical Manual of Mental Disorders, 4th Edition, Text Revision. Washington, DC, American Psychiatric Association, 2000

American Psychiatric Association: American Psychiatric Association Practice Guidelines for the Treatment of Psychiatric Disorders, Compendium 2006. Washington, DC, American Psychiatric Association, 2006

Blanchard EB, Jones-Alexander J, Buckley TC, et al: Psychometric properties of the PTSD Checklist (PCL). Behav Res Ther 34:669–673, 1996

Bombardier CH, Fann JR, Temkin N, et al: Posttraumatic stress disorder symptoms during the first six months after traumatic brain injury. J Neuropsychiatry Clin Neurosci 18:501–508, 2006

Brady KT, Killeen TK, Brewerton T, et al: Comorbidity of psychiatric disorders and posttraumatic stress disorder. J Clin Psychiatry 61(suppl):22–32, 2000

Brailey K, Vasterling JJ, Proctor SP, et al: PTSD symptoms, life events, and unit cohesion in U.S. soldiers: baseline findings from the neurocognition deployment health study. J Trauma Stress 20:495–503, 2007

Brenner LA, Ladley-O'Brien SE, Harwood JE, et al: An exploratory study of neuroimaging, neurologic, and neuropsychological findings in veterans with traumatic brain injury and/or posttraumatic stress disorder. Mil Med 174:347–352, 2009

Breslau N: Outcomes of posttraumatic stress disorder. J Clin Psychiatry 62(suppl):55–59, 2001

Briere J, Elliott DM, Harris K, et al: Trauma Symptom Inventory: psychometrics and association with childhood and adult victimization in clinical samples. J Interpers Violence 10:387–401, 1995

Bryant RA, Marosszeky JE, Crooks J, et al: Posttraumatic stress disorder after severe traumatic brain injury. Am J Psychiatry 157:629–631, 2000

Bryant RA, Marosszeky JE, Crooks J, et al: Posttraumatic stress disorder and psychosocial functioning after severe traumatic brain injury. J Nerv Ment Dis 189:109–113, 2001

Bryant RA, Moulds M, Guthrie R, et al: Treating acute stress disorder following mild traumatic brain injury. Am J Psychiatry 160:585–587, 2003

Bryant RA, Creamer M, O'Donnell M, et al: Post-traumatic amnesia and the nature of post-traumatic stress disorder after mild traumatic brain injury. J Int Neuropsychol Soc 15:862–867, 2009

Cantu RC: Chronic traumatic encephalopathy in the National Football League. Neurosurgery 61:223–225, 2007

Carlson KF, Nelson D, Orazem RJ, et al: Psychiatric diagnoses among Iraq and Afghanistan war veterans screened for deployment-related traumatic brain injury. J Trauma Stress 23:17–24, 2010

Carlson KF, Kehle SM, Meis LA, et al: Prevalence, assessment, and treatment of mild traumatic brain injury and posttraumatic stress disorder: a systematic review of the evidence. J Head Trauma Rehabil 26:103–115, 2011

Carroll LJ, Cassidy JD, Peloso PM, et al: Prognosis for mild traumatic brain injury: results of the WHO Collaborating Centre Task Force on Mild Traumatic Brain Injury. J Rehabil Med 43(suppl):84–105, 2004

Casson IR, Pellman EJ, Viano DC: Chronic traumatic encephalopathy in a National Football League player (letter). Neurosurgery 59:E11, 2006

Chard KM, Schumm JA, McIlvain SM, et al: Exploring the efficacy of a residential treatment program incorporating cognitive processing therapy-cognitive for veterans with PTSD and traumatic brain injury. J Trauma Stress 24:347–351, 2011

Cooper DB, Kennedy JE, Cullen MA, et al: Association between combat stress and post-concussive symptom reporting in OEF/OIF service members with mild traumatic brain injuries. Brain Inj 25:1–7, 2011

Corneil W, Beaton R, Murphy S, et al: Exposure to traumatic incidents and prevalence of posttraumatic stress symptomatology in urban firefighters in two countries. J Occup Health Psychol 4:131–141, 1999

Ehlers A, Clark DM: A cognitive model of posttraumatic stress disorder. Behav Res Ther 38:319–345, 2000

Golding H, Bass E, Percy A, et al: Understanding recent estimates of PTSD and TBI from Operations Iraqi Freedom and Enduring Freedom. J Rehabil Res Dev 46:vii–xiv, 2009

Harvey A, Kopelman MD, Brewin C: PTSD and traumatic brain injury, in Neuropsychology of PTSD: Biological, Cognitive, and Clinical Perspectives. Edited by Vasterling JJ, Brewin C. New York, Guilford, 2005, pp 230–246

Hidalgo RB, Davidson JR: Posttraumatic stress disorder: epidemiology and health-related considerations. J Clin Psychiatry 61(suppl):5–13, 2000

Hoffman SW, Harrison C: The interaction between psychological health and traumatic brain injury: a neuroscience perspective. Clin Neuropsychol 23:1400–1415, 2009

Hoge CW, Terhakopian A, Castro CA, et al: Association of posttraumatic stress disorder with somatic symptoms, health care visits, and absenteeism among Iraq war veterans. Am J Psychiatry 164:150–153, 2007

Hoge CW, McGurk D, Thomas JL, et al: Mild traumatic brain injury in U.S. soldiers returning from Iraq. N Engl J Med 358:453–463, 2008

Jackson GL, Hamilton NS, Tupler LA: Detecting traumatic brain injury among veterans of Operations Enduring and Iraqi Freedom. NC Med J 69:43–47, 2008

Johansen VA, Wahl AK, Eilertsen DE, et al: The predictive value of post-traumatic stress disorder symptoms for quality of life: a longitudinal study of physically injured victims of non-domestic violence. Health Qual Life Outcomes 5:26, 2007

Karatsoreos IN, McEwen BS: Psychobiological allostasis: resistance, resilience and vulnerability. Trends Cogn Sci 15:576–584, 2011

Kennedy JE, Jaffee MS, Leskin GA, et al: Posttraumatic stress disorder and posttraumatic stress disorder-like symptoms and mild traumatic brain injury. J Rehabil Res Dev 44:895–920, 2007

Kennedy JE, Cullen MA, Amador RR, et al: Symptoms in military service members after blast mTBI with and without associated injuries. NeuroRehabilitation 26:191–197, 2010

Kessler RC: Posttraumatic stress disorder: the burden to the individual and to society. J Clin Psychiatry 61(suppl):4–12, discussion 13–14, 2000

Kessler RC, Sonnega A, Bromet E, et al: Posttraumatic stress disorder in the National Comorbidity Survey. Arch Gen Psychiatry 52:1048–1060, 1995

Lew HL, Vanderploeg RD, Moore DF, et al: Overlap of mild TBI and mental health conditions in returning OIF/OEF service members and veterans. J Rehabil Res Dev 45:xi–xvi, 2008

Ling G, Bandak F, Armonda R, et al: Explosive blast neurotrauma. J Neurotrauma 26:815–825, 2009

MacGregor AJ, Shaffer RA, Dougherty AL, et al: Prevalence and psychological correlates of traumatic brain injury in Operation Iraqi Freedom. J Head Trauma Rehabil 25:1–8, 2010

McAllister TW: Psychopharmacological issues in the treatment of TBI and PTSD. Clin Neuropsychol 23:1338–1367, 2009

McCrea M, Iverson GL, McAllister TW, et al: An integrated review of recovery after mild traumatic brain injury (MTBI): implications for clinical management. Clin Neuropsychol 23:1368–1390, 2009

McCrory P: Boxing and the brain: revisiting chronic traumatic encephalopathy (editorial). Br J Sports Med 36:2, 2002

McKee AC, Cantu RC, Nowinski CJ, et al: Chronic traumatic encephalopathy in athletes: progressive tauopathy after repetitive head injury. J Neuropathol Exp Neurol 68:709–735, 2009

Milliken CS, Auchterlonie JL, Hoge CW: Longitudinal assessment of mental health problems among active and reserve component soldiers returning from the Iraq war. JAMA 298:2141–2148, 2007

Moore EL, Terryberry-Spohr L, Hope DA: Mild traumatic brain injury and anxiety sequelae: a review of the literature. Brain Inj 20:117–132, 2006

Omalu BI, DeKosky ST, Hamilton RL, et al: Chronic traumatic encephalopathy in a National Football League player: part II. Neurosurgery 59:1086–1092, discussion 1092–1093, 2006

Omalu B, Bailes J, Hamilton RL, et al: Emerging histomorphologic phenotypes of chronic traumatic encephalopathy in American athletes. Neurosurgery 69:173–183, discussion 183, 2011

Prigerson HG, Maciejewski PK, Rosenheck RA: Combat trauma: trauma with highest risk of delayed onset and unresolved posttraumatic stress disorder symptoms, unemployment, and abuse among men. J Nerv Ment Dis 189:99–108, 2001

Prins A, Ouimette P, Kimerling R, et al: The Primary Care PTSD Screen (PC-PTSD): development and operating characteristics. Primary Care Psychiatry 9:9–14, 2003

Rattok J, Boake C, Bontke CF: Do patients with mild brain injuries have posttraumatic stress disorder, too? J Head Trauma Rehabil 11:95–102, 1996

Sayer NA, Rettmann NA, Carlson KF, et al: Veterans with history of mild traumatic brain injury and posttraumatic stress disorder: challenges from provider perspective. J Rehabil Res Dev 46:703–716, 2009

Solomon Z, Mikulincer M: Trajectories of PTSD: a 20-year longitudinal study. Am J Psychiatry 163:659–666, 2006

Southwick SM, Rasmusson A, Barron J, et al: Neurobiological and neurocognitive alterations in PTSD, in Neuropsychology of PTSD: Biological, Cognitive, and Clinical Perspectives. Edited by Vasterling JJ, Brewin C. New York, Guilford, 2005, pp 27–58

Stein MB, McAllister TW: Exploring the convergence of posttraumatic stress disorder and mild traumatic brain injury. Am J Psychiatry 166:768–776, 2009

Terrio H, Brenner LA, Ivins BJ, et al: Traumatic brain injury screening: preliminary findings in a US Army Brigade Combat Team. J Head Trauma Rehabil 24:14–23, 2009

Vasterling JJ, Proctor SP, Amoroso P, et al: Neuropsychological outcomes of army personnel following deployment to the Iraq war. JAMA 296:519–529, 2006

Vasterling JJ, Verfaellie M, Sullivan KD: Mild traumatic brain injury and posttraumatic stress disorder in returning veterans: perspectives from cognitive neuroscience. Clin Psychol Rev 29:674–684, 2009

Walilko T, North C, Young LA, et al: Head injury as a PTSD predictor among Oklahoma City bombing survivors. J Trauma 67:1311–1319, 2009

Wild J, Gur RC: Verbal memory and treatment response in post-traumatic stress disorder. Br J Psychiatry 193:254–255, 2008

Yehuda R: Risk and resilience in posttraumatic stress disorder. J Clin Psychiatry 65(suppl):29–36, 2004

◆

# CHAPTER 9

# Posttraumatic Psychosis

*Perminder S. Sachdev, M.B.B.S., M.D., Ph.D.*

*Psychosis* is a broad term, usually referring to any psychiatric disorder in which there is a loss of reality testing, which is generally reflected by the presence of delusions, hallucinations, and/or severe thought disorder and may entail serious behavioral disturbances. In individuals with traumatic brain injury (TBI), reports of psychosis have included cases that would meet criteria for delirium, schizophrenia, schizophreniform disorder, delusional disorder, bipolar disorder, or major depression. The greatest interest, however, has been generated by the association between TBI and schizophrenia-like psychosis (Krafft-Ebing 1868), and this is the focus of this chapter. The most important question is whether TBI predisposes an individual to schizophrenia or schizophrenia-like psychosis. If this association can be unequivocally established, a number of other issues become relevant, such as the prevalence of schizophrenia-like psychosis following TBI, its clinical features, risk factors, and prognosis. An important corollary is whether the study of schizophrenia-like psychosis following TBI can advance the understanding of the etiopathogenesis of schizophrenia.

## EPIDEMIOLOGY

The evidence for an association between schizophrenia-like psychosis and TBI has come from a number of sources, and the related issues are indeed complex, due to the differing definitions of TBI and schizophrenia-like psychosis used and the varying methods of ascertainment. The most definitive study would be a longitudinal cohort design, in which a large number of individuals with TBI across a wide age range, matched to a group of individuals without TBI, are followed up prospectively using standard instruments and well-defined diagnostic criteria. Because this ideal study does not exist, the evidence must be pooled from a variety of sources.

## Case Reports

Fujii and Ahmed (2002) systematically reviewed 39 reports from 1971 to 1994 and found 69 cases in which psychosis with hallucinations or delusions was considered a direct consequence of TBI and not accounted for by another mental disorder or delirium. The "direct consequence" criterion was satisfied if there was a temporal association (i.e., TBI preceded schizophrenia-like psychosis, generally by a short interval but with no upper time limit), the patient had no prepsychotic symptoms at the time of TBI, and the patient had no family history of psychosis. The type of brain injury was taken into consideration; as suggested by neuroimaging and/or cognitive assessment, the injury had to be frontotemporal and not exclusively parietal or occipital. Unfortunately, because the anatomical and neuropsychological deficits in schizophrenia are not specific, clinical "judgment" is generally relied upon in making the determination. Anecdotal reports of schizophrenia-like psychosis following TBI do not and cannot provide strong evidence for the association because of the likelihood of chance association and the subjective nature of the determination. However, schizophrenia-like psychosis and TBI have prompted more systematic studies.

## Cross-Sectional Surveys

In the U.S. national Epidemiologic Catchment Area study (Silver et al. 2001), of the 361 individuals with a history of head injury leading to loss of consciousness or confusion, 3.4% were diagnosed with schizophrenia (compared with 1.9% of controls without head injury), a statistically nonsignificant result. Although this was a large population-based study and the ascertainment of schizophrenia used a standard instrument, albeit one whose validity has been questioned, the ascertainment of head injury was crude and relied on self-report alone. Moreover, the cross-sectional nature of the study could not discount the possibility of "reverse causality"—that is, that individuals predisposed to schizophrenia were behaviorally more predisposed to a head injury due to personality features or prepsychotic symptoms.

## Cohort Studies

The earliest attempt to review cohort studies was by Davison and Bagley (1969), who examined eight studies published between 1917 and 1964, seven of which were of war veterans, with follow-up periods of 10–20 years (except two studies that followed patients for 2 years or less). The cumulative incidence of schizophrenia in the subjects with TBI ranged from 0.07% to 9.8%, with a median figure of 1.35%. Using a comparison figure of 0.8% incidence of schizophrenia over 25 years in the general population, the authors concluded that the increased risk in the TBI group was two- to threefold. The limitations resulting from heterogeneity of diagnostic criteria applied and from the use of a population-based incidence figure derived by different methodology are obvious.

In a large study from Finland, 3,552 Finnish veterans of World War II were followed for 22–26 years, and their hospital records were examined for history of psychosis (Achté et al. 1969). Almost all of the subjects (98.8%) had injuries from bullets or shrapnel and 42% of the injuries were open, making them atypical of peacetime injuries. Defined broadly, 317 (8.9%) of the individuals had onset of psychosis following TBI. Of these, 2.1% had schizophrenic psychoses and another 2.0% had paranoid psychoses, resulting in an incidence of schizophrenia-like psychosis of about 4.1%. A significant proportion (42%) had the onset of psychosis more than 10 years after the injury.

In a Belgian study, De Mol et al. (1987) retrospectively studied 530 persons with TBI who were assessed at a neuropsychological center and followed for 1–10 years. Eighteen were diagnosed with a major psychiatric disorder, mostly (83%) within 6 months of the injury, and 12 (2.3%) of this subgroup had DSM-III (American Psychiatric Association 1980) schizophrenia or schizophreniform disorder.

Roberts (1979) attempted to follow up, 10 to 24 years later, with 479 patients with severe TBI (defined as posttraumatic amnesia for longer than 1 week) who had been admitted to the Radcliffe Infirmary, Oxford, England. Of the 291 survivors with sufficient clinical data, seven had been diagnosed with "paranoid dementia" and two with schizophrenia-like psychosis (9/291=3.09%). In the two with schizophrenia-like psychosis, the onset occurred 9 or 17 years postinjury and affective symptoms were prominent.

Ota (1969) studied 1,168 adults who were admitted to the hospital following TBI and reported that 2.7% had psychosis, which could be either "functional" or "organic." Miller and Stern (1965), in a long-term follow-up of 100 subjects with TBI, found 10 with psychosis, all of whom suffered from dementia. Using contemporary diagnostic criteria in assessing 670 patients with penetrating TBI, Lishman (1968) identified only five patients with schizophrenia-like illness.

A more recent historical cohort study (Fann et al. 2004) included 939 adults diagnosed with TBI in an emergency department during 1993; their medical records were searched from 1 year before to 3 years after the injury for psychiatric diagnoses or treatment. An unexpected finding was that patients with TBI had a higher rate of preexisting psychosis (odds ratio [OR] of 10.0 for moderate to severe TBI, and of 1.7 for mild TBI). Among patients with no preexisting psychiatric disorder ($n=85$), the risk of psychosis was significantly elevated by moderate to severe TBI in the second year (OR 5.9, 95% confidence interval [CI] 1.6–22.1) and third year (OR 3.6, 95% CI 1.0–1.3) of follow-up. The limitations of this study include the reliance on case notes for diagnosis, the short preinjury period covered, and the relatively small sample size.

The diversity of the evidence from cohort studies makes for a difficult synthesis, but the conservative conclusion is that population-based studies suggest that civilian TBI leads to only a small increase in the risk of schizophrenia-like psychosis, if at all, and the evidence for this is not consistent. The association may be stronger in those with a genetic vulnerability to schizophrenia or the presence of preinjury psychopathology. War-related brain injury may be a special case that cannot be generalized to civilian populations, and the reported increase of risk may well be due to psychological rather than neurological factors.

## Case-Control Studies

*Studies examining strength of association between TBI and schizophrenia.* Evidence has been presented (Dalman et al. 1999; Lewis and Murray 1987) that implicates pregnancy and delivery complications, some of which result in TBI, as an increased risk for the development of schizophrenia.

In a large case-control study, Wilcox and Nasrallah (1987) used medical records of patients admitted to a university hospital between 1934 and 1944 with schizophrenia ($n=200$), depression ($n=203$), or mania ($n=122$) and "surgical" controls ($n=134$) to examine the prevalence of head injury before age 10. The OR for schizophrenia for those with childhood head injury was 16.6 (95% CI 2.6–689), a highly significant result. The odds for bipolar disorder (OR 6.9, 95% CI 0.8–321) and depression (OR 2.0, 95% CI 0.2–10.5) were nonsignificantly elevated. These authors did not find any significant relationship with a particular injury location.

Gureje et al. (1994), in a case-control study in a Nigerian sample, also found an association between childhood brain trauma and schizophrenia. These patients also had mixed laterality in adulthood, possibly attributable to left hemisphere damage.

The major limitation of studies that rely on historical information is recall bias. Subjects with schizophrenia and their family members may be more likely than matched controls to report past TBI. There is also a possibility of observer bias, in that a clinician may be more likely to inquire about and record an episode of TBI in a neuropsychiatric patient than in a control patient. The issue of a suitable control population is another consideration. These limitations have been overcome by two case register linkage studies from countries in which population-based case registers are maintained and most medical encounters occur in the public sector.

Nielsen et al. (2002), in a nested case-control study, identified 8,288 individuals with schizophrenia (diagnosed using ICD-8) who had been admitted to a Danish psychiatric hospital between 1978 and 1993. Each case was matched to 10 controls from the general population based on the Central Persons Register. The subjects were linked to the National Patient Register to identify any admission secondary to TBI between 1978 and the date of the index psychiatric admission. The authors also noted the occurrence of fractures affecting other parts of the body in this period, as an index of proneness to accidents and injury. Overall, there was no excess of concussion or severe TBI in the patients with schizophrenia compared with the general population (OR 0.94 vs. 0.89, not a significant result). Individuals with schizophrenia were less likely to have had another fracture (OR 0.71, $P<0.01$) and, when this was corrected for, TBI was slightly but significantly more likely to be associated with schizophrenia (OR 1.37 and 1.29, respectively, $P<0.01$). The interpretation of fewer fractures in patients with schizophrenia is problematic, appearing to suggest that in the prodromal phase of schizophrenia, the patients' behavior such as social withdrawal made them less likely to sustain fractures. This finding was further complicated by the fact that the rates of fractures differed depending on the lag periods between injury and psychosis.

Nielsen et al. (2002) also examined the risk in relation to the interval between TBI and schizophrenia, and reported that TBI was more likely in the schizophrenia group in the 12 months preceding the index admission (OR 2.0 and 1.84, respectively, $P<0.01$) and less likely beyond the 1-year interval. Although this study should be considered to be largely negative, it does not rule out a small but significant increase in the risk of schizophrenia in the year following TBI. The study, through the linkage of registers, overcame recall bias. However, observer bias is not ruled out, because it is possible that the history of TBI prompted the clinicians to make a diagnosis of an "organic" psychosis rather than schizophrenia, leading to an underestimate of the association, something the retrospective design does not pick up.

A nested case-control study by Harrison et al. (2006) used a large birth cohort ($N$=785,051), from which 748 cases of schizophrenia and 14,960 matched controls were identified, and a TBI history documented through linkage with the various health registers in Sweden. This study found no increase in schizophrenia after TBI (OR 1.10, 95% CI 0.82–1.47) and only a small increase in nonschizophrenic, nonaffective psychosis (OR 1.37, 95% CI 1.14–1.66); the latter occurred only in association with TBI sustained during adolescence or later. The association was not appreciably influenced by including in the model various confounding factors (year of birth, highest parental income, highest parental education, highest parental occupation, area of birth, family history of psychosis, Apgar score at 5 minutes, gestational age, paternal age, birth weight, birth length). This is the largest case-control study in this field, and its reliance on record linkage and a birth cohort gives it much strength. However, it suffers from the same limitation as the Danish study (Nielsen et al. 2002) in terms of the diagnoses being made in different centers with lack of diagnostic standardization. Overall, this excellent study, in combination with the previous literature, shows that a strong link between TBI and schizophrenia is very unlikely, although a weak association cannot be excluded entirely.

Two other studies used the case-control method with the goal of determining whether TBI increased the risk of schizophrenia in individuals with a genetically increased risk of the disorder. Corcoran and Malaspina (2001) used the Diagnostic Interview for Genetic Studies to inquire about a history of significant head injury in individuals from multiplex schizophrenia pedigrees ($n=561$) and multiplex bipolar disorder pedigrees ($n=1,271$) participating in a genetics study. Overall, the individuals with schizophrenia were more than three times as likely to report a previous TBI as were unaffected individuals. This risk increased with the genetic risk of schizophrenia. In the bipolar pedigree, there was no increased risk, but the risk was fourfold in those with a high genetic risk for schizophrenia (OR 4.27, 95% CI 1.40–13.0). The authors did not test for an interaction effect, and therefore it is unclear whether the increased risk is specific to the group with a high genetic risk for schizophrenia. In a Canadian study, AbdelMalik et al. (2003) also used the case-control design in 23 multiply affected families with schizophrenia and reported that patients with schizophrenia had an excess of TBIs sustained before age 10 years (OR 2.34, 95% CI 1.03–5.03) or before age 17 years (OR 1.90, 95% CI 0.95–3.79), the former being statistically significant.

In summary, the case-control studies provide strong evidence that TBI does not substantially increase the risk of schizophrenia in the general population, although a small increase cannot be ruled out. In individuals with a genetic risk for schizophrenia, the increase in risk may be greater, although the retrospective nature of the studies makes the data prone to bias.

*Risk factors for schizophrenia-like psychosis after TBI.*
Some case-control studies have examined risk factors for schizophrenia-like psychosis following TBI, with a focus on the nature and extent of the injury and the demographic and family history characteristics. In their study, Sachdev et al. (2001) included 45 patients with schizophrenia-like psychosis following TBI, who had been referred for a medicolegal opinion and were so determined by the authors, and matched them with 45 persons with TBI and no schizophrenia-like psychosis or other psychiatric disorder. The authors found that a family history of schizophrenia was a risk factor for schizophrenia-like psychosis, but the nature and degree of TBI did not produce a significant effect, although the study was not powered for subtle effects. Although temporal lobe injury has been reported to be especially important (Achté et al. 1969), this anatomical risk factor was not observed in this study. In a similar case-control study, Fujii and Ahmed (2001) included 25 cases of psychosis secondary to TBI

and 25 controls, and reported that those patients with psychosis had a history of prior head injury or evidence of neurological disorder, suggesting brain damage as a source of vulnerability. The small size of the study and the broad and heterogeneous nature of brain damage make the results inconclusive. Moreover, the authors excluded patients who had a family history of psychosis, thereby making it impossible to examine an interaction with genetic vulnerability. As stated near the end of the previous subsection, two case-control studies (AbdelMalik et al. 2003; Corcoran and Malaspina 2001) reported that genetic vulnerability to schizophrenia, as suggested by a positive family history, was an important risk factor for the development of schizophrenia-like psychosis following TBI. The cohort studies have suggested similar risk factors. De Mol et al. (1987) reported high rates of premorbid psychopathology and suggested that the injury aggravated or precipitated, rather than caused, a preexisting condition. Premorbid psychiatric disorder was also considered to be important by Fann et al. (2004).

## CLINICAL FEATURES

Because the increase in risk of schizophrenia-like psychosis following TBI, albeit small, cannot be dismissed, it is important to examine whether putative posttraumatic schizophrenia-like psychosis is distinct from schizophrenia in its phenomenology, clinical associations, and prognosis. The description here is based primarily on the review by Davison and Bagley (1969) and two more recent reports of schizophrenia-like psychosis after TBI (Buckley et al. 1993; Fujii and Ahmed 2002), one of which was an analysis of 69 published cases (Fujii and Ahmed 2002).

The majority of the subjects in the case reports were young, with a male preponderance. The mean ages at onset of psychosis were 26.3 (SD 10.2) years and 33.4 (SD 15.4) years in the two studies, with 80% and 90% being men (Buckley et al. 1993; Fujii and Ahmed 2002). Because TBI is more common in young men, it is uncertain whether the schizophrenia-like psychosis rates merely reflect this. Fujii and Ahmed (2002) suggested that men may be overrepresented after accounting for the base rates for TBI, but this is far from established. In the large Danish study, in which the authors examined the effect of sex, the mean intervals between TBI and the development of psychosis were 4.6 (Sachdev et al. 2001) and 4.1 (Fujii and Ahmed 2002) years, with a wide range (0–34 years). Although most civilian TBIs are due to motor vehicle accidents, other causes such as assaults, gunshot injuries, and falls are represented in these data sets.

# Characteristics of Traumatic Brain Injury

The TBI associated with schizophrenia-like psychosis is more likely to be nonpenetrating than penetrating; contrary to some suggestions (Achté et al. 1969), penetrating TBI does not appear to be protective against the development of psychosis. The severity of the TBI associated with schizophrenia-like psychosis is usually moderate to severe. Although many schizophrenia-like psychoses occur after TBI in childhood, early TBI was not overrepresented in one large study (Sachdev et al. 2001). In about 40% of cases in this study, TBI was followed by personality or behavioral change, the main characteristics of which were impulsivity, aggressiveness, loss of social graces, moodiness, and, less commonly, apathy (Sachdev et al. 2001). Neuroimaging, clinical, and neuropsychological data provided evidence for brain damage in the temporal, parietal, and frontal lobes, more often unilateral than bilateral. Compared with the control group, the subjects with TBI and schizophrenia-like psychosis had more widespread neuropsychological deficits (Sachdev et al. 2001).

# Psychopathology

Prodromal symptoms are common among persons who develop schizophrenia-like psychosis after TBI. These prodromal symptoms include bizarre or antisocial behavior, social withdrawal, affective instability, and deterioration in work, often lasting for months. Depressive symptoms are often present at the time of presentation, but confusional symptoms at onset are unusual. The psychosis is generally delusional-hallucinatory in nature. A range of delusional symptoms, similar to those seen in schizophrenia, are present and include first-rank schneiderian symptoms. In the study by Sachdev et al. (2001), one or more delusions were present in all subjects, with persecutory (55.5%), referential (22.2%), control (22.2%), grandiose (20%), and religious (15.4%) delusions being the most common types. Delusions of thought alienation, insertion, withdrawal, or broadcast were present in six (13.3%) and somatic passivity in three (6.7%) subjects. The review by Fujii and Ahmed (2002) emphasized the presence of persecutory delusions. Organic themes, described by Cutting (1987), were absent in the Sachdev et al. (2001) study; however, the review of published cases (Fujii and Ahmed 2002) did find five cases with the Capgras delusion and three cases each with reduplicative paramnesia, erotomania, and stealing. Delusions relating to misidentification, stealing, or hiding, which are prone to occur in dementia patients with psychosis, are not generally seen in schizophrenia-like psychosis after TBI. These do occur, however, in patients who develop psychotic symptoms during the period of posttraumatic delirium (Marshall et al. 1995). Hallucinations are predominantly auditory or visual, with the former being more likely. Formal thought disorder and catatonic features are usually absent. Derealization as a basis of delusions has been reported in some cases (Young et al. 1992). The psychosis is therefore predominantly a positive syndrome, with only 22% and 15% of patients demonstrating negative symptoms such as flattening of affect, avolition, or asociality in the two studies. Agitation and aggressive behavior are common.

## Psychotic Symptoms Associated With Mood Disturbances

Disturbances of mood and affect are common among persons with schizophrenia-like psychosis after TBI. Additionally, psychotic symptoms have been reported to be common in patients who develop depression following TBI. Symonds (1937) reported that psychotic symptoms followed soon after the recovery from posttraumatic confusion. Hibbard et al. (1998) surveyed 100 community-dwelling patients about 1–7 years after TBI and reported that 23% of those diagnosed with major depression had psychotic symptoms. Psychotic symptoms in the setting of mania have also been reported in a series of case reports (Shukla et al. 1987; Starkstein et al. 1988).

## Course

The long-term course of schizophrenia-like psychosis after TBI is not well established. Fujii and Ahmed (2002) found some follow-up information on 39 of the 69 cases reviewed. Of these, 25 patients were reported to have improved, 11 had not improved, and 3 were worse. Sachdev et al. (2001) did not follow patients systematically, but it is not unusual for clinicians to encounter TBI-related psychosis that, despite its prominence of positive symptoms, responds poorly to antipsychotic medications.

# Risk Factors and Pathophysiology

*Neuroanatomical substrates.* Psychosis following focal brain injury is a relatively rare event, but several consistent observations relating right brain dysfunction to delusional disorders have emerged. Anatomically, lesions of the temporoparietal region are associated with the highest frequency of lesion-related psychosis (Cutting 1987). The data on anatomical localization in relation to TBI have not been consistent, and no convincing theoretical framework has emerged. In the study by Sachdev et al. (2001), the comparison of neuroimaging data from the subjects with TBI and schizophrenia-like psychosis and data from the control group suggested greater damage in the former group in the left temporal and right parietal regions, but the differences were not significant after Bonferroni correction. Fujii and Ahmed's (2002) review suggested a trend toward focal lesions affecting, in particular, the frontal and temporal lobes. Despite positive findings on computed tomography or magnetic resonance imaging scans for 65% of cases, no brain region emerged as being necessarily affected in patients with schizophrenia-like psychosis. Similarly, laterality has not emerged as a significant factor in the development of psychosis, although a suggestion has been made that left temporal lesions may be more common in those who develop schizophrenia-like psychosis (Sachdev et al. 2001).

*Cognition.* Cognitive deficits have the potential of providing continuity between the brain damage of TBI and the development of psychosis. If the cognitive deficits of schizophrenia-like psychosis among persons with TBI resemble those observed among persons with schizophrenia, and differ from the deficits seen in TBI patients who do not develop psychosis, an argument relating to their specificity can be supported. The question of what constitute core deficits in schizophrenia is still in dispute, although attention, memory, and executive deficits are broadly recognized as being characteristic. In the study by Sachdev et al. (2001), TBI subjects with schizophrenia-like psychosis were more likely to have abnormalities on measures of verbal and nonverbal memory and frontal executive functioning than were TBI subjects without psychosis; however, the former group also tended to have more of a disturbance in language and parietal lobe functioning, suggesting a diffuse impairment in neuropsychological functioning in comparison with the latter group. In the review by Fujii and Ahmed (2002), 88% of cases reported impairments on neuropsychological testing. The most common impaired function was memory, followed by executive and visuospatial functions. Clearly, more work is necessary to establish the salience and specificity of some neurocognitive deficits in the development of schizophrenia-like psychosis.

*Preinjury factors.* In the study by Corcoran and Malaspina (2001), no increase in risk for schizophrenia after TBI was found in the members of bipolar pedigrees (OR 0.75, 95% CI 0.10–5.93), but a fourfold increase was found in families with two or more first-degree relatives with schizophrenia (OR 4.27, 95% CI 1.40–13.0). The authors did not, however, test for interaction effects to confirm that this difference was greater than a chance effect. In the Sachdev et al. (2001) study, the most significant risk factor for schizophrenia-like psychosis after TBI was a genetic vulnerability to psychosis as reflected in the family history, even though this history was present in only a fraction of patients.

Family history has been used as a marker of genetic predisposition for schizophrenia and other psychiatric disorders. For schizophrenia, the lifetime risks of psychosis reported for first-degree relatives have varied from 3.1% to 16.9% (American Psychiatric Association 2000). The Sachdev et al. (2001) finding of 24% risk in first-degree relatives, compared to 3% for controls, is therefore high, even if an upward reporting bias in the schizophrenia-like psychosis group is considered as a factor. In a study of schizophrenia secondary to a variety of neurological disorders, Feinstein and Ron (1998) found a positive family history in only 3.8% of subjects. Among epilepsy patients with chronic schizophrenia-like psychosis, the risk of schizophrenia in first-degree relatives was reported by Slater et al. (1963, 1965) to be no higher than in the general population. It is possible that head injury brings out a vulnerability to schizophrenia due to genetic or other factors in at least some patients. Furthermore, AbdelMalik et al. (2003) reported that in those with a family history of schizophrenia, TBI before age 10 years was related to an earlier age at onset of schizophrenia.

*Epilepsy.* Some patients, depending on the location and severity of TBI, have seizures during the acute period after the trauma (see Chapter 14, "Seizures and Epilepsy"). The rate of epilepsy reported by Fujii and Ahmed (2002), in their review of schizophrenia-like psychosis secondary to TBI, was 34%, which is an overrepresentation (Fujii and Ahmed 1996). On the other hand, in the case-control study presented by Sachdev et al. (2001), the subjects with schizophrenia-like psychosis had a nonsignificant lower epilepsy rate, and epilepsy in these patients was well controlled, unlike in those TBI patients who were not psychotic and who had medication-resistant epilepsy. Sachdev et al. speculated that epileptic seizures might, in some way, be protective against the development of psychosis. An interesting observation from the Fujii and Ahmed (2002) review was that schizophrenia-like psychosis patients with epilepsy were less likely to have delusions than were those without epilepsy.

*Age at time of injury.* The schizophrenia literature suggests that brain injury early in childhood may be important in relation to the risk for schizophrenia (Dalman et al. 1999; Lewis and Murray 1987), because the brain injury is likely to disrupt normal neurodevelopment. The literature on schizophrenia-like psychosis after TBI does not consistently support this conclusion, however, and TBI in the individuals studied occurred across a wide age span, including childhood, adolescence, and adulthood. Wilcox and Nasrallah (1987) and Gureje et al. (1994) designed studies specifically to examine the effect of TBI in childhood and reported a strong association with schizophrenia-like psychosis. In a Canadian study of multiply affected families, injury before age 10 years was overrepresented in the schizophrenia cases (OR 2.34, 95% CI 1.03–5.36) (AbdelMalik et al. 2003). However, in the large Swedish case-control study by Harrison et al. (2006), the small increase in the incidence of nonschizophrenic, nonaffective psychosis occurred only in those incurring injury during adolescence or later. In the study by Sachdev et al. (2001), childhood injury was not overrepresented.

The proposal that pregnancy and birth complications are associated with an increased risk of schizophrenia has been extensively studied and is generally accepted despite some controversy (Lewis and Murray 1987). Wilcox and Nasrallah (1987) concluded that childhood head trauma before age 5 years was more likely to have occurred in patients with schizophrenia. Gureje et al. (1994), in another retrospective study, also found an association between childhood brain trauma and schizophrenia. The markers used to indicate these perinatal insults include low birth weight, prematurity, preeclampsia, prolonged labor, hypoxia, and fetal distress (McGrath and Murray 1995). The overall effect of perinatal accidents when calculated is small, increasing the risk of disease by only 1%. The evidence, therefore, points only to an association and not to causality.

# TREATMENT

The treatment of psychosis in the setting of TBI has not received systematic empirical investigation, and the evidence comprises anecdotal reports and expert opinion only. In general, the management of schizophrenia-like psychosis following TBI is not very different from that of a similar disorder in the absence of brain injury. Comprehensive neuropsychiatric assessment of preinjury history, injury characteristics, and postinjury course and outcomes is essential; the topics addressed in the preceding sections of this chapter serve as a useful guide to the areas on which the clinical evaluation should focus.

Treatment is principally pharmacological but also requires patient and family education, supportive counseling, and other rehabilitative (including vocational) interventions. A multidisciplinary team approach is frequently required, and following established practice guidelines for the psychiatric assessment of adults and the treatment of psychotic disorders is encouraged (American Psychiatric Association 2006).

Specific reports on the treatment of psychosis following TBI describe the use of risperidone (Arciniegas et al. 2003; Schreiber et al. 1998; Silver et al. 2005) and clozapine (Burke et al. 1999; Michals et al. 1993); however, no evidence is available to suggest that these agents are more effective or otherwise preferable to the other atypical (second-generation) or typical (first-generation) antipsychotics. Many clinicians recommend lower dosages of antipsychotic drugs when treating psychosis in individuals with brain injuries. First-generation antipsychotics are useful in many cases but may carry a somewhat higher risk of extrapyramidal side effects. Drugs with greater anticholinergic properties, such as olanzapine, clozapine, and chlorpromazine, also run a higher risk of worsening confusion or memory impairment. If affective instability is a feature and a mood stabilizer is being considered, sodium valproate is generally preferred over lithium because the latter has been reported to worsen ataxia and confusion and lower the seizure threshold (Silver et al. 2005). Clinicians should follow the dictum to "start low and go slow" when prescribing any drugs for these patients.

The patient may be experiencing, in addition to psychosis, other consequences of brain injury, in particular cognitive impairment, that may need attention using rehabilitative strategies and occasionally treatment with cholinomimetic drugs for memory impairment (Arciniegas 2011). Behavioral problems, especially agitation and aggression, in individuals with brain injuries and psychosis may be particularly challenging and will need independent attention.

The treatment of patients with comorbid psychosis, epilepsy, and TBI presents a particular challenge. Many antipsychotics may lower seizure threshold, and therefore treatment of psychosis with any of these drugs risks provoking seizures. This concern is particularly salient with clozapine, which lowers seizure threshold in a dose-dependent fashion. When psychosis remains refractory to other antipsychotics in a patient who also has epilepsy and TBI, combined treatment with sodium valproate with clozapine (Michals et al. 1993) may reduce the risk of treatment-induced seizures; however, no consensus has been reached on this strategy.

# MEDICOLEGAL CONSIDERATIONS

When TBI occurs in settings such as traffic or work-related accidents and produces persistent impairments and functional disability, such injuries are deemed compensable and may entail litigation. The occurrence of psychosis following a head injury can complicate the determination of TBI-related damages, especially when there is a delay of many years between the TBI and the onset of psychosis. Although the evidence of the association is not overwhelming, the argument that TBI contributes to the development of schizophrenia cannot be dismissed entirely. Medicolegal determination, therefore, must be made on a case-by-case basis, after consideration of the premorbid status of the individual, the nature of the TBI, the psychological trauma and social factors related to the injury, neuropsychological and anatomical deficits from the injury, and the nature of the psychosis that follows.

The level of evidence needed for medicolegal purposes differs from that required for scientific inquiry, and it is possible that some injuries may be compensable, at least partially, due to the subsequent development of schizophrenia-like psychosis. Such cases are often contentious because of lack of consensus, the great variability in both the TBI and the psychosis, and the need to obtain a categorical response for the court when a medical determination of relative risk would be more appropriate in light of the available data.

# CONCLUSION

Psychotic symptoms, including delusions and hallucinations, may occur in the early and late periods following TBI. In the early postinjury period, psychotic symptoms are most commonly manifestations of posttraumatic delirium. In the late postinjury period, these symptoms may be part of a schizophrenia-like psychosis, which is usually delusion predominant, or be associated features of a mood disorder. The role of TBI in the genesis of schizophrenia-like psychotic disorders is a matter of considerable debate. The best available epidemiological evidence suggests that TBI confers a modest increased risk for schizophrenia-like psychosis. Family history of a psychotic disorder appears to increase the risk for this outcome. Although evidence suggests that schizophrenia-like psychosis can be associated with male gender, TBI in childhood, nonpenetrating TBI, posttraumatic epilepsy, cognitive impairments, and focal lesions in frontal, temporal, and parietal areas, the available evidence does not permit definitive conclusions about their role as risk factors for this condition. All of these conditions merit consideration in the evaluation of persons with late postinjury psychotic disorders, and are important targets of treatment. The treatment of the psychosis itself is modeled after treatment provided to persons with idiopathic psychotic disorders, especially schizophrenia. Pharmacotherapy is the cornerstone of treatment and is complemented by patient and family education, supportive counseling, and vocational and rehabilitative interventions.

## *Key Clinical Points*

- Although anecdotal case reports and cohort studies have argued for an increased incidence of schizophrenia-like psychosis following TBI, case-control studies suggest that TBI does not substantially increase the risk of psychosis, although a small increase cannot be ruled out.

- The presence of genetic vulnerability, as evidenced by positive family history of schizophrenia, appears to increase the risk of schizophrenia-like psychosis following TBI.

- Other risk factors may include diffuse and severe injuries, especially those involving the temporal and frontal lobes, TBI early in life, cognitive impairments, and the presence of epilepsy. However, the evidence regarding the risk for schizophrenia-like psychosis conferred by these factors is mixed.

- The clinical presentation is similar to that seen in non-injury-related psychosis, but with the prominence of persecutory delusions, other delusions, and auditory hallucinations, and a dearth of negative symptoms.

# REFERENCES

AbdelMalik P, Husted J, Chow EW, et al: Childhood head injury and expression of schizophrenia in multiply affected families. Arch Gen Psychiatry 60:231–236, 2003

Achté KA, Hillbom E, Aalberg V: Psychoses following war brain injuries. Acta Psychiatr Scand 45:1–18, 1969

American Psychiatric Association: Diagnostic and Statistical Manual of Mental Disorders, 3rd Edition. Washington, DC, American Psychiatric Association, 1980

American Psychiatric Association: Diagnostic and Statistical Manual of Mental Disorders, 4th Edition, Text Revision. Washington, DC, American Psychiatric Association, 2000

American Psychiatric Association: American Psychiatric Association Practice Guidelines for the Treatment of Psychiatric Disorders, Compendium 2006. Washington, DC, American Psychiatric Association, 2006

Arciniegas DB: Cholinergic dysfunction and cognitive impairment after traumatic brain injury, part 2: evidence from basic and clinical investigations. J Head Trauma Rehabil 26:319–323, 2011

Arciniegas DB, Harris SN, Brousseau KM: Psychosis following traumatic brain injury. Int Rev Psychiatry 15:328–340, 2003

Buckley P, Stack JP, Madigan C, et al: Magnetic resonance imaging of schizophrenia-like psychoses associated with cerebral trauma: clinicopathological correlates. Am J Psychiatry 150:146–148, 1993

Burke JG, Dursun SM, Reveley MA: Refractory symptomatic schizophrenia resulting from frontal lobe lesion: response to clozapine. J Psychiatry Neurosci 24:456–461, 1999

Corcoran C, Malaspina D: Traumatic brain injury and risk for schizophrenia. Int J Ment Health 30:17–32, 2001

Cutting J: The phenomenology of acute organic psychosis: comparison with acute schizophrenia. Br J Psychiatry 151:324–332, 1987

Dalman C, Allebeck P, Cullberg J, et al: Obstetric complications and the risk of schizophrenia: a longitudinal study of a national birth cohort. Arch Gen Psychiatry 56:234–240, 1999

Davison K, Bagley CR: Schizophrenia-like psychosis associated with organic disorders of the central nervous system: a review of the literature, in Current Problems in Neuropsychiatry: Schizophrenia, Epilepsy, the Temporal Lobe. Edited by Herrington RN, Royal Medico-Psychological Association, and Glasgow Postgraduate Medical Board. London, Headley Bros, 1969, pp 1–89

De Mol J, Violon A, Brihaye J: Post-traumatic psychoses: a retrospective study of 18 cases. Archivio di Psicologia, Neurologia e Psichiatria 48:336–350, 1987

Fann JR, Burington B, Leonetti A, et al: Psychiatric illness following traumatic brain injury in an adult health maintenance organization population. Arch Gen Psychiatry 61:53–61, 2004

Feinstein A, Ron M: A longitudinal study of psychosis due to a general medical (neurological) condition: establishing predictive and construct validity. J Neuropsychiatry Clin Neurosci 10:448–452, 1998

Fujii D, Ahmed I: Psychosis secondary to traumatic brain injury. Neuropsychiatry Neuropsychol Behav Neurol 9:133–138, 1996

Fujii DE, Ahmed I: Risk factors in psychosis secondary to traumatic brain injury. J Neuropsychiatry Clin Neurosci 13:61–69, 2001

Fujii D, Ahmed I: Characteristics of psychotic disorder due to traumatic brain injury: an analysis of case studies in the literature. J Neuropsychiatry Clin Neurosci 14:130–140, 2002

Gureje O, Bamidele R, Raji O: Early brain trauma and schizophrenia in Nigerian patients. Am J Psychiatry 151:368–371, 1994

Harrison G, Whitley E, Rasmussen F, et al: Risk of schizophrenia and other non-affective psychosis among individuals exposed to head injury: case control study. Schizophr Res 88:119–126, 2006

Hibbard MR, Uysal S, Kepler K, et al: Axis I psychopathology in individuals with traumatic brain injury. J Head Trauma Rehabil 13:24–39, 1998

Krafft-Ebing RV: Ueber die durch Gehirnerschütterung und Kopfverletzung hervorgerufenen psychischen Krankheiten. Erlangen, Germany, F Enke, 1868

Lewis SW, Murray RM: Obstetric complications, neurodevelopmental deviance, and risk of schizophrenia. J Psychiatr Res 21:413–421, 1987

Lishman WA: Brain damage in relation to psychiatric disability after head injury. Br J Psychiatry 114:373–410, 1968

Marshall JC, Halligan PW, Wade DT: Reduplication of an event after head injury? A cautionary case report. Cortex 31:183–190, 1995

McGrath J, Murray RM: Risk factors for schizophrenia: from conception to birth, in Schizophrenia. Edited by Hirsch SR, Weinberger DR. Cambridge, MA, Blackwell Science, 1995, pp 187–205

Michals ML, Crismon ML, Roberts S, et al: Clozapine response and adverse effects in nine brain-injured patients. J Clin Psychopharmacol 13:198–203, 1993

Miller H, Stern G: The long-term prognosis of severe head injury. Lancet 1:225–229, 1965

Nielsen AS, Mortensen PB, O'Callaghan E, et al: Is head injury a risk factor for schizophrenia? Schizophr Res 55:93–98, 2002

Ota Y: Psychiatric studies on civilian head injuries, in The Late Effects of Head Injury. Edited by Walker AE, Caveness WF, Critchley M, et al. Springfield, IL, Charles C Thomas, 1969, pp 110–119

Roberts AH: Severe Accidental Head Injury: An Assessment of Long-Term Prognosis. London, Macmillan, 1979

Sachdev P, Smith JS, Cathcart S: Schizophrenia-like psychosis following traumatic brain injury: a chart-based descriptive and case-control study. Psychol Med 31:231–239, 2001

Schreiber S, Klag E, Gross Y, et al: Beneficial effect of risperidone on sleep disturbance and psychosis following traumatic brain injury. Int Clin Psychopharmacol 13:273–275, 1998

Shukla S, Cook BL, Mukherjee S, et al: Mania following head trauma. Am J Psychiatry 144:93–96, 1987

Silver J, Kramer R, Greenwald S, et al: The association between head injuries and psychiatric disorders: findings from the New Haven NIMH Epidemiologic Catchment Area study. Brain Inj 15:935–945, 2001

Silver J, Arciniegas DB, Yudofsky SC: Psychopharmacology, in Textbook of Traumatic Brain Injury. Edited by Silver JM, McAllister TW, Yudofsky SC. Washington, DC, American Psychiatric Publishing, 2005, pp 259–278

Slater E, Beard AW, Glithero E: The schizophrenialike psychoses of epilepsy. Br J Psychiatry 109:95–150, 1963

Slater E, Beard AW, Glithero E: Schizophrenia-like psychoses of epilepsy. Int J Psychiatry 1:6–30, 1965

Starkstein SE, Boston JD, Robinson RG: Mechanisms of mania after brain injury: 12 case reports and review of the literature. J Nerv Ment Dis 176:87–100, 1988

Symonds CP: Mental disorder following head injury. Proc R Soc Med 30:1081–1094, 1937

Wilcox JA, Nasrallah HA: Childhood head trauma and psychosis. Psychiatry Res 21:303–306, 1987

Young AW, Robertson IH, Hellawell DJ, et al: Cotard delusion after brain injury. Psychol Med 22:799–804, 1992

CHAPTER 10

# Aggressive Disorders

Stuart C. Yudofsky, M.D.
Jonathan M. Silver, M.D.
Karen E. Anderson, M.D.

**The onset of disorders** such as stroke and traumatic brain injury (TBI) is often sudden but is frequently followed by persistent and disabling long-term neuropsychiatric consequences. Few posttraumatic neuropsychiatric symptoms and syndromes are more disruptive to interpersonal familial, societal, educational, and occupational functioning and activities than agitation, aggression, and violent behaviors. Agitation and irritability that occur in a patient during the acute stages of recovery from TBI not only endanger the safety of the patient and his or her caregivers but also predict increased lengths of hospital stay and impaired cognition (Bogner et al. 2001). As recovery continues, low frustration tolerance and explosive behavior may develop in response to minimal provocation or sometimes may occur without any warning at all. These behaviors may be limited to irritability or may include violent outbursts resulting in damage to property or assaults on others. In severe cases, it may be unsafe for individuals with aggressive disorders to remain in the community or with their families, and referral to long-term psychiatric or neurobehavioral facilities is sometimes required. All clinicians, and especially mental health professionals, need to be knowledgeable about and able to evaluate and treat neurologically induced agitation, irritability, aggression, and violence among their patients with TBI.

# DEFINITIONS

The definitions of *aggression* and *agitation* have long been plagued by inconsistency, imprecision, and ambiguity. These problems lead to confusion of nosology and measurement and, consequently, diminish the quality of data used to determine diagnosis, prognosis, and treatment. In an effort to ameliorate this problem, two of us (S.C.Y. and J.M.S.), in association with devoted research colleagues, developed, validated, and established the reliability of the Overt Aggression Scale (OAS; Yudofsky et al. 1986) and the Overt Agitation Severity Scale (OASS; Yudofsky et al. 1997). These measures were designed to provide operationalized definitions and objective measurements of aggression and agitation, respectively. The scale authors conceptualized aggressive disorders as occurring along an objective-to-subjective continuum, from aggression to agitation to anxiety. This conceptualization and these scales have gained widespread use and application in both the research and clinical communities, particularly in neuropsychiatry. For the purposes of this chapter, then, the definitions of aggression and agitation comprise meeting the criteria for these as measured by the OAS and the OASS. Both scales are included in their entirety below in "Documenting Aggressive Behavior."

# EPIDEMIOLOGY

Several prospective studies of the occurrence of aggression, agitation, or restlessness following TBI used objective rating instruments such as the OAS. In a prospective study of 100 patients admitted to a regional Level I trauma center who had a Glasgow Coma Scale score of less than 8, had more than 1 hour of coma, and required more than 1 week of hospitalization, only 11 patients exhibited agitated behavior (Brooke et al. 1992). Three patients manifested these behaviors for more than 1 week; however, 35 were observed to be restless but not agitated during this period of observation. In a study of 89 patients assessed during the first 6 months after TBI, aggressive behavior developed in 33.7% of individuals with TBI, compared with 11.5% of patients with multiple trauma but without TBI (Tateno et al. 2003). In a prospective study of 67 patients after TBI, 28.4% exhibited aggressive behavior that was limited, in all but one patient, to verbal aggression (Rao et al. 2009).

In a survey of all skilled nursing facilities in Connecticut, 45% had individuals with a primary diagnosis of TBI who met the definition of agitation (Wolf et al. 1996). In a series of 67 patients admitted with mild to moderate TBI who were studied prospectively, restlessness occurred in 40% and agitation in 19% (van der Naalt et al. 2000). In a study of psychiatric disorders in 100 self-referred individuals who had had TBI several years earlier, 34% admitted to symptoms of irritability (i.e., increased number of arguments/fights, making quick impulsive decisions, complaining, cursing at self, feeling impatient, or threatening to hurt self), and 14% admitted to aggressive behavior (i.e., cursing at others, screaming/yelling, breaking/throwing things, being arrested, hitting/pushing others, threatening to hurt others) (Hibbard et al. 1998). In follow-up periods ranging from 1 to 15 years after injury, these behaviors occurred in 31%–71% of patients who experienced severe TBI.

Studies of mild TBI have evaluated individuals for much briefer periods of time: 1-year estimates of irritability, temper, or agitation from these studies range from 5% to 70%. A small study of death row inmates found that 75% had a history of TBI (Freedman and Hemenway 2000). Irritability also appears to increase with repeated injuries (Carlsson et al. 1987). Of the men who had no head injuries with loss of consciousness, 21% reported irritability, whereas 31% of men with one injury with loss of consciousness and 33% of men with two or more injuries with loss of consciousness admitted to this symptom. In an evaluation of 60 subjects in a county jail, those with TBI in the prior year had significantly worse anger and aggression and trended toward poorer cognition and more psychiatric disorders (Slaughter et al. 2003). In a group of 458 research subjects, aggression was elevated as a function of TBI and personality disorder (Ferguson and Coccaro 2009).

Predicting who will develop aggressive behaviors after brain injury is challenging. Risk factors may include male gender, younger age at injury, lower preinjury intellectual function, preinjury history of aggression, preinjury alcohol and substance abuse, poor premorbid social functioning, frontal lobe lesions, and/or postinjury major depression, irritability, impulsivity, other physical illnesses, psychosocial dysfunction, and low life satisfaction (Baguley et al. 2006; Hammond et al. 2006; Jorge et al. 2004; Rao et al. 2009; Tateno et al. 2003; Wood and Liossi 2006). Neuropsychological performance does not consistently predict propensity toward violence in those who have experienced brain injury (Greve et al. 2001). However, impaired verbal memory and visuospatial abilities have been associated with posttraumatic aggression (Wood and Liossi 2006).

# CLINICAL ASSESSMENT

In the acute phase after brain injury, patients often experience a period of agitation and confusion that may last from days to months. In our clinical experience, after the acute recovery phase has resolved, continuing aggressive outbursts have typical characteristics (Table 10–1). These episodes may occur in the presence of other emotional changes or neurological disorders that occur secondary to brain injury, such as affective lability or seizures.

Certain behavioral syndromes have been related to damage to specific areas of the frontal lobe. Orbitofrontal syndrome is associated with behavioral excesses such as impulsivity, disinhibition, hyperactivity, distractibility, and emotional lability. Outbursts of rage and violent behavior occur after damage to the inferior orbital surface of the frontal lobe and anterior temporal lobes. The diagnostic category that captures such problems in DSM-IV-TR is "personality change due to a general medical condition" (Table 10–2) (American Psychiatric Association 2000). Patients with aggressive behavior would be specified as "aggressive type," whereas those with emotional lability would be specified as "labile type."

**TABLE 10–1.**   Characteristic features of aggression after brain injury

| TYPE | FEATURES |
| --- | --- |
| Reactive | Triggered by modest or trivial stimuli. |
| Nonreflective | Usually does not involve premeditation or planning. |
| Nonpurposeful | Aggression serves no obvious long-term aims or goals. |
| Explosive | Buildup is *not* gradual. |
| Periodic | Brief outbursts of rage and aggression punctuated by long periods of relative calm. |
| Ego-dystonic | After outbursts, patients are upset, concerned, and/or embarrassed, as opposed to blaming others or justifying behavior. |

---

**TABLE 10–2.** DSM-IV-TR criteria for personality change due to a general medical condition

---

A. A persistent personality disturbance that represents a change from the individual's previous characteristic personality pattern. (In children, the disturbance involves a marked deviation from normal development or a significant change in the child's usual behavior patterns lasting at least 1 year.)

B. There is evidence from the history, physical examination, or laboratory findings that the disturbance is the direct physiological consequence of a general medical condition.

C. The disturbance is not better accounted for by another mental disorder (including other mental disorders due to a general medical condition).

D. The disturbance does not occur exclusively during the course of a delirium.

E. The disturbance causes clinically significant distress or impairment in social, occupational, or other important areas of functioning.

*Specify* type:

**Labile type:** if the predominant feature is affective lability

**Disinhibited type:** if the predominant feature is poor impulse control as evidenced by sexual indiscretions, etc.

**Aggressive type:** if the predominant feature is aggressive behavior

**Apathetic type:** if the predominant feature is marked apathy and indifference

**Paranoid type:** if the predominant feature is suspiciousness or paranoid ideation

**Other type:** if the presentation is not characterized by any of the above subtypes

**Combined type:** if more than one feature predominates in the clinical picture

**Unspecified type**

---

*Source.* Reprinted from *Diagnostic and Statistical Manual of Mental Disorders,* 4th Edition, Text Revision. Washington, DC, American Psychiatric Association, 2000. Used with permission. © 2000 American Psychiatric Association.

During the time period of emergence from coma, agitated behaviors can occur as the result of delirium. The usual clinical picture is one of restlessness, confusion, and disorientation. For patients who become aggressive after TBI, it is important to systematically assess for the presence of concurrent neurological and neuropsychiatric disorders because findings from such assessments guide treatment.

When aggressive behavior occurs during the later stages of recovery from posttraumatic encephalopathy, the question of whether aggressivity and impulsivity antedated, were caused by, or were aggravated by the brain injury becomes particularly relevant. Many patients are able to differentiate between the aggressivity exhibited before brain injury and postinjury dyscontrol, the latter of which tends to be less purposeful and amenable to control than the former. Additionally, other preinjury and postinjury neuropsychiatric problems may cause or exacerbate posttraumatic aggression. Therefore, assessment in this context also emphasizes identification of learning disabilities, attention-deficit/hyperactivity disorder, behavioral problems, personality disorders, substance abuse, and co-occurring anxiety and depressive disorders.

Medication effects and side effects commonly result in disinhibition or irritability (Table 10–3). The drug most commonly associated with aggression is alcohol, including intoxication and withdrawal. Stimulating drugs such as cocaine and amphetamines, as well as the stimulating antidepressants, may produce severe anxiety and agitation in patients with or without brain lesions. Antipsychotic medications often increase agitation through anticholinergic side effects, and agitation and irritability usually accompany severe akathisia. Many other drugs may produce confusional states, especially anticholinergic medications that cause agitated delirium. Drugs such as the tricyclic antidepressants and the aliphatic phenothiazine antipsychotic drugs (e.g., chlorpromazine and thioridazine) are well known to have potent anticholinergic effects. Other drugs that have anticholinergic properties that are less commonly recognized include digoxin, ranitidine, cimetidine, theophylline, nifedipine, codeine, and furosemide (Tune et al. 1992).

Patients with TBI are susceptible to developing other medical disorders that may increase aggressive behaviors, and comorbidity must always be considered in the individual who exhibits agitation after TBI (Table 10–4). The clinician should not assume a priori that the brain injury is the cause of the aggressivity but rather should assess the patient for the presence of other common etiologies of aggression. Because patients with neurological disorders are more susceptible to accidents, falls, and other sources of brain disorders, another, comorbid neurological disorder may be the underlying condition that results in TBI. When exacerbations or recurrences of aggressive behavior occur in a patient who has been in good control, an investi-

**TABLE 10–3.** Medications associated with aggression

| MEDICATIONS | ASSOCIATION WITH AGGRESSION |
| --- | --- |
| Alcohol | Aggression during intoxication and withdrawal states |
| Sedative-hypnotic medications (benzodiazepines, benzodiazepine-like agents, barbiturates) | Aggression during intoxication and withdrawal states |
| Opiate analgesics and other narcotics | Aggression during intoxication and withdrawal states |
| Corticosteroids and anabolic steroids | Aggression from acute or chronic administration |
| Antidepressants | Aggression during initial phases of treatment |
| Central nervous system stimulants | Excitement-related aggression in early stages of use/abuse, and paranoia-related aggression in later stages of use/abuse/dependence |
| Antipsychotics | Akathisia-related aggression |
| Anticholinergic medications | Delirium-related aggression |

**TABLE 10–4.** Common etiologies of aggression in individuals with traumatic brain injury

Medications, alcohol and other abused substances, and over-the-counter drugs

Delirium (e.g., hypoxia, electrolyte imbalance, anesthesia and surgery, uremia)

Alzheimer disease

Infectious diseases (encephalitis, meningitis, pneumonia, urinary tract infections)

Epilepsy (ictal, postictal, interictal)

Metabolic disorders (e.g., hyperthyroidism or hypothyroidism, hypoglycemia, vitamin deficiencies)

gation must be completed to search for other etiologies, such as depression, anxiety, posttraumatic stress disorder, pain, infection, medication effects, delirium, and/or changes or problems in social circumstances (including interactions with caregivers).

Epilepsy is sometimes associated with postictal or interictal hostility, irritability, and aggression (Mendez et al. 1986; Robertson et al. 1987; Weiger and Bear 1988). Ictal or postictal aggression is generally nondirected and associated with altered consciousness (i.e., postictal confusion), and these features are not characteristic of interictal aggression. Temporal lobe epilepsy–associated aggression appears more likely with early age at onset of seizures, a long duration of behavioral problems, and male gender, but not with electroencephalographic or neuroimaging abnormalities or a history of psychosis (Herzberg and Fenwick 1988; Stevens and Hermann 1981).

Psychosocial factors are important in the expression of aggressive behavior among individuals with TBI who are sensitive to changes in their environment or to variations in emotional support. Social conditions, disability, and support networks that existed before the injury affect the symptoms and course of recovery (Brown et al. 1981; Rao et al. 2009). Some patients become aggressive only in specific circumstances, such as in the presence of particular family members. This pattern of context-specific or interpersonal interaction–dependent aggression suggests that the individual may have some level of control over aggressive behaviors that can be used as a foundation for behavioral interventions designed to increase that control. Most families require professional support to adjust to the impulsive behavior of a violent relative with posttraumatic aggression. Frequently, efforts to avoid triggering a rageful or violent episode lead families to withdraw from a patient. This can result in a paradox: the patient learns to gain attention by being aggressive. Thus, the unwanted behavior is unwittingly reinforced by familial withdrawal.

# DOCUMENTING AGGRESSIVE BEHAVIOR

Before initiating therapeutic intervention to treat violent behavior, the clinician should document the baseline frequency of these behaviors. Aggression can spontaneously fluctuate from day to day and week to week and, like some mood disorders, may have cyclic exacerbations. These patterns are difficult to identify and interpret without prospective documentation (Silver and Yudofsky 1987, 1991). Objective documentation of aggressive episodes also is used to monitor the efficacy of interventions and to designate specific time frames for the initiation and discontinuation of pharmacotherapy for acute episodes and for the initiation of pharmacotherapy for chronic aggressive behavior.

The OAS (Figure 10–1) is an operationalized instrument of proven reliability and validity that can be used easily and effectively to rate aggressive behavior in patients with a wide range of disorders (Silver and Yudofsky 1987, 1991; Yudofsky et al. 1986). The scale includes items that assess verbal aggression, as well as physical aggression against objects, self, and others. Each category of aggression has four levels of severity that are defined by objective criteria. An aggression score can be derived by obtaining the sum of the most severe ratings of each type of aggressive behavior over a particular time course. Aggressive behavior can be monitored by staff or family members using the OAS. Documentation of agitation can be objectively rated with the OASS (Figure 10–2) (Kopecky et al. 1998; Yudofsky et al. 1997).

# TREATMENT

Aggressive and agitated behaviors may be treated in a variety of settings, ranging from the acute brain injury unit in a general hospital, to a "neurobehavioral" unit in a rehabilitation facility, to outpatient environments including the home setting. A multifactorial, multidisciplinary, collaborative approach to treatment is necessary in most cases. The continuation of family treatments, psychopharmacological interventions, and psychotherapeutic approaches is also usually appropriate. When establishing a treatment plan for patients with agitation or aggression, the overarching principle guiding its development is that diagnosis comes before treatment. History taking, organized within a biopsychosocial framework, is usually the most critical part of the evaluation. It is essential to determine the patient's mental status before the agitated or aggressive event, the physical and social environment in which the behavior occurs, any identifiable precipitant (external or internal to the patient), the ways in which the event is mitigated, and the primary and secondary gains related to agitation and aggression.

Although no medication has been approved by the U.S. Food and Drug Administration (FDA) specifically for the treatment of aggression, medications are widely used (and commonly misused) in the

| OVERT AGGRESSION SCALE (OAS) | | |
|---|---|---|
| Stuart Yudofsky, M.D., Jonathan Silver, M.D., Wynn Jackson, M.D., and Jean Endicott, Ph.D. | | |

**IDENTIFYING DATA**

| Name of Patient | Name of Rater |
|---|---|
| Sex of Patient:  1 Male    2 Female | Date    /    /    (month/day/year)<br>Shift:  1 Night    2 Day    3 Evening |

❏ No aggressive incidents (verbal or physical) against self, others, or objects during the shift. (check here)

**AGGRESSIVE BEHAVIOR** (check all that apply)

| VERBAL AGGRESSION | PHYSICAL AGGRESSION AGAINST SELF |
|---|---|
| ❏ Makes loud noises, shouts angrily | ❏ Picks or scratches skin, hits self, pulls hair (with no or minor injury only) |
| ❏ Yells mild personal insults (e.g., "You're stupid!") | ❏ Bangs head, hits fist into objects, throws self onto floor or into objects (hurts self without serious injury) |
| ❏ Curses viciously, uses foul language in anger, makes moderate threats to others or self | ❏ Small cuts or bruises, minor burns |
| ❏ Makes clear threats of violence toward others or self (e.g., "I'm going to kill you") or requests to help to control self | ❏ Mutilates self, makes deep cuts, bites that bleed, internal injury, fracture, loss of consciousness, loss of teeth |

| PHYSICAL AGGRESSION AGAINST OBJECTS | PHYSICAL AGGRESSION AGAINST OTHER PEOPLE |
|---|---|
| ❏ Slams door, scatters clothing, makes a mess | ❏ Makes threatening gesture, swings at people, grabs at clothes |
| ❏ Throws objects down, kicks furniture without breaking it, marks the wall | ❏ Strikes, kicks, pushes, pulls hair (without injury to them) |
| ❏ Breaks objects, smashes windows | ❏ Attacks others causing mild–moderate physical injury (bruises, sprains, welts) |
| ❏ Sets fires, throws objects dangerously | ❏ Attacks others causing severe physical injury (broken bones, deep lacerations, internal injury) |

| Time incident began: ____:____ A.M./P.M. | Duration of incident: ____:____ (hours/minutes) |
|---|---|

**INTERVENTION** (check all that apply)

| | | |
|---|---|---|
| ❏ None | ❏ Immediate medication given by mouth | ❏ Use of restraints |
| ❏ Talking to patient | ❏ Immediate medication given by injection | ❏ Injury requires immediate medical treatment for patient |
| ❏ Closer observation | ❏ Isolation without seclusion (time-out) | ❏ Injury requires immediate treatment for another person |
| ❏ Holding patient | ❏ Seclusion | |

**COMMENTS**

|  |
|---|
|  |

**FIGURE 10–1.** The Overt Aggression Scale.

*Source.* Reprinted from Yudofsky SC, Silver JM, Jackson W, et al.: "The Overt Aggression Scale for the Objective Rating of Verbal and Physical Aggression." *American Journal of Psychiatry* 143:35–39, 1986. Used with permission.

acute and chronic management of patients with aggressive disorders. The reported effectiveness of these medications is highly variable, as are the reported rationales for their prescription. Some of these medications are offered to inhibit excessive activity in temporolimbic areas (e.g., anticonvulsants), to reduce "hyperactive" limbic monoaminergic

| Overt Agitation Severity Scale (OASS) | | | | | | |
|---|---|---|---|---|---|---|
| | | Frequency (F) | | | | |
| Intensity (I) | Behavior | Not present | Rarely | Some of the time | Most of the time | Always present | Severity score (SS) (I x F = SS) |
| **A** | **Vocalizations and oral/facial movements** | | | | | |
| 1 | Whimpering, whining, moaning, grunting, crying | 0 | 1 | 2 | 3 | 4 | = ____ |
| 2 | Smacking or licking of lips, chewing, clenching jaws, licking, grimacing, spitting | 0 | 1 | 2 | 3 | 4 | = ____ |
| 3 | Rocking, twisting, banging of head | 0 | 1 | 2 | 3 | 4 | = ____ |
| 4 | Vocal perseverating, screaming, cursing, threatening, wailing | 0 | 1 | 2 | 3 | 4 | = ____ |
| **B** | **Upper torso and upper extremity movements** | | | | | |
| 1 | Tapping fingers, fidgeting, wringing of hands, swinging or flailing arms | 0 | 1 | 2 | 3 | 4 | = ____ |
| 2 | Task perseverating (e.g., opening and closing drawers, folding and unfolding clothes, picking at objects, clothes, or self) | 0 | 1 | 2 | 3 | 4 | = ____ |
| 3 | Rocking (back and forth), bobbing (up and down), twisting or writhing of torso, rubbing or masturbating self | 0 | 1 | 2 | 3 | 4 | = ____ |
| 4 | Slapping, swatting, hitting at objects or others | 0 | 1 | 2 | 3 | 4 | = ____ |
| **C** | **Lower extremity movements** | | | | | |
| 1 | Tapping toes, clenching toes, tapping heel, extending, flexing, or twisting foot | 0 | 1 | 2 | 3 | 4 | = ____ |
| 2 | Shaking legs, tapping knees and/or thighs, thrusting pelvis, stomping | 0 | 1 | 2 | 3 | 4 | = ____ |
| 3 | Pacing, wandering | 0 | 1 | 2 | 3 | 4 | = ____ |
| 4 | Thrashing legs, kicking at objects or others | 0 | 1 | 2 | 3 | 4 | = ____ |
| | | | | | Total OASS | = ____ |
| | | | | | Subtract baseline OASS | = ____ |
| | | | | | Revised OASS | = ____ |

**Instructions for Completing Form**

Step one: For each behavior, circle the corresponding frequency.

Step two: For every behavior *exhibited*, multiply the intensity score (I) by the frequency (F) and record as the severity score (SS).

Step three: For the Overt Agitation Severity Score (OASS), total all severity scores and record as total OASS.

Step four: Does this patient have a neuromuscular disorder (i.e., Parkinson's disease, tardive dyskinesia) affecting total OASS? Yes    No

Step five: If yes, please establish a baseline OASS in nonagitated state and subtract from above total OASS for revised OASS.

Comments: _____

Diagnosis: _____    Name of rater: _____

Sex of patient:   Male (1)   Female (2)    Time of observation: _____

Age: _____    Date: _____

Current medication:

| | | |
|---|---|---|
| Name: _____ | Dose: _____ | Frequency: _____ |
| Name: _____ | Dose: _____ | Frequency: _____ |
| Name: _____ | Dose: _____ | Frequency: _____ |
| Name: _____ | Dose: _____ | Frequency: _____ |

**FIGURE 10–2.** The Overt Agitation Severity Scale.

*Source.* Reprinted from Yudofsky SC, Kopecky HJ, Kunik ME, et al.: "The Overt Agitation Severity Scale for the Objective Rating of Agitation." *Journal of Neuropsychiatry and Clinical Neurosciences* 9:541–548, 1997. Used with permission.

neurotransmission (e.g., noradrenergic blockade with propranolol, dopaminergic blockade with haloperidol), to augment orbitofrontal and/or dorsolateral prefrontal cortical activity with monoaminergic agonists (e.g., amantadine, methylphenidate, or perhaps buspirone, or to increase serotonergic input (i.e., selective serotonin reuptake inhibitors [SSRIs]). Unfortunately, few rigorous, double-blind, placebo-controlled studies or prospective cohort studies are available to guide clinicians in the use of pharmacological interventions (Warden et al. 2006).

The approach to treatment that we suggest starts with appropriate assessment of possible etiologies of these behaviors. Treatment is directed first and foremost at comorbid neuropsychiatric conditions (e.g., depression, psychosis, insomnia, anxiety, delirium). Concurrent behavioral and pharmacological management of aggression may be necessary, especially when aggression presents a risk of harm to the patient, others, or the patient's environment. When other contributors to aggressive behavior are not present, then aggression-specific behavioral and pharmacological treatments may be appropriate. In this chapter, we provide a brief overview of the most commonly used and practical treatments. Detailed reviews of the literature supporting these treatments are presented elsewhere (Warden et al. 2006).

## Nonpharmacological Interventions

Psychological, behavioral, and environmental assessment and management are essential elements of the treatment of persons with aggressive disorders following TBI. A few approaches about which clinicians should be aware are described here.

*Psychotherapy.* Supportive counseling provided to patients and/or their caregivers aims to develop a therapeutic alliance, engage the patient and others in treatment, provide education about TBI and behaviors, develop effective coping skills that reduce the frequency and severity of aggressive behaviors, and address barriers to and/or facilitators of treatment success. For patients with the cognitive and communication skills required for treatment with other types of psychotherapy, cognitive-behavioral therapy, dialectical behavior therapy, interpersonal therapy, and group (including family) therapy also may be useful (Anson and Ponsford 2006; Cicerone et al. 2008; Coetzer 2007; Delmonico et al. 1998; Ponsford et al. 2003). Cognitive-behavioral therapies appear to be particularly useful for improving coping skills and increasing frustration tolerance, and may concurrently diminish depressive, anxious, and anger symptoms that contribute to agitation and aggression (Burg et al. 2000; Tiersky et al. 2005).

A critical element of the use of psychotherapy for persons with TBI is matching the techniques to each patient's cognitive abilities. In general, a neutral or passive approach is likely to be less useful than one that is active and, for patients with cognitive impairment, gently and supportively directive. It also is helpful to extend the psychotherapeutic process to caregivers, family members, and others with whom the patient routinely interacts; such extensions include education and support, coping skill development, behavioral analysis (described in the next section), and realistic problem solving.

Even when patients present with severe cognitive impairments, transferences may arise to the treating clinician and the settings in which treatments occur. Although offering transference interpretations to a patient with severe cognitive impairments may not be useful or appropriate, remaining mindful of the influence of transference on behavior and treatment response may help identify precipitants for behaviors and potential avenues of intervention (including necessary changes in caregiving styles, caregivers, and/or the environment) that otherwise might go unrecognized during treatment. Countertransferences, including potentially countertherapeutic reactions, to aggressive patients and/or their caregivers also arise commonly during treatment. Identifying and managing these responses may help minimize their potentially adverse effects on treatment selection and delivery.

*Behavioral analysis and environmental interventions.*
Behavioral and environmental interventions are the cornerstones of the treatment of aggressive disorders following TBI. Behavioral analysis in this context is most simply approached using the ABC (antecedents, behaviors, and consequences) method (Alpert and Spillmann 1997).

*Antecedents* to problematic behaviors or neuropsychiatric symptoms are identified through assiduous history taking and observation. Common causes of problematic behaviors include previously unrecognized or undertreated medical, neurological, psychiatric (especially mood), or substance use disorders; communication difficulties between patient and caregivers; and environmental factors (e.g., poor fit between patient and residence, including persons with whom the patient resides or interacts). Suspicion for problems in the interaction between the patient and the usual caregivers, companions, and/or environment must be particularly high when the patient fails to demonstrate agitated or aggressive behaviors when separated from them (e.g., upon hospitalization, following a change in caregivers or roommate). Once such a history is identified, treatment is directed at eliminating or modifying antecedents to problematic behaviors. This type of treatment may not obviate pharmacotherapy, especially for patients with severe cognitive impairments or easily provoked behaviors. However, pharmacotherapy (short of severe sedation) is unlikely to reduce problematic behaviors when their reliable triggers are not addressed.

*Behaviors* require characterization with regard to their types and severities as well as their possible meanings. Agitation and aggression may be symptoms of psychosis, depression, mania, anxiety, or other neuropsychiatric disturbances; among patients unable to express themselves verbally or effectively, problematic behaviors may be the principal means by which the patients communicate neuropsychiatric distress generated by such conditions. Similarly, agitation and aggression may be manifestations of distress over losses, interpersonal conflicts, or other social or psychological stressors (Block 1987; Persinger 1993), especially when the patient's understanding of such events is limited by cognitive impairments. Pain, physical discomfort, or other physical feelings (e.g., akathisia) also may produce agitation, aggression, or both.

In some cases, agitation and aggression are problems in their own right and carry no intrinsic meaning; however, repeated episodes of agitation and aggression may lead to self-understandings (i.e., "I can't control my behavior," "I'm a dangerous [or bad] person") that imbue these behaviors with meaning for the patient and/or others. With these and other considerations in mind, the clinician evaluating a patient's behaviors must attempt to understand them in neurobiological, medical, psychological, and environmental terms. Although clinical formulations about the meaning of problematic behaviors often must remain speculative, the hypotheses they yield guide nonpharmacological and pharmacological management of agitation and aggression toward their underlying causes.

The *consequences* of a patient's behaviors also require identification. Misunderstanding the meaning of agitation and/or aggression may lead caregivers or others to provide consequences that not only fail to effectively reduce these behaviors but also inadvertently reinforce them. For example, if agitation reflects pain, fatigue, hunger, the need to urinate or defecate, or environmental overstimulation, then responding to that behavior with limit setting or redirection should not be expected to reduce the behavior. In fact, these consequences may lead to an escalation of the behavior when the need driving it continues both to go unmet and to engender increasingly harsh responses from others. Conversely, if a patient receives caregiving only in response to agitation or aggression, those behaviors are reinforced, are likely to recur, and may escalate over time. Operant conditioning—in which behavior X is followed by consequence Y, thereby reinforcing (positively or negatively) behavior X—powerfully affects behavior for better and for worse. When the methods of operation are taken into account, conditioning provides an approach both to the elimination of consequences that are unintentionally reinforcing problematic behaviors and to facilitating their replacement by ones that are more adaptive.

## Pharmacotherapy of Acute Aggression

*Antipsychotic medications.* Antipsychotics are the most commonly used medications in the treatment of aggression. Although these agents are appropriate and effective when aggression is derivative of active psychosis, the use of antipsychotic agents to treat chronic aggression, especially chronic aggression secondary to TBI, is often ineffective and may entail serious medical and neurological complications. In general, the use of these medications, which is predicated on their sedative side effects rather than their antipsychotic properties, serves only to mask the aggression with sedation. Often, patients develop tolerance to the sedative effects and therefore require increasing dosages of these agents. When treatment involves first-generation antipsychotic medications, such increases often produce extrapyramidal side effects and anticholinergic-related cognitive and other physical side effects. Paradoxically (and frequently), and usually because of the development of akathisia, the patient may become more agitated and restless as the dosage of neuroleptic is increased, especially when a high-potency antipsychotic such as haloperidol is administered. Akathisia is often mistaken for increased irritability and agitation, and this mistake precipitates a cycle of increasing neuroleptics and worsening akathisias. Although this cycle is less common with most of the second-generation antipsychotic medications, their use for the treatment of chronic aggression leads to risks of significant weight gain and the metabolic syndrome. Hence, their use for this purpose is best avoided.

Some evidence suggests that medications that potently antagonize dopamine type 2 ($D_2$) receptors interfere with recovery from brain injury (Hoffman et al. 2008; Kline et al. 2007, 2008). Possibly, the effect of decreasing dopamine and inhibiting neuronal function, which may be the mechanism of action to treat aggression, may have other detrimental effects on recovery, may delay it, or both (Rao et al. 1985). The effect of atypical antipsychotics (which, in general, are less potent antagonists of $D_2$ receptors) on recovery after TBI is less clear, and may vary with the specific receptor profiles of each agent. However, the available evidence raises important potential risk-benefit concerns that must be considered before antipsychotic medications are used to treat aggressive behaviors of persons with TBI.

When an antipsychotic medication is used for the treatment of acute aggression for persons with TBI, we recommend starting an atypical antipsychotic medication (e.g., risperidone 0.5 mg orally) and repeating administration of the agent every hour until control of aggression is achieved. If several administrations of the atypical antipsychotic do not reduce aggression, then the hourly dose may be increased until the patient is so sedated that he or she no longer exhibits agitation or violence. After 48 hours of behavioral improvement, the daily dosage of the medication should be decreased gradually (i.e., by 25% per day) to ascertain whether aggressive behavior will reemerge. If it does, then consideration must be given to increasing the dosage of the antipsychotic and/or initiating treatment with a more specific antiaggressive drug.

*Benzodiazepines.* Reports of the effects of benzodiazepines in the treatment of aggression following TBI are inconsistent. The sedative properties of benzodiazepines are especially helpful in the management of acute agitation and aggression, most likely because of the amplifying effect of benzodiazepines on the inhibitory neurotransmitter γ-aminobutyric acid (GABA). Paradoxically, several studies report increased hostility and aggression and the induction of rage in patients treated with benzodiazepines (Smith 1995). Although this paradoxical effect seems to be rare, it presents very substantial management challenges. Benzodiazepines reliably impair cognition and motor function, including coordination and balance, in healthy individuals as well as in persons with TBI (Bleiberg et al. 1993). For these reasons, in the treatment of acute aggression in patients with TBI, we prefer to avoid, or to limit as much as possible, the use of benzodiazepines.

# Pharmacotherapy of Chronic Aggression

For patients who exhibit agitation or aggression for several weeks or more and/or whose responses to nonpharmacological interventions are suboptimal, medications specifically targeting aggression should be initiated to prevent further episodes from occurring. No medication is approved by the FDA for treatment of aggression. Accordingly, all pharmacotherapies for chronic aggression are off-label uses (i.e., the drugs have been approved for other uses such as hypertension, depression, or seizure disorders).

*Antihypertensive medications:* β*-blockers.* Since the first report, in 1977, of the use of β-adrenergic receptor antagonists (β-blockers) in the treatment of acute aggression, over 25 articles have appeared in the neurological and psychiatric literature reporting experience in using β-blockers with over 200 patients with aggression (Yudofsky et al. 1998). These studies provide stronger evidence for β-blockers as treatments for post-TBI aggression than is available for any other agent (Warden et al. 2006). Most of these patients had been unsuccessfully treated with antipsychotics, minor tranquilizers, lithium, and/or anticonvulsants before treatment with β-blockers. The β-blockers that have been investigated in controlled prospective studies include propranolol, nadolol, and pindolol, which appear to be effective treatments of brain injury–related chronic aggression (Alpert et al. 1990; Brooke et al. 1992; Greendyke and Kanter 1986; Greendyke et al. 1986).

When a β-blocker is used to treat post-TBI aggression, we recommend propranolol. Treatment begins with 60 mg/day, and dosage can be increased by that amount every 3–4 days with appropriate monitoring of pulse and blood pressure. Dosages of greater than 640 mg/day usually are not required. When a patient requires the use of a once-daily medication because of compliance difficulties, long-acting propranolol or nadolol can be used. When patients develop bradycardia that prevents prescribing therapeutic dosages of propranolol, pindolol can be substituted, using one-tenth the dosage of propranolol. Pindolol's intrinsic sympathomimetic activity stimulates the β-receptor and restricts the development of bradycardia. However, patients may have decreased ability for aerobic exercise due to β-receptor blockade.

The major side effect of β-blockers when they are used to treat aggression is the lowering of blood pressure and pulse rate. Because peripheral β-receptors are fully occupied at dosages of 300–400 mg/day, further decreases in these vital signs usually do not occur, even when dosages are increased to much higher levels. Despite reports of depression with the use of β-blockers, controlled trials and our experience indicate that it is a rare occurrence (Ko et al. 2002; Yudofsky 1992). Because the use of propranolol is associated with significant increases in plasma levels of thioridazine, which has an absolute dosage ceiling of 800 mg/day, the combination of these two medications should be avoided whenever possible.

*Antidepressants.* The antidepressants that have been reported to control aggressive behavior include those that act on serotonin preferentially (i.e., amitriptyline) or specifically (i.e., trazodone, sertraline, fluoxetine). We suggest using an SSRI such as sertraline, citalopram, or escitalopram as the initial medication from the antidepressant category. The dosages used are similar to those for the treatment of depression and affective lability. We generally avoid paroxetine in light of its nontrivial anticholinergic effects and potential for producing cognitive impairment (Schmitt et al. 2001).

We have evaluated and treated many patients with affective lability who present with comorbid irritability, agitation, and aggression. These patients, whose diagnosis according to DSM-IV-TR would be personality change, labile type, due to traumatic brain injury, also appear to respond well to SSRIs.

*Anticonvulsant medications.* The anticonvulsant carbamazepine has been shown to be effective for the treatment of bipolar disorders and has also been advocated for the control of aggression in populations both with and without epilepsy. Unfortunately, no controlled trials have been reported of this or other anticonvulsant medications for the treatment of aggression following TBI.

In our experience and that of others, the anticonvulsant valproic acid may also be helpful to some patients with chronic aggression after TBI and tends to be relatively neutral with respect to its effects on cognition (see Chapter 14, "Seizures and Epilepsy"). One case report describes beneficial effects of lamotrigine on post-TBI aggression (Pachet et al. 2003). Uncontrolled studies suggest that carbamazepine may decrease aggressive behavior associated with developmental disabilities and schizophrenia as well as other neurological disorders (Yudofsky et al. 1998).

For patients with aggression and posttraumatic epilepsy whose seizures are being treated with anticonvulsant drugs such as phenytoin or phenobarbital, switching to carbamazepine or to valproic acid may treat both conditions. Oxcarbazepine may be an alternative to carbamazepine, although no reports have been published describing the treatment of chronic posttraumatic aggression with oxcarbazepine.

**Antimanic medications.** Lithium is known to be effective in controlling aggression related to manic excitement. It also may have a role in the treatment of aggression in selected, nonbipolar patient populations, including individuals with mental retardation who exhibit self-injurious or aggressive behavior, children and adolescents with behavioral disorders, prison inmates, and individuals with other neurological disorders (Yudofsky et al. 1998). Because of lithium's potential for neurotoxicity, to which persons with neurological disorders may be more vulnerable, we limit the use of lithium in patients whose aggression is related to manic effects and in patients whose recurrent irritability is related to cyclic mood disorders.

**Antianxiety medications.** In preliminary open-label case studies, buspirone, a serotonin 5-HT$_{1A}$ receptor partial agonist, was effective in the management of aggression and agitation for patients with brain injury. In rare instances, we have found that some patients become more aggressive when treated with buspirone. Its advantages are ease of use and tolerability. When this agent is used, we recommend that buspirone be initiated at low dosages (i.e., 7.5 mg twice daily) and increased to 15 mg bid after 1 week. Dosages of 45–60 mg/day may be required before improvement in aggressive behavior results, although improvements may occur more rapidly.

Clonazepam may be effective in the long-term management of aggression, although evidence is restricted to case reports. We use clonazepam when pronounced aggression and anxiety occur together, or when aggression occurs in association with neurologically induced tics and similarly disinhibited motor behaviors. Clonazepam for these purposes should be initiated at 0.5 mg twice daily and may be increased to as high as 2–4 mg twice daily. Unfortunately, cognitive, sedative, and motor side effects are relatively common and may be treatment limiting.

**Stimulants.** Several studies have examined medications that directly or indirectly augment cerebral catecholaminergic function, such as methylphenidate (Mooney and Haas 1993) and amantadine (Hammond 2010), as treatments for chronic agitation and aggression following TBI. In principle, the use of such agents relies on relative preservation of lateral orbitofrontal-subcortical circuits whose function might be enhanced by augmenting cerebral catecholamines. For persons lacking the prefrontal targets of this intervention, such treatments may exacerbate chronic agitation and aggression. Careful evaluation of the neuroanatomy of injury and behavior is warranted before using stimulants and related agents to treat chronic aggression of a person with TBI.

*Antipsychotic medications.* If, after thorough clinical evaluation, the clinician determines that an individual's aggressive episodes result from psychosis, such as paranoid delusions or command hallucinations, then antipsychotic medications are the treatment of choice. Although no controlled studies have been reported of antipsychotic medications for the treatment of aggression (or psychosis) after TBI, case series (Kim and Bijlani 2006) and common clinical experience suggest that the atypical antipsychotics may be useful for this purpose. Their relatively lower rates of adverse motor and cognitive effects make these agents preferable to typical antipsychotics for persons with TBI, who tend to be more susceptible to the adverse motor effects of these medications. When these agents are used, however, pretreatment weight, metabolic, and cardiac assessments are necessary, and serial monitoring for treatment-related metabolic and other adverse systemic effects is imperative.

# CONCLUSION

Aggressive behavior after TBI is common and can be highly disabling. Aggression often significantly impedes appropriate rehabilitation and reintegration into the community. Many neurobiological factors can lead to aggressive behavior after injury. After appropriate evaluation and assessment of possible etiologies, treatment begins with documentation of the aggressive episodes. Psychopharmacological strategies differ according to whether the medication is for the treatment of acute aggression or for the prevention of episodes in the patient with chronic aggression. Although the treatment of acute aggression involves the judicious use of sedation, the treatment of chronic aggression is guided by underlying diagnoses and symptomatologies. Behavioral strategies remain an important component in the comprehensive treatment of aggression. With this comprehensive approach, aggression can be controlled with minimal adverse cognitive sequelae.

# *Key Clinical Points*

- Agitation and aggression are common in the early and late post-TBI periods.

- There is a broad differential diagnosis for agitation and aggression after TBI, including other neuropsychiatric disorders, substance intoxication and withdrawal, focal lesions to ventral prefrontal systems, pain and other physical conditions, medications, psychological health disturbances, interpersonal problems, and environmental factors.

- Careful assessment of agitated or aggressive behaviors, as well as identification of their antecedents and consequences, is required for the development of a rational treatment plan.

- Standardized assessment of agitation and aggression before and serially during treatment is essential. The Overt Agitation Severity Scale and Overt Aggression Scale are recommended for this purpose.

- Psychotherapeutic, behavioral, and environmental management for persons with posttraumatic aggression, those with whom they interact, and their environments are essential components of the treatment.

- Medications may be useful adjuncts to nonpharmacological treatments of post-TBI behavioral disturbances. Clinicians need to keep in mind both that the pharmacotherapies differ for acute versus chronic agitation and/or aggression and that the evidence base required for risk-benefit analyses of these pharmacotherapies is underdeveloped.

# REFERENCES

Alpert JE, Spillmann MK: Psychotherapeutic approaches to aggressive and violent patients. Psychiatr Clin North Am 20:453–472, 1997

Alpert M, Allan ER, Citrome L, et al: A double-blind, placebo-controlled study of adjunctive nadolol in the management of violent psychiatric patients. Psychopharmacol Bull 26:367–371, 1990

American Psychiatric Association: Diagnostic and Statistical Manual of Mental Disorders, 4th Edition, Text Revision. Washington, DC, American Psychiatric Association, 2000

Anson K, Ponsford J: Coping and emotional adjustment following traumatic brain injury. J Head Trauma Rehabil 21:248–259, 2006

Baguley IJ, Cooper J, Felmingham K: Aggressive behavior following traumatic brain injury: how common is common? J Head Trauma Rehabil 21:45–56, 2006

Bleiberg J, Garmoe W, Cederquist J, et al: Effects of Dexedrine on performance consistency following brain injury: a double-blind placebo crossover case study. Neuropsychiatry Neuropsychol Behav Neurol 6:245–248, 1993

Block SH: Psychotherapy of the individual with brain injury. Brain Inj 1:203–206, 1987

Bogner JA, Corrigan JD, Fugate L, et al: Role of agitation in prediction of outcomes after traumatic brain injury. Am J Phys Med Rehabil 80:636–644, 2001

Brooke MM, Questad KA, Patterson DR, et al: Agitation and restlessness after closed head injury: a prospective study of 100 consecutive admissions. Arch Phys Med Rehabil 73:320–323, 1992

Brown G, Chadwick O, Shaffer D, et al: A prospective study of children with head injuries, III: psychiatric sequelae. Psychol Med 11:63–78, 1981

Burg JS, Williams R, Burright RG, et al: Psychiatric treatment outcome following traumatic brain injury. Brain Inj 14:513–533, 2000

Carlsson GS, Svärdsudd K, Welin L: Long-term effects of head injuries sustained during life in three male populations. J Neurosurg 67:197–205, 1987

Cicerone KD, Mott T, Azulay J, et al: A randomized controlled trial of holistic neuropsychologic rehabilitation after traumatic brain injury. Arch Phys Med Rehabil 89:2239–2249, 2008

Coetzer R: Psychotherapy following traumatic brain injury: integrating theory and practice. J Head Trauma Rehabil 22:39–47, 2007

Delmonico RL, Hanley-Peterson P, Englander J: Group psychotherapy for persons with traumatic brain injury: management of frustration and substance abuse. J Head Trauma Rehabil 13:10–22, 1998

Ferguson SD, Coccaro EF: History of mild to moderate traumatic brain injury and aggression in physically healthy participants with and without personality disorder. J Pers Disord 23:230–239, 2009

Freedman D, Hemenway D: Precursors of lethal violence: a death row sample. Soc Sci Med 50:1757–1770, 2000

Greendyke RM, Kanter DR: Therapeutic effects of pindolol on behavioral disturbances associated with organic brain disease: a double-blind study. J Clin Psychiatry 47:423–426, 1986

Greendyke RM, Kanter DR, Schuster DB, et al: Propranolol treatment of assaultive patients with organic brain disease: a double-blind crossover, placebo-controlled study. J Nerv Ment Dis 174:290–294, 1986

Greve KW, Sherwin E, Stanford MS, et al: Personality and neurocognitive correlates of impulsive aggression in long-term survivors of severe traumatic brain injury. Brain Inj 15:255–262, 2001

Hammond F: Use of amantadine hydrochloride in the treatment of irritability and aggression in chronic traumatic brain injury: a randomized, controlled trial. J Neuropsychiatry Clin Neurosci 22:244–246, 2010

Hammond F, Knotts A, Hirsch M, et al: Posttraumatic irritability and related factors. J Head Trauma Rehabil 21:412–413, 2006

Herzberg JL, Fenwick PB: The aetiology of aggression in temporal-lobe epilepsy. Br J Psychiatry 153:50–55, 1988

Hibbard MR, Uysal S, Kepler K, et al: Axis I psychopathology in individuals with traumatic brain injury. J Head Trauma Rehabil 13:24–39, 1998

Hoffman AN, Cheng JP, Zafonte RD, et al: Administration of haloperidol and risperidone after neurobehavioral testing hinders the recovery of traumatic brain injury–induced deficits. Life Sci 83:602–607, 2008

Jorge RE, Robinson RG, Moser D, et al: Major depression following traumatic brain injury. Arch Gen Psychiatry 61:42–50, 2004

Kim E, Bijlani M: A pilot study of quetiapine treatment of aggression due to traumatic brain injury. J Neuropsychiatry Clin Neurosci 18:547–549, 2006

Kline AE, Massucci JL, Zafonte RD, et al: Differential effects of single versus multiple administrations of haloperidol and risperidone on functional outcome after experimental brain trauma. Crit Care Med 35:919–924, 2007

Kline AE, Hoffman AN, Cheng JP, et al: Chronic administration of antipsychotics impedes behavioral recovery after experimental traumatic brain injury. Neurosci Lett 448:263–267, 2008

Ko DT, Hebert PR, Coffey CS, et al: Beta-blocker therapy and symptoms of depression, fatigue, and sexual dysfunction. JAMA 288:351–357, 2002

Kopecky HJ, Kopecky CR, Yudofsky SC: Reliability and validity of the Overt Agitation Severity Scale in adult psychiatric inpatients. Psychiatr Q 69:301–323, 1998

Mendez MF, Cummings JL, Benson DF: Depression in epilepsy: significance and phenomenology. Arch Neurol 43:766–770, 1986

Mooney GF, Haas LJ: Effect of methylphenidate on brain injury–related anger. Arch Phys Med Rehabil 74:153–160, 1993

Pachet A, Friesen S, Winklaar D, et al: Beneficial behavioural effects of lamotrigine in traumatic brain injury. Brain Inj 17:715–722, 2003

Persinger MA: Personality changes following brain injury as a grief response to the loss of sense of self: phenomenological themes as indices of local lability and neurocognitive structuring as psychotherapy. Psychol Rep 72:1059–1068, 1993

Ponsford J, Olver J, Ponsford M, et al: Long-term adjustment of families following traumatic brain injury where comprehensive rehabilitation has been provided. Brain Inj 17:453–468, 2003

Rao N, Jellinek HM, Woolston DC: Agitation in closed head injury: haloperidol effects on rehabilitation outcome. Arch Phys Med Rehabil 66:30–34, 1985

Rao V, Rosenberg P, Bertrand M, et al: Aggression after traumatic brain injury: prevalence and correlates. J Neuropsychiatry Clin Neurosci 21:420–429, 2009

Robertson MM, Trimble MR, Townsend HR: Phenomenology of depression in epilepsy. Epilepsia 28:364–372, 1987

Schmitt JA, Kruizinga MJ, Riedel WJ: Non-serotonergic pharmacological profiles and associated cognitive effects of serotonin reuptake inhibitors. J Psychopharmacol 15:173–179, 2001

Silver JM, Yudofsky SC: Documentation of aggression in the assessment of the violent patient. Psychiatr Ann 17:375–384, 1987

Silver JM, Yudofsky SC: The Overt Aggression Scale: overview and guiding principles. J Neuropsychiatry Clin Neurosci 3:S22–S29, 1991

Slaughter B, Fann JR, Ehde D: Traumatic brain injury in a county jail population: prevalence, neuropsychological functioning and psychiatric disorders. Brain Inj 17:731–741, 2003

Smith VM: Paradoxical reactions to diazepam. Gastrointest Endosc 41:182–183, 1995

Stevens JR, Hermann BP: Temporal lobe epilepsy, psychopathology, and violence: the state of the evidence. Neurology 31:1127–1132, 1981

Tateno A, Jorge RE, Robinson RG: Clinical correlates of aggressive behavior after traumatic brain injury. J Neuropsychiatry Clin Neurosci 15:155–160, 2003

Tiersky LA, Anselmi V, Johnston MV, et al: A trial of neuropsychologic rehabilitation in mild-spectrum traumatic brain injury. Arch Phys Med Rehabil 86:1565–1574, 2005

Tune L, Carr S, Hoag E, et al: Anticholinergic effects of drugs commonly prescribed for the elderly: potential means for assessing risk of delirium. Am J Psychiatry 149:1393–1394, 1992

van der Naalt J, van Zomeren AH, Sluiter WJ, et al: Acute behavioural disturbances related to imaging studies and outcome in mild-to-moderate head injury. Brain Inj 14:781–788, 2000

Warden DL, Gordon B, McAllister TW, et al: Guidelines for the pharmacologic treatment of neurobehavioral sequelae of traumatic brain injury. J Neurotrauma 23:1468–1501, 2006

Weiger WA, Bear DM: An approach to the neurology of aggression. J Psychiatr Res 22:85–98, 1988

Wolf AP, Gleckman AD, Cifu DX, et al: The prevalence of agitation and brain injury in skilled nursing facilities: a survey. Brain Inj 10:241–245, 1996

Wood RL, Liossi C: Neuropsychological and neurobehavioral correlates of aggression following traumatic brain injury. J Neuropsychiatry Clin Neurosci 18:333–341, 2006

Yudofsky SC: Beta-blockers and depression: the clinician's dilemma. JAMA 267:1826–1827, 1992

Yudofsky SC, Silver JM, Jackson W, et al: The Overt Aggression Scale for the objective rating of verbal and physical aggression. Am J Psychiatry 143:35–39, 1986

Yudofsky SC, Kopecky HJ, Kunik M, et al: The Overt Agitation Severity Scale for the objective rating of agitation. J Neuropsychiatry Clin Neurosci 9:541–548, 1997

Yudofsky SC, Silver J, Hales R: Treatment of agitation and aggression, in The American Psychiatric Press Textbook of Psychopharmacology, 2nd Edition. Edited by Schatzberg AF, Nemeroff CB. Washington, DC, American Psychiatric Press, 1998, pp 881–900

# CHAPTER 11

## Apathy

*Robert van Reekum, M.D.*
*Emma van Reekum, B.S.*

**Apathy,** or the apathy syndrome, is a common neuropsychiatric consequence of traumatic brain injury (TBI) and is associated with poor response to treatment, poor prognosis for the associated condition, family and caregiver distress, and poor functional recovery (van Reekum et al. 2005). Post-TBI apathy has not received research attention adequate to allow consensus as to its definition, measurement, prevalence, or treatment, and therefore apathy in other conditions (e.g., Alzheimer disease, Parkinson disease) is often used as a model for understanding and managing apathy after TBI. The validity of such cross-condition analogies is tenuous, so appropriate caution must be exercised when considering the findings and recommendations regarding post-TBI apathy discussed in this chapter.

## DEFINITIONS

Psychiatric nosology (e.g., DSM-IV-TR; American Psychiatric Association 2000) has not considered apathy to be a distinct syndrome or disorder. Rather, psychiatrists and mental health clinicians recognize apathy as a symptom of various other disorders. For example, the criteria for schizophrenia include negative symptoms such as affective flattening and avolition. These negative symptoms resemble the apathy syndrome associated with TBI (Rao et al. 2007). Similarly, a common feature of major depressive episodes is markedly diminished interest and/or pleasure in all, or almost all, activities (i.e., anhedonia). Despite the resemblance between anhedonia and apathy, apathy and major depression are dissociable (van Reekum et al. 2005)—that is, some, but not all, depressed patients are apathetic and some, but not all, apathetic patients also have depression. Other psychiatric disorders that have apathy as a symptom include schizophrenia, schizoid personality disorder, and autism spectrum disorders. In short, apathy is a common symptom of many of the disorders described in DSM-IV-TR.

In its section on disorders due to general medical conditions, DSM-IV-TR addresses the possibility of apathy as a distinct syndrome. When a person with a medical or neurological condition (e.g., TBI) develops as a result of that condition a personality change in which the predominant feature is marked apathy and indifference, the appropriate diagnosis is personality change due to a general medical condition, apathetic type. Unfortunately, specific definitions of apathy and indifference are not provided in DSM-IV-TR, and the categorization of apathy as a personality change implies that apathy is an aspect of personality rather than a distinct neuropsychiatric syndrome.

Clinicians and investigators in the clinical neurosciences, including some in psychiatry and neuropsychiatry, regard apathy as a syndrome (i.e., a constellation of symptoms and signs) of diminished motivation associated with a large number of neurological disorders (Marin 1990). This syndrome is characterized by diminished goal-directed cognition, emotion, and behavior resulting from a disorder of the brain and not better accounted for by a diminished level of consciousness (i.e., delirium), cognitive impairment, or emotional distress (i.e., a mood disorder) (Marin 1991).

Stuss et al. (2000) suggested that apathy be defined as an absence of responsiveness to stimuli (external or internal) as demonstrated by a lack of self-initiated action. They also suggested that apathy may not be a single syndrome, but instead may involve distinct and separable decreases in cognitive, emotional, or behavioral responsiveness depending on the cortical-subcortical neural systems involved in a given patient. Similarly, Levy and Dubois (2006) conceptualized apathy as a quantifiable reduction in self-generated goal-directed behavior.

We propose a definition of apathy that integrates and adds to these perspectives: the apathy syndrome is characterized by a clinically significant loss of motivation as evidenced by a reduced ability to respond to internal and external stimuli in the initiation and maintenance of a goal-directed response. The goal of such responses is likely to be determined at least in part by the will, or intent, of the individual within his or her social/cultural and experiential milieu. Responses are likely to involve affective, behavioral, and cognitive processes.

This definition has not been previously published, or accepted, but might be useful for clinicians working with TBI populations. Regardless, it is important for clinicians to be aware that most of the clinical research into apathy to date has essentially "defined" apathy on the basis of scores on various assessment scales (discussed below in "Clinical Assessment"). The development of these measures has greatly facilitated and promoted research into apathy. The validity of future research in this area will be facilitated by a "gold standard" and widely accepted definition of apathy and diagnostic criteria for the apathy syndrome. These issues are under consideration for inclusion in DSM-5, and their consideration may yield an approach to these problems that improves research and patient care.

# EPIDEMIOLOGY

Apathy is a common problem across a large variety of conditions (van Reekum et al. 2005). The assessment tools used in the published literature do not appear to strongly influence prevalence estimates, although this issue has not been addressed systematically. The average point prevalence of apathy across four studies of apathy, which, collectively, included 304 adults with TBI, was 61% (Andersson et al. 1999a, 1999b; Kant et al. 1998; Marsh et al. 1998). A single study of children with TBI reported a point prevalence of apathy of 14% (Max et al. 2001). The prevalence of apathy among persons with focal frontal lesions and basal ganglia lesions also is high (60% and 41%, respectively) (van Reekum et al. 2005). Findings from a study of a small group of patients ($n=14$) who suffered anoxic brain injury suggests that such injury causes a high risk for apathy (point prevalence of 79%). The available data also suggest that apathy is common in many neurological conditions and psychiatric disorders, including major depression and schizophrenia. A very high point prevalence of apathy was observed among nursing home residents (84.1%); although this high rate of apathy may reflect the severity of illness that results in nursing home placement, factors intrinsic to nursing homes also may contribute to the development of apathy.

Subsequent findings generally are consistent with, and hence supportive of, these conclusions. Apathy is common in many neurological conditions (Aalten et al. 2005; Borroni et al. 2008a, 2008b; Diehl-Schmid et al. 2006; Figved et al. 2005; Glodzik-Sobanska et al. 2005; Kirsch-Darrow et al. 2006; Landes et al. 2005; Robert et al. 2006; Rozzini et al. 2008; Srikanth et al. 2005) and is a clinically relevant problem when it develops (van Reekum et al. 2005). Apathy is associated with adverse outcomes, including decreased functional level, more severe depression, more rapid rate of decline in Alzheimer disease, attenuated responses to treatments directed at the condition underlying apathy, poor prognosis for future functioning, and other behavioral problems (Aalten et al. 2005; de Vugt et al. 2006; Hama et al. 2007; Landes et al. 2005; Robert et al. 2006; Starkstein et al. 2006; Tam et al. 2008). Among persons with severe TBI, apathy is also associated with increased caregiver burden and is rated by caregivers as one of the most problematic behaviors with which they contend (Marsh et al. 1998).

Little research into the clinical outcomes associated with apathy in TBI has been completed to date. Furthermore, the direction of causality involved in the associations between apathy and functional status has not yet been established. For example, apathy might cause a worsening of functioning, but it also might be the case that poor functioning causes or contributes to apathy. Both causal relationships might be operative in some patients (e.g., apathy contributing to poor functioning and, in turn, poor functioning contributing to worsening of apathy). Alternatively, some third factor (e.g., TBI severity) might underlie the associations between apathy and functional status. Regardless, the available evidence suggests that identification and treatment of apathy is important in the care and rehabilitation of individuals with TBI.

# CLINICAL ASSESSMENT

The first step in the clinical assessment of apathy among persons with TBI is recognizing it as an identifiable and clinically significant problem. Although persons with TBI sometimes present for evaluation with a complaint related to apathy, it is more common that apathy itself is not a concern of the apathetic person. Instead, common clini-

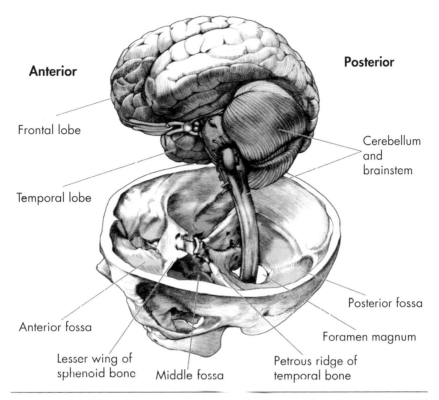

**Anterior**

**Posterior**

Frontal lobe

Cerebellum and brainstem

Temporal lobe

Posterior fossa

Anterior fossa

Foramen magnum

Lesser wing of sphenoid bone

Middle fossa

Petrous ridge of temporal bone

**PLATE 1.** (*Figure 1–1*) Anterior, middle, and posterior cranial fossae in relation to the base of the brain, highlighting areas vulnerable to compression and contusion when biomechanical forces are applied to the head.

*Source.* Reprinted from Blumenfeld H: *Neuroanatomy Through Clinical Cases,* 2nd Edition. Sunderland, MA, Sinauer Associates, © 2010. Used with permission.

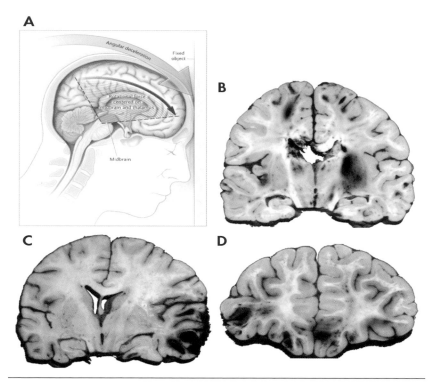

**PLATE 2.** *(Figure 1–2)* Illustration of traumatic brain injury (TBI) biomechanics and postmortem coronal sections of brain.

*Panel A:* Movement of the brain in response to biomechanical force application. *Panels B, C, and D:* Specimens obtained from patients who sustained TBI in road traffic accidents who died shortly thereafter. Hemorrhagic lesions are seen in the corpus callosum, midline structures, and basal ganglia *(B)*, at the lateral aspect of the right temporal lobe *(C)*, and on the inferior aspects of the frontal lobes *(D)*. The near midline hemorrhagic loci are characteristic of traumatic axonal injury.

*Source.* Panel A reprinted from Ropper AH, Gorson KC: "Clinical Practice: Concussion." *New England Journal of Medicine* 356:166–172, 2007. Used with permission of the Massachusetts Medical Society. Panels B, C, and D reprinted from Graham DI, Nicoll JAR, Bone I: *Introduction to Neuropathology.* London, Hodder Education Publishing, 2006. Used with permission.

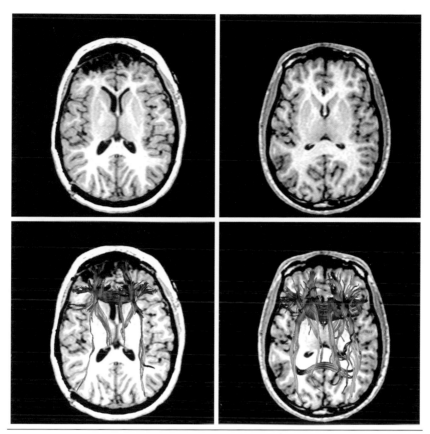

**PLATE 3.** *(Figure 1–4)* Atrophy of association and commissural tracts of the anterior of the corpus callosum associated with frontal lobe lesion demonstrated by T1-weighted axial magnetic resonance imaging and diffusion tensor imaging in an individual with traumatic brain injury *(left column)* compared to a healthy age-matched individual *(right column).*

*Source.* From Oni MB, Wilde EA, Bigler ED, et al: "Diffusion Tensor Imaging Analysis of Frontal Lobes in Pediatric Traumatic Brain Injury." *Journal of Child Neurology* 25:976–984, 2010. © 2010 by Sage Publications. Reprinted with permission of Sage Publications.

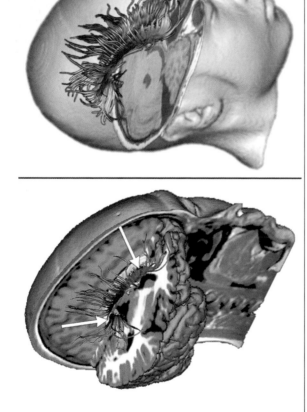

**PLATE 4.** *(Figure 1–5)* Diffusion tensor imaging (DTI) of the corpus callosum and the consequences of severe TBI-induced callosal damage on interhemispheric connectivity.

On the *right* is a three-dimensional reconstruction of normal-appearing callosal projection fibers derived from DTI tractography. On the *left* is a three-dimensional reconstruction of a magnetic resonance image from an individual who sustained a severe traumatic brain injury (TBI) showing a partial sagittal view of the medial aspect of the left hemisphere in which the corpus callosum is identified in white and TBI-related callosal thinning and loss of projecting fibers are indicated by the *white arrows.*

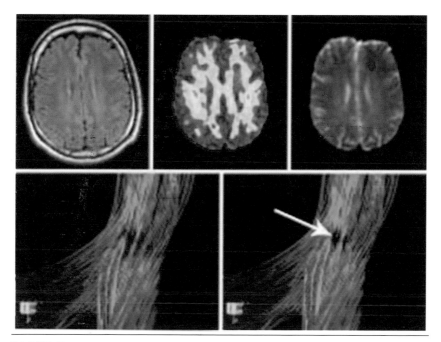

**PLATE 5.** *(Figure 1–6)* Diffusion tensor imaging (DTI) tractography demonstrating discontinuity of white matter tracts crossing the anterior aspect of the corpus callosum and interfacing with tracts within the region of the frontal forceps.

Fluid-attenuated inversion recovery image in the *top upper left* shows no abnormalities. Analysis of the fractional anisotropy (FA) map *(top middle)* identifies a region with reduced FA in the white matter of the left frontal lobe, also indicated on the T2-weighted image *(top right)*. That region of interest includes fibers within the forceps minor and fronto-temporo-occipital fibers *(bottom left, superior oblique view)*, the respective fibers of which are discontinuous *(arrow, bottom right image)*.

*Source.* Reprinted from Rutgers DR, Toulgoat F, Cazejust J, et al: "White Matter Abnormalities in Mild Traumatic Brain Injury: A Diffusion Tensor Imaging Study." *American Journal of Neuroradiology* 29:514–519, 2008. © 2008. Used with permission of American Society of Neuroradiology.

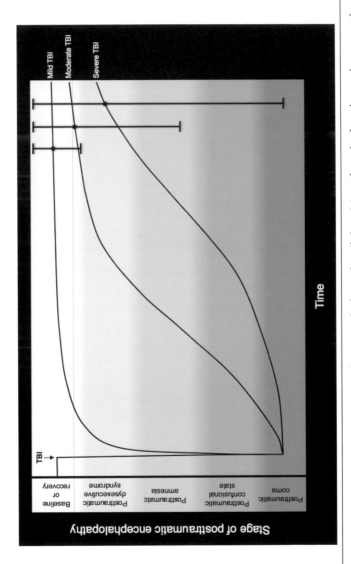

**PLATE 6.** *(Figure 5–1)* Stages of posttraumatic encephalopathy *(left axis)* and typical trajectories over time *(bottom axis)* associated with mild, moderate, or severe traumatic brain injury (TBI), with typical ranges of outcomes *(whisker bars)*.

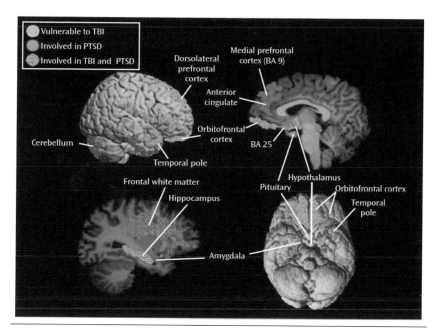

**PLATE 7.** *(Figure 8–2)* Relationship between regional alterations of brain structure associated with posttraumatic stress disorder (PTSD) and traumatic brain injury (TBI).

Several brain regions have been consistently implicated in PTSD *(green)*, including the amygdala, the hippocampus, the orbitofrontal cortex, and the dorsolateral and dorsomedial prefrontal cortex. Several brain regions are vulnerable to the typical biomechanical forces associated with TBI *(red)*, including the orbitofrontal cortex, the dorsolateral prefrontal cortex, the temporal pole, and the hippocampus. Overlap areas *(blue)* include the orbitofrontal cortex, the dorsolateral prefrontal cortex, and the hippocampus. In addition, tracts connecting the amygdala and the medial prefrontal cortex course through the subfrontal white matter and are thus vulnerable to disruption by TBI. BA = Brodmann area.

*Source.* Reprinted from Stein MB, McAllister TW: "Exploring the Convergence of Posttraumatic Stress Disorder and Mild Traumatic Brain Injury." *American Journal of Psychiatry* 166:768–776, 2009. © American Psychiatric Association. Used with permission.

cal experience suggests that others involved with a patient are more likely to make apathy a focus of clinical attention or that it becomes recognized as a problem when the clinician specifically inquires about goal-directed behavior (i.e., motivation). Caregivers, family members, support workers, and rehabilitation providers often are distressed and frustrated by a patient's apathy; however, they rarely offer complaints about apathy specifically. Instead, they describe concerns about an individual's lack of initiative or interest, "spark," or participation in usual and/or expected activities. They may describe the patient as a couch potato or may state that the patient's "get up and go got up and went." Complaints that the patient is "not the same anymore" or that the person's "personality has changed" suggest the possibility of apathy and the need for further inquiry about motivation. The relatively high prevalence rates of apathy among persons with TBI suggest that routine screening for apathy is appropriate; however, the clinical usefulness of this approach has not yet been studied. For the present, we suggest that clinicians remain vigilant for apathy among persons with TBI and maintain a low threshold for initiating a detailed assessment for this problem.

When apathy is suspected, formal diagnostic assessment is the second step in the evaluation process. Unfortunately, and as discussed above in "Definitions," no consensus has been reached as to the appropriate diagnostic criteria for the apathy syndrome. Most research on this subject employs formal assessment tools such as the Apathy Evaluation Scale (AES; Marin et al. 1991); a brief version of the AES called the Apathy Scale (AS; Starkstein et al. 1992); the Neuropsychiatric Inventory (NPI; Cummings et al. 1994); and a number of measures used primarily in disease-specific research (Clarke et al. 2011). Using these scales in clinical practice helps to verify that the patient being assessed resembles the participants included in the research studies to date, and it may improve the reliability and validity of clinical diagnosis.

Unfortunately, there is no accepted clinical gold-standard diagnosis for the apathy syndrome, and the most clinically appropriate scale cutoff scores with which to identify a clinically important level of apathy have not been established. The potential disadvantages of using these scales include costs (for those that are proprietary), the need for specialized training in their administration and scoring, increases in the length of clinical assessments, and the potential for patient and/or informant intolerance of the assessment.

When the assessment for apathy is undertaken, the clinician should seek and interview a reliable informant (e.g., friend, family member, therapist). Informant-based interview about apathy appears to yield more reliable diagnostic information than does patient interview (Clarke et al. 2007). The data sought from an informant include history regarding motivational behaviors, observed signs of apathy (e.g., flat affect, lack of initiation, lack of interest and participation in activities), and the presence of symptoms of (i.e., subjective complaints about) apathy. The clinical interview of the person with apathy should also be undertaken, with a focus on history and symptom assessment; however, the amount of data yielded by direct interview of an apathetic patient may be limited. By contrast, observations made by the clinician during the interview may be quite informative.

The apathy syndrome often involves changes in affect, behavior, and cognition (Stuss et al. 2000). When specifically asked, patients and/or their caregivers may report a "blah," "monotone," and/or nonreactive mood; a lack of behavioral initiation and/or maintenance of activities (e.g., requiring "cueing" or "pushing" to engage, and having limited ability to sustain activities once initiated); and a general loss of interest in previously enjoyed activities as well as detachment from individuals of previous importance.

The third step in the assessment of an individual with apathy is the identification of all the possible contributors. These include the neurological problem that may be producing apathy (i.e., its neurological substrate); other biological, medical, and psychiatric factors; and possible psychosocial contributors.

## Neurobiological Substrates

The neuropathophysiology of apathy has been investigated using autopsy, structural neuroimaging (e.g., computed tomography, magnetic resonance imaging [MRI]), functional neuroimaging (e.g., functional MRI, single-photon emission computed tomography, positron emission tomography), electrophysiological techniques (e.g., electroencephalography, evoked potentials), and neuropsychological testing. Findings from these studies suggest that the apathy syndrome involves dysfunction in cortical-subcortical circuits involving at least the anterior cingulate gyrus, dorsolateral prefrontal cortex, anterior temporal cortex, thalamus, limbic striatum, and connecting white matter tracts (Marin and Wilkosz 2005; van Reekum et al. 2005). Dopamine and acetylcholine appear to be the primary neurotransmitters involved. At the cognitive level, apathy is associated primarily with frontal system, or executive, impairments. Impairments in verbal fluency, insight, facial emotion awareness, working memory, interference tasks, naming, problem solving, and attention to novel stimuli are common. Among persons with TBI, apathy is associated with altered response to novel stimuli, alterations in physiological responsivity to stimuli (Andersson et al. 1999b), and reduced emotional responsivity (Andersson et al. 1999a).

The findings from these various studies suggest the need for an increased index of concern in patients with TBI who present with neuroimaging or neuropsychological testing abnormalities consistent with the known neurobiological substrates of apathy, and further suggest that neurobiological and neuropsychological assessments might usefully inform the diagnosis and/or management of apathy. On the other hand, the diffuse nature of the pathophysiology of TBI, the apparently high baseline prevalence rates of apathy in TBI, the lack of sensitivity of many diagnostic tests in TBI, and the current lack of evidence for a clinical role for these types of data in the management of apathy in TBI collectively argue that at least at present, clinicians should neither rely on nor routinely perform these types of investigations. Diagnosis of the apathy syndrome rests primarily on clinical signs and symptoms. However, understanding that apathy has a neurological basis and having the ability to explain its neurobiological substrates are important for clinicians; communicating this information to patients and caregivers reduces blaming and a rush to discharge and encourages the development of therapeutic interventions directed toward apathy.

## Medical and Psychiatric Factors

Non-neurological biopsychosocial factors may play a role in the development of apathy and/or influence its course after TBI. Little research is available regarding the medical and psychiatric illness factors that influence apathy, but clinical and personal experience strongly suggests that such factors are relevant. Most people have experienced a loss of motivation when ill, tired, or in pain. Comorbid illnesses (e.g., infections), hormonal disturbances (e.g., hypothyroidism), sleep disturbances and fatigue, seizure disorders, sensory impairments, deconditioning, chronic pain, and some postconcussion symptoms may contribute to apathy. Persons with TBI also are at increased risk for certain psychiatric illnesses, including major depression (van Reekum et al. 2000), that may cause or exacerbate apathy. The data relating apathy to psychosis in schizophrenia suggest that the prudent course of action is to be vigilant for apathy among persons with psychosis following TBI. Also, individuals with TBI often take prescribed medications that have the potential to cause or exacerbate apathy. These medications include opiate analgesics, sedative-hypnotics, agents with anticholinergic properties, first- and second-generation antipsychotics, anticonvulsants, and selective serotonin reuptake inhibitors (SSRIs) (Barnhart et al. 2004; Wongpakaran et al. 2007). Some individuals with TBI also may abuse or become dependent on substances with the potential to induce or exacerbate apathy (e.g., marijuana, alcohol, opiates). The clinical assessment of persons with apathy following TBI therefore requires identifying potential medical and psychiatric causes of or contributors to this syndrome.

## Psychosocial Factors

Little research has been done into the role of psychosocial factors that produce or contribute to apathy. Persons with TBI commonly experience loss of relationships, changes in social roles, diminished self-esteem and sense of self-worth, and loss of hope. Stresses are common, and they include frustration with new and unwelcome circumstances, the need for multiple assessments and interventions, and concern for health and future, among others. Environmental changes, including change in residence and cohabitants, institutionalization (with associated reduction in environmental stimulation), and decreased community access also are common. The influence of these and other psychosocial factors on apathy is uncertain. However, it is reasonable to consider the role of these factors in initiating, maintaining, and exacerbating apathy among persons with TBI during the clinical assessment and, where possible, to direct treatments toward them. Such interventions may serve many useful purposes for a patient with TBI, including the removal of possible psychosocial contributors to the apathy syndrome.

## TREATMENT

There is a a paucity of evidence regarding the safety of pharmacological interventions in apathy associated with TBI. Pharmacotherapies entail risks, including those that are intrinsic to the medication employed (e.g., increased risk of seizures), others that are due to interactions with risks entailed by TBI itself (e.g., increased risk of seizure, behavioral dyscontrol), and some that are related to the neuropathophysiology of apathy in TBI. Apathy is associated with disturbances in the structure and function of frontal-subcortical circuits, which serve executive function, comportment and social cognition, motivation, oculomotor function, and voluntary movement. Consistent with the anatomy of apathy, persons with this problem after TBI also are often impulsive, disinhibited, and affectively labile. In some cases, these other problems are masked or ameliorated by the apathy. Pharmacologically treating apathy, however, may lead to an apparent worsening of impulsivity, disinhibition, affective lability, and other aberrant behaviors and cognitions. Caregivers anxious to see reductions in apathy in their loved ones or clients may be dismayed to find that pharmacologically induced improvements in apathy are associated with affects and behaviors that are equally, and sometimes more, difficult to manage or that pose significant safety concerns.

Therefore, an appropriate first step in treatment is to address apathy through elimination or reduction of its medical, psychiatric, and psychosocial contributors. For example, reducing motivation-impairing pain treatments (e.g., opiates) and improving sleep disturbances may effect improvements in motivation. Identifying and treating medical and psychiatric illnesses such as depression, treating hormonal disturbances (e.g., hypothyroidism), reducing doses of and/or eliminating medications that may produce apathy (e.g., SSRIs and tricyclic antidepressants), and removing access to illicit substances also may be useful. Additionally, development of rehabilitation and psychosocial interventions designed to address issues of stress, loss, and environmental factors associated with apathy should be undertaken.

When apathy persists despite these efforts, disrupts everyday function, and/or produces substantial caregiver distress or burden, then specific interventions targeting this problem may be considered.

## Psychological and Behavioral Interventions

Lane-Brown and Tate (2009a) performed a systematic review of the literature describing the nonpharmacological treatment of apathy associated with acquired brain dysfunction among persons age 16 years and older. Four studies of psychological and behavioral interventions identified in this review are directly relevant to the management of apathy associated with TBI. Providing checklists of tasks to be sequentially completed and offering verbal cues for actions needed to complete tasks may mitigate the functional consequences of apathy (Burke et al. 1991; DePoy et al. 1990; Sohlberg et al. 1988). Problem-solving training, rather than memory training, also may improve goal-directed ideation (von Cramon et al. 1991). The latter observation has led some to suggest that rehabilitation of apathy be guided by associated cognitive impairments (Marin and Wilkosz 2005) and include elements such as cueing to initiate tasks among persons unable to initiate activity independently, sequential guidance among those with planning and sequencing impairments, and so forth. This approach, at face value, seems reasonable; however, additional studies systematically evaluating it are needed.

In their systematic review, Lane-Brown and Tate (2009a) also evaluated psychological and behavioral interventions for apathy associated with dementia. Among subjects with severe or mixed levels of functional impairment, various activity-based therapies (e.g., music therapy, singing, structured activity kits) and multisensory stimulation environments appeared to improve apathy. Among those with mild to moderate functional impairments, cognitive interventions improved motivational behaviors. Also noted in this review were interventions that do not appear to improve apathy, including emotion-oriented care and memory notebooks.

Kragt et al. (1997) employed a blinded and controlled (usual care) crossover design with 16 apathetic nursing home residents over a 3-day trial period and found significantly reduced apathy with multisensory (Snoezelen) therapy. Salazar et al. (2000) studied 120 active-duty military personnel who had experienced a TBI resulting in a Glasgow Coma Scale score of 13 or less; the researchers randomized participants to receive an intensive, 8-week inpatient cognitive rehabilitation program or a limited home rehabilitation program with weekly telephone support from a psychiatric nurse. At 1-year follow-up, there was no difference in return-to-work rates and no difference in scores on an apathy scale. In a randomized controlled trial of 92 elderly persons with cognitive impairment, Hopman-Rock et al. (1999) found that psychomotor therapy (relaxation and activities such as games) did not benefit subjects' apathy.

Overall, the evidence base for psychological and behavioral interventions for apathy associated with TBI is limited. Some of the interventions may be useful, including verbal cueing, task checklists, computer retraining, cognitive interventions (including problem solving), music therapies, structured activity kits, and multisensory stimulation environments. Although the evidence base supporting the clinical use of these interventions is underdeveloped, their use entails fewer safety risks than does pharmacotherapy. Accordingly, these interventions warrant consideration and application in the treatment of posttraumatic apathy that is functionally impairing and/ or producing caregiver distress or burden.

## Pharmacological Interventions

Dopaminergic agents, including bromocriptine (Catsman-Berrevoets and von Harskamp 1988; Crismon et al. 1988; Parks et al. 1992; Powell et al. 1996; Watanabe et al. 1995) and the indirectly dopaminergic uncompetitive *N*-methyl-D-aspartate antagonist amantadine (Erkulwater and Pillai 1989; Horiguchi et al. 1990; Kraus and Maki 1997a, 1997b), are reported to improve apathy among persons with TBI. In the reports describing their use for this purpose, these agents were observed to improve motivation, participation, spontaneity, and/or function. These observations were made in single-case studies or open-label case series, and apathy was usually only one of several targets of pharmacotherapy. In a single-subject placebo-controlled study, van Reekum et al. (1995) observed amantadine-induced improvements in a profoundly apathetic TBI inpatient; over three paired sets of blinded observations, treatment with this medication improved rehabilitation participation when compared to placebo.

Methylphenidate, and to a lesser extent D-amphetamine, also may improve apathy associated with neurological disorders (Cantello et al. 1989; Clark and Mankikar 1979; Galynker et al. 1997; Kaplitz 1975; Maletta and Winegarden 1993; Padala et al. 2005; Watanabe et al. 1995). These medications reduced apathy, as evidenced by increased motivation, socialization, participation, hygiene, and psychic activation, as well as decreased negative symptoms. Unfortunately, these studies did not employ randomized controlled designs.

The efficacy of treatment with atypical antipsychotics, including risperidone, olanzapine, and clozapine, for the negative symptoms of schizophrenia has been studied in at least six randomized controlled trials, in which 3,182 subjects were studied (see van Reekum et al. 2005 for review). Decreased negative symptoms, including avolition, were reported with atypical antipsychotic medications in five of these six studies.

Acetylcholinesterase inhibitors, including donepezil, rivastigmine, and galantamine, improve apathy and other neuropsychiatric disturbances associated with neurodegenerative dementias (Cummings et al. 2008; Drijgers et al. 2009; Figiel and Sadowsky 2008; Rodda et al. 2009). These agents are not typically prescribed specifically for this purpose, however, and most of the studies in this area evaluated the medications' effects on apathy and other neuropsychiatric disturbances as post hoc analyses of data derived from multicenter randomized controlled trials. One uncontrolled trial of donepezil examined apathy as an outcome in four persons with TBI. Improvements in apathy were observed, compared with baseline, as assessed by the NPI (Masanic et al. 2001).

Selegiline is a selective irreversible monoamine oxidase (MAO) inhibitor that at low dosages is selective for MAO-B and at high dosages also inhibits MAO-A. In a study of selegiline at moderate to high dosages for the treatment of apathy among four subjects with TBI who had not tolerated treatment with methylphenidate, Newburn and Newburn (2005) observed treatment-related improvements in apathy, as assessed by the AES, as well as daily functioning.

In summary, relatively few studies have been published of pharmacotherapies for apathy associated with TBI. The literature evaluating the effects of pharmacotherapies on apathy associated with neurodegenerative dementias is more fully, but still incompletely, developed. However, generalizing from studies of apathy-targeted pharmacotherapies performed in other neurological or psychiatric populations to the treatment of persons with TBI must be undertaken with caution. Pharmacotherapy entails risks for side effects and may present safety risks (e.g., seizures, disinhibition, aggression). In general, medication interventions for apathy among persons with TBI are best regarded as treatments of last resort; however, pharmacotherapy may be considered when nonpharmacological and caregiver interventions do not provide adequate improvement in apathy and when apathy is producing significant functional disturbances and/or caregiver distress and burden.

When pharmacotherapy is undertaken, the medications presented in Table 11–1 may be considered. Before prescribing these or any other medications, clinicians are encouraged to refer to each medication's product information sheet as well as other reference materials

**TABLE 11–1.** Medications used to treat apathy and related disorders of diminished motivation

| MEDICATION | TOTAL DAILY DOSAGE RANGE |
|---|---|
| Methylphenidate | 5–80 mg (target: 0.5 mg/kg twice daily) |
| Dextroamphetamine | 5–80 mg (target: 0.5 mg/kg twice daily) |
| Modafinil | 100–400 mg |
| Bromocriptine | 2.5–90 mg |
| Carbidopa-levodopa | 25/100-mg tablet, 1–2 tablets three to four times daily |
| Amantadine | 50–200 mg |
| Bupropion XL or SR | 150–450 mg |
| Venlafaxine XR | 37.5–225 mg |
| Protriptyline | 20–60 mg |
| Selegiline | 5–20 mg |
| Donepezil | 5–10 mg |
| Rivastigmine | 1.5–12 mg |
| Galantamine ER | 8–24 mg |

*Note.* The evidence base supporting the use of these medications as treatment for apathy among persons with traumatic brain injury is limited. ER=extended release; SR=sustained release; XL=extended release; XR=extended release.

for complete reviews of dosing, side effects, drug-drug interactions, treatment risks, and treatment contraindications. In general, the treatment of apathy associated with TBI employs stimulants, dopaminergic agents, and other medications that augment cerebral catecholaminergic function. Cholinesterase inhibitors may be a useful alternative when catecholamine-enhancing agents are not tolerated and/or when cognitive impairments are being concurrently treated with a procholinergic approach. Informed consent requires discussion of the limitations of the evidence supporting these interventions, and careful monitoring of treatment-related benefits and adverse effects is essential. If treatment is successful, trials of discontinuation of medications should be considered periodically, especially among persons receiving treatment during the early period following TBI (i.e., when spontaneous recovery occurs). The use of atypical antipsychotics for the treatment of apathy is appropriately considered only for patients experiencing positive psychotic symptoms.

## Other Treatments

Lane-Brown and Tate (2009b) prepared a Cochrane review of interventions for apathy in TBI. Extensive literature searches were conducted using multiple databases. Only one randomized controlled trial that specifically targeted apathy in TBI was found (Smith et al. 1994). Twenty-one subjects residing in a care facility after TBI were treated with cranial electrotherapy stimulation (CES). Reductions in inertia were observed in the CES group, whereas no change in inertia was observed in the sham and no-treatment groups. No between-group comparisons were provided, leading Lane-Brown and Tate to conclude that it is not possible to determine whether CES led to more significant improvements than did control interventions.

Other treatment strategies for apathy in TBI have not been studied to date. Given that the issue of motivational behavior is relevant to fields outside of medicine (e.g., education, social sciences), perhaps much can be learned about potential treatment strategies for apathy from these disciplines. A systematic review of the research external to medicine is beyond the scope of this chapter. As an example, however, Ryan and Deci (2000), writing from the perspective of educational psychology, describe intrinsic and extrinsic types of motivation and note that self-determination theory and extensive research predict that interventions geared toward improving an individual's competence, autonomy, and relatedness are likely to enhance self-motivation and mental health.

## CONCLUSION

*Apathy* refers to a clinically significant loss of motivation as evidenced by a reduced ability to respond to internal and external stimuli in the initiation and maintenance of goal-directed cognitive, emotional, and behavioral responses. It is a common problem in the early period following TBI and may become a chronic problem in some cases. The point prevalence of apathy varies with initial injury severity, time since injury, and the context in which the assessment is made. This syndrome arises as a function of a complex interaction between the neurobiology of TBI and a broad array of medical, psychiatric, medication, substance use, and psychosocial contributors. In most cases, the etiology of the apathy syndrome is likely multifactorial. Regardless of its origins, apathy following TBI is associated with poor response to rehabilitative and other treatments, impaired function, and family and caregiver distress.

The treatment of apathy among persons with TBI is most productively directed at its underlying causes. When such treatment fails to adequately improve apathy, then nonpharmacological interventions may be undertaken. The evidence base supporting their use is limited. However, these interventions present little risk of harm and therefore are reasonable to be undertaken as treatments for apathy following TBI. Pharmacotherapy of apathy is best reserved for patients who do not respond adequately to all other interventions and for use only when apathy produces marked functional limitations and/or caregiver distress and burden. Medications that directly or indirectly augment cerebral catecholaminergic function are used most commonly in this population. When these agents are ineffective or poorly tolerated, or when cognitive impairments are targeted with a procholinergic strategy, cholinesterase inhibitors may be alternative treatments for apathy following TBI.

# *Key Clinical Points*

- Apathy is a syndrome characterized by a clinically significant loss of motivation as evidenced by a reduced ability to respond to internal and external stimuli in the initiation and maintenance of goal-directed cognitive, emotional, and behavioral responses.

- The apathy syndrome has multiple psychosocial contributors, and the point prevalence of apathy among adults with TBI may be as high as 60%.

- Apathy is associated with poor response to rehabilitative and other treatments, impaired function, and family and caregiver distress.

- Treatment is most effective when it is directed at the underlying cause of apathy, as well as its medical, psychiatric, medication, substance use, and psychosocial contributors.

- Nonpharmacological interventions may be of limited effectiveness, but because they are low risk, they are reasonable elements of the treatment plan for persons with apathy following TBI.

- Pharmacotherapy of apathy among persons with TBI may be considered when nonpharmacological and caregiver interventions do not provide adequate improvement in apathy and when apathy is producing significant functional disturbances and/or caregiver distress and burden.

# REFERENCES

Aalten P, de Vugt ME, Jaspers N, et al: The course of neuropsychiatric symptoms in dementia, part I: findings from the two-year longitudinal Maasbed study. Int J Geriatr Psychiatry 20:523–530, 2005

American Psychiatric Association: Diagnostic and Statistical Manual of Mental Disorders, 4th Edition, Text Revision. Washington, DC, American Psychiatric Association, 2000

Andersson S, Gundersen PM, Finset A: Emotional activation during therapeutic interaction in traumatic brain injury: effect of apathy, self-awareness and implications for rehabilitation. Brain Inj 13:393–404, 1999a

Andersson S, Krogstad JM, Finset A: Apathy and depressed mood in acquired brain damage: relationship to lesion localization and psychophysiological reactivity. Psychol Med 29:447–456, 1999b

Barnhart WJ, Makela EH, Latocha MJ: SSRI-induced apathy syndrome: a clinical review. J Psychiatr Pract 10:196–199, 2004

Borroni B, Agosti C, Padovani A: Behavioral and psychological symptoms in dementia with Lewy-bodies (DLB): frequency and relationship with disease severity and motor impairment. Arch Gerontol Geriatr 46:101–106, 2008a

Borroni B, Turla M, Bertasi V, et al: Cognitive and behavioral assessment in the early stages of neurodegenerative extrapyramidal syndromes. Arch Gerontol Geriatr 47:53–61, 2008b

Burke WH, Zencius AH, Wesolowski MD, et al: Improving executive function disorders in brain-injured clients. Brain Inj 5:241–252, 1991

Cantello R, Aguggia M, Gilli M, et al: Major depression in Parkinson's disease and the mood response to intravenous methylphenidate: possible role of the "hedonic" dopamine synapse. J Neurol Neurosurg Psychiatry 52:724–731, 1989

Catsman-Berrevoets CE, von Harskamp F: Compulsive pre-sleep behavior and apathy due to bilateral thalamic stroke: response to bromocriptine. Neurology 38:647–649, 1988

Clark AN, Mankikar GD: D-Amphetamine in elderly patients refractory to rehabilitation procedures. J Am Geriatr Soc 27:174–177, 1979

Clarke DE, Reekum R, Simard M, et al: Apathy in dementia: an examination of the psychometric properties of the Apathy Evaluation Scale. J Neuropsychiatry Clin Neurosci 19:57–64, 2007

Clarke DE, Ko JY, Kuhl EA, et al: Are the available apathy measures reliable and valid? A review of the psychometric evidence. J Psychosom Res 70:73–97, 2011

Crismon ML, Childs A, Wilcox RE, et al: The effect of bromocriptine on speech dysfunction in patients with diffuse brain injury (akinetic mutism). Clin Neuropharmacol 11:462–466, 1988

Cummings JL, Mega M, Gray K, et al: The Neuropsychiatric Inventory: comprehensive assessment of psychopathology in dementia. Neurology 44:2308–2314, 1994

Cummings JL, Mackell J, Kaufer D: Behavioral effects of current Alzheimer's disease treatments: a descriptive review. Alzheimers Dement 4:49–60, 2008

DePoy E, Maley K, Stranraugh J: Executive function and cognitive remediation: a study of activity preference. Occupational Therapy in Health Care 7:101–114, 1990

de Vugt ME, Riedijk SR, Aalten P, et al: Impact of behavioural problems on spousal caregivers: a comparison between Alzheimer's disease and frontotemporal dementia. Dement Geriatr Cogn Disord 22:35–41, 2006

Diehl-Schmid J, Pohl C, Perneczky R, et al: Behavioral disturbances in the course of frontotemporal dementia. Dement Geriatr Cogn Disord 22:352–357, 2006

Drijgers RL, Aalten P, Winogrodzka A, et al: Pharmacological treatment of apathy in neurodegenerative diseases: a systematic review. Dement Geriatr Cogn Disord 28:13–22, 2009

Erkulwater S, Pillai R: Amantadine and the end-stage dementia of Alzheimer's type. South Med J 82:550–554, 1989

Figiel G, Sadowsky C: A systematic review of the effectiveness of rivastigmine for the treatment of behavioral disturbances in dementia and other neurological disorders. Curr Med Res Opin 24:157–166, 2008

Figved N, Klevan G, Myhr KM, et al: Neuropsychiatric symptoms in patients with multiple sclerosis. Acta Psychiatr Scand 112:463–468, 2005

Galynker I, Ieronimo C, Miner C, et al: Methylphenidate treatment of negative symptoms in patients with dementia. J Neuropsychiatry Clin Neurosci 9:231–239, 1997

Glodzik-Sobanska L, Slowik A, Kieltyka A, et al: Reduced prefrontal N-acetylaspartate in stroke patients with apathy. J Neurol Sci 238:19–24, 2005

Hama S, Yamashita H, Shigenobu M, et al: Depression or apathy and functional recovery after stroke. Int J Geriatr Psychiatry 22:1046–1051, 2007

Hopman-Rock M, Staats PG, Tak EC, et al: The effects of a psychomotor activation programme for use in groups of cognitively impaired people in homes for the elderly. Int J Geriatr Psychiatry 14:633–642, 1999

Horiguchi J, Inami Y, Shoda T: Effects of long-term amantadine treatment on clinical symptoms and EEG of a patient in a vegetative state. Clin Neuropharmacol 13:84–88, 1990

Kant R, Duffy JD, Pivovarnik A: Prevalence of apathy following head injury. Brain Inj 12:87–92, 1998

Kaplitz SE: Withdrawn, apathetic geriatric patients responsive to methylphenidate. J Am Geriatr Soc 23:271–276, 1975

Kirsch-Darrow L, Fernandez HH, Marsiske M, et al: Dissociating apathy and depression in Parkinson disease. Neurology 67:33–38, 2006

Kragt K, Holtkamp CC, van Dongen MC, et al: The effect of sensory stimulation in the sensory stimulation room on the well-being of demented elderly: a cross-over trial in residents of the R.C. Care Center Bernardus in Amsterdam [in Dutch]. Verpleegkunde 12:227–236, 1997

Kraus MF, Maki P: The combined use of amantadine and L-dopa/carbidopa in the treatment of chronic brain injury. Brain Inj 11:455–460, 1997a

Kraus MF, Maki PM: Effect of amantadine hydrochloride on symptoms of frontal lobe dysfunction in brain injury: case studies and review. J Neuropsychiatry Clin Neurosci 9:222–230, 1997b

Landes AM, Sperry SD, Strauss ME: Prevalence of apathy, dysphoria, and depression in relation to dementia severity in Alzheimer's disease. J Neuropsychiatry Clin Neurosci 17:342–349, 2005

Lane-Brown AT, Tate RL: Apathy after acquired brain impairment: a systematic review of non-pharmacological interventions. Neuropsychol Rehabil 19:481–516, 2009a

Lane-Brown A, Tate R: Interventions for apathy after traumatic brain injury. Cochrane Database Syst Rev 2009b, Issue 2, Art. No.: CD006341. DOI: 10.1002/14651858.CD006341.pub2.

Levy R, Dubois B: Apathy and the functional anatomy of the prefrontal cortex–basal ganglia circuits. Cereb Cortex 16:916–928, 2006

Maletta GJ, Winegarden T: Reversal of anorexia by methylphenidate in apathetic, severely demented nursing home patients. Am J Geriatr Psychiatry 1:234–243, 1993

Marin RS: Differential diagnosis and classification of apathy. Am J Psychiatry 147:22–30, 1990

Marin RS: Apathy: a neuropsychiatric syndrome. J Neuropsychiatry Clin Neurosci 3:243–254, 1991

Marin RS, Wilkosz PA: Disorders of diminished motivation. J Head Trauma Rehabil 20:377–388, 2005

Marin RS, Biedrzycki RC, Firinciogullari S: Reliability and validity of the Apathy Evaluation Scale. Psychiatry Res 38:143–162, 1991

Marsh NV, Kersel DA, Havill JH, et al: Caregiver burden at 1 year following severe traumatic brain injury. Brain Inj 12:1045–1059, 1998

Masanic CA, Bayley MT, van Reekum R, et al: Open-label study of donepezil in traumatic brain injury. Arch Phys Med Rehabil 82:896–901, 2001

Max JE, Robertson BA, Lansing AE: The phenomenology of personality change due to traumatic brain injury in children and adolescents. J Neuropsychiatry Clin Neurosci 13:161–170, 2001

Newburn G, Newburn D: Selegiline in the management of apathy following traumatic brain injury. Brain Inj 19:149–154, 2005

Padala PR, Petty F, Bhatia SC: Methylphenidate may treat apathy independent of depression. Ann Pharmacother 39:1947–1949, 2005

Parks RW, Crockett DJ, Manji HK, et al: Assessment of bromocriptine intervention for the treatment of frontal lobe syndrome: a case study. J Neuropsychiatry Clin Neurosci 4:109–111, 1992

Powell JH, al-Adawi S, Morgan J, et al: Motivational deficits after brain injury: effects of bromocriptine in 11 patients. J Neurol Neurosurg Psychiatry 60:416–421, 1996

Rao V, Spiro JR, Schretlen DJ, et al: Apathy syndrome after traumatic brain injury compared with deficits in schizophrenia. Psychosomatics 48:217–222, 2007

Robert PH, Berr C, Volteau M, et al: Neuropsychological performance in mild cognitive impairment with and without apathy. Dement Geriatr Cogn Disord 21:192–197, 2006

Rodda J, Morgan S, Walker Z: Are cholinesterase inhibitors effective in the management of the behavioral and psychological symptoms of dementia in Alzheimer's disease? A systematic review of randomized, placebo-controlled trials of donepezil, rivastigmine and galantamine. Int Psychogeriatr 21:813–824, 2009

Rozzini L, Chilovi BV, Bertoletti E, et al: Mild parkinsonian signs and psycho-behavioral symptoms in subjects with mild cognitive impairment. Int Psychogeriatr 20:86–95, 2008

Ryan RM, Deci EL: Intrinsic and extrinsic motivations: classic definitions and new directions. Contemp Educ Psychol 25:54–67, 2000

Salazar AM, Warden DL, Schwab K, et al: Cognitive rehabilitation for traumatic brain injury: a randomized trial. Defense and Veterans Head Injury Program (DVHIP) Study Group. JAMA 283:3075–3081, 2000

Smith RB, Tiberi A, Marshall J: The use of cranial electrotherapy stimulation in the treatment of closed-head-injured patients. Brain Inj 8:357–361, 1994

Sohlberg MM, Sprunk H, Metzelaar K: Efficacy of an external cuing system in an individual with severe frontal lobe damage. Cogn Rehabil 6:36–41, 1988

Srikanth S, Nagaraja AV, Ratnavalli E: Neuropsychiatric symptoms in dementia-frequency, relationship to dementia severity and comparison in Alzheimer's disease, vascular dementia and frontotemporal dementia. J Neurol Sci 236:43–48, 2005

Starkstein SE, Mayberg HS, Preziosi TJ, et al: Reliability, validity, and clinical correlates of apathy in Parkinson's disease. J Neuropsychiatry Clin Neurosci 4:134–139, 1992

Starkstein SE, Jorge R, Mizrahi R, et al: A prospective longitudinal study of apathy in Alzheimer's disease. J Neurol Neurosurg Psychiatry 77:8–11, 2006

Stuss DT, van Reekum R, Murphy KJ: Differentiation of states and causes of apathy, in The Neuropsychology of Emotion. Edited by Borod JC. New York, Oxford University Press, 2000, pp 340–363

Tam CW, Lam LC, Lui VW, et al: Clinical correlates of functional performance in community-dwelling Chinese older persons with mild cognitive impairment. Int Psychogeriatr 20:1059–1070, 2008

van Reekum R, Bayley M, Garner S, et al: N of 1 study: amantadine for the amotivational syndrome in a patient with traumatic brain injury. Brain Inj 9:49–53, 1995

van Reekum R, Cohen T, Wong J: Can traumatic brain injury cause psychiatric disorders? J Neuropsychiatry Clin Neurosci 12:316–327, 2000

van Reekum R, Stuss DT, Ostrander L: Apathy: why care? J Neuropsychiatry Clin Neurosci 17:7–19, 2005 von Cramon DY, Matthes-von Cramon G, Mai N: Problem-solving deficits in brain-injured patients: a therapeutic approach. Neuropsychol Rehabil 1:45–64, 1991

Watanabe MD, Martin EM, DeLeon OA, et al: Successful methylphenidate treatment of apathy after subcortical infarcts. J Neuropsychiatry Clin Neurosci 7:502–504, 1995

Wongpakaran N, van Reekum R, Wongpakaran T, et al: Selective serotonin reuptake inhibitor use associates with apathy among depressed elderly: a case-control study. Ann Gen Psychiatry 6:7, 2007

# CHAPTER 12

## Substance Use Disorders

*Jennifer Bogner, Ph.D.*

**The co-occurrence** of traumatic brain injury (TBI) and substance use disorder can result in more adverse outcomes than either disorder in isolation. Growing neurophysiological, neuropsychological, and neuroimaging evidence suggests that more impaired functioning occurs in persons who have a history of both TBI and substance use disorders (Baguley et al. 1997; Jorge et al. 2005; Wilde et al. 2004). A history of substance abuse prior to the index TBI is associated with decreased productivity, lower life satisfaction, and increased likelihood of psychiatric problems at follow-up (Bogner et al. 2001; Brenner et al. 2008; Jorge et al. 2005).

Compounded deficits in self-regulation—that is, in the ability to make choices and execute behaviors that are consistent with one's long-term goals and self-interests—may be one of the sources of poorer long-term outcomes. Due to the mechanism of injury, the majority of individuals with TBI experience damage to the frontal lobe, the mediator of self-regulation (Barkley 2001). Likewise, substance use disorders are thought to be caused by, as well as to contribute to, difficulties with self-regulation (Justus et al. 2001; Petry et al. 1998). Because of deficient self-regulation associated with the co-occurring disorders, the ability to maintain control of alcohol or other drug use

303

may be reduced, and the effects of use on health and functioning may be intensified. Careful screening to identify these disorders must be conducted, and treatment methods must be adjusted to accommodate for deficits in cognition, including executive functioning.

# DEFINITIONS

DSM-IV-TR (American Psychiatric Association 2000) and ICD-10 (World Health Organization 1992/2010) define *harmful substance use, abuse,* and *dependence* (Table 12–1). In the absence of a diagnosable substance use disorder, the health care professional should also be concerned with *hazardous use,* which is defined as the use of alcohol or other drugs that can increase the risk of physical, mental, or social consequences. The National Institute on Alcohol Abuse and Alcoholism (2010) provides guidelines for the identification of alcohol misuse in the absence of an alcohol use disorder (Box 12–1). These guidelines not only indicate the amount of alcohol consumption considered to be unhealthy for the majority of the population, but also specify that use is contraindicated for persons with some health conditions. Although no clear guidelines exist regarding the use of alcohol or other drugs following TBI, the deleterious outcomes associated with substance use lend support to the recommendation to abstain from alcohol and other drug use after TBI.

# EPIDEMIOLOGY

Studies of the rate of co-occurring TBI and substance use disorders—from subject samples selected on the basis of TBI as well as samples of persons receiving substance abuse treatment—suggest that approximately one-third to two-thirds of individuals with either condition have the other as a comorbidity (Alterman and Tarter 1985; Corrigan 1995; Hillbom and Holm 1986; Malloy et al. 1990; Parry-Jones et al. 2006). Rates may be even higher in populations of persons who also have a severe mental health disorder (Corrigan and Deutschle 2008). Although some studies have suggested that substance abuse may initially decline in individuals following TBI, those individuals with a history of substance abuse are at increased risk for eventually resuming substance abuse (Bombardier et al. 2003), suggesting that without successful intervention, the co-occurrence of TBI and substance use disorders will continue to be problematic.

**TABLE 12–1.** Diagnostic criteria for harmful substance use, abuse, and dependence

| CONDITION | DEFINITION |
|---|---|
| Harmful substance use (ICD-10) | Pattern of use observed throughout past month or repeatedly during past year for which there is evidence that it has substantially contributed to damage to physical or mental health; may not be diagnosed if criteria for substance dependence are met |
| Substance abuse (DSM-IV-TR) | Pattern of use during past 12 months, leading to impairment, as manifested by at least one of the following: failure to fulfill major role obligations, use in physically hazardous situations, recurrent legal problems, persistent or recurrent negative social consequences |
| Substance dependence (DSM-IV-TR) | At any time in the same 12 month period, a maladaptive pattern of substance use consisting of at least three of the following: tolerance; withdrawal; using substance in larger amounts or for longer than intended; persistent desire or unsuccessful efforts to cut down or control substance use; devotion of time to obtaining, using, or recovering from effects of substance use; giving up important activities because of substance use; continued substance use despite knowledge that it is adversely affecting physical or psychological health |

*Source.* American Psychiatric Association 2000; World Health Organization 1992/2010.

# CLINICAL ASSESSMENT

Screening for substance use disorders can be conducted by any health care provider with training in the signs and symptoms of substance misuse. Although a number of tools are available, careful clinical interview is likely to remain the key method for ascertaining the extent and effects of an individual's substance use history. Clinicians who develop therapeutic rapport with the individual and use a nonjudgmental approach, open-ended questions, and reflective listening are more likely to engage the person and obtain a comprehensive history than are clinicians who rely strictly on answers from questionnaires or toxicology screens.

Standardized assessment tools can be used to supplement the clinical interview (in some settings, the standardized tools are required).

---

**BOX 12–1.**  NATIONAL INSTITUTE ON ALCOHOL ABUSE AND
ALCOHOLISM DEFINITION OF ALCOHOL MISUSE

- For healthy men <65 years, more than four drinks in a day or 14 drinks in a week

- For healthy men ≥65 years and for healthy women of any age, more than three drinks in a day or seven drinks in a week

- Use by individuals with medical conditions that contraindicate alcohol use or who are taking certain medications

*Source.*  Adapted from National Institute on Alcohol Abuse and Alcoholism: Moderate & Binge Drinking. Available at: http://www.niaaa.nih.gov/alcohol-health/overview-alcohol-consumption/moderate-binge-drinking. Accessed October 29, 2012.

---

The American College of Surgeons Committee on Trauma (2006) recommends the CAGE questionnaire (Ewing 1984) paired with questions on the amount of consumption, the Alcohol Use Disorders Identification Test (AUDIT; Babor et al. 2001), and the CRAFFT (Knight et al. 2002) for screening of adolescents. A more recent tool developed by the World Health Organization, the Alcohol, Smoking and Substance Involvement Screening Test (ASSIST; Humeniuk et al. 2010), also may be useful. The ASSIST has not been specifically studied with persons with TBI, but it is similar to other tools and has been validated in nine countries. The ASSIST allows for an assessment of risk and the level of intervention required for the full range of substances, rather than being limited specifically to alcohol or to other drugs. An ASSIST-linked brief intervention has also been tested and found to be efficacious in an international randomized controlled trial. The National Institute on Drug Abuse has modified the ASSIST slightly, adding additional information to evaluate alcohol consumption, additional probes, and more guidance on methods of intervention.

Measurement of blood alcohol concentration (BAC) also may be used for screening for alcohol use at the time of the index injury, although a positive result does not necessarily indicate a history of substance abuse. Maximum accuracy is obtained when the blood is drawn immediately after TBI; however, the American College of Surgeons has provided an algorithm to estimate the level at the time of injury if the blood is drawn hours later. In 2000, the U.S. Congress passed the Department of Transportation Appropriations Act for fiscal year 2001 and adopted a BAC of 0.08% (percentage by volume) as the national legal threshold that indicates impaired driving, although lower BACs are associated with cognitive and motor impairments (Chamberlain and Solomon 2002). Extremely high levels suggest tolerance, an indicator of alcohol dependence. A toxicology screen to detect other drugs can also be conducted but results should be cautiously interpreted because the window of detection differs for various drugs; a negative result indicates only that the threshold was not met, and not that the drug was not ingested; and standard toxicology screens do not test for all drugs.

# TREATMENT

## Psychological and Behavioral Interventions

Corrigan (2005, 2007) proposed a four-quadrant model for conceptualizing behavioral interventions for substance use disorder and TBI. Differences in severity for each of the co-occurring conditions are thought to have implications for treatment. As shown in Figure 12–1, dichotomizing the severity of each condition as either high or low defines four quadrants. The resulting quadrants identify the service delivery systems in which individuals are likely to be found, as well as the most appropriate treatment tools for the setting and population.

Persons with lower-severity substance use disorders (e.g., hazardous use or abuse but not substance dependence) and less severe TBI are most likely to be seen in primary care or emergency (acute medical) settings (Figure 12–1, Quadrant I). The encounter in these settings may represent a unique moment in a person's life when he or she may be more open to change, because many of these individuals will have just experienced a substance-related injury or received a medical diagnosis related to substance use. Screening and brief interventions are the most feasible and effective tools in this setting, given the need to also provide primary or emergency care in a restricted amount of time. The goal of a brief intervention is to raise awareness of the person's level of risk associated with substance misuse and to encourage behavioral change. Advice and assistance are tailored to the individual's level of risk and readiness for change (Table 12–2)

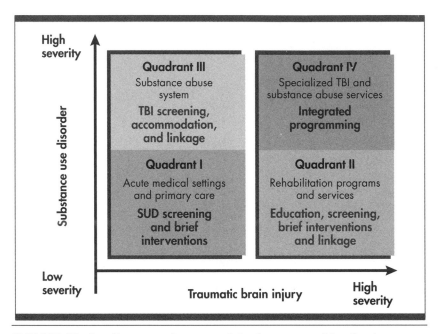

**FIGURE 12–1.**   Four-quadrant model of opportunities for intervention with co-occurring substance abuse and traumatic brain injury.

*Note.*   SUD=substance use disorder; TBI=traumatic brain injury.

(Prochaska and DiClemente 1982). Individuals who are at low risk and abstainers are advised not to increase use, those who are at risk or moderate users are provided advice regarding their risk and assistance based on their readiness to change, and those who exhibit signs of more severe substance use disorders are encouraged to accept a referral for treatment. One of the most widely used and evaluated brief interventions for alcohol problems is the FRAMES model; as shown in Table 12–3, FRAMES comprises Feedback, Responsibility, Advice to change, Menu of options, Empathy, and Self-efficacy (Bien et al. 1993; Gentilello et al. 1999).

Individuals who sustain more severe TBI ideally receive rehabilitation (Figure 12–1, Quadrant II), providing another opportunity for intervention in the context of a life-changing event. Rehabilitation provides a climate for behavioral change; if the rehabilitation team provides a consistent message regarding the risks of substance use following injury, that message has a greater chance to be received. All rehabilitation patients should be screened for a history of substance use disorders, and those with such histories should receive education,

**TABLE 12–2.** Stages of change

| STAGE | DESCRIPTION |
| --- | --- |
| Precontemplation | Person does not recognize that substance use is a problem and does not currently intend to change behavior. |
| Contemplation | Person has begun to recognize that substance use is a problem. Person may be weighing pros and cons of discontinuing use, and could be underestimating the pros or overestimating the cons. |
| Preparation | Person is making plans for a change but has not yet set a firm goal. |
| Action | Person is changing behavior to abstain or reduce substance use. Person may make environmental alterations to support the goal. |
| Maintenance | Person has sustained successful change for 6 months or more but may be challenged by urges to use. Person is working to consolidate changes into a sustainable lifestyle to prevent relapse. |

**TABLE 12–3.** FRAMES model of intervention

| COMPONENT | DESCRIPTION |
| --- | --- |
| **F**eedback | Using results of screening, compare level of use to recommended levels (none may be recommended for persons with TBI) and describe risks of use at that level. |
| **R**esponsibility | Emphasize personal control and responsibility for making changes. |
| **A**dvice to change | Provide specific recommendations to reduce or eliminate substance use. |
| **M**enu of options | Provide a choice of strategies to facilitate behavior change (e.g., identifying triggers for use; keeping a drinking diary). |
| **E**mpathy | Use a nonjudgmental, nonconfrontational approach. |
| **S**elf-efficacy | Instill confidence, optimism, and hope that the individual can make the necessary changes. |

brief intervention, and a referral for treatment. Education is provided to those without a history of substance use disorders in an effort to prevent the development of substance misuse or other substance use disorders.

The goal of education is to increase the individual's awareness of reasons not to use alcohol or other drugs, and to debunk or lessen the influence of the individual's reasons for continued use (Box 12–2).

---

**BOX 12–2.** EDUCATIONAL MESSAGES REGARDING SUBSTANCE USE
AFTER TRAUMATIC BRAIN INJURY

- People who use alcohol or other drugs after they have a brain injury don't recover as much.

- Brain injuries cause problems in balance, walking, or talking that get worse when a person uses alcohol or other drugs.

- People who have had a brain injury often say or do things without thinking first, a problem that is made worse by using alcohol and other drugs.

- Brain injuries cause problems with thinking, like concentration or memory, and using alcohol or other drugs makes these problems worse.

- After brain injury, alcohol and other drugs have a more powerful effect.

- People who have had a brain injury are more likely to have times that they feel low or depressed, and drinking alcohol and getting high on other drugs makes this worse.

- After a brain injury, drinking alcohol or using other drugs can cause a seizure.

- People who drink alcohol or use other drugs after a brain injury are more likely to have another brain injury.

*Source.*   Reprinted from *User's Manual for Faster More Reliable Operation of a Brain After Injury.* © Ohio Valley Center for Brain Injury Prevention and Rehabilitation, 1996, 2005. Used with permission.

Notably, some individuals will present as "converts," expressing the feeling that they have learned from their experience and will never use alcohol or other drugs again. These individuals do not feel as if they need additional assistance, because they have already made the decision to cease use. Although their intentions are to be commended and reinforced, converts are frequently unaware of the difficulties that they may encounter with sustaining abstinence after they leave the protected hospital environment. Therefore, family members and others in the person's environment should also be educated on the dangers of continued substance use and on how to assist with sustaining change after discharge. Education can be provided individually and/or in a group format (preferably both) and should utilize multiple forms of media.

Brief intervention may also be provided in the rehabilitation setting. Unfortunately, although a substantial body of literature has accumulated attesting to the effectiveness of brief interventions, studies have generally excluded persons with significant cognitive deficits due to more severe TBI, usually because the individuals were unable to provide consent or participate in the intervention (Corrigan et al. 2010). Currently, the best option is to provide brief interventions with accommodations for cognitive deficits (Table 12–4), link individuals with more severe substance use disorders with ongoing treatment, and follow up with individuals after discharge.

Individuals with TBI who show signs of a substance use disorder or who are at risk for hazardous substance use should be referred for ongoing intervention (Figure 12–1, Quadrants III and IV). A substance use disorder treatment specialist can conduct a comprehensive diagnostic assessment and recommend a course for treatment. A designated rehabilitation team member plays a critical role not only in identifying and linking the patient to the appropriate provider, preferably within the individual's home community, but also in reducing barriers to appointment attendance that might arise from deficient executive functioning or tangible resources. The rehabilitation team member can assist with scheduling the appointment and with addressing other preparatory activities (e.g., arranging transportation, child care, funding). A reminder call has been found to greatly facilitate appointment attendance. Assuming that a release is obtained from the patient, the substance use disorder treatment provider should be given information about TBI, with recommendations for accommodations specific to the individual. The rehabilitation team

**TABLE 12–4.** Suggestions for substance use disorder treatment providers working with persons who have limitations in cognitive abilities

| OBJECTIVE | METHODS |
| --- | --- |
| Determine the person's unique communication and learning styles | Ask how well the person reads and writes; or evaluate via samples. |
| | Evaluate whether the individual is able to comprehend both written and spoken language. |
| | If someone is not able to speak (or speak easily), inquire as to alternate methods of expression (e.g., writing or gestures). |
| | Both ask about and observe a person's attention span; be attuned to whether attention seems to change in busy versus quiet environments. |
| | Both ask about and observe a person's capacity for new learning; inquire as to strengths and weaknesses or seek consultation to determine optimum approaches. |
| Assist the individual to compensate for a unique learning style | Modify written material to make it concise and to the point. |
| | Paraphrase concepts, use concrete examples, incorporate visual aids, or otherwise present an idea in more than one way. |
| | If it helps, allow the individual to take notes or at least write down key points for later review and recall. |
| | Encourage the use of a calendar or planner; if the treatment program includes a daily schedule, make sure a "pocket version" is kept for easy reference. |
| | Make sure homework assignments are written down. |
| | After group sessions, meet individually to review main points. |
| | Provide assistance with homework or worksheets; allow more time and take into account reading or writing abilities. |
| | Enlist family, friends, or other service providers to reinforce goals. |
| | Do not take for granted that something learned in one situation will be generalized to another. |
| | Repeat, review, rehearse, repeat, review, rehearse. |

**TABLE 12–4.** Suggestions for substance use disorder treatment providers working with persons who have limitations in cognitive abilities *(continued)*

| OBJECTIVE | METHODS |
|---|---|
| Provide direct feedback regarding inappropriate behaviors | Let a person know a behavior is inappropriate; do not assume the individual knows and is choosing to do so anyway.<br>Provide straightforward feedback about when and where behaviors are appropriate.<br>Redirect tangential or excessive speech, including use of a predetermined method of signaling in groups. |
| Be cautious when making inferences about motivation based on observed behaviors | Do not presume that noncompliance arises from lack of motivation or resistance; check it out.<br>Be aware that unawareness of deficits can arise as a result of specific damage to the brain and may not always be due to denial.<br>Confrontation shuts down thinking and elicits rigidity; roll with resistance.<br>Do not just discharge for noncompliance; follow up and find out why someone has no-showed or otherwise not followed through. |

*Source.* Reprinted from *User's Manual for Faster More Reliable Operation of a Brain After Injury.* © Ohio Valley Center for Brain Injury Prevention and Rehabilitation, 1998, 2010. Used with permission.

member should follow up to determine whether the appointment was attended, and should provide additional assistance as needed. Ideally, the rehabilitation and substance use disorder treatment providers will continue to work together to achieve optimal outcomes in both treatment settings.

The limited research on substance users with cognitive impairments (Bates et al. 2006) as well as clinical observations of persons with TBI in treatment suggests that individuals with co-occurring TBI and substance use disorders have greater difficulties with treatment adherence than do persons with substance use disorders alone; treatment compliance and retention in treatment are key factors in predicting outcomes (Simpson et al. 1997). Greater difficulties with treatment compliance may be due to compounded deficits in self-regulation. Although both substance use disorders and TBI are associated with impulsive behaviors, clinical observations suggest a greater disconnect between behavior and long-term goals and intentions among individuals with the co-occurring disorders. When deficits in self-regulation are combined with difficulties with organization and memory, it is not surprising that persons with TBI and substance use disorders fail to attend appointments or follow a treatment plan. In addition, disinhibition and deficits in social pragmatics can disrupt individual and group sessions, affecting relationships with fellow patients as well as counselors. Furthermore, deficits in attention and new learning can slow the acquisition of new skills and behaviors.

The behaviors associated with deficient cognitive and executive functioning can easily be misinterpreted as resistance to treatment, and this can undermine the therapeutic relationship. Awareness on the part of the provider regarding the complexities of deficits associated with TBI, combined with the use of accommodations for cognitive and executive functioning deficits, can serve to facilitate more effective treatment.

Ideally, persons with more severe TBI combined with substance abuse or dependence should receive treatment in specialized, integrated community-based treatment programs administered by teams of providers with expertise in TBI and substance use disorders (Figure 12–1, Quadrant IV). Such programs should include education and skill building for consumers, intensive case management embracing a holistic approach, and interprofessional consultation and education for treatment providers (Corrigan 2007; Corrigan et al. 1995; Langley et al. 1990; Vungkhanching et al. 2007). Unfortunately, few integrated, comprehensive programs exist, making it necessary to adapt services that are available to best meet the needs of persons with co-occurring disorders. To that end, collaborative, ad hoc treatment teams that include providers from both the substance abuse treatment and rehabilitation service systems may represent the best alternative.

In addition to the provision of appropriate accommodations, the effectiveness of substance use disorder treatment depends on engaging and retaining the individual in treatment until goals are met. Recent substance use disorder treatment approaches employ motivational incentives (Higgins et al. 2002; Petry et al. 2000), usually as an adjunct to other treatment methodologies; these approaches also appear to be effective for persons with TBI and substance use disorders (Corrigan and Bogner 2007; Corrigan et al. 2005). For example, at intake individuals can be informed that if they attend all of their appointments during the next month, they will receive a fifteen dollar gift certificate (or another nominal amount). Studies using a similar incentive plan have found that individuals are more likely not only to attend the first month's appointments, but also to stay in treatment until goals are met, without additional financial incentives (Corrigan and Bogner 2007; Corrigan et al. 2005). Individuals do not tend to identify the incentive as their reason for attending treatment. Although the mechanism of action is still not fully understood, the financial incentive may provide an early, salient, and concrete goal that might be needed by persons with significant deficiencies in self-regulation, particularly during the early phases of treatment.

# Pharmacotherapy

Pharmacotherapy may be a useful adjunct to psychological and behavioral treatments for some individuals with substance use disorders, and particularly for those with alcohol use disorders. Naltrexone, acamprosate, and disulfiram are approved by the U.S. Food and Drug Administration (FDA) for treatment of alcohol dependence. Topiramate also may be an effective treatment for alcohol dependence, but it does not have FDA approval for this use as of this writing. However, the effectiveness of these agents specifically for individuals with TBI is not known. The mechanisms of action for at least some of the agents involve the reward-processing neural circuitry located in areas frequently damaged following TBI; accordingly, the effects of medications acting on these circuits also may be altered.

Patient adherence to treatment is essential to achieving maximum benefits from pharmacotherapy. Adherence may be especially difficult to achieve in persons with memory and organizational deficits. For these reasons, adherence to prescribed treatment needs to be monitored closely, and pharmacotherapy needs to be provided in conjunction with psychological and/or behavioral therapies. The National Institute on Alcohol Abuse and Alcoholism recommends that the provider incorporate brief intervention methodology into regular follow-ups with the patient. Patients may also benefit from assistance with the development of compensatory strategies to support treatment adherence, for which consultation with a rehabilitation therapist may be required.

# CONCLUSION

Co-occurring TBI and substance use disorders are frequently observed and challenging to treat. Deficiencies in self-regulation common to both disorders most likely serve to perpetuate their dual presentation and can significantly interfere with treatment and rehabilitation. All individuals with TBI should be carefully screened for substance misuse and, regardless of history of substance use, provided with education regarding the effects of substance use in conjunction with TBI. For persons at risk for substance misuse, additional treatment will be required. Most importantly, accommodations for deficits in cognitive functioning and self-regulation should be incorporated into all treatment methodologies. Given that the behaviors associated with deficient cognitive and executive functioning can easily be misinterpreted as resistance to treatment, care should be taken to identify and address the effects of a TBI early in the treatment relationship. Careful screening to identify these disorders must be conducted, and treatment methods must be adjusted to accommodate for deficits in cognition, including executive functioning. Treatment rests principally on psychological and behavioral interventions; the four-quadrant model presented in this chapter is a particularly useful heuristic for the treatment of comorbid TBI and substance use disorders.

## *Key Clinical Points*

- The co-occurrence of TBI and substance use disorder can potentially result in more adverse outcomes than either disorder in isolation.
- Given that this comorbidity adversely affects outcomes associated with either condition, that no "safe" amount of use in this population has been identified, and that control of use can be more difficult for persons with deficits in self-regulation, it is recommended that persons with TBI abstain from alcohol and other drug use.
- Screening, intervention, and education are most effective when conducted by an informed health care professional using an open and accessible interactional style and when the clinical approach is adjusted to accommodate for cognitive and behavioral deficits related to TBI and/or substance use disorder.
- The behaviors associated with deficient cognitive and executive functioning can easily be misinterpreted as resistance to treatment, and this can seriously undermine the therapeutic relationship.

# REFERENCES

Alterman AI, Tarter RE: Relationship between familial alcoholism and head injury. J Stud Alcohol 46:256–258, 1985

American College of Surgeons Committee on Trauma: Resources for Optimal Care of the Injured Patient. Chicago, IL, American College of Surgeons Committee on Trauma, 2006

American Psychiatric Association: Diagnostic and Statistical Manual of Mental Disorders, 4th Edition, Text Revision. Washington, DC, American Psychiatric Association, 2000

Babor TF, Higgins-Biddle JC, Saunders JB, et al: Alcohol Use Disorders Identification Test (AUDIT): Guidelines for Use in Primary Care. Geneva, World Health Organization, 2001

Baguley IJ, Felmingham KL, Lahz S, et al: Alcohol abuse and traumatic brain injury: effect on event-related potentials. Arch Phys Med Rehabil 78:1248–1253, 1997

Barkley RA: The executive functions and self-regulation: an evolutionary neuropsychological perspective. Neuropsychol Rev 11:1–29, 2001

Bates ME, Pawlak AP, Tonigan JS, et al: Cognitive impairment influences drinking outcome by altering therapeutic mechanisms of change. Psychol Addict Behav 20:241–253, 2006

Bien TH, Miller WR, Tonigan JS: Brief interventions for alcohol problems: a review. Addiction 88:315–335, 1993

Bogner JA, Corrigan JD, Mysiw WJ, et al: A comparison of substance abuse and violence in the prediction of long-term rehabilitation outcomes after traumatic brain injury. Arch Phys Med Rehabil 82:571–577, 2001

Bombardier CH, Temkin NR, Machamer J, et al: The natural history of drinking and alcohol-related problems after traumatic brain injury. Arch Phys Med Rehabil 84:185–191, 2003

Brenner LA, Harwood JEE, Homaifar BY, et al: Psychiatric hospitalization and veterans with traumatic brain injury: a retrospective study. J Head Trauma Rehabil 23:401–406, 2008

Chamberlain E, Solomon R: The case for a 0.05% criminal law blood alcohol concentration limit for driving. Inj Prev 8 (suppl 3):iii1–iii17, 2002

Corrigan JD: Substance abuse as a mediating factor in outcome from traumatic brain injury. Arch Phys Med Rehabil 76:302–309, 1995

Corrigan JD: Substance abuse, in Rehabilitation for Traumatic Brain Injury. Edited by High WM Jr, Sander AM, Struchen MA, et al. New York, Oxford University Press, 2005, pp 133–155

Corrigan JD: The treatment of substance abuse, in Brain Injury Medicine: Principles and Practice. Edited by Zasler ND, Katz DI, Zafonte RD. New York, Demos, 2007, pp 1105–1115

Corrigan JD, Bogner J: Interventions to promote retention in substance abuse treatment. Brain Inj 21:343–356, 2007

Corrigan JD, Deutschle JJ Jr: The presence and impact of traumatic brain injury among clients in treatment for co-occurring mental illness and substance abuse. Brain Inj 22:223–231, 2008

Corrigan JD, Lamb-Hart GL, Rust E: A programme of intervention for substance abuse following traumatic brain injury. Brain Inj 9:221–236, 1995

Corrigan JD, Bogner J, Lamb-Hart G, et al: Increasing substance abuse treatment compliance for persons with traumatic brain injury. Psychol Addict Behav 19:131–139, 2005

Corrigan JD, Bogner J, Hungerford DW, et al: Screening and brief intervention for substance misuse among patients with traumatic brain injury. J Trauma 69:722–726, 2010

Ewing JA: Detecting alcoholism: the CAGE questionnaire. JAMA 252:1905–1907, 1984

Gentilello LM, Rivara FP, Donovan DM, et al: Alcohol interventions in a trauma center as a means of reducing the risk of injury recurrence. Ann Surg 230:473–480, discussion 480–483, 1999

Higgins ST, Alessi SM, Dantona RL: Voucher-based incentives: a substance abuse treatment innovation. Addict Behav 27:887–910, 2002

Hillbom M, Holm L: Contribution of traumatic head injury to neuropsychological deficits in alcoholics. J Neurol Neurosurg Psychiatry 49:1348–1353, 1986

Humeniuk RE, Henry-Edwards S, Ali RL, et al: The Alcohol, Smoking and Substance Involvement Screening Test (ASSIST): Manual for Use in Primary Care. Geneva, World Health Organization, 2010

Jorge RE, Starkstein SE, Arndt S, et al: Alcohol misuse and mood disorders following traumatic brain injury. Arch Gen Psychiatry 62:742–749, 2005

Justus AN, Finn PR, Steinmetz JE: P300, disinhibited personality, and early onset alcohol problems. Alcohol Clin Exp Res 25:1457–1466, 2001

Knight JR, Sherritt L, Shrier LA, et al: Validity of the CRAFFT substance abuse screening test among adolescent clinic patients. Arch Pediatr Adolesc Med 156:607–614, 2002

Langley MJ, Lindsay WP, Lam CS, et al: A comprehensive alcohol abuse treatment programme for persons with traumatic brain injury. Brain Inj 4:77–86, 1990

Malloy P, Noel N, Longabaugh R, et al: Determinants of neuropsychological impairment in antisocial substance abusers. Addict Behav 15:431–438, 1990

National Institute on Alcohol Abuse and Alcoholism: Moderate & Binge Drinking. 2012. Available at: http://www.niaaa.nih.gov/alcohol-health/overview-alcohol-consumption/moderate-binge-drinking. Accessed October 29, 2012.

National Institute on Drug Abuse: NM ASSIST: Screening for Tobacco, Alcohol and Other Drug Use. Available at: http://www.drugabuse.gov/nidamed/nm-assist-screening-tobacco-alcohol-other-drug-use. Accessed October 29, 2012.

Parry-Jones BL, Vaughan FL, Miles Cox W: Traumatic brain injury and substance misuse: a systematic review of prevalence and outcomes research (1994–2004). Neuropsychol Rehabil 16:537–560, 2006

Petry NM, Bickel WK, Arnett M: Shortened time horizons and insensitivity to future consequences in heroin addicts. Addiction 93:729–738, 1998

Petry NM, Martin B, Cooney JL, et al: Give them prizes, and they will come: contingency management for treatment of alcohol dependence. J Consult Clin Psychol 68:250–257, 2000

Prochaska JO, DiClemente CC: Trans-theoretical therapy: toward a more integrative model of change. Psychotherapy: Theory Research and Practice 19:276–288, 1982

Simpson DD, Joe GW, Rowan-Szal GA, et al: Drug abuse treatment process components that improve retention. J Subst Abuse Treat 14:565–572, 1997

Vungkhanching M, Heinemann AW, Langley MJ, et al: Feasibility of a skills-based substance abuse prevention program following traumatic brain injury. J Head Trauma Rehabil 22:167–176, 2007

Wilde EA, Bigler ED, Gandhi PV, et al: Alcohol abuse and traumatic brain injury: quantitative magnetic resonance imaging and neuropsychological outcome. J Neurotrauma 21:137–147, 2004

World Health Organization: The ICD-10 Classification of Mental and Behavioural Disorders: Clinical Descriptions and Diagnostic Guidelines. Geneva, World Health Organization, 1992/2010

# POSTTRAUMATIC SOMATIC PROBLEMS

# CHAPTER 13

# Headache

*Robert L. Ruff, M.D., Ph.D.*
*Ronald G. Riechers II, M.D.*
*Mark F. Walker, M.D.*
*Suzanne Ruff, Ph.D.*

**Headache is a common** problem following traumatic brain injury (TBI) as well as head or neck trauma. It is especially common in the early postinjury period but may persist for months or years thereafter. Although headache is often associated with other postconcussive symptoms, it may dominate the clinical picture in some individuals. Whether as the presenting symptom or a key comorbidity in a patient with multiple acute or persistent postconcussive symptoms, headache contributes importantly to distress and functional limitations among persons with TBI. In this chapter, we offer a brief review of posttraumatic headaches, beginning with the definition, epidemiology, and pathophysiology of this condition. We then describe the assessment and management of posttraumatic headache, with special focus on the management of headache among Veterans with polytrauma and persons with severe TBI, including those with communication impairments.

# DEFINITION

The classification system of the International Headache Society (Headache Classification Subcommittee of the International Headache Society 2004) has a distinct category for posttraumatic headaches, which encompasses headaches associated with head and neck trauma. This classification system is based on a medical model and may not fully capture the complexity of posttraumatic headaches (Zasler 1999). Posttraumatic headaches usually develop within 7 days of head trauma or return of consciousness following TBI. Occasionally, the onset of headaches may be delayed by weeks to months. The most frequent types of civilian head trauma also injure the cervical spinal cord and neck musculature. Pain can originate from both the head and the neck.

Posttraumatic headaches often have features of other headache types. The most common patterns of posttraumatic headaches resemble tension, cervicogenic, and migraine headaches. Other less common headache types that will not be further discussed include epilepsy-related headache; cluster headache; paroxysmal hemicrania; dysautonomic headache; cavernous sinus headache; carotid artery cavernous sinus fistula headache; tension pneumocephalus headache; posttraumatic sinus headache; retro-orbital headache; and other headache types associated with upper cervical pathology producing myofascial injury or occipital nerve injury (Zasler 1999). Posttraumatic headaches can have a pattern of mixed headaches, with features of more than one primary type of headache.

The majority of civilian posttraumatic headaches can be classified as tension-type or cervicogenic headaches, with the fraction of tension headaches being as high as 85% (Evans 2004). Tension headaches meet at least two of the following four criteria: 1) bilateral pain, 2) pain that is pressing or tightening but not pulsating, 3) mild to moderate pain intensity, or 4) pain that is not aggravated or is only minimally aggravated by physical activity. Tension headaches are not accompanied by nausea or vomiting. Tension headaches may be accompanied by either phonophobia or photophobia, but not both. (Note that in this chapter, we refer only to photophobia rather than photosensitivity; the latter describes an aversion to light, whereas photophobia also can include a sensation of eye pain.) During a tension headache, patients may have tenderness of pericranial muscles. Among individuals who experienced tension headaches prior to head trauma, posttraumatic tension headaches are associated with an increase in headache frequency or intensity or a change in the pain pattern following head trauma. Most headaches resolve within 3 months, but the condition will persist indefinitely for a significant minority of individuals (McCrea and American Academy of Clinical Neuropsychology 2008).

Cervicogenic pain is focused in the neck and occipital region of the head. It is often associated with palpable contraction of posterior cervical muscles and can be partially alleviated by cervical massage or heat applied to the neck. In our experience, topical treatments that may increase blood flow to skin and underlying muscle can reduce pain. Cervicogenic pain can be increased by neck movement, particularly extreme forward flexion or rotation. In contrast, tension headaches have a pattern of pain that is bandlike and temporal, or perceived as behind the eyes. Tension headaches can also be perceived as a holocephalic pressure or as if a belt or cap is tightening about the head. Both cervicogenic and tension headaches are usually characterized by a dull, aching type of pain. Individuals with head and neck trauma may have features of both cervicogenic pain and tension headaches.

Most cases of posttraumatic migraine headaches resemble migraine without aura (common migraine). The criteria for migraine are recurrent episodes of pain lasting 4–72 hours with at least two of the following four characteristics: 1) unilateral pain, 2) pulsating quality, 3) moderate or severe intensity, or 4) exacerbation caused by or causing avoidance of routine physical activity. In addition, migraines have at least one of the following characteristics: 1) nausea, vomiting, or both, or 2) phonophobia or photophobia. Among individuals who experienced migraine headaches prior to head trauma, posttraumatic migraine headaches are associated with a definite increase in headache frequency or intensity or change in the pain pattern following head trauma. In civilian populations, posttraumatic migraine headaches typically resolve within 3 months (McCrea and American Academy of Clinical Neuropsychology 2008). Mixed migraine tension headaches have features of both headache types. Headaches associated with combat-acquired TBI are often mixed migraine tension headaches in character and complicated by coexistent stress disorders, such as posttraumatic stress disorder (PTSD), depression, and sleep disorders (Ruff et al. 2008, 2009).

# EPIDEMIOLOGY

The prevalence of posttraumatic headaches differs for TBI in a civilian setting versus TBI in a combat setting. Among civilians, 15.34%

with mild TBI (mTBI) had persistent posttraumatic headache at 3 months compared to 2.2% among controls with minor non-TBI injury (Faux and Sheedy 2008). In contrast, 52%–55% of combat Veterans had headaches more than 1 year after combat-related TBI (Lew et al. 2009; Ruff et al. 2008).

Among civilians and Veterans, prevalence of pain, particularly posttraumatic headache, is inversely related to TBI severity (Theeler and Erickson 2009). Uomoto and Esselman (1993) found that 95% of individuals with mTBI reported pain, predominantly headaches, whereas only 22% of those with moderate to severe TBI did so. Patients with poor cognitive recovery may have a lower incidence of headaches because pain perception is related to the integrity of cognitive function (Formisano et al. 2009). Additionally, pain may be underrecognized in people with poor cognition. Skull fracture or meningeal laceration predisposes to headache (Clark et al. 2009; Gironda et al. 2009; Lew et al. 2009).

The character of posttraumatic headaches differs between civilian-sustained TBI and combat-acquired TBI associated with Operation Iraqi Freedom (OIF)/Operation Enduring Freedom (OEF). Posttraumatic headaches associated with mTBI acquired in a civilian setting are usually tension or cervicogenic headaches, whereas headaches following mTBI in combat have features of migraine in 60% of individuals (Ruff et al. 2008; Theeler and Erickson 2009).

Posttraumatic headache prevalence varies with time after the injury. At 1 month following injury, rates of headaches range from 31.3% (Keidel and Diener 1997) to 90% (Rutherford et al. 1979). At 3 months postinjury, which corresponds to the threshold criterion for diagnosis of chronic posttraumatic headache (Headache Classification Subcommittee of the International Headache Society 2004), the rates have been found to be as high as 78%. At 6 months, prevalence ranged up to 44% (De Benedittis and De Santis 1983). Four years following injury, 20%–24% of civilians with TBI still reported headaches (Keidel and Diener 1997). Civilians with prolonged posttraumatic headaches often have complex psychosocial problems that compromise recovery (Martelli et al. 1999).

Combat TBI differs from civilian TBI in several ways. Current combat TBI is often caused by explosions that produce injuries to multiple body areas (i.e., polytrauma). Blast-associated injuries can include sequels of pressure-wave exposure, shrapnel injuries, traumatic amputation, and physical displacement injuries. Concurrent nociceptive and neuropathic pain conditions are common (Clark et al. 2009). Nociceptive pain results from tissue injury, whereas neuropathic pain results from alterations to the central or peripheral nervous systems involved in pain transmission or modulation. Neuropathic pain can have an electric-like character. OIF/OEF soldiers injured by combat-related blasts had less improvement in pain intensity than did soldiers with other types of combat injuries or those injured in noncombat situations, despite equivalence in TBI frequency and severity (Clark et al. 2009). Additionally, combat troops who do not experience physical trauma as a consequence of blast exposure may be subjected to repeated blasts throughout their tours of duty, possibly incurring unidentified mTBIs.

The psychosocial context in which injuries occur can affect the consequences of TBI. Comorbid psychiatric conditions, particularly PTSD, develop in association with combat TBI (Clark et al. 2009; Lew et al. 2009; Ruff et al. 2008, 2009). Comorbid PTSD occurred in about 40% of military personnel and Veterans with combat-acquired mTBI (Gironda et al. 2009; Lew et al. 2009), in contrast to about 6% of civilians with mTBI (Bryant et al. 2010). Soldiers with mTBI were more likely to report persisting headache than were soldiers with other injuries (Hoge et al. 2008). Combat TBI and PTSD challenge reintegration into society (Roberts 2008). Individuals with psychiatric conditions are known to experience higher levels of pain-related disability and poorer outcomes (Breslau et al. 2003).

# PATHOPHYSIOLOGY

The pathophysiology of headaches is poorly understood. Cervicogenic head and neck pain is associated with injuries to cervical paraspinal muscles and vertebrae (Kaniecki 2003). Posttraumatic headaches may be associated with the existence of hypersensitivity of central pain processing networks. Patients with tension headaches experience more intense pain in response to noxious stimulation to the face and have lower pain thresholds (Ashina 2004), and central sensitization is implicated at the level of the upper cervical spinal dorsal horns and trigeminal nuclei (Bendtsen 2000). Brain trauma may precipitate tension headaches by injuring the central pain modulation pathways that disrupt normal mechanisms for suppressing pain.

The impact of nervous system trauma on the genesis of pain has been most extensively studied in spinal cord injury, which may provide insight into TBI pain. Classes of neuronal sodium ($Na^+$) channels differ in their properties. Increasing Nav1.3 channel expression causes neuronal hyperexcitability. Trauma upregulates Nav1.3 channels in thalamic neurons involved in pain transmission and pain modulation (Waxman and Hains 2006). Maintenance of pain after trauma and upregulation of Nav1.3 channels result from activation of microglia that produce prostaglandin ($PGE_2$) (Zhao et al. 2007). Decreasing $PGE_2$ production reduces Nav1.3 channel expression and diminishes pain (Zhao et al. 2007).

TBI may trigger or rekindle migraine due to damage to meningeal blood vessels or injury-induced neuronal hyperexcitability. Migraine is currently seen as a neurovascular disorder with the primary dysfunction in the central nervous system. Altered cerebral activity changes the activation of pain-producing intracranial meningeal structures that give rise to headache pain (Hargreaves and Shepheard 1999). Episodes of migraine are associated with trigeminal nerve activation of pain-sensitive meningeal structures (Bolay et al. 2002). TBI also may injure the meninges and alter the trigeminal communication with the meninges. By mechanisms similar to those of tension headaches, injury to excitable elements of the meninges may produce a hyperexcitable state, leading to migraine.

Migraine is also associated with cortical hyperexcitability to auditory and visual stimuli (Coppola et al. 2007). The phenomenon of cortical spreading depression entails a wave of cortical excitation moving over the cortex, followed by reduced cortical excitability (Mulleners et al. 2001). Spreading depression is most prominent in the occipital cortex. The occipital poles are particularly vulnerable to injury due to TBI, and perhaps injury-induced hyperexcitability facilitates spreading depression. Thalamocortical traffic is increased during attacks of migraine (Coppola et al. 2007). Thalamocortical activity is associated with pathological trigeminal stimulation of the meninges. The trigeminal sensory fibers release substance P, which is a small neuropeptide that is both a neurotransmitter and a proinflammatory agent. Meningeal inflammation contributes to migraine pain (Bolay et al. 2002).

## CLINICAL ASSESSMENT

A diagnosis of posttraumatic headache requires a standard comprehensive clinical interview (Sherman et al. 2006). When a patient complains about headache, the history taking should focus on eliciting details about the character of the headache pain, its speed of onset, location(s), and duration, as well as factors that exacerbate or relieve it. The acronym COLDER—for character, onset, location, duration, exacerbation, and relief—may serve as a useful reminder of these elements of the headache history (Zafonte and Horn 1999). History taking also seeks to identify environmental triggers or other antecedents to the headache, prodromal symptoms, and headache-associated symptoms (e.g., photosensitivity or sonosensitivity, photophobia or sonophobia, eye pain, tearing, nausea, vomiting, dizziness, fatigue). The frequency of headaches, their course, and their relationship to TBI are noted as well.

Other conditions that may exacerbate headaches, including sleep disturbances, depression, and anxiety, among others, should be identified. Although headaches are the primary pain condition following combat-acquired TBI (Clark et al. 2009; Gironda et al. 2009; Lew et al. 2009), they commonly are accompanied by other postconcussive symptoms, such as fatigue; memory, attention/concentration, and executive functioning deficits; and emotional distress (Clark et al. 2009; Ofek and Defrin 2007). Premorbid personal and family headache histories also may be diagnostically informative.

A thorough physical examination is an essential element of the headache assessment (Zafonte and Horn 1999). The examination focuses first on observation and palpation of the head, face (including temporomandibular joints), mouth, neck, and shoulder girdle. The posture in which the head, jaw, neck, and shoulders are held is observed, and the range of motion of the head, jaw, and neck is assessed. Cranial nerve examination, including assessment of vision and hearing and all relevant reflexes, and auscultation of the blood vessels of the neck are performed. This problem-focused examination is followed by a thorough general physical and neurological examination.

Although neuroimaging or laboratory studies are commonly obtained in the evaluation of headache, they generally are not necessary (Silberstein 2000). History or examination findings suggesting headache of cervicogenic or musculoskeletal origin may be evaluated further using plain radiographs of the cervical spine. Among patients with nonacute presentations, clinical findings that increase the likelihood of abnormalities on neuroimaging studies (i.e., magnetic resonance imaging), and hence support their performance, include headaches with atypical features or characteristics that do not conform to the strict definitions of primary headache disorders; the presence of a comorbid medical condition that increases the risk for central nervous system abnormalities (i.e., immune deficiency, autoimmune disorder); rapidly increasing headache frequency; history of headache causing awakening from sleep; and, either by history or examination, unexplained focal neurological signs and/or impaired coordination (Silberstein 2000). Among patients with acute headache presentations, focal or progressive elemental neurological signs or symptoms, altered consciousness, increasing or extreme severity, nausea and/or vomiting, or nighttime occurrence suggests the need for neuroimaging evaluation (Sherman et al. 2006; Zafonte and Horn 1999).

The definitions of headache types described earlier in the section "Definition" are used to diagnose posttraumatic headache(s); Table 13–1 describes the characteristics of tension-like, migraine-like, and cervicogenic posttraumatic headaches. When the history and examination do not lead to a clear headache diagnosis, it may be useful for patients to develop a headache diary to record the frequency, intensity, duration, prodromal signs, and triggers of headaches. Use of this diary during treatment also should be encouraged, and individuals with cognitive deficits should be provided with assistance with this task.

# TREATMENT

## Pharmacotherapy

*Episodic tension or cervicogenic headaches.* Episodic tension headaches usually respond to nonsteroidal anti-inflammatory drugs (NSAIDs). Pain treatment is more likely to be successful if the medication is taken at headache onset. Occasionally, opioid medications are required to treat severe tension headache; however, repeated use of opioid medication can lead to problems associated with dependence and may exacerbate cognitive and behavioral manifestations of TBI. Aspirin and acetaminophen are often combined with caffeine or a sedative drug in a single medication. Combination drugs may be more effective than NSAIDs or acetaminophen alone, but persistent usage may lead to rebound headaches and chronic daily headaches. Combinations of acetaminophen or aspirin and an opioid should be used with caution.

**TABLE 13–1.** Criteria for characterizing posttraumatic headaches as tension, cervicogenic, or migraine headaches

| HEADACHE FEATURE | HEADACHE TYPE | | |
| --- | --- | --- | --- |
| | TENSION | CERVICOGENIC | MIGRAINE |
| Pain intensity | Mild to moderate | Mild to moderate | Often severe or debilitating |
| Pain character | Dull, aching, or pressure; sharp pain possibly present, but not predominant | Similar to tension headaches | Throbbing or pulsatile; can also be sharp/stabbing or electric-like |
| Duration | Less than 4 hours | Less than 4 hours | Can last longer than 4 hours |
| Phonophobia or photophobia | One but not both may be present | Usually neither is present | One or both often present |
| Able to carry out routine activities or work | Usually | Usually | Usually not |
| Location | Bilateral—frontal, retro-orbital, temporal, or holocephalic | Cervical and occipital | Usually unilateral and may vary in location among episodes |
| Nausea or malaise | Not present | Not present | May be present |
| Palpable muscle tenderness | Pericranial muscles including temporalis, masseter, pterygoid, sternocleidomastoid, splenius, or trapezius | Posterior neck muscles | Localized muscle tenderness not typical; possible muscle tenderness with long-duration headaches |

*Note.* Posttraumatic headaches can have features of more than one primary headache type.

Individuals with more than three tension headaches per week may benefit from preventive treatments (Table 13–2). Medications useful in reducing tension headache frequency include tricyclic antidepressants, NSAIDs, and acetaminophen; if the headaches are associated with anxiety, then anxiolytic medications also may be useful. Persistent usage of NSAIDs or acetaminophen may result in rebound headaches. Although other agents such as anticonvulsants have been used to prevent tension headaches, they have not been evaluated in controlled clinical trials. Poorly controlled tension headaches may indicate that attention should be directed to physical or psychological factors triggering headaches.

*Migraine-like headache.* Treatments for migraine headaches include both abortive and preventive approaches. Medications used commonly for prophylaxis against recurrent migraine headaches are described in Table 13–3. One of the authors of this chapter (R.L.R.) has observed β-blockers and topiramate to be the best prophylactic agents for posttraumatic migraine or mixed headaches in Veterans of OIF/OEF. These agents can improve the life quality of individuals with migraines (Garcia-Monco et al. 2007). β-Blockers are useful when headaches are associated with anxiety, and these medications typically do not impair cognition. There is anecdotal concern that β-blockers may worsen depression; however, careful analysis suggests that they do not cause depression (Huffman and Stern 2007). Because β-blockers may worsen sleep disorders and may intensify nightmares, sleep should be carefully monitored. If β-blockers are effective in reducing the frequency and intensity of headaches, but are associated with nightmares, the nightmares can be treated using prazosin (Raskind et al. 2007). Topiramate may be the first choice for Veterans with impaired sleep. The dose of topiramate needs to be increased slowly to minimize daytime somnolence and impaired cognition. Topiramate may potentiate neural repair (Follett et al. 2004). Weight loss, a potential side effect of topiramate, may benefit some patients.

Effective abortive treatment (Table 13–4) requires that individuals recognize their own headache warning signs. These may include a classic aura or prodromal symptoms such as changes in mood, onset of fatigue, sensory sensitivity, and difficulty with attention or concentration. Abortive treatment is more successful if treatment begins at headache onset. Prompt initiation of acute treatment also reduces the need for opioid medications to "rescue" patients from severe pain. If acute treatment is not effective, rescue treatments may be

**TABLE 13–2.** Medications that may reduce the frequency of tension or cervicogenic headaches

| MEDICATION | TYPICAL DOSING | SIDE EFFECTS | COMMENTS |
|---|---|---|---|
| Tricyclic antidepressants | Amitriptyline 10–75 mg at bedtime | Weight gain, dry mouth, daytime somnolence | Most effective, but side effects limit utility |
| | Nortriptyline 10–50 mg at bedtime | Somnolence, dry mouth | Fewer side effects, but may not be as effective as amitriptyline |
| Antianxiety agents | Lorazepam 25–50 mg twice daily Clonazepam 10 mg two to four times daily | Sedation and habituation; possibility of dependency | Should be used on a time-limited basis for periods up to 4 weeks |
| Nonsteroidal anti-inflammatory drugs | Choline-magnesium-trisalicylate 750 mg three times daily | Potential for gastrointestinal upset | Rebound headaches possible with regular usage, particularly of combination medications containing caffeine |
| | Ibuprofen 400–600 mg three to four times daily | Renal damage possible from excessive use | |
| Acetaminophen | 250–500 mg three to four times daily | Liver damage can result from excessive use; avoid use in patients with hepatitis | Rebound headaches possible, particularly if agent combined with caffeine |
| Anticonvulsant medications | Topiramate 100–200 mg/day in two divided doses | Sedation, impaired cognition | Not shown to be effective for tension headaches; best used for headaches with migraine features |
| | Valproate 100–250 mg three times daily | Sedation, impaired cognition, and ataxia | |

**TABLE 13–3.**   Medications used to prevent migraine headaches

| MEDICATION | COMMENT |
|---|---|
| Amitriptyline 10–50 mg at bedtime, upper limit of 150 mg/day | Side effects include dry mouth, weight gain, and next-day sedation. Some side effects can be minimized by very gradually increasing the dosage. |
| Timolol 10–30 mg/day or propranolol 20–160 mg/day | Side effects include fatigue, lightheadedness, insomnia, bradycardia or exercise intolerance, depression, and sexual dysfunction. Agent should be avoided in patients with asthma, severe cardiovascular disease, insulin-dependent diabetes mellitus, and Raynaud disease. In Veterans with PTSD, β-blockers may worsen nightmares. These agents are particularly useful when headache onset is associated with episodes of anxiety. Some literature suggests that β-blockers can worsen depression, but more recent data suggest that β-blockers do not trigger or worsen existing depression. |
| Topiramate 50–150 mg/day | Side effects are similar to those of divalproex, but in our experience, topiramate is better tolerated by Veterans with TBI. Side effects can be minimized by starting with 25 mg/day and increasing by 25 mg/day at weekly intervals up to 50–100 mg twice daily or until headaches are controlled. |
| Divalproex sodium 125–200 mg/day | Side effects of potential cognitive impairment and tremor can limit acceptability of this medication. |
| Methysergide 4–8 mg/day | Agent is rarely used due to concern about the side effect of retroperitoneal fibrosis. This side effect can be avoided if the medication is stopped for 1 month after 11 months of use. Advantage of this agent is that it is well tolerated aside from the potential serious side effect of retroperitoneal fibrosis. |

*Note.*   Medications are presented on the basis of evidence of their medium to high efficacy and mild to moderate side effects. PTSD=posttraumatic stress disorder; TBI=traumatic brain injury.

**TABLE 13–4.** Acute migraine interventions

| TYPE OF INTERVENTION | SPECIFIC AGENTS USED | COMMENT |
|---|---|---|
| Medications | NSAIDs alone or combined with caffeine, isometheptene, or a sedative | These can be useful for moderate-intensity infrequent headaches. Repeated use may lead to rebound headaches. |
| | Triptans | These are currently the first-line acute treatment, with several different preparations available. They may be combined with an antiemetic. |
| | Ergotamines (includes dihydroergotamine) | Some individuals get good response from injectable ergotamine. |
| | Tramadol | This agent is a mild agonist of the μ opioid receptor. It is not a controlled substance. Sedation can limit utility. Some individuals respond well to tramadol alone or combined with acetaminophen. |
| Oxygen inhalation | Typically provided as 2–4 L/minute via nasal prongs or mask | This is an effective intervention for some people with migraine. It is safe and has few side effects and will not induce rebound or overuse headaches. The limitation is that the individual may not have access to oxygen when a headache starts. |

*Note.* In general, medications should be provided orally whenever possible. In cases of nausea and/or vomiting, medication administration via injection, suppository, or orally dissolving preparation is appropriate. NSAID=nonsteroidal anti-inflammatory drug.

**TABLE 13–5.**   Rescue interventions for migraine

| Type of intervention | Specific agents used | Comment |
| --- | --- | --- |
| Medications | Ketorolac | Gastric protection against ulceration should be used because ketorolac can cause gastric ulceration. |
| | Triptans or ergotamines | These agents are available in parenteral formulations, but may be ineffective for an advanced migraine attack. |
| | Tramadol | The side effect of sedation can be useful because migraine attacks can abate with sleep. |
| | Divalproex sodium | Intravenous administration of 500 mg can break a migraine. |
| | Butorphanol | The nasal inhalation formulation may abort a migraine attack. |
| | Opioids | Morphine sulfate 2–4 mg (or comparable dose of another parenteral opioid) can be useful in breaking a migraine attack. Regular usage can lead to habituation. These are restricted medications. |
| Oxygen inhalation | Typically provided as 2–4 L/minute via nasal prongs or mask | This treatment can be given in conjunction with other interventions. |

*Note.*   In general, medications should be provided orally whenever possible. If nausea and/or vomiting are present, then medication administration via injection, suppository, or orally dissolving preparation is appropriate.

required to break the migraine (Table 13–5). If rescue therapy is required on a regular basis, then prophylactic treatment is needed.

Acute migraine treatment must be used prudently to avoid inducing overuse or rebound headaches. Overuse headaches are typically tension-like. Overuse of opioid medication may contribute to the transformation from episodic to chronic migraine (Bigal and Lipton 2009). Treatment of medication-overuse headaches requires stopping daily use of acute treatments, which often results in withdrawal symptoms that include rebound headaches. In many cases, patients fall into a pattern of continued medication overuse in an effort to avoid rebound headaches. Headache diaries may reveal overuse. When patients are caught in a pattern of medication overuse, headaches are usually refractory to preventive medications. In most cases, headaches improve after an analgesic washout period. It is important to educate patients that acute migraine medication should be limited to three treatments per week.

# Psychological and Behavioral Interventions

*Tension and cervicogenic headaches.* Tension and cervicogenic headaches associated with TBI may be resistant to medication alone. Patients may achieve better pain relief if medication is coupled with other treatments. Cognitive-behavioral interventions such as relaxation training and biofeedback can help individuals learn to identify tension and relax the muscles contributing to the tension headache. Physical therapy can be used to exercise neck muscles and maintain appropriate range of motion. Physical activity can reduce the frequency and intensity of tension headaches. Improving other psychiatric conditions, including depression and PTSD, also may reduce the frequency and/or perceived severity of headaches (Fann et al. 2000; Griffith 2009; Peterlin et al. 2009).

Cognitive-behavioral interventions for headache conditions produce headache relief comparable to that from medication (Holroyd et al. 2009). Education regarding headaches and wellness may help to correct pain-related cognitive distortions, encourage proactive self-management, and promote an increased sense of control over the headache conditions. Finally, because individuals with recent onset of posttraumatic headache are at risk for transformation to treatment-resistant chronic daily headache conditions, patients should be educated about analgesic overuse.

Spinal manipulation can be used to treat cervicogenic pain if the neck is mechanically stable. A review of nine studies that tested spinal manipulative therapy for tension headaches concluded that spinal manipulation is comparable in benefit to medications used for the prevention of tension headaches (Bove and Nilsson 1998).

*Migraine headaches.* Effective treatment for posttraumatic migraine headaches typically requires the use of a combination of acute and preventive medications and nonpharmacological prevention strategies, including lifestyle regulation, stimulant reduction, and trigger avoidance. Cognitive-behavioral migraine intervention should include a focus on identification and avoidance of migraine triggers. Common headache risk factors and triggers include sleep disruption; increased time between meals; stress; and specific foods, beverages, and odors. Other nonpharmacological treatments commonly employed are extracranial pressure and cold compresses. Regular exercise, sleep, and meal schedules are also an important part of the treatment regimen. Oxygen inhalation can also be used to abort an acute migraine or as a migraine rescue treatment (see Tables 13–4 and 13–5).

*Sleep problems.* Obtaining deep, restful sleep may be particularly important for individuals with posttraumatic headache. Sleep disorders commonly develop after TBI. For individuals with moderate to severe TBI, sleep disorders include hypersomnia, insomnia, and impaired breathing during sleep, including sleep apnea (Orff et al. 2009). Individuals with mTBI may suffer from interrupted sleep in association with posttraumatic stress reactions, including PTSD (Ruff et al. 2009). Prazosin successfully blocks nightmares and other sleep interruptions caused by PTSD (Raskind et al. 2007). In an observational study of OIF/OEF Veterans with mTBI due to combat explosions, prazosin treatment combined with sleep hygiene counseling was able to reduce headache frequency and severity (Ruff et al. 2009). Healthy sleep patterns facilitate synaptic homeostasis (Tononi and Cirelli 2003) and other processes that contribute to cerebral plasticity (Jha et al. 2005), which will enhance the ability of the brain to adapt after traumatic injury.

# HEADACHE MANAGEMENT IN PATIENTS WITH COMMUNICATION IMPAIRMENTS

The assessment of pain in patients with communication impairments is challenging (Weiner and Herr 2002). Patients with impaired cognition and communication due to TBI may not be able to convey pain complaints. The interaction between pain and cognitive symptoms may exacerbate functional impairments and impede response to treatment (Ivanhoe and Hartman 2004). Pain assessment in patients with severe brain injury has received little attention. One may adopt assessment techniques used to assess pain in people with dementia (Collett et al. 2007).

Initial effort should be directed toward determining whether a patient can use some form of self-report to communicate the existence of pain and its intensity. Neuropsychological and speech-language testing can be used to assess a patient's abilities to provide self-report, to identify specific deficits to consider in the assessment, and to recommend strategies for obtaining valid information. Patients with mild to moderate cognitive impairment often can respond reliably to standard measures of pain intensity (Chibnall and Tait 2001). Reliability of self-report scales can improve with practice. Clinicians should question patients specifically about headaches because patients may not report having headaches when asked only about their experience of "pain."

Behavioral observation can validate a patient's self-report and help assess pain when the patient is unable to reliably provide self-report information. Family members or caregivers familiar with the patient's behavior can recognize behavioral changes that indicate pain (Weiner and Herr 2002). Behavior patterns include facial expressions, verbalizations or vocalizations, body movements, changes in interpersonal interactions, changes in activity patterns or routines, and mental status changes.

Empirical trials of analgesic medication can be used to assess pain. These trials should be done in conjunction with other methods of assessment to evaluate whether the behaviors indicate appreciable pain (Gallagher et al. 2006). Some analgesics can negatively impact cognitive status, and this risk should be evaluated throughout the course of a trial to minimize effects on overall treatment. Unfortunately, no consensus exists on the best pain assessment tools to use for individuals with cognitive impairment.

# CONCLUSION

Posttraumatic headaches are among the most common acute and chronic problems experienced by persons with TBI. These headaches may be associated with other postconcussive symptoms or may be the principal feature of the patient's clinical presentation. Posttraumatic headaches contribute importantly to distress and functional limitations among persons with TBI, and are an important focus of treatment. Clinical assessment includes detailed history taking and headache characterization. Examination of the head, neck, and shoulder regions is complemented by physical and neurological examination and, in selected cases, neuroimaging and other laboratory studies. The treatment of posttraumatic headaches is organized according to their clinical phenotypes, the most common of which are tension, cervicogenic, and migraine headaches. Treatments include pharmacotherapy as well as psychological and behavioral interventions that target headaches and associated comorbidities (e.g., depression, anxiety, PTSD, sleep disturbances). The assessment and management of posttraumatic headaches may require modification to meet the needs of individuals with polytrauma as well as persons with severe TBI.

## *Key Clinical Points*

- Posttraumatic headaches represent a secondary headache disorder developing with a temporal relationship to head trauma, and may have the typical clinical features of tension headache, cervicogenic headache, migraine headache, or a mixed type including features of different headache syndromes.

- Epidemiological studies have demonstrated that posttraumatic headaches have a higher incidence in Veteran populations compared with civilian injured populations; regardless of the setting of injury, headaches are more common after mild TBI than moderate or severe TBI.

- The pathophysiologies of posttraumatic headaches are not fully elucidated; however, peripheral mechanisms (e.g., injury to cervical paraspinal muscles) and central mechanisms (e.g., altered vascular reactivity, increased expression of hyperexcitable sodium channels in the thalamus) are suspected.

- Selection of the appropriate pharmacological agent to treat posttraumatic headaches is guided by the clinical characteristics of the headache (e.g., migraine, tension-type, cervicogenic). Care must be taken to avoid excessive use of headache-abortive agents, which may precipitate analgesic rebound headache.

- Cognitive-behavioral therapies for patients with posttraumatic headache focus on education about lifestyle factors affecting headaches, evaluation and identification of triggers, addressing stress and its impact on headaches, and, perhaps most importantly, addressing sleep hygiene issues.

# REFERENCES

Ashina M: Neurobiology of chronic tension-type headache. Cephalalgia 24:161–172, 2004

Bendtsen L: Central sensitization in tension-type headache: possible pathophysiological mechanisms. Cephalalgia 20:486–508, 2000

Bigal ME, Lipton RB: Excessive opioid use and the development of chronic migraine. Pain 142:179–182, 2009

Bolay H, Reuter U, Dunn AK, et al: Intrinsic brain activity triggers trigeminal meningeal afferents in a migraine model. Nat Med 8:136–142, 2002

Bove G, Nilsson N: Spinal manipulation in the treatment of episodic tension-type headache: a randomized controlled trial. JAMA 280:1576–1579, 1998

Breslau N, Lipton RB, Stewart WF, et al: Comorbidity of migraine and depression: investigating potential etiology and prognosis. Neurology 60:1308–1312, 2003

Bryant RA, O'Donnell ML, Creamer M, et al: The psychiatric sequelae of traumatic injury. Am J Psychiatry 167:312–320, 2010

Chibnall JT, Tait RC: Pain assessment in cognitively impaired and unimpaired older adults: a comparison of four scales. Pain 92:173–186, 2001

Clark ME, Scholten JD, Walker RL, et al: Assessment and treatment of pain associated with combat-related polytrauma. Pain Med 10:456–469, 2009

Collett B, O'Mahony S, Schofield P, et al: The Assessment of Pain in Older People: National Guidelines (Concise Guidance to Good Practice Series, No. 8). London, Royal College of Physicians, October 2007

Coppola G, Pierelli F, Schoenen J: Is the cerebral cortex hyperexcitable or hyperresponsive in migraine? Cephalalgia 27:1427–1439, 2007

De Benedittis G, De Santis A: Chronic post-traumatic headache: clinical, psychopathological features and outcome determinants. J Neurosurg Sci 27:177–186, 1983

Evans RW: Post-traumatic headaches. Neurol Clin 22:237–249, viii, 2004

Fann JR, Uomoto JM, Katon WJ: Sertraline in the treatment of major depression following mild traumatic brain injury. J Neuropsychiatry Clin Neurosci 12:226–232, 2000

Faux S, Sheedy J: A prospective controlled study in the prevalence of post-traumatic headache following mild traumatic brain injury. Pain Med 9:1001–1011, 2008

Follett PL, Deng W, Dai W, et al: Glutamate receptor–mediated oligodendrocyte toxicity in periventricular leukomalacia: a protective role for topiramate. J Neurosci 24:4412–4420, 2004

Formisano R, Bivona U, Catani S, et al: Post-traumatic headache: facts and doubts. J Headache Pain 10:145–152, 2009

Gallagher R, Drance E, Higginbotham S: Finding the person behind the pain: chronic pain management in a patient with traumatic brain injury. J Am Med Dir Assoc 7:432–434, 2006

Garcia-Monco JC, Foncea N, Bilbao A, et al: Impact of preventive therapy with nadolol and topiramate on the quality of life of migraine patients. Cephalalgia 27:920–928, 2007

Gironda RJ, Clark ME, Ruff RL, et al: Traumatic brain injury, polytrauma, and pain: challenges and treatment strategies for the polytrauma rehabilitation. Rehabil Psychol 54:247–258, 2009

Griffith JL: Posttraumatic stress disorder in headache patients: implications for treatment. Headache 49:552–554, 2009

Hargreaves RJ, Shepheard SL: Pathophysiology of migraine: new insights. Can J Neurol Sci 26 (suppl 3):S12–S19, 1999

Headache Classification Subcommittee of the International Headache Society: The International Classification of Headache Disorders, 2nd edition. Cephalalgia 24(suppl):9–160, 2004

Hoge CW, McGurk D, Thomas JL, et al: Mild traumatic brain injury in U.S. soldiers returning from Iraq. N Engl J Med 358:453–463, 2008

Holroyd KA, Labus JS, Carlson B: Moderation and mediation in the psychological and drug treatment of chronic tension-type headache: the role of disorder severity and psychiatric comorbidity. Pain 143:213–222, 2009

Huffman JC, Stern TA: Neuropsychiatric consequences of cardiovascular medications. Dialogues Clin Neurosci 9:29–45, 2007

Ivanhoe CB, Hartman ET: Clinical caveats on medical assessment and treatment of pain after TBI. J Head Trauma Rehabil 19:29–39, 2004

Jha SK, Jones BE, Coleman T, et al: Sleep-dependent plasticity requires cortical activity. J Neurosci 25:9266–9274, 2005

Kaniecki R: Headache assessment and management. JAMA 289:1430–1433, 2003

Keidel M, Diener HC: Post-traumatic headache [in German]. Nervenarzt 68:769–777, 1997

Lew HL, Otis JD, Tun C, et al: Prevalence of chronic pain, posttraumatic stress disorder, and persistent postconcussive symptoms in OIF/OEF veterans: polytrauma clinical triad. J Rehabil Res Dev 46:697–702, 2009

Martelli MF, Grayson RL, Zasler ND: Posttraumatic headache: neuropsychological and psychological effects and treatment implications. J Head Trauma Rehabil 14:49–69, 1999

McCrea M, American Academy of Clinical Neuropsychology: Mild Traumatic Brain Injury and Postconcussion Syndrome: The New Evidence Base for Diagnosis and Treatment. New York, Oxford University Press, 2008

Mulleners WM, Chronicle EP, Palmer JE, et al: Visual cortex excitability in migraine with and without aura. Headache 41:565–572, 2001

Ofek H, Defrin R: The characteristics of chronic central pain after traumatic brain injury. Pain 131:330–340, 2007

Orff HJ, Ayalon L, Drummond SP: Traumatic brain injury and sleep disturbance: a review of current research. J Head Trauma Rehabil 24:155–165, 2009

Peterlin BL, Tietjen GE, Brandes JL, et al: Posttraumatic stress disorder in migraine. Headache 49:541–551, 2009

Raskind MA, Peskind ER, Hoff DJ, et al: A parallel group placebo controlled study of prazosin for trauma nightmares and sleep disturbance in combat veterans with post-traumatic stress disorder. Biol Psychiatry 61:928–934, 2007

Roberts R: Impact on the brain. Scientific American Mind 19:51–57, 2008

Ruff RL, Ruff SS, Wang XF: Headaches among Operation Iraqi Freedom/Operation Enduring Freedom veterans with mild traumatic brain injury associated with exposures to explosions. J Rehabil Res Dev 45:941–952, 2008

Ruff RL, Ruff SS, Wang XF: Improving sleep: initial headache treatment in OIF/OEF veterans with blast-induced mild traumatic brain injury. J Rehabil Res Dev 46:1071–1084, 2009

Rutherford WH, Merrett JD, McDonald JR: Symptoms at one year following concussion from minor head injuries. Injury 10:225–230, 1979

Sherman KB, Goldberg M, Bell KR: Traumatic brain injury and pain. Phys Med Rehabil Clin N Am 17:473–490, viii, 2006

Silberstein SD: Practice parameter: evidence-based guidelines for migraine headache (an evidence-based review): report of the Quality Standards Subcommittee of the American Academy of Neurology. Neurology 55:754–762, 2000

Theeler BJ, Erickson JC: Mild head trauma and chronic headaches in returning US soldiers. Headache 49:529–534, 2009

Tononi G, Cirelli C: Sleep and synaptic homeostasis: a hypothesis. Brain Res Bull 62:143–150, 2003

Uomoto JM, Esselman PC: Traumatic brain injury and chronic pain: differential types and rates by head injury severity. Arch Phys Med Rehabil 74:61–64, 1993

Waxman SG, Hains BC: Fire and phantoms after spinal cord injury: $Na^+$ channels and central pain. Trends Neurosci 29:207–215, 2006

Weiner DK, Herr K: Comprehensive interdisciplinary assessment and treatment planning: an integrative overview, in Persistent Pain in Older Adults: An Interdisciplinary Guide for Treatment. Edited by Weiner DK, Herr K, Rudy TE. New York, Springer, 2002, pp 18–57

Zafonte RD, Horn LJ: Clinical assessment of posttraumatic headaches. J Head Trauma Rehabil 14:22–33, 1999

Zasler ND: Posttraumatic headache: caveats and controversies. J Head Trauma Rehabil 14:1–8, 1999

Zhao P, Waxman SG, Hains BC: Extracellular signal-regulated kinase-regulated microglia-neuron signaling by prostaglandin E2 contributes to pain after spinal cord injury. J Neurosci 27:2357–2368, 2007

CHAPTER 14

# Seizures and Epilepsy

*Lauren Frey, M.D.*

*The occurrence of seizures* after head injury is a recognized complication of traumatic brain injury (TBI) and worsens functional outcome after TBI (Asikainen et al. 1999). This chapter provides a review of the definition, incidence, natural history, clinical assessment, and treatment options for patients with posttraumatic epilepsy (PTE).

## DEFINITIONS

### Seizure

During a seizure, the brain produces abnormal, sustained, and highly synchronous electrical discharges that disrupt otherwise normal brain activity. A patient's experiential and behavioral manifestations of the brain's abnormal electrical activity depend on where the abnormal discharge starts in the brain and how far the discharge spreads within the brain. For example, a typical complex partial seizure of mesial temporal or hippocampal onset may begin with the patient experiencing a sensation of déjà vu or an unpleasant smell. As the seizure progresses and the abnormal electrical activity spreads within the brain, the patient may stare and may have involuntary lip smacking or make picking movements with his or her hands. If the seizure discharge spreads to involve the whole brain, a generalized tonic-clonic convulsion may occur. A list of common clinical manifestations of seizures, according to region of onset, is presented in Table 14–1.

## Types of Posttraumatic Seizures

Posttraumatic seizures are usually divided into three categories: immediate seizures, early seizures, and late seizures. Immediate seizures are those that occur at the time of or within minutes after TBI. The pathophysiology of immediate seizures and their long-term clinical significance are unclear. As a result, they are often excluded from epidemiological studies of PTE. Early seizures are those occurring while the patient is still experiencing the direct effects of head injury, a period commonly defined as 1 week after TBI (Jennett 1975). Approximately 90% of early seizures develop during this first postinjury week (Jennett 1975). These seizures appear to result from transient dysregulation of inhibitory function in the brain due to injury-related cell loss. Late posttraumatic seizures (or PTE) are usually defined as those seizures occurring more than 1 week after injury. These seizures appear to reflect the development of longer-term, and possibly permanent, aberrant neuronal network function.

# EPIDEMIOLOGY

## Incidence and Natural History of Posttraumatic Seizures

Approximately 5%–30% of adult patients with TBI develop posttraumatic seizures; the rates of posttraumatic seizures vary with initial injury severity (Frey 2003). Notably, a single, even unprovoked, posttraumatic seizure does not define PTE; instead, PTE requires recurrent (i.e., two or more) unprovoked seizures. Because many studies of PTE have not used this definition and instead assign this diagnosis to an individual experiencing only a single unprovoked seizure, the incidence of PTE is not clearly established. Most patients who experience a second unprovoked late posttraumatic seizure do so during the first 2 years after their first late posttraumatic seizure. Haltiner et al. (1997) reported that up to 86% of TBI survivors with a first posttraumatic seizure will also have a second seizure within the following 2 years.

**TABLE 14–1.** Common clinical manifestations of seizures and associated typical seizure onset localizations

| Seizure focus | Clinical manifestations |
|---|---|
| Mesial temporal (hippocampal) lobe | May begin with an aura of a rising epigastric sensation, fear, environmental distortion (déjà vu, micropsia), or unpleasant olfactory hallucinations; usually progresses to a blank stare with simple or reactive manual automatisms and oral automatisms |
| Lateral temporal lobe | May begin with an aura of vertigo, simple or complex auditory hallucinations, receptive aphasia, or motor or sensory involvement of the contralateral face or arm; usually progresses to a blank stare with simple or reactive manual automatisms and oral automatisms |
| Secondary motor association cortex | Asymmetric tonic limb posturing, vocalizations, clouding of consciousness; person may have minimal postictal confusion |
| Posterior cingulate gyrus | Prominent motor activity, bimanual/bipedal movements, vocalizations, aversive/fencing postures, largely nocturnal occurrence; minimal postictal confusion |
| Anterior cingulate gyrus | Complex motor activity, vocalizations, urinary incontinence, clouding of consciousness; may rapidly secondarily generalize |
| Orbitofrontal lobe | Prominent autonomic signs/symptoms, olfactory hallucinations |
| Primary motor or sensory cortex | Focal tonic or clonic motor movements; numbness or paresthesias (rarely painful); frequently secondarily generalizes |
| Parietal lobe | Somatosensory experiences, vertigo, aphasia, choking/sinking sensation, feeling of absence of body/body part |
| Occipital lobe | Visual hallucinations (usually simple), visual loss, micropsia, palinopsia, metamorphopsia; often spreads to ipsilateral temporal lobe |

By any definition, then, the risk of PTE is greatest during the first 3 years following TBI (Haltiner et al. 1997; Salazar et al. 1985) and remains elevated for many years thereafter (Annegers et al. 1998). The burden of evidence suggests that there is no significant relationship between the latency to first seizure and seizure duration or recurrence (Caveness et al. 1979; Salazar et al. 1985). However, patients with frequent seizures in the first postinjury year often continue to have frequent seizures and have a smaller chance of seizure freedom over time (Salazar et al. 1985). Intractable PTE develops in a nontrivial minority of patients, with a pooled estimate suggesting a frequency of 13.3% despite aggressive anticonvulsant treatment (Temkin 2009).

# Risk Factors for Posttraumatic Epilepsy

Injury factors, preinjury factors, and postinjury factors may contribute to the risk of PTE. Specific factors that confer increased risk for PTE include greater initial injury severity, acute intracerebral hematoma, higher-risk site of injury, metal fragment retention (in the brain), occurrence of early posttraumatic seizures, skull fracture, residual cortical neurological deficits, chronic alcohol use, older age, and persistent focal abnormalities on an electroencephalogram (EEG) more than 1 month after injury.

Severely injured patients are at the highest risk of developing PTE, and this risk remains higher in this subgroup over the long term than among more mildly injured patients (Angeleri et al. 1999; Annegers et al. 1980, 1998; Appleton and Demellweek 2002; Caveness 1976; Caveness et al. 1962, 1979; Englander et al. 2003; Hendrick and Harris 1968; Walker and Erculei 1970; Weiss et al. 1983). In the most comprehensive population-based study of PTE after civilian TBI, Annegers et al. (1998) determined that the standardized incidence ratio for the occurrence of PTE was 1.5 in mildly injured patients, 2.9 in moderately injured patients, and 17.0 in severely injured patients.

Subdural hematoma and brain contusion are thought to be the strongest independent clinical predictors of PTE risk and may confer up to a 10-fold increase in risk (Annegers et al. 1998; D'Alessandro et al. 1988; Englander et al. 2003; Heikkinen et al. 1990; Jennett 1975; Salazar et al. 1985). Indirect evidence also suggests that the site of injury may influence the risk of development of PTE. As seen on computed tomography (CT), a single lesion in the temporal or frontal regions (as opposed to other brain regions, such as the parietal or occipital lobes) is associated with an increased risk of PTE (relative risk=3.43) in univariate analyses; however, this risk does not survive multivariate analyses (Angeleri et al. 1999).

The occurrence of early posttraumatic seizures is the most consistently significant risk factor for the development of PTE in the literature, although the strength of this association is variable. If this is a significant risk factor for PTE, then it appears to be one regardless of the number of early posttraumatic seizures an individual experiences (Jennett 1975).

Premorbid chronic alcoholism likely increases the risk of development of PTE. Chronic alcohol use is also an independent risk factor for the development of epilepsy from any cause (Hauser et al. 1988; Kollevold 1979; Ng et al. 1988). Other risk factors for the development of PTE, such as older age at the time of injury, metal fragment retention in the brain, skull fracture, residual cortical neurological deficits, and persistent focal abnormalities on the EEG more than 1 month after injury, may simply be proxies for TBI severity (Angeleri et al. 1999; Annegers et al. 1998; Asikainen et al. 1999; Englander et al. 2003; Heikkinen et al. 1990; Salazar et al. 1985).

## Genetics and Posttraumatic Epilepsy

The role of genetics in PTE risk is uncertain. The majority of studies find that a family history of epilepsy is not a significant risk factor for the development of seizures after head injury. Findings suggest that variability in the development of seizures, as well as epilepsy, after TBI is not principally a function of genetic susceptibility (Ottman et al. 1996; Salazar et al. 1985; Schaumann et al. 1994).

# CLINICAL ASSESSMENT

## Identifying Seizures

One of the first clinical questions that must be answered when an adult TBI survivor presents with new-onset episodic neurological dysfunction is whether the patient had (or is having) a seizure. The differential diagnosis for new-onset episodic neurological dysfunction also includes syncope (an abrupt and transient loss of consciousness due to a sudden decrease in global cerebral perfusion), transient global amnesia (the sudden onset of complete anterograde amnesia without clouding of consciousness or loss of personal identity), transient ischemic attack (transient interruption of the vascular supply to a specific part of the brain), and complicated migraine headache

(Table 14–2). The history focuses on identifying precipitating factors and prodromal symptoms, if any, before the event in question. Characterizing the event itself usually requires interviewing any witnesses and should include the patient's mental status (responsiveness, orientation, language, memory), motor function (presence or absence of abnormal motor activity, sequence of events, any focality to the movements), and sensory function (numbness, tingling, experiential phenomena), as well as the duration of the event. Information about the patient's recovery from the event, including how much time was required to recover and whether there were any persistent neurological deficits, is diagnostically helpful as well.

# Neurodiagnostic Assessments

History taking and clinical examination sometimes do not provide information sufficient to determine whether a patient is having posttraumatic seizures. Electroencephalography and/or magnetic resonance imaging (MRI) can be useful in the clinical assessment of episodic neurological dysfunction in a patient with TBI.

*Electroencephalography.* Electroencephalography is a graphical depiction of summated cortical electrical activity, usually recorded from electrodes stuck to the individual's scalp with conductive paste. Electroencephalography can be performed in the inpatient or outpatient setting. Because the ideal EEG samples the patient's awake, drowsy, and asleep brain activity, many patients are asked to be sleep deprived before their test to ensure that they sleep during their EEG. Drowsiness and sleep are relatively hypersynchronous brain states; therefore, more epileptiform abnormalities are seen on EEG during drowsiness or sleep than in a waking record. In addition, sleep deprivation, like other physiological stressors, tends to lower seizure threshold and may bring out abnormal electroencephalographic rhythms.

Although many different electroencephalographic abnormalities are possible after TBI, the most useful diagnostic finding in this setting is the presence of interictal epileptiform discharges (IEDs). IEDs, or interictal "spikes," are transient waveforms on the EEG and serve as markers of abnormal neuronal network excitation (Prince and Connors 1986). IEDs are associated with an increased risk for spontaneous seizures, and the presence of IEDs on the EEG of a patient with spells after TBI should raise suspicion that these spells are,

**TABLE 14–2.** Differential diagnosis of complex partial seizures

| EVENT | COMPLEX PARTIAL SEIZURE | SYNCOPE | TRANSIENT GLOBAL AMNESIA | TRANSIENT ISCHEMIC ATTACK | COMPLICATED MIGRAINE HEADACHE |
|---|---|---|---|---|---|
| Before | Patients will often have an aura or warning, such as a sensation in face, arm, or leg; déjà vu; rising nausea; rising epigastric sensation; or a particular smell or taste. These warnings are always stereotyped, but are not always remembered after the seizure. | Prodromal symptoms are common, including nausea, feeling clammy, looking pale, blurry or gray or black vision, tunnel vision, lightheadedness, dizziness (not vertigo), and tinnitus. Precipitating factors include prolonged standing, orthostasis, fright or sudden pain, dehydration, or medications that induce hypotension or orthostasis. Patients often have a personal or family history of syncope. | Precipitating factors include physical or emotional stress, sexual intercourse, driving an automobile, or swimming in cold water. | A history of similar symptoms prior is not unusual. Risk factors include cerebral atherosclerosis, advanced age, hypertension, dyslipidemia, diabetes mellitus, smoking; or recent neck trauma or manipulation. | A history of similar symptoms prior is not unusual. Patients often have a personal or family history of migraine headache. |

**TABLE 14–2.** Differential diagnosis of complex partial seizures (continued)

| EVENT | COMPLEX PARTIAL SEIZURE | SYNCOPE | TRANSIENT GLOBAL AMNESIA | TRANSIENT ISCHEMIC ATTACK | COMPLICATED MIGRAINE HEADACHE |
|---|---|---|---|---|---|
| During | Hallmark is an alteration in level of awareness, which may be accompanied by aphasia, nonsensical speech, confusion, eye blinking, staring, chewing or other oral automatisms (lip smacking), nonpurposeful and/or repetitive limb movements, or wandering. The expected duration of these phenomena is generally less than 2 minutes. | Patient looks pale and sweaty; may have mydriasis, tachypnea, bradycardia, reduced muscle tone, or Bell's phenomenon (eyes roll upward); might fall; may jerk or tonically posture during hypoxic-ischemic phase. If present, jerks are usually multifocal and are rarely rhythmic, prolonged, or of high amplitude. Injury, incontinence, and tongue biting are rare but possible. Episode continues until cerebral blood flow and oxygenation are restored. | Patient may have dense time and place disorientation with preserved remote episodic and semantic memory. Patients frequently ask repetitive questions. Symptoms do not include alteration or loss of consciousness, focal neurological signs, apraxia, or aphasia. Episode may last for several hours. | Vertigo is a prominent symptom, and patients may report a swimming or swaying sensation. Other common symptoms include diplopia, nystagmus, facial numbness and/or paresthesias, dysphagia, dysarthria, limb numbness, ataxia (in limb or trunk), loss of consciousness, aphasia, or focal motor signs. Episode may last minutes to hours. | Visual scotoma is very common. When present, other associated neurological symptoms are negative (i.e., loss of function) rather than positive (excess or distortion of function). Headache develops within 10–20 minutes after symptom onset. |

**TABLE 14–2.** Differential diagnosis of complex partial seizures *(continued)*

| EVENT | COMPLEX PARTIAL SEIZURE | SYNCOPE | TRANSIENT GLOBAL AMNESIA | TRANSIENT ISCHEMIC ATTACK | COMPLICATED MIGRAINE HEADACHE |
|---|---|---|---|---|---|
| After | A brief period of postictal confusion is expected and occasionally may be prolonged; patient may have amnesia for ictal state. Rarely, neurological deficits (e.g., aphasia, motor deficits) may persist for up to 2 days after seizure (Todd's phenomenon). | Upon restoration of cerebral blood flow and oxygenation, recovery is rapid. Brief period of malaise, confusion, drowsiness, and event-related amnesia sometimes occurs. | Patient returns to baseline memory function. | Neurological symptoms resolve completely. Failure of symptoms to resolve indicates stroke rather than transient ischemic attack. | Neurological symptoms typically resolve completely. |

in fact, seizures. Although no TBI-specific data exist, in their series of unselected patients with a first-time spell and a likely clinical diagnosis of seizure, Neufeld et al. (2000) found that 69% of the patients had abnormal EEGs and 21% had clear epileptiform abnormalities.

Studies of interictal spiking, however, do not consistently support the thesis that spiking patterns predict seizure occurrence, even among patients with established epilepsy. In other words, the identification of such electroencephalographic abnormalities in the absence of clinical events that are consistent with seizures is insufficient to diagnose PTE. The identification of these abnormalities is also of very limited value as a predictor of PTE. Electroencephalography also is of limited usefulness in identification of other conditions in the differential diagnosis for seizures.

When a patient presents with spells suggestive of epilepsy and with an EEG that is normal, and clinical suspicion still exists that a patient's spells are seizures, then the clinician has several options for continued evaluation and management. Repeating the outpatient EEG is sometimes useful, because a single EEG provides a relatively narrow view of a patient's neurophysiological function (i.e., it samples only the brief period of time during which the patient is connected to the recording electrodes). In several large studies of adults with established epilepsy diagnoses, only 29%–55% of initial EEGs yielded IEDs; an increased yield generally is observed with repeated EEGs, with some studies demonstrating abnormalities in up to 90% of individuals with established epilepsy diagnoses by the fourth EEG (Ebersole and Pedley 2003). Referring the patient for inpatient video-EEG monitoring may also be useful. Long-term (days to weeks) EEG monitoring provides a much longer sample of a patient's brain activity and, as such, will increase the yield for epileptiform abnormalities (if present). Additionally, such a study may be able to capture a patient's spells and characterize the electrical activity of the brain during such events. Even if these additional assessments are undertaken, it sometimes is appropriate to empirically initiate pharmacotherapy with an anticonvulsant (i.e., antiepileptic drug, or AED). For patients with a clinical history that is strongly suggestive of seizures, waiting for a confirmatory diagnostic test may not be necessary, or even preferable, because waiting may result in delays in instituting treatment.

*Neuroimaging.* Brain imaging studies, especially MRI, are also useful in the clinical assessment of possible PTE. Brain imaging studies provide a structural rather than functional assessment of the brain and, therefore, can provide information about possible structural correlates of risk of PTE. Both CT and MRI can provide information about acute or chronic sequelae of injury-related hemorrhage, metal fragment retention, and skull fracture, all risk factors for the occurrence of PTE. In one series that prospectively assessed persons with TBI for new-onset seizures, the presence of cortical or subcortical T2 hyperintense areas on MRI at 1 year after injury conferred an increased risk for PTE (Angeleri et al. 1999). The odds of developing PTE may also be increased by the presence of gliotic scarring around injury-related hemosiderin deposits, but not by the presence of the hemosiderin itself (Angeleri et al. 1999). Gliotic scarring around areas of hemosiderin (but, again, not the hemosiderin deposits themselves) also is associated with medical refractoriness in established patients with PTE (Angeleri et al. 1999; Kumar et al. 2003; Lowenstein 2009).

# TREATMENT

## Pharmacotherapy

Pharmacological treatment is the mainstay of therapy for patients with PTE. Because PTE is a partial-onset epilepsy, a wide range of AEDs are potential therapies. Importantly, no medication has been shown to be unequivocally the "best" for improving seizure control. However, AEDs vary with respect to tolerability, making potential adverse effects of drug treatment an important consideration in choosing a medication. In general, agents that have known efficacy and minimal adverse effects and that are affordable are appropriate initial treatments. Table 14–3 lists many of the commonly used AEDs and briefly summarizes their pharmacological properties; Table 14–4 describes the common effects, side effects, and risks associated with these AEDs (Brailowsky et al. 1986; Brunbech and Sabers 2002; Dikmen et al. 1991, 2000; Ketter et al. 1999; Massagli 1991; Meador et al. 1993, 2001; Yablon 1993; Zaccara et al. 2008). These tables are not intended to be exhaustive references regarding these agents; before prescribing any of these AEDs, clinicians should review the manufacturer's prescribing information for each medication.

Many of the central nervous system effects of the AEDs derive from reports generated during efficacy trials. Because relatively few studies have directly compared the adverse effects of AEDs, definitive state-

**TABLE 14–3.** Pharmacological properties of commonly used anticonvulsant medications

| Medication | Mechanism of action | Protein binding | Elimination | Drug-drug interactions |
|---|---|---|---|---|
| Lamotrigine | Prolongs voltage-sensitive sodium channel inactivation, inhibits synaptic glutamate release | 55% | Hepatic conjugation | Does not appear to significantly affect other AEDs, although anecdotal evidence suggests that levels of the 10,11-epoxide of carbamazepine may be increased when LTG is added. OXC, CBZ, PHT, and PB decrease LTG levels, and VPA increases LTG levels. |
| Topiramate | Inhibits voltage-dependent sodium channels and glutamatergic AMPA receptor-mediated sodium currents, potentiates GABA receptor-associated chloride currents, mildly inhibits carbonic anhydrase | 13% | Renal excretion, hepatic oxidation | Slows metabolism and increases levels of PHT, and has minor effects on other AEDs. Enzyme inducers (CBZ, PHT, PB) decrease TPM levels. |
| Zonisamide | Blocks excitatory T-type calcium channels (thalamus), prolongs sodium channel inactivation, somewhat inhibits carbonic anhydrase | 38%–49% | Hepatic conjugation, oxidation | May increase CBZ and PHT levels. Enzyme-inducing AEDs (CBZ, PHT, PB) decrease ZNS levels. |

**TABLE 14–3.** Pharmacological properties of commonly used anticonvulsant medications *(continued)*

| MEDICATION | MECHANISM OF ACTION | PROTEIN BINDING | ELIMINATION | DRUG-DRUG INTERACTIONS |
|---|---|---|---|---|
| Oxcarbazepine | Blocks voltage-sensitive sodium channels by active 10-monohydroxy metabolite | 40% | Hepatic conjugation, renal excretion | Increases PHT (40%) and PB (15%) levels. Enzyme-inducing AEDs (CBZ, PHT, PB) lower serum levels of OXC. |
| Levetiracetam | Alters synaptic release and trafficking of excitatory neurotransmitters | Minimal | Renal excretion, hepatic hydrolysis | No known interactions with other AEDs. |
| Pregabalin | Modulates calcium channel function | Minimal | Renal excretion | No known interactions with other AEDs. |
| Lacosamide | Enhances slow inactivation of voltage-gated sodium channels | <15% | Renal excretion, hepatic demethylation | No known interactions with other AEDs. |
| Gabapentin | Uncertain; may modulate GABA and glutamate synthesis | <3% | Renal excretion | No known interactions with other AEDs. |
| Phenytoin | Acts on voltage-dependent sodium channels | 75%–93% | Hepatic metabolism, renal excretion | Interacts with many other AEDs; analysis of potential interactions requires case-by-case assessment. |

**TABLE 14–3.** Pharmacological properties of commonly used anticonvulsant medications (continued)

| MEDICATION | MECHANISM OF ACTION | PROTEIN BINDING | ELIMINATION | DRUG-DRUG INTERACTIONS |
|---|---|---|---|---|
| Valproic acid | Blocks sodium channel, activates calcium-dependent potassium conductance, inhibits T-type calcium current, and may have GABA-based effects | 80%–95% | Hepatic metabolism, renal excretion | Interacts with many other AEDs; analysis of potential interactions requires case-by-case assessment. |
| Carbamazepine | Acts on voltage-dependent sodium channels; its principal metabolite, carbamazepine-10,11-epoxide, also has anticonvulsant activity | 76% | Hepatic metabolism, renal excretion | Induces its own hepatic metabolism, requiring dose adjustments to maintain serum levels during early period of treatment with CBZ. Interacts with many other AEDs; analysis of potential interactions requires case-by-case assessment. |

*Note.*  AED=antiepileptic drug; AMPA=α-amino-3-hydroxy-5-methyl-4-isoxazole-propionate; CBZ=carbamazepine; GABA=γ-aminobutyric acid; LTG=lamotrigine; OXC=oxcarbazepine; PB=phenobarbital; PHT=phenytoin; TPM=topiramate; VPA=valproic acid; ZNS=zonisamide.

**TABLE 14–4.** Common effects, side effects, and risks associated with anticonvulsant medications

| MEDICATION | COMMENTS |
|---|---|
| Lamotrigine | Has no clear risk of somnolence, fatigue, cognitive impairment, or weight gain; may have antidepressant effects; may improve arousal among patients with disorders of consciousness; is associated with dose-related dizziness; ataxia and diplopia may occur; may worsen headaches. OCPs may reduce LTG levels, and LTG may reduce the effectiveness of OCPs. Pregnancy increases LTG dose requirements and necessitates close monitoring of drug levels. Severe hypersensitivity reactions (rash, Stevens-Johnson syndrome) may occur in up to 10% of patients, especially children and with more rapid dose titration or altered metabolism/elimination. |
| Topiramate | May cause somnolence, cognitive impairment (especially word-finding difficulties, memory impairment), psychosis, dizziness, fatigue, weight loss, nausea, urolithiasis, paresthesias, and change in taste of carbonated beverages. Increases insulin efficacy, and lessens OCP efficacy. Responder rates plateau, and dropout rates, due to adverse effects, increase at dosages greater than 400 mg/day. Dosage should be reduced by half among patients with renal impairment. |
| Zonisamide | May cause somnolence, impaired attention, dizziness, anorexia, nausea, urolithiasis, paresthesias, and alterations in taste. Severe hypersensitivity reactions (rash, Stevens-Johnson syndrome) may occur and are likely related to sulfa moiety. |
| Oxcarbazepine | Has relatively few adverse cognitive effects; may cause headache, dizziness, fatigue, and ataxia. May decrease efficacy of OCPs. May cause hyponatremia (which occurs more frequently during treatment with OXC than with CBZ and is more common in elderly persons). Severe hypersensitivity reactions (rash, Stevens-Johnson syndrome) may occur. There is a 25%–30% cross-reactivity with CBZ. Dosage should be reduced in patients with renal impairment. |

**TABLE 14–4.**   Common effects, side effects, and risks associated with anticonvulsant medications *(continued)*

| MEDICATION | COMMENTS |
| --- | --- |
| Levetiracetam | Has relatively few adverse cognitive effects; may cause somnolence, an effect that does not appear to be dose related; may cause anxiety, depression, emotional lability, psychosis, and agitation; may cause weight gain; and may cause transient leukopenia. Lower dosages recommended for patients with renal impairment, those taking high-dose NSAIDs, and the elderly. Absorption improved if taken with an empty stomach. |
| Pregabalin | Dose-related somnolence, dizziness, and ataxia are well established. May cause fatigue, which is not dose related; may cause peripheral edema, weight gain, blurred vision, and PR interval prolongation on ECG. Abrupt withdrawal may cause increase in seizure frequency, necessitating gradual tapering (over at least 1 week). Angioedema and hypersensitivity reactions may occur, especially when pregabalin is combined with other AEDs. Combining pregabalin with thiazolidinedione antidiabetic agents can cause fluid retention. Lower dosages recommended for patients with renal impairment and for elderly patients. |
| Lacosamide | May cause nausea, dizziness, ataxia, and diplopia; may cause cardiac rhythm or conduction abnormalities, especially among patients with known heart disease or diabetes. Slower titrations may improve initial drug tolerability. Dosages ≤ 300 mg/day are recommended for patients with end-stage renal disease or mild to moderate liver disease. |
| Gabapentin | May impair attention and processing speed; may have anxiolytic effects; commonly causes somnolence and dizziness; somnolence risk increases at dosages of > 600 mg/day; may cause weight gain; may cause peripheral edema, especially in the elderly. Dosages should be adjusted downward in patients with impaired renal function and in elderly patients. |

**TABLE 14–4.** Common effects, side effects, and risks associated with anticonvulsant medications *(continued)*

| MEDICATION | COMMENTS |
|---|---|
| Phenytoin | Adverse cognitive effects are well established among adults with epilepsy and among persons with TBI receiving PHT prophylactically. May cause somnolence, psychomotor slowing, hyperactivity, irritability, and rarely psychosis; produces motor impairments and may interfere with neurological recovery. Long-term use may cause hirsutism, gingival hyperplasia, peripheral neuropathy, osteopenia, and cerebellar dysfunction. Absorption may improve with twice-daily dosing in patients taking ≥ 400 mg/day. Small dosage changes may result in large increases in active drug concentration. May cause hepatotoxicity and blood dyscrasias. Risk of serious dermatological reaction is increased among persons with HLA-B*1502 genotype. |
| Valproic acid | May cause somnolence, fatigue, weight gain, hair loss, tremor, dizziness, and secondary parkinsonism. Has relatively benign cognitive side-effect profile; occasional cognitive impairment may occur, but less commonly than with PHT or CBZ. Has well-established antimanic and mood-stabilizing effects; may also have anxiolytic and aggression-reducing effects. May cause thrombocytopenia, platelet dysfunction, hepatotoxicity, or pancreatitis. VPA-related hepatotoxicity risk is greatest in children under age 2 years given AED polytherapy. VPA should not be used in women of childbearing age, due to treatment-associated risk of fetal neural tube defects. |
| Carbamazepine | Adverse cognitive effects are common, including among persons with TBI; has well-established antimanic and mood-stabilizing effects; may cause somnolence, fatigue, modest diplopia, hyponatremia, hepatotoxicity, and blood dyscrasias (including agranulocytosis and aplastic anemia). Risk of serious dermatological reaction is increased among persons with HLA-B*1502 genotype. |

*Note.* AED=antiepileptic drug; CBZ=carbamazepine; ECG=electrocardiogram; LTG=lamotrigine; NSAID=nonsteroidal anti-inflammatory drug; OCP=oral contraceptive pill; OXC=oxcarbazepine; PHT=phenytoin; TBI=traumatic brain injury; VPA=valproic acid.

ments about the relative tolerability of these agents are not possible. Additionally, analyses performed by the U.S. Food and Drug Administration (2008) demonstrate increased risk of suicidal ideation or behavior with all of the AEDs studied, including many of those in Table 14–3, when compared with placebo (Patorno et al. 2010). Clinicians should caution patients about this increased risk and assess for symptoms of depression, including suicidal ideation, as a part of routine patient care.

*Considerations in treatment failure or success with anti-epileptic drugs.* Although treatment with AEDs is essential, it is not always successful. Empirical treatment with AEDs may fail for several reasons. The initial AED may afford only partial control of seizures. If a patient is failing the first-choice AED because of either poor tolerability or poor seizure control, the next step is to try a different AED in monotherapy. Many epilepsy patients will have seizure control with a single agent; however, up to 30%–50% will require two or more agents to achieve effective seizure control. If a patient has failed two drugs in monotherapy at respectable dosages for reasons of poor seizure control, but not tolerability, addition of a second AED should be considered. Potential advantages of a dual-therapy regimen include the possibility of an improvement in seizure control. Potential disadvantages include higher cost, higher drug burden, more risk of adverse effects, more risk of drug-drug interactions, and reduced compliance with more complex drug regimens. Principles of rational polypharmacy can help with adjunct medication selection (Leppik 1990). Ideally, compared to the first agent, a second AED should have a different mechanism of action, a low risk of drug-drug interactions, and a low potential for expanding the patient's adverse effects profile (see Table 14–3). The same principles would apply to the selection of a third medication, if needed.

Empirical treatment with an AED also may fail because that agent produces intolerable side effects and requires dosage adjustment or replacement with another medication. The principles of medication selection described in the preceding paragraph may facilitate identification of an adjunctive or alternative medication that will improve the tolerability of treatment.

Treatment also fails when patients are misdiagnosed with PTE. In such circumstances, treatment with an AED should not be expected to reduce the frequency of spells. If there is any question about whether a patient's events are epileptic seizures, referral to an epilepsy center for long-term video-EEG monitoring and formal event characterization is warranted.

Once complete seizure control has been established, many epileptologists will consider weaning a patient from AEDs if he or she has remained free of seizures for several years while taking stable drug dosages. An analysis of 53 studies of drug withdrawal presented by the American Academy of Neurology found that an overall weighted average of 31.2% of seizure-free children and 39.4% of seizure-free adults had recurrent seizures after medication withdrawal. Several clinical factors were then identified that correlated with a higher chance of continued seizure freedom while not taking AEDs. These included being free of seizures while taking AEDs for 2–5 years, having a single type of partial or generalized seizure, having a normal neurological examination and normal IQ, and having a normal EEG after AED treatment. Adults fitting this clinical profile can expect to have at least a 61% chance of remaining seizure-free after drug withdrawal. Children meeting this profile have at least a 69% chance of a successful drug withdrawal (Quality Standards Subcommittee of the American Academy of Neurology 1996). Although this analysis was performed on studies of unselected populations of epilepsy patients, the results can be considered useful in the care of patients with PTE, especially in the absence of any PTE-specific studies. Attempting drug withdrawal in patients not fitting this clinical profile may also be appropriate, although the risk of seizure recurrence may be higher. In each case, it is critical to counsel the patient about the risk of seizure recurrence; the social and emotional consequences of seizure recurrence; and the institution of peri-withdrawal limitations on activities such as driving. The actual schedule for AED withdrawal often depends on the patient and the medication. The American Academy of Physical Medicine and Rehabilitation suggests dose reductions of no more than 20% of the total daily dose every five drug half-lives (Brain Injury Special Interest Group of the American Academy of Physical Medicine and Rehabilitation 1998; Yablon 1993). For patients whose risk of seizure recurrence after drug withdrawal is unacceptably high or who never achieve seizure freedom, the expectation is that they will need lifelong AED therapy.

*Prophylactic use of antiepileptic drugs after TBI.* Empirical use of AEDs after TBI has been studied as a means of preventing seizure-associated acceleration of secondary brain injury and/or preventing the development of PTE. A 1997 Cochrane review of 10 studies meeting strict inclusion criteria found that prophylactic treatment with phenytoin, carbamazepine, or phenobarbital reduced the risk of seizures within the first week after injury but did not affect the rates of PTE or death, or the degree of residual injury-related neurological disability (Schierhout and Roberts 2001/2012). Subsequently, additional medications, such as valproic acid and glucocorticoids have undergone trials to test their efficacy in the prevention of PTE; these interventions also were without benefit (Temkin 2001; Watson et al. 2004).

In recent years, multiple comprehensive practice parameters have been published by the Brain Injury Special Interest Group of the American Academy of Physical Medicine and Rehabilitation (1998), the Brain Trauma Foundation (Bratton et al. 2007), and the American Academy of Neurology (Chang and Lowenstein 2003). These parameters agree that AEDs (most often phenytoin) may be used as a treatment option for the prevention of early posttraumatic seizures in the first week after injury in patients at high risk of seizures after either penetrating or nonpenetrating TBI. The parameters also are clear in recommending against the prophylactic use of AEDs after the first postinjury week among patients without a history of seizures, regardless of whether the TBI in question is penetrating or nonpenetrating.

## Psychological, Behavioral, and Complementary Therapies

Studies of complementary and alternative medical therapies in the treatment of epilepsy, in general, are applicable to patients with PTE. Although space prohibits a comprehensive review in this chapter, a large number of complementary therapies have been studied in persons with epilepsy, including herbal medicines, acupuncture, conscious behavioral inhibition of symptoms at seizure onset, other cognitive-behavioral therapies, relaxation techniques (including yoga and meditation), and homeopathy. Interested readers are encouraged to read recent reviews on the subject (Schachter 2008, 2009). Recent studies have confirmed the widespread, anecdotally successful use of complementary therapies by patients with epilepsy (Liow et al. 2007). In many epilepsy practices, patient-initiated use of complementary therapies is encouraged, especially if the patient perceives an improvement in his or her seizures or overall well-being.

However, all patients must be cautioned about the potential for interactions between AEDs and herbal or homeopathic medications, because many interactions do exist.

Of the available complementary and alternative medical therapies used in the treatment of patients with epilepsy, quantitative EEG (QEEG)–guided neurofeedback has the longest history of use and likely the strongest clinical support. QEEG-guided neurofeedback seeks to alter or normalize the underlying neurophysiology of the brain through operant conditioning. The inherent neuroplasticity of the brain responds to the repeated, trained production of "healthier" brain rhythms by making these rhythms more clinically dominant (Sterman and Egner 2006). A meta-analysis of QEEG-guided neurofeedback done in groups of patients with pharmacologically intractable seizures from multiple causes (including TBI) found a clear reduction in seizure frequency with sensorimotor rhythm (SMR)–based training protocols (Tan et al. 2009). These findings are of particular clinical importance considering that QEEG-guided neurofeedback has also been used successfully to improve residual deficits in the TBI rehabilitation setting (Thornton and Carmody 2009).

## Other Treatments

Other possible treatments for epilepsy include vagus nerve stimulation or resective epilepsy surgery. The vagus nerve stimulator (VNS) is a small pacemaker-like device that is implanted under the pectoral muscle in the left chest. A small wire is then tunneled under the skin from the device to the left vagus nerve in the neck. The stimulator is programmed to deliver around-the-clock intermittent stimulation to the vagus nerve and has been shown to result in a significant reduction in seizure frequency in many (but not all) patients with intractable partial-onset seizures. Potential risks of the VNS include the risks of the implant surgery itself (e.g., risks of general anesthesia, risks of bleeding or infection, risks associated with the implantation of a bio-foreign object). In addition, rare patients continue to feel discomfort at the chest or neck site, even after healing should have been complete.

Resective epilepsy surgery involves the identification and then removal of the seizure-onset zone and, like the VNS, is used in patients with pharmacologically intractable partial-onset seizures. The benefit of surgical resection of mesial temporal lobe seizure foci has been clearly established. In their study of 80 patients with intractable mesial temporal lobe epilepsy, Wiebe et al. (2001) found that 58% of postsurgical patients were free from seizures that impaired awareness, compared to only 8% of medically treated patients ($P<0.001$). Thirty-eight percent of postsurgical patients experienced complete seizure freedom, compared to 3% of medically treated patients ($P<0.001$). The authors also found significant differences in scores on the Quality of Life in Epilepsy (QOLIE-89) inventory between surgical and medical patients at 12 months, as well as a trend toward better rates of employment and school attendance at 1 year in the surgically treated group. Some of the patients in this study had PTE. Other potential benefits of surgical resection include reduction in AED requirement and reduction in the risk of injury or death that is associated with continued frequent seizures. Potential risks of resective epilepsy surgery include the risks of neurosurgery itself (e.g., risks of general anesthesia, risks of bleeding or infection, risks of transient or permanent neurological damage). Counseling regarding and/or an evaluation for either VNS placement or surgical eligibility can be arranged through referral to an established epilepsy surgery program and should be considered for all patients with pharmacologically intractable PTE.

## Community Resources

Although some TBI support groups and foundations offer information about PTE and treatment options, additional information can be found through associations such as the Epilepsy Foundation of America or the American Epilepsy Society, both of which maintain active Web-based educational content.

# CONCLUSION

Seizures are common immediate, early, and late consequences of TBI and adversely affect functional outcome. The frequency of seizures, including recurrent unprovoked seizures (PTE), varies with initial injury severity. There is a broad differential diagnosis for spells and other paroxysmal neurobehavioral events among persons with TBI; knowledge of seizure semiology and brain-behavior relationships is necessary to guide history taking and distinguish between epileptic and nonepileptic causes of such spells. Clinical examination and neurodiagnostic testing, including electroencephalography and neuro-imaging, contribute usefully to the evaluation of persons with suspected seizures. Pharmacotherapy, the first-line treatment of PTE, should be coupled with educational and supportive interventions for persons with PTE and their families. Among persons with pharmacologically intractable PTE, consultation with a tertiary care epilepsy program is encouraged.

## *Key Clinical Points*

---

- A seizure is the occurrence of an abnormal, sustained, and highly synchronous electrical discharge that disrupts otherwise normal brain activity. A posttraumatic seizure is a seizure that occurs after head trauma and that is thought to be causally related to the trauma itself.

- Approximately 5%–30% of adult patients with TBI will develop posttraumatic epilepsy; the rates vary with initial injury severity.

- A patient's experiential and behavioral manifestations of the brain's abnormal electrical activity depend on where the abnormal discharge starts in the brain and how far the discharge spreads within the brain.

- Support for the diagnosis of posttraumatic seizures (as opposed to other causes for episodic neurological dysfunction) can be obtained from thorough history and examination, as well as through ancillary studies, such as electroencephalography or magnetic resonance imaging.

- Pharmacological treatment with antiepileptic drugs is the mainstay of therapy for patients with posttraumatic epilepsy.

- Consultation with an established epilepsy care program should be considered for all patients with pharmacologically intractable posttraumatic epilepsy.

---

# REFERENCES

Angeleri F, Majkowski J, Cacchio G, et al: Posttraumatic epilepsy risk factors: one-year prospective study after head injury. Epilepsia 40:1222–1230, 1999

Annegers JF, Grabow JD, Groover RV, et al: Seizures after head trauma: a population study. Neurology 30:683–689, 1980

Annegers JF, Hauser WA, Coan SP, et al: A population-based study of seizures after traumatic brain injuries. N Engl J Med 338:20–24, 1998

Appleton RE, Demellweek C: Post-traumatic epilepsy in children requiring inpatient rehabilitation following head injury. J Neurol Neurosurg Psychiatry 72:669–672, 2002

Asikainen I, Kaste M, Sarna S: Early and late posttraumatic seizures in traumatic brain injury rehabilitation patients: brain injury factors causing late seizures and influence of seizures on long-term outcome. Epilepsia 40:584–589, 1999

Brailowsky S, Knight RT, Efron R: Phenytoin increases the severity of cortical hemiplegia in rats. Brain Res 376:71–77, 1986

Brain Injury Special Interest Group of the American Academy of Physical Medicine and Rehabilitation: Practice parameter: antiepileptic drug treatment of posttraumatic seizures. Arch Phys Med Rehabil 79:594–597, 1998

Bratton SL, Chestnut RM, Ghajar J, et al: Guidelines for the management of severe traumatic brain injury, XIII: antiseizure prophylaxis. J Neurotrauma 24(suppl):S83–S86, 2007

Brunbech L, Sabers A: Effect of antiepileptic drugs on cognitive function in individuals with epilepsy: a comparative review of newer versus older agents. Drugs 62:593–604, 2002

Caveness WF: Epilepsy, a product of trauma in our time. Epilepsia 17:207–215, 1976

Caveness WF, Walker AE, Ascroft PB: Incidence of posttraumatic epilepsy in Korean veterans as compared with those from World War I and World War II. J Neurosurg 19:122–129, 1962

Caveness WF, Meirowsky AM, Rish BL, et al: The nature of posttraumatic epilepsy. J Neurosurg 50:545–553, 1979

Chang BS, Lowenstein DH: Practice parameter: antiepileptic drug prophylaxis in severe traumatic brain injury: report of the Quality Standards Subcommittee of the American Academy of Neurology. Neurology 60:10–16, 2003

D'Alessandro R, Ferrara R, Benassi G, et al: Computed tomographic scans in posttraumatic epilepsy. Arch Neurol 45:42–43, 1988

Dikmen SS, Temkin NR, Miller B, et al: Neurobehavioral effects of phenytoin prophylaxis of posttraumatic seizures. JAMA 265:1271–1277, 1991

Dikmen SS, Machamer JE, Winn HR, et al: Neuropsychological effects of valproate in traumatic brain injury: a randomized trial. Neurology 54:895–902, 2000

Ebersole J, Pedley T: Current Practice of Clinical Electroencephalography, 3rd Edition. Philadelphia, PA, Lippincott Williams & Wilkins, 2003

Englander J, Bushnik T, Duong TT, et al: Analyzing risk factors for late posttraumatic seizures: a prospective, multicenter investigation. Arch Phys Med Rehabil 84:365–373, 2003

Frey LC: Epidemiology of posttraumatic epilepsy: a critical review. Epilepsia 44(suppl):11–17, 2003

Haltiner AM, Temkin NR, Dikmen SS: Risk of seizure recurrence after the first late posttraumatic seizure. Arch Phys Med Rehabil 78:835–840, 1997

Hauser WA, Ng SK, Brust JC: Alcohol, seizures, and epilepsy. Epilepsia 29(suppl):S66–S78, 1988

Heikkinen ER, Ronty HS, Tolonen U, et al: Development of posttraumatic epilepsy. Stereotact Funct Neurosurg 54–55:25–33, 1990

Hendrick EB, Harris L: Post-traumatic epilepsy in children. J Trauma 8:547–556, 1968

Jennett B: Epilepsy after Non-Missile Head Injuries, 2nd Edition. London, Heinemann Medical, 1975

Ketter TA, Post RM, Theodore WH: Positive and negative psychiatric effects of antiepileptic drugs in patients with seizure disorders. Neurology 53(suppl):S53–S67, 1999

Kollevold T: Immediate and early cerebral seizures after head injuries, part IV. J Oslo City Hosp 29:35–47, 1979

Kumar R, Gupta RK, Husain M, et al: Magnetization transfer MR imaging in patients with posttraumatic epilepsy. AJNR Am J Neuroradiol 24:218–224, 2003

Leppik IE: How to get patients with epilepsy to take their medication: the problem of noncompliance. Postgrad Med 88:253–256, 1990

Liow K, Ablah E, Nguyen JC, et al: Pattern and frequency of use of complementary and alternative medicine among patients with epilepsy in the midwestern United States. Epilepsy Behav 10:576–582, 2007

Lowenstein DH: Epilepsy after head injury: an overview. Epilepsia 50(suppl):4–9, 2009

Massagli TL: Neurobehavioral effects of phenytoin, carbamazepine, and valproic acid: implications for use in traumatic brain injury. Arch Phys Med Rehabil 72:219–226, 1991

Meador KJ, Loring DW, Abney OL, et al: Effects of carbamazepine and phenytoin on EEG and memory in healthy adults. Epilepsia 34:153–157, 1993

Meador KJ, Loring DW, Ray PG, et al: Differential cognitive and behavioral effects of carbamazepine and lamotrigine. Neurology 56:1177–1182, 2001

Neufeld MY, Chistik V, Vishne TH, et al: The diagnostic aid of routine EEG findings in patients presenting with a presumed first-ever unprovoked seizure. Epilepsy Res 42:197–202, 2000

Ng SK, Hauser WA, Brust JC, et al: Alcohol consumption and withdrawal in new-onset seizures. N Engl J Med 319:666–673, 1988

Ottman R, Lee JH, Risch N, et al: Clinical indicators of genetic susceptibility to epilepsy. Epilepsia 37:353–361, 1996

Patorno E, Bohn RL, Wahl PM, et al: Anticonvulsant medications and the risk of suicide, attempted suicide, or violent death. JAMA 303:1401–1409, 2010

Prince DA, Connors BW: Mechanisms of interictal epileptogenesis. Adv Neurol 44:275–299, 1986

Quality Standards Subcommittee of the American Academy of Neurology: Practice parameter: a guideline for discontinuing antiepileptic drugs in seizure-free patients—summary statement. Neurology 47:600–602, 1996

Salazar AM, Jabbari B, Vance SC, et al: Epilepsy after penetrating head injury, I: clinical correlates: a report of the Vietnam Head Injury Study. Neurology 35:1406–1414, 1985

Schachter SC: Complementary and alternative medical therapies. Curr Opin Neurol 21:184–189, 2008

Schachter SC: Botanicals and herbs: a traditional approach to treating epilepsy. Neurotherapeutics 6:415–420, 2009

Schaumann BA, Annegers JF, Johnson SB, et al: Family history of seizures in posttraumatic and alcohol-associated seizure disorders. Epilepsia 35:48–52, 1994

Schierhout G, Roberts I: Anti-epileptic drugs for preventing seizures following acute traumatic brain injury. Cochrane Database Syst Rev (4):CD000173, 2001/2012. DOI: 10.1002/14651858.CD000173.pub2 ("other versions" tab).

Sterman MB, Egner T: Foundation and practice of neurofeedback for the treatment of epilepsy. Appl Psychophysiol Biofeedback 31:21–35, 2006

Tan G, Thornby J, Hammond DC, et al: Meta-analysis of EEG biofeedback in treating epilepsy. Clin EEG Neurosci 40:173–179, 2009

Temkin NR: Antiepileptogenesis and seizure prevention trials with antiepileptic drugs: meta-analysis of controlled trials. Epilepsia 42:515–524, 2001

Temkin NR: Preventing and treating posttraumatic seizures: the human experience. Epilepsia 50(suppl):10–13, 2009

Thornton KE, Carmody DP: Traumatic brain injury rehabilitation: QEEG biofeedback treatment protocols. Appl Psychophysiol Biofeedback 34:59–68, 2009

U.S. Food and Drug Administration: Statistical Review and Evaluation: Antiepileptic Drugs and Suicidality. Rockville, MD, U.S. Department of Health and Human Services, 2008

Walker AE, Erculei F: Post-traumatic epilepsy 15 years later. Epilepsia 11:17–26, 1970

Watson NF, Barber JK, Doherty MJ, et al: Does glucocorticoid administration prevent late seizures after head injury? Epilepsia 45:690–694, 2004

Weiss GH, Feeney DM, Caveness WF, et al: Prognostic factors for the occurrence of posttraumatic epilepsy. Arch Neurol 40:7–10, 1983

Wiebe S, Blume WT, Girvin JP, et al: A randomized, controlled trial of surgery for temporal-lobe epilepsy. N Engl J Med 345:311–318, 2001

Yablon SA: Posttraumatic seizures. Arch Phys Med Rehabil 74:983–1001, 1993

Zaccara G, Gangemi PF, Cincotta M: Central nervous system adverse effects of new antiepileptic drugs: a meta-analysis of placebo-controlled studies. Seizure 17:405–421, 2008

# CHAPTER 15

# Sleep and Fatigue

*Sandeep Vaishnavi, M.D., Ph.D.*
*Una McCann, M.D.*
*Vani Rao, M.D.*

**Sleep problems and fatigue** are common after traumatic brain injury (TBI). The etiology of these disturbances is multifactorial. Sleep disturbance and fatigue after TBI can be a result of the trauma itself or can be secondary to medical problems, pain, neuropsychiatric disturbances, and/or side effects of medications. Because sleep disturbance is common in the general population, the clinician needs to differentiate between premorbid sleep problems and those that are temporally related to TBI.

The complex relationship between sleep and TBI can be understood as a series of mutually independent processes. First, acute brain injury can lead to disrupted levels of consciousness and a disrupted sleep process. A second and distinct type of sleep disruption often develops in the chronic phase of recovery; during this phase, severity of injury is often another factor that influences the type and nature of sleep problems experienced by patients. Finally, subjective and objective measures of sleep disturbance may be discordant, in that subjective complaints may occur without objective evidence, and vice versa (Orff et al. 2009).

The relationship between sleep disturbances and psychiatric disorders is also complex. The neural mechanisms that mediate sleep also have a role in the regulation and stabilization of mood. Dysfunction of these neural circuits after TBI can, therefore, cause both mood and sleep problems. In addition, psychotropics can exacerbate sleep problems, and sleep disturbances can precipitate psychiatric symptoms, such as anxiety and dysphoria.

Fatigue is a nonspecific and highly subjective symptom that is often reported in patients with TBI. It is described as a feeling of exhaustion, tiredness, or weakness. In many ways, sleep disturbances after TBI are better defined and understood than symptoms of fatigue. Therefore, in this chapter, we first discuss the normal sleep cycle, and then the prevalence, pathophysiology, and types of posttraumatic sleep disorders, followed by the evaluation and treatment of these sleep disturbances. We then focus on fatigue after TBI. Although sleep disturbances and fatigue overlap, we treat them as separate entities, for clarity. We briefly review the literature and make practical suggestions for the management of sleep and fatigue following TBI. A more detailed description of TBI sleep disturbances can be found in the chapter "Fatigue and Sleep Problems" in the *Textbook of Traumatic Brain Injury* (Rao et al. 2005).

# NORMAL SLEEP CYCLE

Sleep is an active, complex, and vital brain process, with multiple regulating factors. Multiple discrete brain centers, including the brain stem, basal forebrain, and hypothalamus, modulate sleep production and wakefulness. Serotonin and acetylcholine are two neurotransmitters that are known to be key sleep modulators, although other hormones and endogenous products, as well as norepinephrine, also play important roles. Table 15–1 describes the two sleep states, rapid eye movement (REM) and non–rapid eye movement (NREM) sleep, and Table 15–2 describes the four stages of NREM sleep. Readers interested in a more detailed review of normal sleep are referred to standard textbooks on this subject (Kryger et al. 2000).

# POSTTRAUMATIC SLEEP DISORDERS

## Prevalence of Posttraumatic Sleep Disorders

Sleep disturbance is common in the early period after TBI, with prevalence rates ranging from 42% to 70% (Fichtenberg et al. 2002; Mak-

**TABLE 15–1.** Sleep states

| STATE | GENERAL CHARACTERISTICS |
|---|---|
| Rapid eye movement (REM) sleep | Increased levels of brain activity |
| | Presence of intermittent bursts of REM |
| | Dreaming and vivid recall of dreams |
| | Absence of body movements but partial or full penile erection |
| | Increase in pulse rate, blood pressure, and respiratory rate |
| | Electroencephalogram reveals low-voltage mixed-frequency waves |
| Non–rapid eye movement (NREM) sleep | Decreased levels of brain activity |
| | No REM activity |
| | Slight decrease in pulse rate, blood pressure, and respiratory rate |
| | Intermittent involuntary body movement |
| | Three stages present, with arousal threshold lowest in stage 1 and highest in stage 3/4 |

**TABLE 15–2.** Stages of non–rapid eye movement sleep

| STAGE | GENERAL CHARACTERISTICS | ELECTROENCEPHALOGRAPHIC FINDINGS |
|---|---|---|
| 1 | Light sleep, lasts for a brief period, occupies about 5% of total sleep | 4–7 cycles/second, low-voltage mixed-frequency waves |
| 2 | Occupies about 50% of total sleep | Spindle-shaped tracings at 12–14 cycles/second, with occasional sleep spindles and K complexes |
| 3/4 | Slow-wave sleep | High-voltage delta waves at 1–4 cycles/second |

ley et al. 2008). Cohen et al. (1992) suggested that sleep complaints may vary temporally: difficulty in initiating and maintaining sleep is more common soon after injury, whereas excessive daytime somnolence is more common in the late postinjury period. In their study of individuals several months post-TBI, 81% had difficulty in initiating and maintaining sleep (early and middle insomnia) and 14% had excessive daytime sleepiness. By comparison, among individuals 2–3 years post-TBI, 73% complained of excessive daytime sleepiness and only 8% complained of difficulty in initiating and maintaining sleep. Castriotta et al. (2007) observed abnormal polysomnographic findings among 47% of individuals who were at least 3 months post-TBI, and excessive daytime sleepiness (as defined by abnormal Multiple Sleep Latency Test [MSLT] scores) was present in 25% of this sample. Interestingly, no correlation was found between subjective scores (Epworth Sleepiness Scale) and MSLT scores in this study.

## Pathophysiology

The hypothesized pathophysiology of sleep disturbance following TBI is based on knowledge of the neuropathology of TBI and the physiology of the sleep-wake cycle. Sleep disturbance following acute TBI can result directly from brain trauma, because sleep is dependent on the proper functioning of multiple levels of the central nervous system, especially the brain stem, basal forebrain, hypothalamus, and frontal-subcortical systems.

To test this hypothesis, Rao et al. (2011) compared sleep polysomnograms and sleep electroencephalogram power spectra (PS) data in seven subjects with mild TBI (mTBI) who were 2 weeks or less postinjury against those of seven age- and race-matched healthy comparison subjects. Despite having similar polysomnograms, the two groups differed significantly on PS measures, suggesting that mTBI leads to alterations in the electrical signals that make up individual sleep stages. These findings suggest that PS measures during sleep may provide a sensitive marker of brain injury. In addition to sleep changes that result from damage to brain structures involved in sleep regulation, sleep disturbance can also be secondary to neuropsychiatric sequelae of TBI, chronic pain, medications, abnormal hypocretin levels, and/or abnormal melatonin levels. A study in persons with moderate and severe TBI reported low cerebrospinal fluid levels of hypocretin-1, an excitatory hypothalamic neuropeptide involved in regulation of sleep-wake cycles and known to be reduced or absent among individuals with narcolepsy (Baumann et al. 2005). A correlation may exist between decreased evening melatonin production and increased slow-wave sleep following TBI (Shekleton et al. 2010), with reductions in the levels of melatonin and hypocretin reflecting the effects of brain injury.

In a study of the psychiatric correlates of sleep disturbances in the first 3 months after TBI, Rao et al. (2008) reported that acute post-TBI anxiety disorder is the most consistent significant risk factor associated with worsening sleep status. Parcell et al. (2008), in a study comparing healthy controls to persons with moderate to severe TBI, made similar observations. Additionally, individuals with TBI had an increase in stage 3/4 sleep, reduced REM sleep, and frequent awakenings at night. No correlations were found between sleep problems and either injury severity or time since injury; this suggests that sleep problems of various forms may serve as general indicators of TBI.

# Types of Posttraumatic Sleep Disturbances

Sleep disturbances after TBI can be broadly divided into insomnia, hypersomnia, sleep-wake cycle disturbance, and parasomnia. Verma et al. (2007) characterized sleep problems that occur in the late postinjury period using both subjective and objective measures, and found a full spectrum of sleep disturbances. Insomnia was reported in 25% of patients; those who had problems initiating sleep were found to have high anxiety scores, and those who had problems maintaining sleep had high depression scores. Excessive daytime sleepiness was the presenting complaint in 50% of patients, and was secondary to sleep apnea, narcolepsy, and periodic leg movements. REM sleep behavior disorder was reported by 25% of this sample. As exemplified by this study and as described in the following subsections on sleep disturbances, problems across at least these three subtypes of sleep disorders are common in this population.

Insomnia. *Insomnia* denotes difficulty in initiating or maintaining sleep, with daytime fatigue or impaired functioning, and is common among persons with recent TBI. The prevalence in this population ranges from 36% (McLean et al. 1984) to approximately 70% (Keshavan et al. 1981). Using DSM-IV (American Psychiatric Association 1994) criteria for insomnia, Fichtenberg et al. (2002) noted a prevalence of 30% among persons in the postacute period following TBI.

Fichtenberg et al. (2000) observed correlations between insomnia, depression, and mTBI. However, insomnia was not associated with age, gender, education, or time since injury. This observation suggests that evaluation of patients with insomnia after TBI, and especially mTBI, should include screening for depression and perhaps other psychiatric disturbances as well.

There are conflicting results concerning the relationship between insomnia and TBI severity. Cohen et al. (1992) reported an increased prevalence of insomnia following severe TBI, whereas Clinchot et al. (1998) and Fichtenberg et al. (2000) noted a decreased prevalence among individuals with such injuries. It is possible, however, that interpretation biases contribute to these discrepancies. Decreased prevalence of insomnia after severe TBI may reflect a tendency in this group to underreport sleep problems (Clinchot et al. 1998). Conversely, or additionally, increased awareness and/or intolerance of symptoms among persons with mTBI (Fichtenberg et al. 2000) may elevate the base rates in this population as compared to those among persons with more severe TBI.

*Hypersomnia.* Hypersomnia is defined by both subjective complaints of excessive daytime sleepiness and an MSLT score of <10. Hypersomnia is a relatively common problem among persons with TBI (Baumann et al. 2007). For example, in a study of 184 patients evaluated 15±5 months postinjury, functionally significant complaints of excessive daytime sleepiness were observed in more than 98% of subjects (Guilleminault et al. 2000). Approximately 82% of the patients were found to have hypersomnia with an MSLT score of <10, and 32% were found to have sleep-disordered breathing problems; extensive evaluation of pretrauma behavior suggested that symptomatic sleep-disordered breathing was associated with TBI. Injury severity was also associated with hypersomnia; coma longer than 24 hours, neurosurgical intervention, pain, and skull fracture were commonly associated with hypersomnia. Among these factors, pain at night also contributed to both nocturnal sleep disruption and excessive daytime sleepiness.

In light of the relatively high frequency of symptomatic sleep-disordered breathing in this population, the prudent action is to evaluate individuals complaining of excessive daytime sleepiness after TBI for sleep apnea. Sleep apnea in TBI may be central, obstructive, or mixed. Central sleep apnea may be secondary to the injury to the brain stem regions that control breathing (Webster et al. 2001), and obstructive sleep apnea could be secondary to injury to the upper airways, cervical cord lesions, and weight gain (Mahowald and Mahowald 1996).

Additionally, narcolepsy is sometimes observed among individuals following TBI. Narcolepsy is a disorder of the central nervous system characterized by excessive daytime sleepiness, cataplexy, sleep paralysis, hypnogogic hallucinations, autonomic behaviors, and fragmented nighttime sleep. This disorder is associated with the human lymphocyte antigen (HLA) DR2 and DQB1*0602 and is associated with hypocretin (orexin) deficiency. Among patients in whom a clinical diagnosis of narcolepsy is suspected, performing formal sleep studies (short mean sleep latency and multiple sleep-onset REM periods), HLA typing, and, if possible, assessment of cerebrospinal fluid hypocretin levels is recommended. However, even if a patient is confirmed not to have either the HLA subtype or low hypocretin levels, the causal association between TBI and narcolepsy remains difficult to establish, at best. Arriving at a decision regarding the relevance of TBI to the symptomatic manifestation of narcolepsy remains a matter of individual clinician judgment.

*Sleep-wake cycle disturbances.* Sleep-wake cycle disturbance, or circadian rhythm sleep disorder, is defined as the inability to go to sleep or to stay awake at a desired clock time. Both the duration and pattern of sleep are normal when patients with this disorder do fall asleep (Kryger et al. 2000). There are several varieties of sleep-wake cycle disturbances, including the delayed, advanced, and disorganized types. The pathogenesis of sleep-wake cycle disturbance remains unclear, although dysfunction of the suprachiasmatic nucleus has been postulated. Although sleep-wake cycle disturbances are common in the general population, the relationship between TBI and this specific subcategory of sleep disturbances—beyond that which may be better accounted for by posttraumatic insomnia or hypersomnia—is not well established presently.

*Parasomnias.* Parasomnias are undesirable motor or behavioral events that occur during sleep; these events may result in physical injuries to the patient and produce substantial distress for those residing with or providing caregiving to affected individuals (Mahowald and Mahowald 1996). Sleepwalking, sleep terrors, REM sleep behavior disorders, and nocturnal seizures are some of the varieties of parasomnias. Other than occasional case studies, little literature is available on the prevalence and clinical presentation of this condition after TBI. In one study (Verma et al. 2007), parasomnias were the presenting complaint among 25% of patients presenting to a sleep disorder specialty clinic following mild, moderate, or severe TBI. Among these individuals, REM sleep behavior disorder was the most common of the parasomnias.

# Evaluation of Sleep Disturbances After TBI

The evaluation of TBI-related sleep disturbances is outlined in Table 15–3. As a general rule, it is important first to perform a thorough evaluation for potential medical causes of (or contributors to) sleep disturbances among persons with TBI; some of the more common causes are idiopathic (i.e., pre-TBI) sleep disorders, chronic viral illness, malignancies, and medication side effects. Next, determining whether sleep symptoms are occurring in isolation or are associated with (or secondary to) other neuropsychiatric disturbances is essential. For both of these tasks, key elements of the evaluation include a detailed interview of the patient and obtaining (with the patient's consent) collateral information from family members and other knowledgeable informants. Additionally, reviewing prior medical records (including, among other purposes, for evaluation of the TBI history) is recommended.

If the sleep disturbance with which the patient presents does not appear to be secondary to another clinical (medical or neuropsychiatric) syndrome, then performing formal sleep studies is recommended. These studies not only help in identifying the type of sleep disturbance, but also may be useful in differentiating fatigue (normal sleep studies) from sleep disturbances. The most commonly used objective tests include the polysomnogram, the MSLT, and actigraphy.

# Treatment of Posttraumatic Sleep Disturbances

Sleep disturbances in persons with TBI can be treated with pharmacological interventions and an array of nonpharmacological interventions, such as sleep hygiene techniques, phototherapy, chronotherapy, and psychotherapy.

*Nonpharmacological interventions.* Nonpharmacological approaches to treatment of post-TBI sleep disturbances include the following:

**Diet and lifestyle**.   Diet, rest, exercise, and sleep hygiene programs should be recommended to patients with sleep disturbance. Patients and their families should also be educated about their symptoms and the treatment options available.

**Phototherapy**.   Circadian rhythm disorders may respond to phototherapy. The actual mechanism of action is unknown, but exposure

---

**TABLE 15–3.** Evaluation of sleep disturbances in traumatic brain injury

---

**Detailed history from patient and collateral informants**

Focus on:

    Nature and severity of brain injury

    Sleep pattern preinjury and postinjury

    Alcohol and substance abuse history preinjury and postinjury

    Current medications and dosages

    Preinjury psychiatric history

    Duration and description of current problems

**Neuropsychiatric evaluation**

    Comprehensive evaluation, including physical, neurological, and mental status examination

**Neuropsychological tests in subjects with cognitive complaints and/or deficits**

**Laboratory tests**

    Brain scans

    Computed tomography and/or magnetic resonance imaging

**Specific sleep studies**

    Polysomnography

    Multiple Sleep Latency Test

    Actigraphy

---

to bright light at strategic times of the sleep-wake cycle produces a shift of the underlying biological rhythm (Mahowald and Mahowald 1996). The timing of light exposure depends on the diagnosis, because morning exposure results in phase advance and evening exposure results in phase delay. Bright light therapy of 10,000 lux is commonly used. The duration of exposure varies from one-half hour to 2–3 hours. Common side effects of phototherapy include headache and eye strain. Light therapy should be avoided in patients with photosensitivity or those who have eye diseases.

**Chronotherapy.** Chronotherapy involves entraining a new sleep schedule by advancing or delaying sleep onset by a few hours every day until the desired sleep onset time is obtained. This requires much determination on the part of the patient, not only to obtain the "new" sleep schedule, but also to maintain it thereafter. Similarly, the setting is also important, because hospitalized patients with strict ward rules may not be able to implement chronotherapy effectively (Mahowald and Mahowald 1996). Systematic studies on the indications and effectiveness of chronotherapy are lacking.

**Psychotherapy.**   Few studies are available on the effectiveness of behavioral therapies, such as progressive deep muscle relaxation, in the treatment of insomnia in the general population. In a study of cognitive-behavioral therapy (CBT) for the treatment of insomnia associated with TBI, Ouellet and Morin (2007) found CBT to be efficacious in terms of reduction in total wake time, and improvement in sleep efficiency and fatigue. The different types of CBT include stimulus control, sleep restriction, cognitive restructuring, sleep hygiene education, and fatigue management (recognizing and revising dysfunctional beliefs about fatigue and rest).

*Pharmacotherapy.* Even though sleep disturbances are common among patients with TBI, there is a paucity of research assessing the safety and efficacy of pharmacological interventions for these problems. In general, pharmacotherapies are best regarded as adjunctive to nonpharmacological interventions. The medications mentioned in the following subsections are based on our knowledge of treatment of primary psychiatric disorders and sleep disturbances in the general population. Table 15–4 provides a description of commonly used medications and their usual therapeutic dosages.

**Antidepressants**.   Trazodone (25–200 mg/day) is used frequently for the treatment of insomnia. Although no trials have used trazodone as a hypnotic in the TBI population, the medication remains a popular choice because of its benign side-effect profile. Some concern has been expressed about the effects of this medication on neuronal recovery in rodent models (Boyeson and Harmon 1993). In our clinical experience, other sedating antidepressants, such as mirtazapine (7.5–30 mg/day) and tricyclic agents, have also been helpful. However, prior to initiation, the potential for cardiac, anticholinergic, and metabolic side effects produced by these agents should be considered carefully; among patients in whom these problems may pose significant health risks, prescription of an alternative pharmacotherapy merits consideration.

**TABLE 15–4.** Medications commonly used to treat sleep disturbances after traumatic brain injury

| MEDICATION | PREFERRED DAILY DOSAGES | CLINICAL USES | MOST COMMON SIDE EFFECTS |
|---|---|---|---|
| Trazodone | 25–200 mg | Insomnia | Daytime sedation, orthostasis |
| Mirtazapine | 7.5–30 mg | Insomnia | Increased appetite, weight gain |
| Amitriptyline | 10–50 mg | Insomnia | Dry mouth, blurred vision, constipation, arrhythmias |
| Zolpidem | 5–10 mg | Insomnia | Confusion, daytime sedation |
| Zaleplon | 5–10 mg | Insomnia | Confusion, daytime sedation |
| Lorazepam | 0.5–2 mg | Insomnia | Confusion, disorientation, daytime sedation, unsteadiness |
| Modafinil | 100–400 mg | Excessive daytime sleepiness Narcolepsy Fatigue | Headaches, anxiety, dizziness, diarrhea |
| Melatonin | 0.3–5 mg | Insomnia | Headache, nausea, vivid dreams, irritability |
| Ramelteon | 8 mg | Initial insomnia | Drowsiness, dizziness, fatigue |

**Nonbenzodiazepine sedative-hypnotics.** Zolpidem (5–10 mg at bedtime) and zaleplon (5–10 mg at bedtime) are nonbenzodiazepines also used in the treatment of transient insomnia. Although structurally different from the benzodiazepines, these agents act (relatively selectively) at type 1 receptors of the benzodiazepine receptor complex. These receptors appear to be particularly important to sleep mediation and play a lesser role in cognitively relevant neural circuits, thereby making these agents potentially attractive pharmacotherapies for sleep disturbance (Damgen and Luddens 1999). Zolpidem and zaleplon are less likely to cause daytime drowsiness than most benzodiazepines. When they do produce such problems, their relatively short half-lives may permit adjustment of the time at which the medications are administered such that their effects on daytime functioning are mitigated substantially. Other common side effects produced by these agents include anxiety, nausea, and dysphoric reactions; rebound insomnia; and anterograde amnesia. In light of these potential problems, these agents are commonly used as second-line to the sedating antidepressants.

**Benzodiazepine sedative-hypnotics.**   The mechanism of action of benzodiazepines in the treatment of insomnia is unclear, although subjective and objective evidence supports their usefulness in improving sleep. However, their potential for causing excessive daytime sleepiness, impairing neuronal recovery, reducing sensorimotor functioning, and producing paradoxical behavioral reactions (e.g., disinhibition, rage outbursts) is concerning and underscores the importance of using caution when prescribing these medications in this population (Larson and Zollman 2010).

Benzodiazepines commonly used as hypnotics include lorazepam (0.5–2.0 mg at bedtime), temazepam (7.5–30.0 mg at bedtime), and clonazepam (0.25–2.0 mg at bedtime). The main indication is for the treatment of transient insomnia or insomnia of short duration. Discontinuation should be gradual to avoid producing a benzodiazepine withdrawal syndrome (including autonomic dysfunction and emotional lability), especially when discontinuing benzodiazepines with relatively short half-lives or those that have been used for relatively long periods of time.

**Modafinil.**   Modafinil has been found to be both safe and efficacious in the treatment of narcolepsy at a dosage of 200–400 mg/day. In patients with liver dysfunction, one-half of the recommended dosage should be provided because there is a rare chance that modafinil will cause liver toxicity (Elovic 2000). Although modafinil appears to be useful in the treatment of hypersomnia, further controlled studies need to be conducted in patients with TBI. A double-blind, placebo-controlled crossover trial did not find any difference between modafinil and placebo in treating patients with TBI (Jha et al. 2008).

**Sodium oxybate.** The U.S. Food and Drug Administration (FDA) has approved sodium oxybate for the treatment of cataplexy and daytime sleepiness in narcolepsy. It is the sodium salt of γ-hydroxybutyrate (GHB) and inhibits the release of several neurotransmitters, including γ-aminobutyric acid (GABA), dopamine, and glutamate. In a number of open-label, double-blind, placebo-controlled trials, sodium oxybate has been found to be effective for the reduction of cataplectic attacks and daytime somnolence in patients with narcolepsy (Zaharna et al. 2010). The usual starting dosage is 4.5 g/night given as two divided doses 2–4 hours apart. Increases can be made by 0.75 g/dose at 2-week intervals to a maximum of 9 g/night. In patients with hepatic impairment, the starting dosage should be 2.25 g/night. Common side effects include dizziness, headache, somnolence, nausea, vomiting, and enuresis.

**Melatonin.** Melatonin, a metabolite of serotonin, is a hormone secreted by the pineal gland. Darkness augments the production of melatonin, and light suppresses its secretion. It plays an important role in maintaining the body's biological rhythm and synchronizing the sleep-wake cycle with the environment. Studies in the general population have shown that exogenous melatonin (0.3–5 mg at bedtime) may be useful in improving the duration and quality of sleep and altering the biological rhythm.

Ramelteon (8 mg at bedtime) is a melatonin agonist that acts on melatonin type 1-and type 2 receptors in the suprachiasmatic nucleus. It has been approved by the FDA for insomnia characterized by difficulty in sleep onset. Advantages of this medication include the absence of excessive sedating effects and reduced abuse liability. There are no studies on the use of ramelteon in patients with TBI.

**Atypical antipsychotics.** Atypical antipsychotics are often used in the context of TBI and sleep disturbance, although studies are limited. In a case study of a patient with TBI, Schreiber et al. (1998) noted the beneficial effects of risperidone for psychosis and sleep disturbance. Quetiapine also has been used for sleep augmentation in various populations and may be helpful, in our clinical experience, for insomnia co-occurring with paranoia or agitation after TBI.

*Miscellaneous therapies.* Cranial electrotherapy stimulation (CES) is a noninvasive technique approved by the FDA for the treatment of anxiety, depression, and insomnia. CES involves transcutaneous application of microcurrent to the brain for 20–60 minutes/day for several days to weeks. Kirsch (2002) has published extensively on the effectiveness of CES for anxiety, depression, and insomnia, and has noted a positive outcome in 89% of 126 published studies. Nevertheless, research in this field is still in the early stage, and no studies have reported the effectiveness of CES for the treatment of TBI-related insomnia.

Audiovisual entrainment (AVE) is a noninvasive neurotherapy that is hypothesized to treat insomnia, anxiety, depression, posttraumatic stress disorder, seasonal affective disorder, and attention-deficit/hyperactivity disorder. AVE involves use of flashing lights and rhythmic tones to specifically synchronize (entrain) brain waves to desired frequencies. In a review of the effects of brainwave entrainment for the treatment of psychiatric problems, Huang and Charyton (2008) noted that it is an effective treatment strategy, but more controlled trials are necessary.

# FATIGUE AFTER TRAUMATIC BRAIN INJURY

The prevalence of fatigue in individuals with TBI ranges from about 40% to 70% (Kreutzer et al. 2001). Despite a trend toward improvement over time, a significant number of TBI survivors still experience fatigue after the first year of injury. Poor sleep quality is the most common clinical variable associated with fatigue. In a study comparing patients with TBI to normal healthy controls, Cantor et al. (2008) found that fatigue was more common in the TBI group and significantly higher in females than males. However, no other demographic or injury variables were associated with fatigue. Even though depression, pain, and sleep were more common in those with fatigue, they accounted for only 23% of the variance in the TBI group, compared with 53% of the variance in the control group, suggesting that fatigue after TBI may be related to the brain injury itself.

## Pathophysiology of Posttraumatic Fatigue

Much less is known about the pathophysiology of fatigue than of sleep disturbances in TBI. Bay and Xie (2009) describe fatigue as a "multidimensional symptom" that affects several components, including physical, emotional, cognitive, motivational, and functional domains. Similarly, the biological and psychological correlates of fatigue are many (Bay and Xie 2009; Cantor et al. 2008) and can be conceptualized as preinjury factors (e.g., female gender), injury factors (e.g., physical and metabolic abnormalities associated with trauma to the brain), and postinjury factors (e.g., cognitive and psychiatric sequelae of TBI, pharmacotherapy for TBI). Several biochemical abnormalities such as hypocortisolemia and immune system dysfunction have also been implicated in the pathogenesis of fatigue (Bay and Xie 2009; Bertolone et al. 1993). The diagnosis of post-TBI fatigue, however, should be one of exclusion and considered after careful evaluation of preinjury and postinjury factors.

## Evaluation of Posttraumatic Fatigue

Fatigue is one of the most common and earliest signs of brain injury, yet there is a paucity of literature on the clinical presentation and evaluation of fatigue in patients with TBI. Because fatigue is a subjective experience, self-report scales are more appropriate for assessing the severity of this symptom, although they have obvious limitations. Commonly used scales include the Fatigue Impact Scale (FIS; Fisk et al. 1994), the Fatigue Severity Scale (FSS; Krupp et al. 1989), the Barrow Neurological Institute (BNI) Fatigue Scale (Borgaro et al. 2004), and the Cause of Fatigue (COF) Questionnaire (Ziino and Ponsford 2005). Both the BNI Fatigue Scale and the COF Questionnaire were developed specifically for patients with TBI and are therefore recommended for use in this population.

The relationship between self-reports of fatigue and objective assessment of fatigue is controversial. Although some studies have reported a positive relationship between subjective fatigue and poor performance on cognitive tests that require sustained effort, such as tests of attention (Ziino and Ponsford 2006), others have not (Cantor et al. 2008). Subjective fatigue is associated with reduced speed, but not reduced accuracy, on cognitive tests.

An endocrine evaluation for patients with TBI complaining of fatigue may be warranted. Bushnik et al. (2007) examined the relationship between fatigue and endocrine factors in a study of 64 subjects with TBI 1 year after injury. Abnormality in at least one domain of the pituitary axis was found in 90% of subjects.

## Treatment of Posttraumatic Fatigue

Management of post-TBI fatigue includes pharmacological and nonpharmacological interventions. Treatment first targets observable symptoms (e.g., sleep disturbance, chronic pain), coexisting medical conditions (e.g., hypothyroidism, diabetes mellitus), psychiatric disorders (e.g., depression), and simplification of the medication regimen, including minimizing the use of sedating agents.

*Nonpharmacological interventions.* Nonpharmacological approaches to treatment of post-TBI fatigue include the following:

**Education.** Patient and family members should be educated about the frequent occurrence of fatigue in persons with TBI as an isolated problem or secondary to other psychiatric disturbances, or both. Often, the patient's self-esteem is enhanced when the patient learns that the "feeling of tiredness" is not a sign of laziness but instead is a common symptom following TBI.

**Diet and lifestyle.** Good nutrition and a balance between regular exercise and adequate rest are important for combating fatigue. Regular exercise is important because it prevents deconditioning and promotes normalization of physical and mental efficiency and performance. The exercise protocol should be individualized because too much or too little exercise can be detrimental. In addition, adequate rest is also important, and patients should be encouraged to practice good sleep hygiene (Table 15–5).

**Psychotherapy.** CBT has been found to be useful in patients with chronic fatigue syndrome (Prins et al. 2001). In a large, multicenter randomized controlled trial, CBT was found to be significantly more effective than control conditions for both fatigue improvement and functional performance. Studies of this approach are lacking for the treatment of fatigue after brain injury.

---

**TABLE 15–5.** Sleep hygiene

Maintain a regular sleep schedule of going to bed and waking around the same time every day (±30 minutes), including holidays and weekends.

Avoid daytime naps.

If unable to fall asleep within 10–20 minutes of lying in bed, get out of bed and do something relaxing and return to bed when sleepy.

Avoid stimulants such as coffee and sodas, alcohol, and strenuous exercise late in the day, because they may be too stimulating and delay sleep.

Avoid bright lights, loud noise, and eating, reading, and watching TV in the bedroom.

Maintain a sleep log, noting duration and quality of sleep.

---

*Pharmacological interventions.* In general, pharmacotherapies are best regarded as adjunctive to nonpharmacological interventions. Only a few studies are available on the treatment of fatigue specifically after TBI.

**Stimulants.** Stimulants increase cerebral catecholaminergic (i.e., dopaminergic and/or noradrenergic) function and sometimes are used to treat impaired arousal, fatigue, inattention, and hypersomnia after brain injury. Methylphenidate (10–60 mg/day) and dextroamphetamine (5–40 mg/day) are the commonly used stimulants. These medications are generally taken twice daily, with the second dose taken at least 6–8 hours before sleep initiation, and more commonly at midday, to avoid medication-induced or medication-exacerbated insomnia. Some patients, however, may need to be dosed more frequently, depending on treatment response. Treatment is usually begun at the lowest dosage and dosage is gradually increased if necessary. Possible side effects include paranoia, dysphoria, agitation, dyskinesia, anorexia, and irritability. Because of a potential for abuse, patients taking these drugs should be closely monitored.

**Dopamine agonists.** Carbidopa-levodopa (10/100 mg/day to 25/100 mg four times daily) and bromocriptine (2.5–10.0 mg/day) are dopamine agonists that have been studied in small, uncontrolled case studies for the treatment of mood, cognition, and behavior problems in patients with TBI (Dobkin and Hanlon 1993; Lal et al. 1988).

**Amantadine.** Amantadine was first used in the treatment of influenza in the 1960s and was later found to have antiparkinsonian effects. It enhances release of dopamine, inhibits reuptake, and increases dopamine activity at the postsynaptic receptors. Amantadine is sometimes used in clinical practice for purposes similar to those of the stimulants and may improve arousal, some aspects of cognition, and motivation among persons with TBI. Its use for posttraumatic fatigue is understudied, but it is sometimes used for this purpose as well. When amantadine is prescribed, usual dosages are 50–200 mg twice daily. Although confusion, hallucinations, pedal edema, and hypotension are reported side effects, these problems are observed relatively infrequently in everyday clinical practice.

**Modafinil.** Modafinil is structurally distinct from the stimulants, but its clinical effects are quite similar to those of agents in that class. Teitelman (2001) conducted an open-label study in patients with TBI who complained of excessive daytime sleepiness and in patients with somnolence secondary to sedating psychiatric drugs. Modafinil was well tolerated at a dosage of 100–400 mg once daily. All patients reported improvement in daytime sleepiness. No adverse effects were encountered. However, modafinil was not found to be efficacious in the treatment of post-TBI fatigue or excessive daytime sleepiness in a double-blind, placebo-controlled crossover trial (Jha et al. 2008). Although modafinil was found to be safe and tolerable, a significantly increased rate of insomnia was reported in the modafinil group. Controlled studies of modafinil for fatigue in patients with multiple sclerosis or Parkinson disease have also been disappointing.

Armodafinil is the *R*-enantiomer of modafinil and has a similar mechanism of action. Although it has not been studied in patients with TBI, armodafinil appears to be modestly effective for the treatment of fatigue, obstructive sleep apnea, and narcolepsy in non-TBI populations. It has no apparent clinical advantage over modafinil, however, and clinicians are advised to remain circumspect about any such advantages pending publication of studies demonstrating them. If this agent is used, the usual dosage is 150–250 mg once daily. Common side effects include headache, dizziness, and insomnia, but there are case reports of angioedema, multiorgan hypersensitivity reactions, and Stevens-Johnson syndrome (Garnock-Jones et al. 2009).

**Creatine.**   In an experimental pilot study, Sakellaris et al. (2008) determined the neuroprotective effect of creatine, in children with moderate to severe TBI, in reducing rates of headache, dizziness, and fatigue soon after discharge from the hospital. Children in the creatine group compared to the placebo group had significantly lower rates of headache, dizziness, and fatigue in the 6-month follow-up period. However, this study is only experimental, and replication with larger patient numbers and a longer duration of follow-up is necessary.

## CONCLUSION

Sleep disturbances and fatigue are common among persons with TBI, but the etiologies and pathophysiologies of these problems require further investigation. Among persons with TBI, fatigue and sleep disturbance may occur as isolated entities or as symptoms of another medical or psychiatric syndrome. When present, comorbid medical and psychiatric conditions should be treated prior to initiating sleep- or fatigue-specific interventions.

The development of posttraumatic sleep disturbances and/or fatigue is most likely multifactorial, reflecting complex contributions of and interactions among biological effects of TBI, psychosocial stressors, non-TBI-related (including preinjury) neuropsychiatric disorders, and environmental factors. Establishing the correct diagnosis is important because treatment differs as a function of diagnosis; however, confidence in clinical diagnosis may not always be possible in this population.

Indeed, the relationship between fatigue and sleep disturbance is both complex and controversial. Although we presented sleep disturbances and fatigue separately in this chapter for the sake of conceptual clarity, it is important to acknowledge that disentangling one from the other in any individual patient is quite challenging. Subjective sleep logs, fatigue scales, and objective laboratory sleep tests such as polysomnograms and MSLT may help clinicians and patients differentiate between these types of conditions and facilitate directing initial treatments toward the problem producing the most distress and/or dysfunction.

In general, management of sleep problems after TBI precedes treatment of fatigue. Comprehensive medical and psychiatric evaluations, including objective assessments (i.e., formal sleep studies) when appropriate and feasible, are prerequisites to the treatment of posttraumatic sleep disturbances. Nonpharmacological strategies such as sleep hygiene and CBT should be initiated simultaneously and prior to pharmacotherapy. Circadian rhythm problems should be managed with light therapy.

Pharmacotherapy for sleep disturbances is considered if nonpharmacological interventions are of limited or no success. We recommend an initial trial of a sedating antidepressant, such as trazodone. If not effective, other sedating antidepressants, such as low-dose mirtazapine or tricyclic agents, can be considered, provided the patient has no contraindications. Ramelteon or melatonin may also be helpful for sleep initiation. If these agents are not helpful, then a trial of nonbenzodiazepine sedative-hypnotics can be initiated. We strongly recommend that these medications be used only for a short period. We keep benzodiazepines and antipsychotics in reserve because of their potential central nervous system side effects.

Management of post-TBI fatigue includes pharmacological and nonpharmacological interventions. Treatment first targets observable symptoms (e.g., sleep disturbance, chronic pain), coexisting medical conditions (e.g., hypothyroidism, diabetes mellitus), psychiatric disorders (e.g., depression), and simplification of the medication regimen, including minimizing the use of sedating agents. Nonpharmacological treatments are first-line thereafter, and include education, diet and lifestyle adaptations, and CBT. When medications are used, stimulants and other agents that directly or indirectly augment cerebral catecholaminergic function may be useful.

## Key Clinical Points

---

- Sleep disturbances and fatigue are common but incompletely understood problems among persons with TBI.

- Identifying and treating other medical or neuropsychiatric causes of (and/or contributors to) posttraumatic sleep disturbances and fatigue are necessary before prescribing treatments specifically for these problems.

- Although posttraumatic sleep disturbances and fatigue commonly co-occur, it is often productive to begin treatment of sleep disturbances prior to initiating specific treatments for fatigue.

- In the management of posttraumatic sleep disorders and/or fatigue, nonpharmacological interventions take precedence over pharmacotherapies.

---

# REFERENCES

American Psychiatric Association: Diagnostic and Statistical Manual of Mental Disorders, 4th Edition. Washington, DC, American Psychiatric Association, 1994

Baumann CR, Stocker R, Imhof HG, et al: Hypocretin-1 (orexin A) deficiency in acute traumatic brain injury. Neurology 65:147–149, 2005

Baumann CR, Werth E, Stocker R, et al: Sleep-wake disturbances 6 months after traumatic brain injury: a prospective study. Brain 130:1873–1883, 2007

Bay E, Xie Y: Psychological and biological correlates of fatigue after mild-to-moderate traumatic brain injury. West J Nurs Res 31:731–747, 2009

Bertolone K, Coyle PK, Krupp LB, et al: Cytokine correlates of fatigue in multiple sclerosis. Neurology 43:A356, 1993

Borgaro SR, Gierok S, Caples H, et al: Fatigue after brain injury: initial reliability study of the BNI Fatigue Scale. Brain Inj 18:685–690, 2004

Boyeson MG, Harmon RL: Effects of trazodone and desipramine on motor recovery in brain-injured rats. Am J Phys Med Rehabil 72:286–293, 1993

Bushnik T, Englander J, Katznelson L: Fatigue after TBI: association with neuroendocrine abnormalities. Brain Inj 21:559–566, 2007

Cantor JB, Ashman T, Gordon W, et al: Fatigue after traumatic brain injury and its impact on participation and quality of life. J Head Trauma Rehabil 23:41–51, 2008

Castriotta RJ, Wilde MC, Lai JM, et al: Prevalence and consequences of sleep disorders in traumatic brain injury. J Clin Sleep Med 3:349–356, 2007

Clinchot DM, Bogner J, Mysiw WJ, et al: Defining sleep disturbance after brain injury. Am J Phys Med Rehabil 77:291–295, 1998

Cohen M, Oksenberg A, Snir D, et al: Temporally related changes of sleep complaints in traumatic brain injured patients. J Neurol Neurosurg Psychiatry 55:313–315, 1992

Damgen K, Luddens H: Zaleplon displays a selectivity to recombinant GABA(A) receptors different from zolpidem, zopiclone and benzodiazepines. Neurosci Res Commun 25:139–148, 1999

Dobkin BH, Hanlon R: Dopamine agonist treatment of antegrade amnesia from a mediobasal forebrain injury. Ann Neurol 33:313–316, 1993

Elovic E: Use of Provigil for underarousal following TBI. J Head Trauma Rehabil 15:1068–1071, 2000

Fichtenberg NL, Millis SR, Mann NR, et al: Factors associated with insomnia among post-acute traumatic brain injury survivors. Brain Inj 14:659–667, 2000

Fichtenberg NL, Zafonte RD, Putnam S, et al: Insomnia in a post-acute brain injury sample. Brain Inj 16:197–206, 2002

Fisk JD, Ritvo PG, Ross L, et al: Measuring the functional impact of fatigue: initial validation of the Fatigue Impact Scale. Clin Infect Dis 18 (suppl 1):S79–S83, 1994

Garnock-Jones KP, Dhillon S, Scott LJ: Armodafinil. CNS Drugs 23:793–803, 2009

Guilleminault C, Yuen KM, Gulevich MG, et al: Hypersomnia after head-neck trauma: a medicolegal dilemma. Neurology 54:653–659, 2000

Huang TL, Charyton C: A comprehensive review of the psychological effects of brainwave entrainment. Altern Ther Health Med 14:38–50, 2008

Jha A, Weintraub A, Allshouse A, et al: A randomized trial of modafinil for the treatment of fatigue and excessive daytime sleepiness in individuals with chronic traumatic brain injury. J Head Trauma Rehabil 23:52–63, 2008

Keshavan MS, Channabasavanna SM, Reddy GN: Post-traumatic psychiatric disturbances: patterns and predictors of outcome. Br J Psychiatry 138:157–160, 1981

Kirsch DL: The Science Behind Cranial Electrotherapy Stimulation, 2nd Edition. Edmonton, AB, Canada, Medical Scope Publishing, 2002

Kreutzer JS, Seel RT, Gourley E: The prevalence and symptom rates of depression after traumatic brain injury: a comprehensive examination. Brain Inj 15:563–576, 2001

Krupp LB, LaRocca NG, Muir-Nash J, et al: The Fatigue Severity Scale: application to patients with multiple sclerosis and systemic lupus erythematosus. Arch Neurol 46:1121–1123, 1989

Kryger MH, Roth T, Dement WC: Principles and Practice of Sleep Medicine, 3rd Edition. Philadelphia, PA, WB Saunders, 2000

Lal S, Merbtiz CP, Grip JC: Modification of function in head-injured patients with Sinemet. Brain Inj 2:225–233, 1988

Larson EB, Zollman FS: The effect of sleep medications on cognitive recovery from traumatic brain injury. J Head Trauma Rehabil 25:61–67, 2010

Mahowald M, Mahowald M: Sleep disorders, in Head Injury and Postconcussive Syndrome. Edited by Rizzo M, Tranel DD. New York, Churchill Livingstone, 1996, pp 285–304

Makley MJ, English JB, Drubach DA, et al: Prevalence of sleep disturbance in closed head injury patients in a rehabilitation unit. Neurorehabil Neural Repair 22:341–347, 2008

McLean A Jr, Dikmen S, Temkin N, et al: Psychosocial functioning at 1 month after head injury. Neurosurgery 14:393–399, 1984

Orff HJ, Ayalon L, Drummond SP: Traumatic brain injury and sleep disturbance: a review of current research. J Head Trauma Rehabil 24:155–165, 2009

Ouellet MC, Morin CM: Efficacy of cognitive-behavioral therapy for insomnia associated with traumatic brain injury: a single-case experimental design. Arch Phys Med Rehabil 88:1581–1592, 2007

Parcell DL, Ponsford JL, Redman JR, et al: Poor sleep quality and changes in objectively recorded sleep after traumatic brain injury: a preliminary study. Arch Phys Med Rehabil 89:843–850, 2008

Prins JB, Bleijenberg G, Bazelmans E, et al: Cognitive behaviour therapy for chronic fatigue syndrome: a multicentre randomised controlled trial. Lancet 357:841–847, 2001

Rao V, Rollings P, Spiro J: Fatigue and sleep problems, in Textbook of Traumatic Brain Injury. Edited by Silver JM, McAllister TW, Yudofsky SC. Washington, DC, American Psychiatric Publishing, 2005, pp 369–384

Rao V, Spiro J, Vaishnavi S, et al: Prevalence and types of sleep disturbances acutely after traumatic brain injury. Brain Inj 22:381–386, 2008

Rao V, Bergey A, Hill H, et al: Sleep disturbance after mild traumatic brain injury: indicator of injury? J Neuropsychiatry Clin Neurosci 23:201–205, 2011

Sakellaris G, Nasis G, Kotsiou M, et al: Prevention of traumatic headache, dizziness and fatigue with creatine administration: a pilot study. Acta Paediatr 97:31–34, 2008

Schreiber S, Klag E, Gross Y, et al: Beneficial effect of risperidone on sleep disturbance and psychosis following traumatic brain injury. Int Clin Psychopharmacol 13:273–275, 1998

Shekleton JA, Parcell DL, Redman JR, et al: Sleep disturbance and melatonin levels following traumatic brain injury. Neurology 74:1732–1738, 2010

Teitelman E: Off-label uses of modafinil (letter). Am J Psychiatry 158:1341, 2001

Verma A, Anand V, Verma NP: Sleep disorders in chronic traumatic brain injury. J Clin Sleep Med 3:357–362, 2007

Webster JB, Bell KR, Hussey JD, et al: Sleep apnea in adults with traumatic brain injury: a preliminary investigation. Arch Phys Med Rehabil 82:316–321, 2001

Zaharna M, Dimitriu A, Guilleminault C: Expert opinion on pharmacotherapy of narcolepsy. Expert Opin Pharmacother 11:1633–1645, 2010

Ziino C, Ponsford J: Measurement and prediction of subjective fatigue following traumatic brain injury. J Int Neuropsychol Soc 11:416–425, 2005

Ziino C, Ponsford J: Selective attention deficits and subjective fatigue following traumatic brain injury. Neuropsychology 20:383–390, 2006

CHAPTER 16

# Posttraumatic Sensory Impairments

*Nathan D. Zasler, M.D.*

**Several types of sensory impairments** are associated with traumatic brain injury (TBI). Some of these impairments are the result of injury to the brain, whereas others reflect the effects of cervical trauma, cranial injury, cranial nerve injury, or cranial-adnexal injury—that is, injury to structures in the head but not the brain itself (Hammond and Masel 2007). Adequate differential diagnosis is crucial to establishing the cause of the sensory complaint and, thereby, directing appropriate clinical management.

Well-documented sensory sequelae of TBI include audiovestibular disorders, such as hearing loss, hyperacusis, and tinnitus, as well as disorders of a more vestibular nature, such as dizziness, imbalance complaints, and frank vertigo. Visual complaints are also common following TBI, as well as after cranial trauma and whiplash. Chemosensory complaints involving smell and taste aberrations have also been reported in the literature, with olfactory impairment being a much more common phenomenon than gustatory impairment. Postural instability is another commonly observed sensory disorder following TBI and is generally considered one of the hallmarks of postconcussive impairment.

Although this chapter cannot, in the space allotted, address all of the sensory impairments associated with TBI, this review is intended to provide readers with an overview of some of the more critical and/ or common clinical issues in this area of post-TBI assessment and care.

# VESTIBULAR DISORDERS

Neuro-otological trauma can involve dysfunction of the inner ear, including the labyrinth and vestibular nerve (Iverson et al. 2007; Tusa and Brown 1996). Benign paroxysmal positional vertigo (BPPV) is one of the more common vestibular disorders following TBI and cranial trauma. This diagnosis is suggested by complaints of transient vertigo that are positionally triggered by head movement. Vertiginous attacks may be intermittent and/or produce longer-lasting periods of disequilibrium. The diagnosis is supported by examination findings of torsional and up-beating nystagmus during the Hallpike-Dix maneuver when the affected ear is positioned inferiorly. Nystagmus associated with BPPV lasts 3–30 seconds and typically habituates (i.e., extinguishes); this is unlike positional vertigo associated with central causes, which is much less common after TBI, and particularly after mild TBI (mTBI) (Barber 1964). BPPV may be the result of cupulolithiasis or canalithiasis; these are conditions in which free-floating calcium crystals, broken off from the utricle (one of two otolith organs in the inner ear), float in the endolymph of the cupula or canal of the posterior semicircular canal of the inner ear. Less frequently, BPPV may occur from calcium debris in the anterior canal; in this circumstance, the nystagmus is torsional and down-beating. BPPV may also involve the horizontal canal; in these cases, the nystagmus is horizontal and directed toward whichever ear is inferior. Generally, BPPV onset is closely temporally linked with the trauma; however, it can have a delayed onset, and prior cranial trauma or TBI may loosen otoconia and increase susceptibility to development of BPPV (Cifu and Caruso 2010). Blast injuries appear to be risk factors for BPPV (Fausti et al. 2009).

Treatment for BPPV depends on the canal involved (Ernst et al. 2005) and generally employs techniques referred to as particle repositioning maneuvers. BPPV due to horizontal canal involvement tends to respond best to repetitive movements of sitting and lying as noted by Brandt and Daroff (1980). For posterior canalithiasis, a single, slow maneuver of the head, as described by Epley (1992), to reposition the debris in the asymptomatic labyrinth is recommended. Alternatively, Semont's maneuver may be employed for posterior cupulolithiasis (Semont et al. 1988). This involves seating the patient on a table and rotating the head 45 degrees toward the unaffected side. The patient is then moved quickly so as to lie on the side toward the affected ear, parallel to the plane of the affected posterior canal. After 4–5 minutes, the patient is rapidly moved through the initial sitting position to the opposite side while the head is still positioned at 45 degrees toward the unaffected side. The patient holds that position for 4–5 minutes and then slowly moves to a sitting position. Newer treatments that allow for self-directed repositioning at home appear promising, including the DizzyFIX device (Bromwich et al. 2010).

Dizziness associated with TBI may also reflect posttraumatic endolymphatic hydrops (ELH), a condition that develops as a delayed complication due to trauma to the membranous labyrinth (Clark and Rees 1977). Posttraumatic ELH with symptom onset delays as long as 5–10 years postinjury is sometimes observed. Posttraumatic ELH (the underlying pathophysiological condition of Ménière's disease) causes episodic tinnitus, sensations of ear fullness, and hearing loss, often associated with vertigo lasting from hours to days, although the presentation can be variable. After repeated attacks, patients typically develop a low-frequency sensorineural hearing loss with tinnitus that is constant. The definitive diagnostic test for this condition remains controversial, although audiogram-confirmed fluctuating hearing loss is often relied upon. Treatment involves dietary sodium restriction, limitation of alcohol and caffeinated products, and potential use of diuretics. When medical management fails, surgical approaches have been used if the disorder is unilateral. Mastoid or subarachnoid shunting is the most "benign" of the surgical procedures, although it is not always effective and/or long lasting. Labyrinthectomy can be considered in patients with disabling attacks for which other interventions have failed. Alternatively, vestibular neurectomy can be considered when hearing is preserved.

Labyrinthine concussion may also occur in association with TBI. The disorder presents with acute vertigo, nausea, hearing loss, and disequilibrium, generally in association with tinnitus. Typically, the symptoms resolve within a few days, and the patient is left with a dynamic deficit that can last for weeks to months, until central compensation occurs. Physical therapy interventions are useful once acute vertigo subsides.

Perilymphatic fistulas (PLFs) are consequences of closed head trauma (not necessarily with accompanying TBI) but may also be seen with other types of trauma, such as barotraumas (Conroy and Erogul 2009). The fistulous communication is typically between the inner and middle ear, with leakage of perilymphatic fluid through the defect. Blast injuries may also be responsible for this type of injury in the context of barotrauma. Barotrauma secondary to blast injuries can cause oval or round window membrane rupture. PLFs typically present with sudden, progressive, or fluctuating hearing loss of a sensorineural nature with associated tinnitus and typically vertigo with disequilibrium (Fukaya and Nomura 1988). Various physical examination techniques have been suggested to be useful in the assessment for PLFs, including Hennebert's sign (i.e., nystagmus or drift of the eyes induced by positive or negative pressure applied through the external auditory canal) and the Valsalva maneuver. However, these two symptom provocation maneuvers are both nonspecific and not particularly sensitive. Other examination techniques that suggest the presence of a PLF include perilymphatic fluid analysis at the time of intraoperative assessment and a specific test involving platform posturography called the platform fistula test. PLFs often resolve spontaneously, but some may remain open and symptomatic. Chronic PLFs can be surgically closed by patching over the leaking oval or round window with a temporal aponeurosis or stapedectomy with interposition (Iverson et al. 2007). After surgical treatment, the most commonly improved symptom seems to be vertigo; resolution of hearing impairments occurs less commonly.

Brain stem and vestibulocerebellar injury can also result in dizziness; however, in everyday clinical practice, injuries to these structures are not common causes of this problem. Seizures may also be associated with dizziness; more specifically, ictal vertigo presents with a sense of rotation. Ictal vertigo has also been termed "tornado epilepsy." Although this is an interesting type of seizure, it is an uncommon epileptic variant. Vertigo, in some patients with partial seizures due to an epileptic focus in the superior temporal gyrus, may present with symptoms similar to ELH without hearing loss. Migraine has been well identified as a consequence of TBI and may be associated with episodic vertigo and disequilibrium. Basilar artery migraine, previously called Bickerstaff's migraine, may develop following whiplash injury; prodromal symptoms of basilar artery migraine are typically associated with posterior circulation insufficiency, and include vertigo and drop attacks (Bickerstaff 1961). Individuals with basilar artery migraine may also have abnormal vestibular testing, as well as abnormal electroencephalographic studies. Pharmacological treatment parallels that for other migrainous disorders, with use of symptomatic, abortive, and prophylactic migraine medications (see Chapter 13, "Headache"). Anticonvulsants generally work well as prophylactic agents in patients with basilar migraine.

Cervicogenic vertigo must also be considered in the context of dizziness complaints in patients with TBI. The mechanism for this disorder has been theorized to be related to aberrations in the afferent input from positional proprioceptors in the cervical and, to a lesser extent, lumbar regions; overexcitation of the cervical sympathetic nerve fibers; and/or compromise of vertebral artery blood flow. Other attempts to explain this phenomenon have been based on cervical proprioceptive mechanisms through autonomic pathways etiologically related to ipsilateral cervical hypertonicity. Myofascial concomitants associated with trigger points must also be considered in the etiology of cervical vertigo (i.e., trigger points in the clavicular branch of the sternocleidomastoid muscle may present with proprioceptive dysfunction, including, but not limited to, postural dizziness, vertigo, syncope, and disequilibrium). Treatment relies on adequate examination and identification of cervical pathology to facilitate directing treatment at those causes (e.g., myofascial referred pain, facet-mediated pain, vertebral somatic dysfunction) (Iverson et al. 2007; Rowlands et al. 2009).

Other etiologies that need to be considered include psychogenic dizziness and iatrogenic causes such as drug-induced dizziness. Depression, anxiety spectrum disorders, and somatization have all been associated with dizziness complaints. Common drugs that have been associated with dizziness include anticonvulsants, antidepressants, antihypertensives, anti-inflammatory drugs, hypnotics, muscle relaxants, and vestibular depressants.

Practitioners should understand that complaints of "dizziness" are often not well delineated by the patient or family member. Obtaining information from the patient or a knowledgeable informant is necessary to understand clearly the nature of the patient's symptoms and to differentiate between true vertigo and other conditions such as disequilibrium, presyncope, motion sickness, and psychogenic dizziness. The duration of the dizziness episode may be a clue to its etiology. Short-duration episodes of dizziness are more common with BPPV; however, migraine and epilepsy can present similarly. Longer-duration episodes of dizziness (i.e., an hour to a day or more) can be seen with ELH, and dizziness with labyrinthine concussion, cervical vertigo, or PLF can be more chronic and persisting. Positional triggering of symptoms provides additional clues about the potential causes of dizziness but is not, in and of itself, pathognomonic of a particular posttraumatic vertigo etiology. Also, certain vestibulopathies are more classically associated with either intermittent or constant hearing loss (e.g., ELH or PLF), whereas others are not (e.g., BPPV) (Fitzgerald 1996).

Typically, with acute vertigo, treatment begins with bed rest for 1–3 days (varying with the severity of symptoms) and may involve prescription of vestibular sedatives. Use of these agents is generally not recommended unless the patient is experiencing functionally disabling vertigo that interferes with mobility and/or is having severe nausea and/or emesis. Chronic use of these agents is not recommended, in light of their interference with central neurohabituation. A computed tomography or magnetic resonance imaging scan should be done if a central deficit is suspected. Subacutely, vestibular exercises should be recommended, ideally with concurrent cessation of vestibular sedatives. As clinically indicated, an audiogram as well as an electronystagmogram (ENG) with caloric and/or rotary chair testing, should be ordered for diagnostic confirmation. Clinicians should remember that an unremarkable ENG with calorics does not rule out the presence of vestibular dysfunction as a cause of posttraumatic dizziness or vertigo. Depending on the nature of the presentation, platform posturography may also be helpful not only in identifying specific balance impairments (Basta et al. 2007) but also in guiding the treating clinician's interventional strategies for modulating such impairments.

In general, individuals with post-TBI vestibular disorders are best served by clinicians with specific training in and experience managing these types of posttraumatic conditions. Such clinicians include physiatrists (physical medicine and rehabilitation physicians), neuro-otologists, audiologists, and physical therapists with expertise in TBI-related disorders. Referral to clinicians of these types is an appropriate element of the evaluation and treatment plan for persons with dizziness and other vestibular function complaints following TBI.

# TINNITUS

Tinnitus is a common complaint and may develop in 30%–70% of persons with histories of head trauma. Tinnitus, as a symptom, is not pathognomonic of any condition. Posttraumatic tinnitus, specifically, most likely reflects an electrophysiological derangement somewhere along the central nervous system hearing pathway; it may involve the cochlea, the eighth cranial nerve, or more proximal (i.e., limbic) dysfunction in the central nervous system (Attias et al. 2005; Eggermont and Roberts 2004; Rauschecker et al. 2010).

Tinnitus has multiple causes and in any given patient may be the result of preexisting nontraumatic problems, including sensorineural hearing loss, age-related hearing loss, and/or prior loud noise exposure in vocational or recreational contexts (e.g., use of firearms, operation of noisy machinery, loud music). Other conditions such as otosclerosis and even earwax buildup can be responsible for tinnitus. Tinnitus also may be caused by posttraumatic conditions, including Ménière's disease, temporomandibular joint disorders, and neck injuries with vascular or myofascial involvement, as well as psychogenic causes such as stress and depression. Additionally, tinnitus may reflect direct TBI-associated dysfunction of the inner ear, acoustic nerve, or primary or secondary hearing centers (Horn and Zasler 1992).

Neuro-otological and audiological assessments such as otoacoustic emissions are indicated in patients with tinnitus (Ceranic et al. 1998; Langguth et al. 2010). When pulsatile tinnitus is reported, it is important for the evaluating physician to rule out posttraumatic vascular conditions such as arterial venous malformations, sinus thrombosis, and aneurysm, as well as carotid dissection, due to their relatively high morbidity (Lerut et al. 2007). Asymptomatic Arnold-Chiari type 1 malformations are described as "triggered" into becoming symptomatic by whiplash-type injuries, and may be associated with tinnitus. Unusual presentations of posttraumatic epilepsy may also present with tinnitus. This type of epilepsy should be suspected particularly when disturbance of consciousness or significant pitch changes and/or complex sounds are associated with the tinnitus. When the cause of tinnitus is unclear, and especially when the patient's clinical presentation is unusual, referral to a physician specializing in the evaluation and management of such conditions (usually a neurologist, neurophysiatrist, or neuro-otologist) is appropriate and encouraged.

Auditory stimulation techniques, both passive and active, have been used to treat tinnitus (Seidman et al. 2010). Jastreboff Tinnitus Retraining Therapy (TRT) is an example of passive auditory stimulation that relies on central habituation (Jastreboff and Jastreboff

2000). Tinnitus masking is a passive auditory stimulation technique that can be total or partial. For example, this technique might involve the use of white noise generators at night for a patient whose tinnitus is interfering with sleep. When this approach to treatment is employed, using the lowest-level masker needed to provide adequate relief is recommended. Another form of passive auditory stimulation used to treat tinnitus is music therapy. Additionally, phase-shift therapies have also been used for tinnitus of cochlear origin (Meeus et al. 2010).

Neuromonics, an Australian-based company, has developed a treatment approach to tinnitus modulation that appears to decrease tinnitus and associated functional disturbance (Goddard et al. 2009). This approach employs a small, lightweight device with headphones that delivers music embedded with a pleasant acoustic neural stimulus. The developers propose that this stimulus, customized for each user's audiological profile, stimulates the auditory pathways to promote neural plastic changes. Over time, these changes help the brain to filter out the tinnitus perception from conscious attention and reduce the associated tinnitus disturbance, providing long-term relief from symptoms. The Neuromonics treatment protocol ranges from 6 to 12 months, although in clinical trials some patients reported immediate relief. Additionally, given that tinnitus may be exacerbated by stress and anxiety, potential interventions recommended to modulate tinnitus symptoms include antidepressant medications, biofeedback, avoidance of stimulants, and proper sleep hygiene.

# HYPERACUSIS

Hyperacusis is a sensory disorder that occurs when an individual perceives an unusual auditory sensitivity to environmental noise or tones. This disorder occurs along a spectrum of severity and entails functional consequences ranging from mild to severe. The incidence or prevalence of this disorder after TBI has not been defined clearly. Audiologically, patients with hyperacusis typically present with a compressed dynamic range on audiogram; higher decibels are necessary for the patients to first hear sound, and sounds at lower decibel levels may be perceived as uncomfortable. Phenomenologically, hyperacusis can be thought of as "super hearing"; the patient may experience more intense perception of sounds within the normal range of hearing or perceive sounds outside the normal range of hearing, resulting in distraction. When hyperacusis is severe, distress and discomfort from sounds that are experienced as excessively loud may occur (Bohnen et al. 1991). Patients with this condition often develop so-called sonophobia, marked by fears of and/or aversions to sounds that individuals with normal hearing tolerate easily and find innocuous. Neuroanatomically, hyperacusis involves not only auditory sensory pathways and auditory cortices but also frontal, parietal, and medial temporal cortices (parahippocampal areas). There are several possible structural and/or functional anatomical contributors to the experience of hyperacusis and, perhaps, plausible associations of this phenomenon with multiple neurological conditions (Hwang et al. 2009).

Hyperacusis is generally described as being of two forms, cochlear and vestibular. Cochlear hyperacusis is associated with feelings of ear discomfort, annoyance, and irritation when certain sounds are heard, especially those that are very soft or high pitched. This type of hyperacusis is often associated with sound avoidance behavior and/or affective responses, including crying, and anxiety reactions such as panic attacks. Cochlear hyperacusis involves a theoretical loss of regulatory function by the system conducting impulses along the auditory neural pathways, although dysfunction of the ossicular chain mechanism has also been hypothesized as contributory.

In contrast, vestibular hyperacusis involves a disturbance of the balance mechanism in response to sound exposure. This condition has also been referred to as Tullio's syndrome or phenomenon, as well as audiogenic seizure disorder (i.e., a type of reflex epilepsy). In vestibular hyperacusis, damage to the nerve cells and the balance system is suspected, possibly secondary to TBI or other influences. Exposure to sound often results in falling or a loss of balance or postural control, and some of the same reactions that occur with cochlear hyperacusis are observed. Other symptoms typically include sudden severe vertigo and nausea. Often, people with this type of disorder will experience cognitive symptoms during episodes. Headache is a common concomitant in both auditory and vestibular types of hyperacusis.

Although hyperacusis can be associated with a number of conditions, TBI is certainly one that has been well identified as a cause. Sonophobia and/or sonosensitivity also are associated with a variety of disorders, including migraine and tension headache. Sonophobia and/or sonosensitivity typically are transient phenomena when they are produced by conditions such as headache disorders; however, they may be persistent problems when they have a primary neurogenic origin, as appears to be the case after TBI (Waddell and Gronwall 1984).

From a diagnostic standpoint, cochlear hyperacusis can be assessed through simple tests such as the loudness discomfort level test and balance screening test using an audiometer and observation. Testing for vestibular hyperacusis is more challenging and best deferred to specialists with expertise in the evaluation of this condition (i.e., otologists, neuro-otologists, audiologists). If the clinical presentation suggests audiogenic seizures, then evaluation by an epileptologist (neurologist specializing in the evaluation and treatment of persons with epilepsy) is strongly recommended.

Although no definitive treatment exists for cochlear hyperacusis, a variety of interventions are described in the literature. The treatment of hyperacusis can include neuromodulation techniques, such as transcranial magnetic stimulation, epidural stimulation with implantable electrodes, and neurofeedback, as well as use of antecedent control (Fluharty and Glassman 2001). Acoustic therapies, including sound generator therapy (starting with subthreshold exposure and gradually increasing sound exposure levels) and Neuromonics tinnitus treatment (described in the preceding section, "Tinnitus"), are also sometimes used; however, little evidence supports the use of these interventions for hyperacusis. "Pink" noise can also be used to treat hyperacusis; this involves exposure to broadband noise at soft levels for a defined period of time each day for the purpose of reestablishing sound tolerance. Music therapy has likewise been advocated as a treatment for hyperacusis. Steroids have also been used to treat hyperacusis acutely (i.e., within 72 hours of onset).

The treatment of vestibular hyperacusis is more controversial. Treatments include a low-salt diet combined with antinausea drugs or introduction of nonsteroidal anti-inflammatory drugs directly into the cochlear/vestibular system using catheters. Therapy of reflex seizures, including audiogenic seizures, involves limiting exposure to the provoking stimulus and prescribing standard antiepileptic drugs.

# HEARING IMPAIRMENTS

Hearing loss following TBI can be associated with brain injury, cranial or cranial-adnexal trauma, or cervical whiplash injury (Iverson et al. 2007; Tranter and Graham 2009). Such an audiological impairment can be associated with conductive dysfunction, sensorineural dysfunction, or both (Abd al-Hady et al. 1990). Mixed hearing loss may also occur. It is unusual to develop hearing loss due to damage to either the eardrums or the ossicular chain within the middle ear without an associated fracture of the skull base (Mishra and Digre 1996). Tympanic membrane perforations can occur from direct blunt trauma or from temporal bone fractures. Trauma may cause hemorrhage or tearing of the tympanic membrane, as well as ossicular chain disruption, through either dislocation or fracture; ossicular chain disruption is commonly associated with longitudinal fractures of the temporal bone. The latter injuries have also been associated with tympanic membrane perforation and ossicular chain fracture or dislocation. Injuries involving the middle ear alone are typically associated with conductive-type hearing losses. Longitudinal fractures, which are often associated with conductive hearing loss, typically result from temporal and parietal blows. Transverse fractures, which are much less common, usually result from frontal or occipital blows (Pedersen and Johansen 1986).

Conductive hearing loss due to tympanic membrane injury typically improves spontaneously; in the uncommon cases where this does not occur, the problem is generally amenable to surgical repair. Ossicular chain disruption, which typically occurs at the incudostapedial joint, is usually amenable to surgical correction and is associated with good audiological functional outcomes.

Sensorineural hearing loss, which is more common than conductive hearing loss, can be caused by a number of different lesions along the auditory pathway. These include disruption of the eighth cranial nerve and central auditory pathways, disruption of the membranous labyrinth from transverse fracture of the temporal bone, PLF, labyrinthine concussion, and end-organ injury (Nolle et al. 2004).

According to the available literature, individuals with TBI more frequently have high-frequency hearing loss than low-frequency hearing loss. Among persons with mTBI, sensorineural hearing loss develops mainly at 4000 Hz. Following more severe TBI, the frequency range of hearing loss is generally wider (Dorman and Morton 1982; Sismanis 1992). Cervical acceleration-deceleration injuries often seen in association with TBI have also been reported to be associated with high-frequency hearing loss. No correlation appears to exist between severity of injury and frequency or severity of hearing loss incurred. Sensorineural hearing loss has a much worse prognosis overall than conductive hearing loss and, if functionally significant, is treated with amplification using hearing aids. Clinicians should be aware that hearing impairment is common in association with other posttraumatic vestibular disorders, including blast injuries, PLFs, labyrinthine concussion, and ELHs. Patients with unilateral hearing loss normally do not require amplification via use of hearing aids; however, patients with bilateral hearing loss may require use of hearing aids and, if their hearing loss is profound, may require cochlear implants (Management of Concussion–Mild Traumatic Brain Injury Working Group 2009). Appropriate assessment and treatment will typically require involvement of a neuro-otologist and audiologist.

# OLFACTORY AND GUSTATORY (CHEMOSENSORY) IMPAIRMENTS

Chemosensory impairments involving smell and taste are often reported following TBI, with reported rates of anosmia (loss of the sense of smell) and hyposmia (impairment of the sense of smell) of 5%–65% depending on the type and severity of TBI (Swann et al. 2006). Although impairments of smell or taste can be subjectively distressing for affected individuals, these impairments are functionally significant as well. A person's safety at home or elsewhere can be compromised, for example, through loss of the ability to perceive the smell of something burning before smoke is visible or the ability to identify spoiled foods by smell or taste prior to ingesting them. Given the frequency and importance of these sensory impairments, it is both noteworthy and unfortunate that practitioners in most clinical settings, including many neurological and TBI specialty clinics, rarely inquire about smell and taste sensation during clinical interviews of patients and families, and infrequently assess these sensations formally or informally.

TBI-related ageusia or dysgeusia (lack or distortion of the sense of taste) may result from direct tongue injury; seventh, ninth, or tenth cranial nerve damage; or brain stem or cortical injury. Given that gustatory function is directly mediated by three cranial nerves (the seventh, ninth, and tenth) and all three nerves are bilateral and well protected by bone, it is rare to see marked impairments of gustatory function arising from injury (Iverson et al. 2007). When persons with TBI experience taste impairments, these usually reflect secondary effects of impaired olfaction on the subjective experience of taste. Prescription as well as over-the-counter drugs should also be considered as potential causes of taste changes, because a variety of agents are notorious for gustatory alterations. Although maxillofacial fractures increase the risk of gustatory dysfunction, the incidence remains well below that of olfactory dysfunction in this patient population (Costanzo and Zasler 1992; Joung et al. 2007).

Focal cortical contusions involving the frontotemporal lobes are associated with anosmia or hyposmia. This association derives largely from the co-occurrence of shearing injury to the first cranial nerve in the anterior cranial fossa (at or near the cribriform plate) due to anterior or posterior force vectors and focal injury to primary and secondary olfactory cortical centers (Haxel et al. 2008). Olfactory impairment following TBI is a spectrum disorder, and impairments may range from minimal perturbations in sense of smell at one end of the spectrum to total anosmia at the other (Collet et al. 2009).

Other conditions may be responsible for impairments of smell (and secondarily taste). These include a number of neurological diseases (e.g., Alzheimer disease, Parkinson disease, diffuse Lewy body disease), trauma-related disturbances of nasal passage airflow, nasal and sinus disease unrelated to TBI, chronic tobacco use, and some psychiatric disorders (e.g., schizophrenia) in which altered smell function also may occur (Joung et al. 2007; Kern et al. 2000).

Olfactory impairments, which may be conductive and/or sensorineural, can be identified by thorough clinical interview and examination. A screening examination for olfactory function is an essential element of the evaluation of all persons with TBI, regardless of whether that evaluation is performed by a neurologist, physiatrist, neuropsychiatrist, or neuropsychologist. Several commercially available smell testing kits may be of use for this purpose. Fortin et al. (2010) compared the University of Pennsylvania Smell Identification Test (UPSIT) and the Alberta Smell Test, which are among the most frequently used in this population. The Alberta Smell Test, which allows for assessment of laterality of smell loss, has been advocated as a good screening test, and the 40-item UPSIT is used to refine the clinical diagnosis due to the availability of a nomogram scoring sheet with malingering cutoffs. Although the UPSIT can be useful in both clinical and forensic contexts, the test does not assess for laterality of loss.

When the history or screening examination suggests the presence of chemosensory impairment, referral for specialty evaluation by an otolaryngologist is recommended; a principal goal of this assessment is to identify and treat reversible causes of olfactory impairment. A number of chemosensory clinics in the United States do formal chemosensory evaluations for both gustation and olfaction (Table 16–1). If local resources are unavailable or personnel are unable to perform these specialized assessments, clinicians may consider contacting one of these specialty centers for additional guidance or referral.

No evidence-based treatments are available to facilitate recovery from anosmia or hyposmia due to TBI, although suggested interventions have included steroids, zinc supplementation, vitamin therapy, and theophylline. Minocycline has been shown to inhibit olfactory sensory neuron death in the face of a potent proapoptotic stimulus and may be efficacious in the management of peripheral olfactory loss as well. Whether these interventions foster recovery beyond that attributable to spontaneous recovery alone remains uncertain. If patients do not recover their smell function within 6 months, the impairment is likely permanent. Compensatory strategies should be recommended, as appropriate, including safety measures such as use of carbon monoxide detectors and smoke detectors, among other interventions (Zasler et al. 1992).

# VISUAL IMPAIRMENTS

A variety of subjective visual complaints can be reported by persons with TBI. Some of these complaints can be difficult to interpret; are not always well quantified by examining physicians; and, occasionally, may not have a well-explained organic basis. As with other sensory impairments, visual complaints are varied in both type and severity and may reflect not only the effects of TBI but also direct or indirect eye trauma (Burke et al. 1992). The literature germane to neuro-ophthalmological and ophthalmological impairments following TBI is somewhat limited, especially considering the overall frequency of this class of impairments in this population. Increasing awareness of these types of impairments due to combat-related injuries, particularly those related to blast phenomena, may lead to additional investigations in this area (Brahm et al. 2009; Dougherty et al. 2011).

Among persons with visual complaints following TBI, neuro-ophthalmological examination includes assessment of visual acuity, color perception, and visual fields (to confrontation); pupillary examination; funduscopic examination; testing of ocular motility, in-

**TABLE 16–1.** Chemosensory clinics in the United States

| CENTER | WEB SITE |
| --- | --- |
| Monell Chemical Senses Center, Philadelphia, Pennsylvania | http://www.monell.org |
| Taste and Smell Center, University of Connecticut Health Center, Farmington, Connecticut | http://uconntasteandsmell.uchc.edu |
| Smell and Taste Disorders Center, Virginia Commonwealth University, Richmond, Virginia | http://www.vcu.edu/ent/clinical/ smelltaste/index.html |
| Nasal Dysfunction Clinic, University of California— San Diego | http://health.ucsd.edu/specialties/ surgery/otolaryngology/areas- expertise/sinus-nasal/Pages/ default.aspx |
| Rocky Mountain Taste and Smell Center, University of Colorado Denver, Aurora, Colorado | http://www.ucdenver.edu/academics/ colleges/medicalschool/centers/ tastesmell/Pages/tastesmell.aspx |
| Health Taste and Smell Center, University of Cincinnati, Cincinnati, Ohio | http://ent.uc.edu/patientcare/ specialties/taste_smell.html |
| University of Florida Center for Smell and Taste, Gainesville, Florida | http://ufcst.mbi.ufl.edu |
| University of Pennsylvania Smell and Taste Center, Philadelphia, Pennsylvania | http://www.med.upenn.edu/stc |

cluding convergence; and slit-lamp examination. Ancillary testing, depending on the scope of the complaints noted, might include formal visual field testing, visual evoked responses, and/or neuroimaging studies (Mishra and Digre 1996).

Among the most serious causes of posttraumatic visual impairments is traumatic optic neuropathy (TON), which may result from either direct or indirect injury to the optic nerve. The main treatment options for TON include systemic corticosteroids and surgical optic nerve decompression, either alone or in combination. Review and analysis of the literature are complicated by the variety of therapeutic approaches and a lack of randomized controlled studies on the use of these modalities for TON (Zoumalan et al. 2010).

Optic chiasm trauma, although infrequent, is usually associated with severe frontal injury and tends to present with bitemporal and junctional scotomas in conjunction with an array of other visual complaints (Savino et al. 1980). Occasionally, see-saw nystagmus is seen in conjunction with scotomatous deficits when injury occurs at the chiasmal level. Patients with this impairment are also at high risk for hypothalamic-pituitary-adrenal axis dysfunction. Treatment of chiasmal injuries includes, as relevant, management of fractures compressing the chiasm, decompression of associated hematomas, and acute steroid treatment.

Optic tract lesions, including those involving optic radiations and occipital cortex, can produce focal lesions resulting in visual field defects, as well as scotomas. Such visual impairments are more common among persons with TBI of relatively greater severity (Uzzell et al. 1988). Rehabilitative treatment may include teaching visual compensatory strategies and use of neuro-optometric interventions to expand the patient's field of vision or the awareness of field of vision.

Traumatic oculomotor cranial neuropathies are quite common after TBI. These are more common among persons with moderate to severe TBI than among those with mTBI (Baker and Epstein 1991). Such injuries often result in complaints of blurry vision and, when more significant, diplopia (double vision). Historically, many ophthalmologists have advocated for use of an eye patch to negate diplopia or blurry vision; however, such an intervention interferes with a substantial part of the visual field as well as binocular vision and depth perception. Treatment, therefore, should focus on preservation of binocular vision, to the greatest extent possible, and employ neuro-optometric treatment interventions such as lenses, prisms that are ground into optical lenses, partial selective occlusion, and (in some cases) vision therapy. Other more aggressive treatment interventions, which are most appropriately undertaken after a plateau in neurological recovery is reached with regard to oculomotor impairment, include botulinum toxin for eye realignment in primary gaze and strabismus surgery.

Prior to making any definitive treatment plan for patients with diplopia, entrapment of extraocular muscle by orbital fractures must be excluded as the cause of the diplopia. When entrapment of extraocular muscle is present, surgical intervention is the treatment of choice. Entrapment can also be associated with ocular changes such as enophthalmos (posterior displacement of the eye) or proptosis (anterior displacement of the eye) in the acute phase, as well as numbness in the distribution of the maxillary branch of the trigeminal nerve.

Convergence insufficiency is also reported occasionally following TBI, and the onset of this problem may be acute (Carroll and Seaber 1974). Patients with convergence insufficiency complain of difficulty reading due to symptoms of eye strain, headache, and blurred vision. Such individuals will often use accommodative convergence to avoid diplopia (Bartiss 2010). Often, this impairment, particularly in association with mTBI, will be transient. The pathoanatomical basis for convergence insufficiency has yet to be clarified, although one possibility is that midbrain control centers are dysfunctional due to the TBI. Treatment of this problem includes vision therapies, such as convergence exercises, as well as plus lenses, prisms, and surgical interventions (with the latter reserved for use in persistent cases of convergence insufficiency).

Divergence paralysis has also been described as a consequence of TBI (Padula et al. 2013; Rutkowski and Burian 1972). Patients with this problem present with uncrossed diplopia at distance and have an esotropic deviation at distance with full abduction and no evidence of associated cranial nerve palsies involving the extraocular musculature. Some patients with this problem experience spontaneous recovery, whereas others do not. Neuro-optometric interventions, including use of prism lenses, may be helpful for the latter group of patients.

Accommodative disorders, including accommodation paresis and accommodative spasm, also may occur following TBI. One should always consider medication side effects as a cause of or contributor to accommodative dysfunction; anticholinergic medications, opiates, and other sedatives tend to be the most common iatrogenic causes of this problem. Treatments of accommodative dysfunction include plus lenses and, more controversially, accommodative vision therapy (American Optometric Association 1998).

Skew deviation is a vertical misalignment of the eyes secondary to either cerebellar or brain stem involvement and typically occurs in only very severely injured patients. The vertical deviation can be either incomitant or comitant and is not associated with either torsion or cyclodeviation (which distinguishes it from a fourth cranial nerve palsy).

Gaze paresis and internuclear ophthalmoplegia are two additional visual impairments associated with TBI. Horizontal gaze paresis is quite rare, but ipsilateral conjugate horizontal gaze paresis may occur with pontine lesions and contralateral voluntary gaze paresis and has been associated with frontal lobe injuries. Internuclear ophthalmoplegia is characterized by absent or slow adducting saccades and associated nystagmus of the abducting eye. Although it is also relatively uncommon, it has been described in patients with TBI.

A substantive literature exists on abnormal eye movements among persons with TBI; these include pathological pursuits, saccades, gaze stabilization, and nystagmus, in addition to abnormalities in visual tracking synchronization (Heitger et al. 2002; Montfoort et al. 2006; Padula et al. 2013). Vertical heterophoria, or difficulty maintaining vertical alignment of the visual axes, is associated with a compensatory head tilt and has been theorized to be associated with various other common posttraumatic sequelae, including dizziness and headaches (Doble et al. 2010). Vertical heterophoria symptoms are typically modulated with appropriate prism treatment.

Photophobia—or more appropriately, photosensitivity (because *photophobia* generally implies eye pain, whereas *photosensitivity* refers to sensitivity to light)—is a commonly reported complaint among persons with TBI (Waddell and Gronwall 1984). Recent research has demonstrated that critical flicker frequency is related to light and motion sensitivity in individuals with mTBI; damage to higher visual pathways is hypothesized as the cause of subjective hypersensitivity to light and motion in the presence of normal critical flicker frequency (Chang et al. 2007). Elevated dark adaptation thresholds have also been noted in persons with TBI (Du et al. 2005). Although photosensitivity may be a manifestation of an underlying neurovascular dysfunction (i.e., migraine variant), no clear evidence supports this position. It also is possible that photosensitivity reflects dissociation of the ambient visual system from the focal or central visual system after TBI, thereby leading to a loss of the regulatory effects of ambient vision on focal vision. Traditionally, photochromatic lenses have been prescribed to accommodate for posttraumatic photosensitivity (Jackowski et al. 1996).

Direct ocular injuries may also occur and produce a variety of problems in and of themselves, including disorders of the vitreous (both prefoveal and foveal). Such problems are commonly associated with retinal traction with resultant subjective symptoms of "floaters." Retinal injuries, including detachment and hemorrhage, may also cause visual symptoms (Iverson et al. 2007).

Lastly, given the mental health focus of this text, I would be remiss not to mention psychogenic visual loss in the context of differential assessment of visual impairments in patients with TBI. Cortical blindness, although rare in practice, may occur following TBI; however, in the absence of neuroimaging correlates to explain such findings, psychogenic causes should be considered. Also, in the absence of concurrent neurological and imaging findings supporting a neurogenic cause, the following should be considered as possibly psychogenic: monocular or binocular visual loss, hemianopic losses, and other more obvious nonorganic presentations such as patchy scotomatous loss or tunnel vision. Functional vision loss may be due to exaggeration, malingering, or psychogenic causes (i.e., conversion or factitious disorder).

When a patient may have any of the aforementioned types of posttraumatic vision disorders, appropriate referral to a qualified neuro-ophthalmologist and/or neuro-optometrist with experience in TBI-related visual disorders is generally the preferred way to proceed. If the presentation has "nonorganic" features, neuro-ophthalmological and/or neuro-optometric evaluation should proceed collaboratively with psychiatric assessment. Although neuro-ophthalmologists may be excellent at neurological assessment and diagnosis of the vision disorder, many clinicians have found that additional consultation with neuro-optometrists may offer more functionally oriented treatment recommendations.

# POSTURAL INSTABILITY

Balance problems experienced by persons with TBI have a variety of causes. Imbalance is a symptom of another underlying problem, such as a proprioceptive deficit, a visual-based impairment, underlying vestibular pathology, motor control problems, or a cerebellar disorder. One of the more interesting and controversial types of balance disorders is postural instability following concussion or mTBI (Riemann and Guskiewicz 2000). This type of postural instability is generally short lived in individuals with isolated (i.e., nonrecurrent) mTBI. The available data suggest that such problems may last anywhere from 72 hours to at least 30 days postinjury, and indicate that heightened vulnerability to brain reinjury may persist during this time as well. During the period of recovery from mTBI, postural instability increases risk for additional TBI and the rare but potentially life-threatening second-impact syndrome. This risk is exaggerated by fatigue following exercise (aerobic or anaerobic) during the early period after mTBI and may not be evident when patients are at rest or not physically challenged by exertion (Fox et al. 2008); therefore, exertional provocation testing is an important element of return-to-play (or return-to-duty) guidelines and should be considered relative to postural stability evaluations and the manner in which they are used to guide reinjury risk assessments (McCrory et al. 2009).

Neurological evaluation is warranted in patients with TBI who complain of balance problems and is best performed by experienced specialists in neurology, neuro-otology, physical medicine and rehabilitation, and/or physical therapy. No gold standard exists for postural instability assessments among persons with TBI, and other testing may complement data derived from these types of balance assessments (Davis et al. 2009). However, specific protocols are available for postural stability assessment (Guskiewicz 2003); techniques that are currently being used include, among others, the Balance Error Scoring System (BESS; Bell et al. 2011), dynamic posturography, the center of pressure measure, the virtual time-to-contact measure, force plate and motion tracking technologies, and less sophisticated clinical balance tests (Shepard et al. 2013; Slobounov et al. 2008). For example, the BESS comprises six different balance conditions—three stance settings, double-leg, single-leg, and tandem—each of which lasts 20 seconds. Assessment is performed on two surfaces, stable (firm) and unstable (a foam pad is used to simulate an unstable surface). The BESS score is assigned based on the number of errors that occur during the different balance conditions, with higher BESS scores reflecting greater disturbances in balance and coordination (Bell et al. 2011).

Treatment of postural instability includes substitution strategies, such as central preprogramming of movement, as well as the use of visual and somatosensory cues. Challenging a patient's balance skills through progression to functionally relevant tasks also is important. This treatment, which includes challenges during activities that require positional change and head movements, continues until the patient is functioning at a level that allows resumption of his or her normal activities.

## CONCLUSION

An adequate breadth of understanding is required not only to identify the presence of sensory disorders following TBI but also to differentiate the cause(s) of these disorders so that appropriate diagnostic testing and treatment can be provided. Knowledge regarding the types of clinicians involved in the traditional assessment and management of the various sensory impairments seen in the TBI population is also clearly important so that patients are directed for appropriate and timely clinical services.

## *Key Clinical Points*

- Dizziness is a symptom, not a diagnosis; given that fact, clinicians must refer patients with complaints of dizziness after TBI to specialists adept at assessing such individuals to determine the exact complaint, etiology, and treatment.

- Tinnitus, like dizziness, is a symptom and is a treatable problem; it has multiple causes, including ones referable to the central nervous system, head and skull injuries, and cervical injuries. Treatment of tinnitus, therefore, depends on its cause.

- Complaints consistent with pulsatile tinnitus necessitate immediate referral to a neuro-otologist to rule out conditions associated with high morbidity and mortality, such as carotid artery dissection.

- Audiological evaluations are a necessary element of the assessment of any patient with hearing loss after TBI. Such evaluations are needed to determine the type of hearing loss and to develop a plan of care that minimizes its functional consequences.

- Olfactory evaluation using a standardized screening test is an essential element of the evaluation of all persons with TBI, given the high frequency of olfactory impairment after TBI, the subjective distress such impairment may cause, the high correlation of smell impairment with frontotemporal contusional injury and associated executive impairment, and the potentially serious safety risks associated with this class of impairments.

- Hyperacusis can be seen as a sensory impairment following TBI and may manifest as two different presentations: cochlear or vestibular. The exact pathophysiological mechanisms involved in these disorders remains in debate. Treatment of these conditions remains poorly established, particularly with regard to vestibular hyperacusis.

- Postural imbalance is a common sensory disorder problem following TBI, including in postconcussive patients. There are now numerous postural stability assessments available to gauge risk of reinjury on return to sports, active duty, and/or work as related to balance impairment. Treatment options include substitution strategies and visuo-somatosensory cueing.

- Visual impairments, including subtle problems such as convergence and accommodative disorders, vertical heterophoria, and other eye movement abnormalities, should always be considered, even when patients present with innocuous-sounding complaints such as "blurry" vision or problems reading.

# REFERENCES

Abd al-Hady MR, Shehata O, el-Mously M, et al: Audiological findings following head trauma. J Laryngol Otol 104:927–936, 1990

American Optometric Association: Care of the Patient With Accommodative and Vergence Dysfunction (Optometric Clinical Practice Guideline, No 18). St. Louis, MO, American Optometric Association, 1998

Attias J, Zwecker-Lazar I, Nageris B, et al: Dysfunction of the auditory efferent system in patients with traumatic brain injuries with tinnitus and hyperacusis. J Basic Clin Physiol Pharmacol 16:117–126, 2005

Baker RS, Epstein AD: Ocular motor abnormalities from head trauma. Surv Ophthalmol 35:245–267, 1991

Barber HO: Positional nystagmus, especially after head injury. Laryngoscope 74:891–944, 1964

Bartiss MJ: Convergence insufficiency. Medscape Reference, 2010. Available at: http://emedicine.medscape.com/article/1199429-overview. Accessed May 12, 2012.

Basta D, Clarke A, Ernst A, et al: Stance performance under different sensorimotor conditions in patients with post-traumatic otolith disorders. J Vestib Res 17:25–31, 2007

Bell DR, Guskiewicz KM, Clark MA, et al: Systematic review of the balance error scoring system. Sports Health 3:287–295, 2011

Bickerstaff E: Basilar artery migraine. Lancet 277:15–17, 1961

Bohnen N, Twijnstra A, Wijnen G, et al: Tolerance for light and sound of patients with persistent post-concussional symptoms 6 months after mild head injury. J Neurol 238:443–446, 1991

Brahm KD, Wilgenburg HM, Kirby J, et al: Visual impairment and dysfunction in combat-injured service members with traumatic brain injury. Optom Vis Sci 86:817–825, 2009

Brandt T, Daroff RB: Physical therapy for benign paroxysmal positional vertigo. Arch Otolaryngol 106:484–485, 1980

Bromwich M, Hughes B, Raymond M, et al: Efficacy of a new home treatment device for benign paroxysmal positional vertigo. Arch Otolaryngol Head Neck Surg 136:682–685, 2010

Burke JP, Orton HP, West J, et al: Whiplash and its effect on the visual system. Graefes Arch Clin Exp Ophthalmol 230:335–339, 1992

Carroll RP, Seaber JH: Acute loss of fusional convergence following head trauma. Am Orthopt J 24:57–59, 1974

Ceranic BJ, Prasher DK, Raglan E, et al: Tinnitus after head injury: evidence from otoacoustic emissions. J Neurol Neurosurg Psychiatry 65:523–529, 1998

Chang TT, Ciuffreda KJ, Kapoor N: Critical flicker frequency and related symptoms in mild traumatic brain injury. Brain Inj 21:1055–1062, 2007

Cifu DX, Caruso D: Traumatic Brain Injury. New York, Demos Medical, 2010

Clark SK, Rees TS: Posttraumatic endolymphatic hydrops. Arch Otolaryngol 103:725–726, 1977

Collet S, Grulois V, Bertrand B, et al: Post-traumatic olfactory dysfunction: a cohort study and update. B-ENT 5 (suppl 13):97–107, 2009

Conroy NE, Erogul M: Perilymph fistula. Medscape Reference, 2009. Available at: URL. Accessed May 12, 2012.

Costanzo RM, Zasler ND: Epidemiology and pathophysiology of olfactory and gustatory dysfunction in head trauma. J Head Trauma Rehabil 7:15–24, 1992

Davis GA, Iverson GL, Guskiewicz KM, et al: Contributions of neuroimaging, balance testing, electrophysiology and blood markers to the assessment of sport-related concussion. Br J Sports Med 43 (suppl 1):i36–i45, 2009

Doble JE, Feinberg DL, Rosner MS, et al: Identification of binocular vision dysfunction (vertical heterophoria) in traumatic brain injury patients and effects of individualized prismatic spectacle lenses in the treatment of postconcussive symptoms: a retrospective analysis. PM R 2:244–253, 2010

Dorman EB, Morton RP: Hearing loss in minor head injury. NZ Med J 95:454–455, 1982

Dougherty AL, MacGregor AJ, Han PP, et al: Visual dysfunction following blast-related traumatic brain injury from the battlefield. Brain Inj 25:8–13, 2011

Du T, Ciuffreda KJ, Kapoor N: Elevated dark adaptation thresholds in traumatic brain injury. Brain Inj 19:1125–1138, 2005

Eggermont JJ, Roberts LE: The neuroscience of tinnitus. Trends Neurosci 27:676–682, 2004

Epley JM: The canalith repositioning procedure: for treatment of benign paroxysmal positional vertigo. Otolaryngol Head Neck Surg 107:399–404, 1992

Ernst A, Basta D, Seidl RO, et al: Management of posttraumatic vertigo. Otolaryngol Head Neck Surg 132:554–558, 2005

Fausti SA, Wilmington DJ, Gallun FJ, et al: Auditory and vestibular dysfunction associated with blast-related traumatic brain injury. J Rehabil Res Dev 46:797–810, 2009

Fitzgerald DC: Head trauma: hearing loss and dizziness. J Trauma 40:488–496, 1996

Fluharty G, Glassman N: Use of antecedent control to improve the outcome of rehabilitation for a client with frontal lobe injury and intolerance for auditory and tactile stimuli. Brain Inj 15:995–1002, 2001

Fortin A, Lefebvre MB, Ptito M: Traumatic brain injury and olfactory deficits: the tale of two smell tests! Brain Inj 24:27–33, 2010

Fox ZG, Mihalik JP, Blackburn JT, et al: Return of postural control to baseline after anaerobic and aerobic exercise protocols. J Athl Train 43:456–463, 2008

Fukaya T, Nomura Y: Audiological aspects of idiopathic perilymphatic fistula. Acta Otolaryngol Suppl 456:68–73, 1988

Goddard JC, Berliner K, Luxford WM: Recent experience with the Neuromonics tinnitus treatment. Int Tinnitus J 15:168–173, 2009

Guskiewicz KM: Assessment of postural stability following sport-related concussion. Curr Sports Med Rep 2:24–30, 2003

Hammond FM, Masel BE: Cranial nerve disorders, in Brain Injury Medicine: Principles and Practice. Edited by Zasler ND, Katz DI, Zafonte RD. New York, Demos, 2007, pp 1529–1544

Haxel BR, Grant L, Mackay-Sim A: Olfactory dysfunction after head injury. J Head Trauma Rehabil 23:407–413, 2008

Heitger MH, Anderson TJ, Jones RD: Saccade sequences as markers for cerebral dysfunction following mild closed head injury. Prog Brain Res 140:433–448, 2002

Horn LJ, Zasler N (eds): Rehabilitation of Post Concussive Disorders. Philadelphia, PA, Hanley & Belfus, 1992

Hwang JH, Chou PH, Wu CW, et al: Brain activation in patients with idiopathic hyperacusis. Am J Otolaryngol 30:432–434, 2009

Iverson GL, Zasler N, Lange RT: Post-concussive disorders, in Brain Injury Medicine: Principles and Practice. Edited by Zasler ND, Katz DI, Zafonte RD. New York, Demos, 2007, pp 1373–1406

Jackowski MM, Sturr JF, Taub HA, et al: Photophobia in patients with traumatic brain injury: uses of light-filtering lenses to enhance contrast sensitivity and reading rate. NeuroRehabilitation 6:193–201, 1996

Jastreboff PJ, Jastreboff MM: Tinnitus Retraining Therapy (TRT) as a method for treatment of tinnitus and hyperacusis patients. J Am Acad Audiol 11:162–177, 2000

Joung YI, Yi HJ, Lee SK, et al: Posttraumatic anosmia and ageusia: incidence and recovery with relevance to the hemorrhage and fracture on the frontal base. J Korean Neurosurg Soc 42:1–5, 2007

Kern RC, Quinn B, Rosseau G, et al: Post-traumatic olfactory dysfunction. Laryngoscope 110:2106–2109, 2000

Langguth B, Biesinger E, Del Bo L, et al: Algorithm for the diagnostic and therapeutic management of tinnitus, in Textbook of Tinnitus. Edited by Moller AR, Langguth B, De Ridder D, et al. New York, Springer Science + Business Media, 2010, pp 381–385

Lerut B, De Vuyst C, Ghekiere J, et al: Post-traumatic pulsatile tinnitus: the hallmark of a direct carotico-cavernous fistula. J Laryngol Otol 121:1103–1107, 2007

Management of Concussion–Mild Traumatic Brain Injury Working Group: VA/DoD Clinical Practice Guideline for Management of Concussion/Mild Traumatic Brain Injury (mTBI). Department of Veterans Affairs and Department of Defense. Washington, DC, Department of Veterans Affairs, Department of Defense, 2009

McCrory P, Meeuwisse W, Johnston K, et al: Consensus statement on concussion in sport: 3rd International Conference on Concussion in Sport held in Zurich, November 2008. Clin J Sport Med 19:185–200, 2009

Meeus O, Heyndrickx K, Lambrechts P, et al: Phase-shift treatment for tinnitus of cochlear origin. Eur Arch Otorhinolaryngol 267:881–888, 2010

Mishra AV, Digre KB: Neuro-ophthalmologic disturbances in head injury, in Head Injury and Postconcussive Syndrome. Edited by Rizzo M, Tranel DD. New York, Churchill Livingstone, 1996, pp 201–226

Montfoort I, Kelders WP, van der Geest JN, et al: Interaction between ocular stabilization reflexes in patients with whiplash injury. Invest Ophthalmol Vis Sci 47:2881–2884, 2006

Nolle C, Todt I, Seidl RO, et al: Pathophysiological changes of the central auditory pathway after blunt trauma of the head. J Neurotrauma 21:251–258, 2004

Padula WV, Singman E, Vicci V, et al: Evaluating and treating visual dysfunction, in Brain Injury Medicine: Principles and Practice, 2nd Edition. Edited by Zasler ND, Katz DI, Zafonte RD. New York, Demos Medical, 2013, pp 750–768

Pedersen CB, Johansen LV: Traumatic lesions of the middle ear: etiology and results of treatment. Clin Otolaryngol 11:93–97, 1986

Rauschecker JP, Leaver AM, Muhlau M: Tuning out the noise: limbic-auditory interactions in tinnitus. Neuron 66:819–826, 2010

Riemann BL, Guskiewicz KM: Effects of mild head injury on postural stability as measured through clinical balance testing. J Athl Train 35:19–25, 2000

Rowlands RG, Campbell IK, Kenyon GS: Otological and vestibular symptoms in patients with low grade (Quebec grades one and two) whiplash injury. J Laryngol Otol 123:182–185, 2009

Rutkowski PC, Burian HM: Divergence paralysis following head trauma. Am J Ophthalmol 73:660–662, 1972

Savino PJ, Glaser JS, Schatz NJ: Traumatic chiasmal syndrome. Neurology 30:963–970, 1980

Seidman MD, Standring RT, Dornhoffer JL: Tinnitus: current understanding and contemporary management. Curr Opin Otolaryngol Head Neck Surg 18:363–368, 2010

Semont A, Freyss G, Vitte E: Curing the BPPV with a liberatory maneuver. Adv Otorhinolaryngol 42:290–293, 1988

Shepard NT, Handelsman JA, Clendaniel RA: Balance and dizziness, in Brain Injury Medicine: Principles and Practice, 2nd Edition. Edited by Zasler ND, Katz DI, Zafonte RD. New York, Demos Medical, 2013, pp 779–793

Sismanis A: Post-concussive neuro-otological disorder, in Rehabilitation of Post Concussive Disorders. Edited by Horn LJ, Zasler N. Philadelphia, PA, Hanley & Belfus, 1992, pp 79–88

Slobounov S, Cao C, Sebastianelli W, et al: Residual deficits from concussion as revealed by virtual time-to-contact measures of postural stability. Clin Neurophysiol 119:281–289, 2008

Swann IJ, Bauza-Rodriguez B, Currans R, et al: The significance of post-traumatic amnesia as a risk factor in the development of olfactory dysfunction following head injury. Emerg Med J 23:618–621, 2006

Tranter RM, Graham JR: A review of the otological aspects of whiplash injury. J Forensic Leg Med 16:53–55, 2009

Tusa RJ, Brown SB: Neuro-otological trauma and dizziness, in Head Injury and Postconcussive Syndrome. Edited by Rizzo M, Tranel DD. New York, Churchill Livingstone, 1996, pp 177–200

Uzzell BP, Dolinskas CA, Langfitt TW: Visual field defects in relation to head injury severity: a neuropsychological study. Arch Neurol 45:420–424, 1988

Waddell PA, Gronwall DM: Sensitivity to light and sound following minor head injury. Acta Neurol Scand 69:270–276, 1984

Zasler N, Martelli MF (eds): Functional Medical Disorders in Rehabilitation Medicine: State of the Art Reviews in Physical Medicine and Rehabilitation. Philadelphia, PA, Hanley & Belfus, 2002

Zasler ND, McNeny R, Heywood PG: Rehabilitative management of olfactory and gustatory dysfunction following brain injury. J Head Trauma Rehabil 7:66–75, 1992

Zoumalan CI, Kim JW, Gigantelli JW: Traumatic optic neuropathy. Medscape Reference, 2010. Available at: http://emedicine.medscape.com/article/868129-overview. Accessed November 14, 2012.

# PART IV

## SPECIAL TOPICS

# CHAPTER 17

# Traumatic Brain Injury in Late Life

*William C. Walker, M.D.*
*David X. Cifu, M.D.*

***The older adult*** or geriatric population includes individuals age 65 years and older. This is the traditional definition used in the federal statutes in the United States (e.g., for Medicare and Social Security eligibility). Although this age cutoff allows group comparison, an important consideration is that the traumatic brain injury (TBI) literature often reports differences in demographics and outcome across the age spectrum in a continuous rather than a categorical (i.e., old vs. young) manner (Englander et al. 2007).

## MEDICAL ISSUES RELEVANT TO OLDER PERSONS WITH TRAUMATIC BRAIN INJURY

### Baseline Functional Status

Older individuals frequently have baseline functional impairments (e.g., problems with walking, transferring, or dressing). These baseline differences may complicate TBI outcomes and may necessitate home and lifestyle modifications, assistive equipment or technology, and caregiver assistance that might not be necessary in the treatment of younger persons with comparably severe TBI.

## Sensory Health

Older individuals often have baseline sensory health issues that may complicate or exacerbate sensory issues imposed by TBI. For example, visual acuity, refractive power, extraocular motion, tear secretion, and corneal and lens function all diminish with age, leading many older individuals to use corrective lenses (Kane et al. 1999). Presbycusis is an age-related, progressive, sensorineural hearing loss that affects 60% of older adults (Kane et al. 1999). Normal aging is also accompanied by a relative decrement of taste acuity and vibratory and touch sensation (Kane et al. 1999).

## TBI Susceptibility

Acute TBI is compounded by the sensitivity of an older brain to disturbances of homeostasis, including altered blood flow or cerebrospinal fluid dynamics, decreased oxygenation, the effects of central-acting medications, and excessive environmental stimuli, among others. With aging, the adult brain becomes more susceptible to traumatic hemorrhages; this appears to be the result of age-related brain atrophy and bridging vein fragility (Englander et al. 2007). Frontal and temporal lobe contusions and subdural hematomas are particularly common in fall-related brain injuries of older adults. Cerebral contusions tend to occur in multiple locations and may not be apparent radiologically until several days after TBI (Rakier et al. 1995).

## Medical Complications

TBI in older adults can introduce medical complications. Older adults are particularly susceptible to cerebrovascular events from trauma-related hypotension. Peritraumatic stroke may also occur in older adults from thromboembolism, thrombosis, or ischemia from cerebral edema. Older individuals also are more susceptible to the adverse neurological effects of acute anemia due to large volume blood loss. Blood transfusions and/or fluid replacement may mitigate these effects, but these treatments present their own risks (e.g., transfusion reactions, iatrogenic blood-borne infection). Neurogenic dysphagia from TBI in older adults is more likely to be complicated by preinjury gastrointestinal conditions or dental problems (Englander et al. 2007).

## Functional Outcomes

Compared with younger adults matched for TBI severity, older adults have poorer short-term functional outcomes and longer acute hospital stays; the influence of age on these outcomes appears to become significant after age 40 years (Braakman et al. 1980; Chesnut et al. 2000; Frankel et al. 2006; Jennett et al. 1979; Katz and Alexander 1994; Langlois et al. 2003; Stablein et al. 1980). The reduced baseline physiological reserves of elderly persons result in both greater damage from the initial injury and less repair (Rothweiler et al. 1998). Analysis of the National Institute on Disability and Rehabilitation Research TBI Model Systems (TBI-MS) data set, which includes adults with moderate or severe TBI who are admitted to participating inpatient rehabilitation centers (TBI Model Systems Database 2010), reveals that adults age 55 and older had longer inpatient rehabilitation lengths of stay, higher costs, lower functional status at hospital discharge, and twice the nursing home placement rate of individuals age 50 and younger (Cifu et al. 1996; Frankel et al. 2006). According to the TBI-MS data, longer-term functional prognosis, as measured by the Glasgow Outcome Scale at 1 and 2 years postinjury, also declines incrementally with increased age (Walker et al. 2010); 52.3% of those under age 65 versus 41.3% of those over age 65 were living independently at 1 year postinjury (TBI Model Systems Database 2010). Nonetheless, almost all elderly individuals receiving rehabilitation in the TBI-MS achieved significant functional improvement, two-thirds achieved discharge placement to a private residence, and 83% were living in private residences 1 year later (Frankel et al. 2006; TBI Model Systems Database 2010).

## Baseline Cognition and Cognitive Recovery

Compared with younger adults matched for TBI severity, older adults experience more frequent and more severe cognitive impairment (Englander et al. 2007). The typical cognitive recovery patterns of the two groups are similar, but older adults recover at a slower rate and with a lower likelihood of returning to baseline (Goldstein and Levin 1995). Lower premorbid cognitive reserve capacity and higher incidence of baseline dementia undoubtedly contribute to the excess burden of cognitive impairment among older persons with TBI. Older individuals also have slower rates of drug metabolism and excretion, which result in a greater propensity for additive cognitive medication side effects such as agitation, somnolence, and increased confusion.

## Health Care Funding

In the United States, the health care of nearly all older adults is supported by Medicare. Medicare Part A helps cover durable medical equipment, inpatient care, and skilled nursing facility rehabilitation services. Medicare Part B helps pay for physician services, home health care, and outpatient therapies. Inpatient rehabilitation services are reimbursed under Part A through a prospective payment system, with payments adjusted for multiple factors, including medical complexity of the person with TBI.

## Health After TBI

Older individuals with a prior TBI who are living in the community have greater perceived health problems than their peers. In an age-matched case control study, individuals over age 55 who had sustained TBI in the past 4 years reported more problems with body temperature changes, skin and hair changes, headaches, speaking and understanding others, sensory changes, movement and spasticity, sleeping, and neck and back pain (Breed et al. 2004). Depression after TBI does not have an identified age bias (Rosenthal et al. 1998).

## Aging With TBI, Apolipoprotein E ε4, and Dementia

Older age is associated with declining cognitive performance (e.g., diminished memory, slower processing speed) in healthy adults, and a similar decline occurs among adults with a prior TBI (Johnstone et al. 1998). Evidence suggests that an individual's genotype also contributes to both cognitive outcome after TBI and the rate of any subsequent age-related cognitive decline. The apolipoprotein E (APOE) molecule is a lipid transporter in the brain and cerebrospinal fluid and is critically important to the process of protecting against oxidative insults to the brain (Coleman et al. 1995). The presence of the APOE ε4 allele is linked with poorer outcome after TBI (Teasdale et al. 1997) and may be associated with an increased risk for Alzheimer disease (Ashman et al. 2008; Mayeux et al. 1993; Mehta et al. 1999).

# EPIDEMIOLOGY

The demographics of individuals with TBI differ across age. Whereas the incidence of TBI in younger adults is much higher in men than in women, this gender bias equalizes after age 65. In adults over age 80, the preponderance of women with TBI most likely reflects their longevity. The overall rate of TBI in adults over age 65 (524 per 100,000 in 2003) closely resembles the rate for all ages combined (538 per 100,000) (Rutland-Brown et al. 2006). Individuals older than age 65 are hospitalized more often for TBI than are younger persons (234 per 100,000 vs. 100 per 100,000) and have twice the mortality rate from TBI (38.4 per 100,000 vs. 17.5 per 100,000) (Rutland-Brown et al. 2006).

## Falls

Falls are the leading cause of medically attended TBI in the United States, and the risk of a fall-related TBI among adults increases with age (Rutland-Brown et al. 2006). Compared with the risk for TBI among adults younger than age 65, the risk is increased threefold among adults ages 65–74, eightfold among adults ages 75–84, and 16-fold among adults age 85 and older (Englander and Cifu 1999). TBI by other causes is declining in response to governmental and other social factors, especially the use of safety restraints in motor vehicles; however, the older adult population that is most at risk for falls continues to proportionally rise over time. The U.S. Census Bureau (2008) estimates that the U.S. population age 65 and older will increase from the current 40 million (13% of the entire U.S. population) to 55 million (16%) by 2020. Given advances in acute medical and trauma care, along with current demographic and longevity trends, the prevalence of TBI among older adults is likely to increase during the next several decades.

Approximately 30% of older adults fall each year, and many of them sustain injuries that necessitate hospitalization (Englander and Cifu 1999). Tinetti and Speechley (1989) stratified adult fall risk factors into four groups: chronic, short term, activity related, and environmental. Chronic fall risk factors include problems such as neurological disease, sensory impairment, and musculoskeletal disease. Short-term fall risk factors include episodic postural hypotension, acute illness, alcohol use, medication effects, and similar transient or episodic conditions or events. Activity-related factors include tripping while walking, climbing ladders, descending stairs, and other activities that place the individual at risk for falling. Environmental factors comprise objects or other elements of the environment whose presence creates obstacles or navigational challenges that increase the risk for falls (e.g., throw rugs, poor lighting, ill-fitting shoes or trousers). These same fall risk factors also predispose elderly people to motor vehicle, pedestrian, and recreational accidents that may result in TBI. Management of these risk factors includes scheduled, consistent, and competent primary health care to minimize medical morbidities, regulate medications, and provide ongoing education. Geriatric rehabilitation programs can address these risk factors more comprehensively.

## Other Mechanisms of Injury

Motor vehicle crashes that injure elderly people tend to be of lower speed than those that injure younger individuals. Diffuse axonal injury, focal contusions, and subdural hematomas are common among older adults involved in motor vehicle crashes, even those of low velocity (Katz and Alexander 1994). Accidents between vehicles and older pedestrians tend to occur at crosswalks and in parking lots, and also can result in diffuse axonal injury, focal contusions, and/or extra-axial lesions, most commonly subdural hematomas. Assault, although more common in middle age, may also cause TBI in elderly individuals (Englander et al. 2007).

## Mortality

Mortality after TBI increases with advanced age; this increase appears to be attributable in large part to increased age-related occurrence of and intolerance for injury-associated hypotension or hypoxia due to limited cardiopulmonary reserve (Englander et al. 2007). Several studies suggest that cardiac, pulmonary, and multisystem organ failures after TBI are more common among older than younger individuals (Englander et al. 2007). Since the 1980s, improved injury prevention strategies and acute medical care have led to a steady decline in the incidence of TBI-related death in all age groups, except those over age 75 (Adekoya et al. 2002; Sosin et al. 1995).

## Multiple Trauma

TBI in the setting of major trauma with multiple injuries occurs disproportionally less often in older adults than in younger age groups. TBI-MS data show lower fracture rates for older adults than younger adults, especially for skull fractures (23% vs. 37%) and pelvis or lower extremity fractures (15% vs. 25%) (Englander et al. 2007), as well as lower rates of combined TBI and spinal cord injury (TBI Model Systems Database 2010).

# POPULATION-SPECIFIC CLINICAL ASSESSMENT ISSUES

## Neuroimaging

For major trauma or suspected severe TBI, brain imaging criteria are not age dependent. However, when an individual presents with a possible concussion or mild TBI (mTBI), age should be considered in the decision whether to obtain head computed tomography (CT) or magnetic resonance imaging (MRI). Older individuals are more likely to have "complicated" mTBI, a classification for patients meeting clinical criteria for mTBI but having abnormal findings on head CT or brain MRI. After a review of 1,448 patients with mTBI seen in the emergency department, Borczuk (1995) recommended CT scanning for all patients age 60 and over who present for evaluation in the immediate injury period; by contrast, CT scanning was recommended for persons younger than age 60 only when they have focal neurological deficits, clinical signs of basilar skull fracture, or cranial soft tissue injuries.

## Medical Evaluation

An assessment of the acute medical and neurological status of the older adult with TBI must take into account medical conditions that may impede or prolong the recovery process; these include significant accumulated chronic comorbidities (e.g., arthritis, cardiopulmonary disease, diabetes, atherosclerosis, renal failure, cancer) as well as any chronic premorbid conditions that could further reduce cerebral functional reserve at baseline (e.g., cerebrovascular disease, chronic alcoholism, advanced liver or renal disease, dementia). The evaluation should also seek to identify all residual or emerging TBI- or trauma-related medical complications and any joint and muscular abnormalities, especially pain. Older individuals are likely to have one or more chronic conditions that may contribute to their experience of pain.

# Medication Review

A thorough review of the older patient's preinjury and current medication routine is essential for optimizing TBI care (Englander et al. 2007). During the acute traumatic period, previously prescribed medications may be inappropriate, not feasible to administer, or unknown to providers. The family should be encouraged to collect all medications that they find in the patient's home and present them to practitioners for review and discussion.

Aging alters gastrointestinal motility and hence medication absorption. Older adults may have more side effects from taking medications commonly used to treat or prevent conditions associated with acute trauma. These medications include histamine type 2 receptor antagonists to prevent stress ulceration, anticonvulsants to prevent seizures, sedatives and/or hypnotics for agitation, antiarrhythmics for transient or chronic cardiac conduction events, narcotics and analgesics for pain control, and antibiotics for infection. Nonprescription medications and supplements must be identified and scrutinized for potential adverse effects or interactions, and in general should be discontinued during inpatient care.

# Medical Rehabilitation Evaluation

A medical rehabilitation evaluation by a physiatrist is recommended for the elderly TBI survivor with significant functional limitations. An initial physiatric evaluation should occur in the intensive care unit (ICU) to determine acute needs and begin long-range planning, and a more comprehensive evaluation should occur after transition to the floor or rehabilitation unit (Englander et al. 2007). Preinjury activity levels, cognitive limitations, behavioral issues, and chronic medical conditions should be ascertained. This information will assist in the determination of an individual's readiness and appropriateness for specific rehabilitation interventions (i.e., specificity, intensity, and goal setting for therapies). The patient's postinjury cognitive and behavioral status, diurnal variations in alertness, and ability to tolerate both physical and mental activities should be determined through patient interview and examination, as well as medical record review.

The existing impairments (e.g., hemiparesis, dysphagia, incontinence, cognitive deficits) and functional level (mobility status, activities of daily living) should be thoroughly delineated and quantified.

## Swallowing and Nutrition Assessment

Unique aspects of the nutritional and swallowing assessment in the older adult after TBI include ascertaining baseline denture wear and nutritional deficits. Dentures may no longer fit properly after they have been removed for even several days during acute care. Up to 20% of ambulatory older individuals have a measurable vitamin deficiency (Kane et al. 1999). Obtaining weekly or biweekly weights and serum albumin levels can help in monitoring nutritional status.

## Bladder Function

Ascertaining preinjury voiding patterns of older adults is helpful in discerning any underlying pathology that is independent of the effects of TBI. Normal aging affects bladder function in several ways (Chutka et al. 1996). Prostate hypertrophy in men with relative bladder outlet obstruction and diminished capacity produces symptoms of increased urinary frequency, hesitancy, and/or diminished stream. Pelvic relaxation in women from uterine prolapse or cystocele results in intermittent stress incontinence. Decreased bladder capacity leads to increased urinary frequency. Decreased capability to suppress bladder contractions at low volumes results in urinary urgency. All of these factors increase the risk of urinary incontinence following TBI in late life. Additionally, older individuals (like young persons) with TBI may develop centrally mediated incontinence as a result of an inability to sense bladder fullness and/or impaired regulation of the pontine micturition center (Opitz et al. 1998).

## Bowel Function

Bowel routines are typically disrupted during hospitalization after trauma and, from the perspective of some health care providers, are a relatively low-priority issue in acute care settings. Among older individuals, disruption of bowel routines can become a significant and highly distressing preoccupation when not properly addressed. Older age, among other variables, is associated with bowel incontinence in the hospital and at 1-year follow-up (Foxx-Orenstein et al. 2003).

Older individuals are also more prone to constipation, which is exacerbated by trauma-related dietary changes, immobility, and narcotic use for pain management (Kane et al. 1999). Ascertaining preinjury bowel routine is necessary to establish goals for a bowel program.

## Social Support

Social support networks for elders with TBI should be comprehensively reviewed. Available formal support systems include federal (Medicare, Social Security), state (Medicaid, department of rehabilitation services, welfare, area agencies on aging), and local (adult day health programs, transportation, Meals on Wheels, aid from religious organizations) resources. Informal supports, such as family and friends, tend to be more limited as an individual advances in age. Because older adults tend to have significant others who are older, disabled, or deceased, they are more likely to have increased involvement of extended families in their systems of support. Daughters are more likely than sons to play a major support role, particularly in hands-on care (Englander et al. 2007). Additionally, practitioners must consider advance directives, congruence of patient and caregiver goals, and religious and cultural factors. Inquiry about alcohol and other substance abuse is often erroneously overlooked in taking social history for older adults. After dementia and anxiety disorders, alcoholism is the third most common mental disorder among elderly men in the United States (Myers et al. 1984).

# TREATMENT OF OLDER ADULTS WITH TRAUMATIC BRAIN INJURY

## Pharmacotherapy

*General approach.* After TBI, an older adult's prescription and nonprescription medications should be regularly reviewed, and all nonessential medications should be stopped or tapered as soon as feasible. Medications that must be continued should be prescribed in the simplest form possible—that is, taken at the lowest frequency with the fewest pills and during typical waking hours based on the person's routine activities. General principles for TBI pharmacology also apply.

*Pain.* Given the higher propensity in older adults for side effects from pain medications, nonpharmacological interventions are the preferred initial pain treatment approach for this population; however, acute trauma pain also commonly requires pharmacotherapy. When pain medications are prescribed, scheduled (rather than as-needed) dosing generally affords better overall pain control and facilitates performance of self-care and rehabilitative activities.

Acetaminophen requires no dosage adjustment in elderly people, is virtually absent of side effects, and has equal analgesic efficacy to nonsteroidal anti-inflammatory drugs (NSAIDs) (Bradley et al. 1991). If the individual has concomitant inflammatory arthritis or heterotopic ossification, then NSAIDs and heterotopic ossification–modifying medications may be indicated. Older individuals are more susceptible to both renal and gastrointestinal side effects of NSAIDs, so appropriate monitoring is required. Narcotic analgesics should be reserved for pain refractory to nonpharmacological interventions and simple analgesics, because these medications are more potent in older individuals and almost invariably cause constipation and lethargy.

When neuropathic pain is present, anticonvulsants or antidepressants are typically more effective than traditional analgesic medications. The cognitive and autonomic side effects of these medications, as well as their potential for systemic toxicity and drug-drug interactions, generally guide the medication selection. Older individuals, particularly those experiencing cognitive impairments before and/or after TBI, are more susceptible to the anticholinergic side effects of antidepressants (e.g., tricyclic antidepressants, paroxetine), including cognitive dysfunctions, postural hypotension, and urinary retention. Within the tricyclic class, anticholinergic side effects are minimal with protriptyline, greatest with amitriptyline, and intermediate with nortriptyline.

**Venous thromboembolism.** The risk of developing venous thromboembolism after trauma is significant, and overwhelming evidence indicates that higher age raises this risk. Chemoprophylaxis with anticoagulants is the mainstay of venous thromboembolism prevention and should be considered in every older adult hospitalized after TBI. Chemoprophylaxis selection and dosing should be based on risk-benefit algorithms that incorporate age along with all other patient risk factors, counterbalancing against any existing contraindications.

**Seizures.** Individuals older than age 65 and adults younger than age 65 are at equal risk for both early and late seizures after TBI (Englander et al. 2003; TBI Model Systems Database 2010). When an older individual develops posttraumatic epilepsy, the choice of antiepileptic medication is predicated on the following principles involved in choosing any medication for long-term usage: side effects, the degree of protein binding, drug interactions, cost, and compliance. Some of the newer antiepileptic drugs, such as oxcarbazepine and levetiracetam, may be better tolerated in older adults, because these medications have fewer interactions, have greater therapeutic windows, and do not require serum monitoring ("Drugs for Epilepsy" 2008; Sirven 2001).

*Arousal and attention deficits.* Arousal and attention deficits can be treated rapidly and safely in medically stable adults after TBI with methylphenidate (short-acting preparation of 0.3 mg/kg twice daily) (Willmott and Ponsford 2009). Methylphenidate minimally raises heart rate and blood pressure (Willmott et al. 2009). However, its use requires caution among patients with coronary artery disease, tachyarrhythmias, or poorly controlled hypertension, all of which are common among older adults. Amantadine and modafinil are safe medications in elderly people; the onset of action of these medications is considerably delayed when compared to that of methylphenidate (Cardenas and McLean 1992). Carbidopa-levodopa may be useful if inattention is accompanied by bradykinesia and rigidity, with results apparent within 1–2 weeks of initiating therapy (Englander et al. 2007).

*Agitation.* Management strategies in older adults with agitation, including pharmacotherapies, are similar to those used with younger individuals (Reyes et al. 1981). Sundowning is an agitation subtype seen almost exclusively in older persons with dementia, but it can also occur in older adults after TBI of any severity, including mTBI. Sundowning is characterized by transient psychotic symptoms at night, along with increased nighttime agitation and disorientation; this phenomenon is most likely due to the effects of aging on circadian physiology (Goldberg 2001). The use of low dosages of risperidone, olanzapine, or quetiapine at bedtime can be helpful in reducing these disturbing symptoms and reestablishing a normal circadian rhythm (Englander et al. 2007), although the use of these agents by elderly people may be associated with an increased risk for cerebrovascular accidents and death (Ballard et al. 2009; Gentile 2010; Mittal et al. 2011).

*Alterations in mood and sleep.* Pharmacological management of mood and sleep disorders in older persons with TBI is similar to that of younger individuals, except that medication interactions and side-effect profiles have greater importance (Zafonte et al. 1999). For depression or anxiety, selective serotonin reuptake inhibitors (SSRIs) are generally the best-tolerated medication class and therefore are a good first choice for older individuals. Nevertheless, SSRI side effects are more likely with older age. One of these side effects, SSRI-induced hyponatremia, occurs exclusively in older individuals.

Benzodiazepines should be avoided in all individuals after TBI, regardless of age. In elderly persons, these agents predictably impair cognition and motor function, increase risk for falls, and may produce paradoxical reactions.

*Bladder function.* Unless infection is present, pharmacotherapy is rarely indicated for urinary incontinence or retention. One exception is the use of local (or systemic) estrogens in postmenopausal older adult females with atrophic urethritis. The mainstay of management for incontinence in older individuals after TBI is a timed toileting program. Postvoid residual measurements should be obtained when incontinence is resistant to toileting efforts, to exclude overflow from underlying retention. Significant retention is best managed with intermittent catheterizations. If retention fails to resolve, pharmacological treatment with α-receptor blockers such as alfuzosin, doxazosin, terazosin, or tamsulosin may facilitate emptying through relaxing the internal and external sphincters.

*Bowel function.* Older persons hospitalized after TBI should routinely receive stool softeners and fiber supplementation. Diarrhea, when occurring, is managed similarly to diarrhea in younger patients, except that older individuals are more likely to suffer dehydration effects and to require intravenous fluids. Fecal impaction can paradoxically present as loose incontinent stool leaking around the impacted area. One-time administration of a laxative, bowel stimulant, and/or suppository often is sufficient to relieve this problem.

# Psychological and Behavioral Interventions

*Substance abuse.* Older individuals often return to drinking alcohol after TBI, but not as commonly as their younger counterparts do. In the TBI-MS cohort, 20.1% of older individuals reported alcohol use at 1 year postinjury; of these individuals, 10.7% reported drinking more than five drinks per day (TBI Model Systems Database 2010). When individuals return to the community after TBI, caretakers or partners must be educated on the consequences of ongoing substance use, and codependency issues must be addressed and confronted directly. For alcohol abuse or dependency, Hurt et al. (1988) recommend equally intense treatment for the older individual as for the younger one. However, most substance abuse programs are designed for younger adults, and the group experience may be less relevant for the older individual.

*Sexuality.* A common misperception in our society is that older adults are asexual. Sexuality encompasses a sense of self; the capacity to show affection, to love, and to maintain relationships; and knowledge of the social context of sexual behavior and gender roles. Although physiological changes in vaginal mucosa and erectile and orgasmic performance often occur in normal aging, sexuality does not diminish with age (Englander et al. 2007). Therefore, older individuals with TBI and their partners should be assessed for sexual and relationship concerns. After TBI, changes in sexual desire in either direction can occur; there may be decreased interest and desire or an egocentric, impulsive, or disinhibited behavior pattern. When concerns are identified, techniques to enhance overall communication and interaction skills between partners are most therapeutic (Herstein-Gervasio and Griffith 1999). Although sildenafil, tadalafil, and vardenafil are effective for erectile dysfunction commonly encountered after TBI, they are often contraindicated in older adults due to concomitant coronary artery disease and hypertension.

*Recreation and vocation.* A thorough survey of an older adult's preinjury recreational pursuits is necessary to explore options after TBI. Sedentary and general fitness activities can usually be resumed with minor modifications. Socialization, often the primary leisure activity for elders, should be encouraged post-TBI to minimize feelings of isolation, unless significant agitation is present. Return-to-work rates are poor for older adults after TBI, so realistic goals should be established with appropriate supports in the workplace (Englander et al. 2007). Often, early retirement or part-time volunteer work is necessary when an individual cannot return to the workplace.

*Driving.* Driving recommendations after TBI should take into account the older adult's preinjury capabilities and new impairments. Interviews and more rigorous testing procedures may be given to those with seizures or cognitive or motor deficits. Some jurisdictions require health care practitioners to report to public health authorities or the department of motor vehicles any physical or cognitive conditions that may alter an individual's driving safety; however, administrative and legal responses to such reports vary by location, even within the same state (Englander et al. 2007).

## Medical Rehabilitation

*Intensive care unit.* For both older and younger adults with severe TBI, rehabilitation interventions, including early controlled mobilization in and out of bed, should begin in the ICU. Older adults with neurological impairment or medical illness usually require more rest periods, so schedules may be required to gradually increase tolerance to out-of-bed activity.

*Acute rehabilitation selection.* After medical and surgical stabilization, older adults with TBI should have access to rehabilitative services in an environment that is appropriate for their capabilities. The chosen rehabilitation pathway(s) will depend on medical and nursing acuity needs, endurance for therapeutic activities, formal and informal support systems, patient and family goals, and funding options. Selection of the appropriate level is best made by a physiatrist, whose training often provides the best understanding of admission and continuing-stay criteria, as well as funding constraints attendant on the various treatment setting options. Older individuals who do not need or cannot tolerate inpatient or day rehabilitation services and can be managed in the community will often benefit from home health or outpatient therapy services. Skilled nursing facility–based subacute rehabilitation services are appropriate for older adults who are unable to tolerate the intensity of acute comprehensive medical rehabilitation or cannot be otherwise managed at home.

*Sensory health.* Adequate lighting is crucial to help older individuals with sensory health impairments safely adapt to their new TBI-related impairments. Easily correctable visual problems, especially the resumption of glaucoma medication or corrective lenses, can greatly aid the rehabilitation process. The use of preinjury prescribed hearing aids is challenging because the injured individual is often the only one familiar with their adjustment. Until hearing aid use can be reestablished, written communication, direct eye contact to facilitate lip reading, gestural communication, and an environment without extraneous noise are helpful alternatives. If the patient is permitted to swallow foods, visitors should be encouraged to bring in the patient's favorite foods to fully ascertain whether any changes in taste or smell will affect the patient's appetite. Older adults with premorbid touch or proprioceptive sensory impairments are more likely to need compensation techniques and assistive devices for safe mobility and self-care (Englander et al. 2007).

*Self-care.* Standard rehabilitation principles should be employed to help the older adult with TBI recover self-care abilities. Older patients, however, often have difficulty being motivated to learn "splinter skills," which are small portions of tasks such as range-of-motion exercises (Englander et al. 2007). Mounting evidence suggests that "whole task" therapy that emphasizes direct living skills is more efficacious for older patients, perhaps because internalized structure and independence generally increase with age (Vanderploeg et al. 2008). Regardless of the approach used, learning an older individual's preinjury habits and routines is vital to organizing relevant therapy. Another useful tactic, which is more important with older patients than with younger patients, is to secure some familiar clothing and grooming utensils, and incorporate them into familiar daily routines in the hospital setting.

*Mobility.* Motor and balance functions tend to recover more slowly following TBI in older adults than in younger adults because of premorbid limitations in cognition, sensation, strength, and balance (Englander et al. 2007). Elderly patients also have decreased tolerance for intensive therapy sessions, due to lower endurance and more joint and muscle pain and stiffness. Comprehensive caregiver education and training are paramount because many elders have a difficult time comprehending and adjusting to mobility limitations and thereby are at a significant safety risk with high fall propensity. Household mobility may be optimized with a home evaluation by members of the rehabilitation team to assess architectural barriers (doorways, stairs, floor coverings), furniture arrangement, and adequacy of natural and artificial lighting, and then to train caregivers on safe mobility practices in the discharge environment.

# CONCLUSION

Older adults are at increased risk for TBI and are more likely than younger adults to experience a variety of neurological, neuropsychiatric, general health, and functional outcomes following TBI. The care of older persons with TBI requires familiarity with the principles of geriatric medicine, neurology, psychiatry, and rehabilitation medicine. Application of these principles to the evaluation and management of older persons with TBI is necessary to provide patient- and family-centered care and to mitigate the impairments and functional consequences of neurotrauma in late life.

## *Key Clinical Points*

- The incidence and prevalence of TBI in older persons, especially older women, are increasing in proportion to the shifting demographics of industrialized countries (i.e., aging of the population).

- Falls are the most common cause of TBI among older adults, followed by auto–pedestrian and low- to moderate-speed motor vehicle accidents.

- The neuropathology of TBI among older adults tends to be more focal than in younger persons, with subdural hematomas and cerebral contusions occurring more commonly at any given level of injury severity.

- Polytrauma is survived less frequently by older adults than younger adults; however, the outcomes associated with such injuries are improved by providing timely and age-adjusted rehabilitation services and affording the time necessary to optimize cognitive, psychiatric, physical, and functional recovery.

- Treatment of the older adult with TBI is guided by the principles of geriatric medicine, neurology, psychiatry, and rehabilitation, with close attention to the timing, setting, and intensity of therapeutic interventions.

- Therapeutic interventions are most effective when they are tailored to the individual's and family's needs and cultural expectations, are adapted to the specific postdischarge environment in which the person with TBI lives, and involve early education and training of caregivers.

# REFERENCES

Adekoya N, Thurman DJ, White DD, et al: Surveillance for traumatic brain injury deaths: United States, 1989–1998. MMWR Surveill Summ 51:1–14, 2002

Ashman TA, Cantor JB, Gordon WA, et al: A comparison of cognitive functioning in older adults with and without traumatic brain injury. J Head Trauma Rehabil 23:139–148, 2008

Ballard C, Corbett A, Chitramohan R, et al: Management of agitation and aggression associated with Alzheimer's disease: controversies and possible solutions. Curr Opin Psychiatry 22:532–540, 2009

Borczuk P: Predictors of intracranial injury in patients with mild head trauma. Ann Emerg Med 25:731–736, 1995

Braakman R, Gelpke GJ, Habbema JD, et al: Systematic selection of prognostic features in patients with severe head injury. Neurosurgery 6:362–370, 1980

Bradley JD, Brandt KD, Katz BP, et al: Comparison of an antiinflammatory dose of ibuprofen, an analgesic dose of ibuprofen, and acetaminophen in the treatment of patients with osteoarthritis of the knee. N Engl J Med 325:87–91, 1991

Breed ST, Flanagan SR, Watson KR: The relationship between age and the self-report of health symptoms in persons with traumatic brain injury. Arch Phys Med Rehabil 85(suppl):S61–S67, 2004

Cardenas DD, McLean A: Psychopharmacologic management of traumatic brain injury. Phys Med Rehabil Clin N Am 3:273–290, 1992

Chesnut RM, Ghajar J, Maas AIR, et al: Part 2: early indicators of prognosis in severe traumatic brain injury. J Neurotrauma 17:555, 2000

Chutka DS, Fleming KC, Evans MP, et al: Urinary incontinence in the elderly population. Mayo Clin Proc 71:93–101, 1996

Cifu DX, Kreutzer JS, Marwitz JH, et al: Functional outcomes of older adults with traumatic brain injury: a prospective, multicenter analysis. Arch Phys Med Rehabil 77:883–888, 1996

Coleman M, Handler M, Martin C: Update on apolipoprotein E state of the art. Hosp Physician 31:22–24, 1995

Drugs for epilepsy. Treat Guidel Med Lett 6:37–46, 2008

Englander J, Cifu DX: The older adult with traumatic brain injury, in Rehabilitation of the Adult and Child With Traumatic Brain Injury, 3rd Edition. Edited by Rosenthal M, Griffith E, Kreutzer JS, et al. Philadelphia, PA, FA Davis, 1999, pp 453–470

Englander J, Bushnik T, Duong TT, et al: Analyzing risk factors for late post-traumatic seizures: a prospective, multicenter investigation. Arch Phys Med Rehabil 84:365–373, 2003

Englander J, Cifu DX, Tran T: The older adult, in Brain Injury Medicine: Principles and Practice. Edited by Zasler ND, Katz DI, Zafonte RD. New York, Demos, 2007, pp 315–332

Foxx-Orenstein A, Kolakowsky-Hayner S, Marwitz JH, et al: Incidence, risk factors, and outcomes of fecal incontinence after acute brain injury: findings from the Traumatic Brain Injury Model Systems national database. Arch Phys Med Rehabil 84:231–237, 2003

Frankel JE, Marwitz JH, Cifu DX, et al: A follow-up study of older adults with traumatic brain injury: taking into account decreasing length of stay. Arch Phys Med Rehabil 87:57–62, 2006

Gentile S: Second-generation antipsychotics in dementia: beyond safety concerns: a clinical, systematic review of efficacy data from randomised controlled trials. Psychopharmacol (Berl) 212:119–129, 2010

Goldberg G: Mild traumatic brain injury and concussion. Physical Medicine and Rehabilitation: State of the Art Reviews 15:363–398, 2001

Goldstein FC, Levin HS: Neurobehavioral outcome of traumatic brain injury in older adults: initial findings. J Head Trauma Rehabil 10:57–73, 1995

Herstein-Gervasio A, Griffith E: Sexuality and sexual dysfunction, in Rehabilitation of the Adult and Child With Traumatic Brain Injury, 3rd Edition. Edited by Rosenthal M, Griffith E, Kreutzer JS, et al. Philadelphia, PA, FA Davis, 1999, pp 479–502

Hurt RD, Finlayson RE, Morse RM, et al: Alcoholism in elderly persons: medical aspects and prognosis of 216 inpatients. Mayo Clin Proc 63:753–760, 1988

Jennett B, Teasdale G, Braakman R, et al: Prognosis of patients with severe head injury. Neurosurgery 4:283–289, 1979

Johnstone B, Childers MK, Hoerner J: The effects of normal ageing on neuropsychological functioning following traumatic brain injury. Brain Inj 12:569–576, 1998

Kane R, Ouslander J, Abrass I: Essentials of Clinical Geriatrics, 4th Edition. New York, McGraw-Hill, 1999

Katz DI, Alexander MP: Traumatic brain injury: predicting course of recovery and outcome for patients admitted to rehabilitation. Arch Neurol 51:661–670, 1994

Langlois JA, Kegler SR, Butler JA, et al: Traumatic brain injury–related hospital discharges: results from a 14-state surveillance system, 1997. MMWR Surveill Summ 52:1–20, 2003

Mayeux R, Ottman R, Tang MX, et al: Genetic susceptibility and head injury as risk factors for Alzheimer's disease among community-dwelling elderly persons and their first-degree relatives. Ann Neurol 33:494–501, 1993

Mehta KM, Ott A, Kalmijn S, et al: Head trauma and risk of dementia and Alzheimer's disease: the Rotterdam study. Neurology 53:1959–1962, 1999

Mittal V, Kurup L, Williamson D, et al: Risk of cerebrovascular adverse events and death in elderly patients with dementia when treated with antipsychotic medications: a literature review of evidence. Am J Alzheimers Dis Other Demen 26:10–28, 2011

Myers JK, Weissman MM, Tischler GL, et al: Six-month prevalence of psychiatric disorders in three communities, 1980 to 1982. Arch Gen Psychiatry 41:959–967, 1984

Opitz J, Thorsteinsson G, Schurt A, et al: Neurogenic bladder and bowel, in Rehabilitation Medicine: Principles and Practice, 3rd Edition. Edited by DeLisa JA, Gans BM. Philadelphia, PA, Lippincott-Raven, 1998, pp 1073–1106

Rakier A, Guilburd JN, Soustiel JF, et al: Head injuries in the elderly. Brain Inj 9:187–193, 1995

Reyes RL, Bhattacharyya AK, Heller D: Traumatic head injury: restlessness and agitation as prognosticators of physical and psychologic improvement in patients. Arch Phys Med Rehabil 62:20–23, 1981

Rosenthal M, Christensen BK, Ross TP: Depression following traumatic brain injury. Arch Phys Med Rehabil 79:90–103, 1998

Rothweiler B, Temkin NR, Dikmen SS: Aging effect on psychosocial outcome in traumatic brain injury. Arch Phys Med Rehabil 79:881–887, 1998

Rutland-Brown W, Langlois JA, Thomas KE, et al: Incidence of traumatic brain injury in the United States, 2003. J Head Trauma Rehabil 21:544–548, 2006

Sirven JI: Acute and chronic seizures in patients older than 60 years. Mayo Clin Proc 76:175–183, 2001

Sosin DM, Sniezek JE, Waxweiler RJ: Trends in death associated with traumatic brain injury, 1979 through 1992: success and failure. JAMA 273:1778–1780, 1995

Stablein DM, Miller JD, Choi SC, et al: Statistical methods for determining prognosis in severe head injury. Neurosurgery 6:243–248, 1980

TBI Model Systems Database. Englewood, CO, Traumatic Brain Injury Model Systems National Data and Statistical Center, 2010. Available at: http://www.tbindsc.org. Accessed October 30, 2012.

Teasdale GM, Nicoll JA, Murray G, et al: Association of apolipoprotein E polymorphism with outcome after head injury. Lancet 350:1069–1071, 1997

Tinetti ME, Speechley M: Prevention of falls among the elderly. N Engl J Med 320:1055–1059, 1989

U.S. Census Bureau, 2008. 2008 National Population Projections. Available at: http://www.census.gov/population/projections/data/national/2008/downloadablefiles.html. Accessed October 30, 2012.

Vanderploeg RD, Schwab K, Walker WC, et al: Rehabilitation of traumatic brain injury in active duty military personnel and veterans: Defense and Veterans Brain Injury Center randomized controlled trial of two rehabilitation approaches. Arch Phys Med Rehabil 89:2227–2238, 2008

Walker WC, Ketchum JM, Marwitz JH, et al: A multicentre study on the clinical utility of post-traumatic amnesia duration in predicting global outcome after moderate-severe traumatic brain injury. J Neurol Neurosurg Psychiatry 81:87–89, 2010

Willmott C, Ponsford J: Efficacy of methylphenidate in the rehabilitation of attention following traumatic brain injury: a randomised, crossover, double blind, placebo controlled inpatient trial. J Neurol Neurosurg Psychiatry 80:552–557, 2009

Willmott C, Ponsford J, Olver J, et al: Safety of methylphenidate following traumatic brain injury: impact on vital signs and side-effects during inpatient rehabilitation. J Rehabil Med 41:585–587, 2009

Zafonte R, Elovic E, Mysiw W, et al: Pharmacology in traumatic brain injury: fundamentals and treatment strategies, in Rehabilitation of the Adult and Child With Traumatic Brain Injury, 3rd Edition. Edited by Rosenthal M, Griffith E, Kreutzer JS, et al. Philadelphia, PA, FA Davis, 1999, pp 544–548

CHAPTER 18

# Athletes and Sports-Related Concussion

*Christopher M. Bailey, Ph.D.*
*Michael A. McCrea, Ph.D.*
*Jeffrey T. Barth, Ph.D.*

*Concussion,* or mild traumatic brain injury (mTBI), is one of the most complex clinical phenomena, as is reflected by long-standing debate over both the defining aspects of the condition and the best methods of clinical management. Since the 1980s, the sports arena has provided a natural laboratory for examining the nature and consequences of mild head injury and, in the process, has revealed a variety of circumstances and characteristics that are unique to sports-related concussion and its management (Barth et al. 2002). In this chapter, we describe the basic and clinical science of concussion, its epidemiology and underlying pathophysiology, and some of the controversy associated with the identification and definition of this injury. We then discuss the unique characteristics of sports-related mTBI and review the current methods for clinical management and treatment of sports-related concussions.

## DEFINITION

The most recent consensus statement on concussion in sports defines concussion as "a complex pathophysiological process affecting the brain, induced by traumatic biomechanical forces" (McCrory et al.

2009, p. 186). Although most definitions reference concepts such as trauma-induced injury and altered mental status, a clear and widely accepted definition of concussion has been a topic of much controversy for decades. As a result, a variety of labels have been proposed to describe a concussion and symptoms associated with relatively mild head trauma, including minor head injury, mTBI, uncomplicated mild head injury, cerebral concussion, and simple or complex concussion (Barth et al. 2002). Table 18–1 presents examples of definitions and common grading systems. The terms *mTBI* and *concussion* are used as synonyms for the purposes of this chapter.

Although differences in definition reflect the imperfect nature of identifying concussion severity, clear similarities exist across definitions. Recent trends by clinicians, however, have been to deemphasize traditional methods for identifying concussion. For example, instead of basing decisions on the long-used Glasgow Coma Scale (GCS; Teasdale and Jennett 1974) scores of 13–15, because of the scores' limited sensitivity, clinicians are increasingly recognizing the multifactorial nature of concussion diagnosis and management. They now recognize variance in concussion outcome, attributable to factors at the time of the acute injury (e.g., duration of loss of consciousness, posttraumatic amnesia, and postconcussive symptoms; repetitive concussions) as well as factors during the postinjury recovery (e.g., pain, sleep disturbance, psychological distress).

# EPIDEMIOLOGY

No matter how it is defined, concussion represents a public health problem. Approximately 1.5 million concussions per year result in emergency department visits (Bazarian et al. 2005). The true prevalence of concussion is unknown given that an estimated 30%–50% of persons with such injuries never receive medical attention (Fife 1987). In the United States, concussion represents 75% of all hospital visits associated with TBI; these injuries cost approximately $17 billion per year in medical care, lost productivity, and litigation (Centers for Disease Control and Prevention 2003). Given the public health problem posed by concussion, a clear need exists for appropriate diagnosis and management.

# PATHOPHYSIOLOGY

Research on the pathophysiology of concussion may better characterize the underlying mechanisms and lead to improved clinical identi-

**TABLE 18–1.** Definitions of mild traumatic brain injury and concussion used commonly in clinical practice and research

| AUTHOR | CRITERIA | | | |
| --- | --- | --- | --- | --- |
| | GCS | LOC | PTA | Other |
| ACRM[a] | 13–15 | <30 min | <24 hours | At least one of the following: LOC, PTA, altered mental status, or focal neurological deficit |
| CDC[b] | | <30 min | <24 hours | Altered mental status, amnesia, and symptoms |
| WHO[c] | 13–15 | <30 min | <24 hours | At least one symptom; rule out other causes |
| **Grades** | | | | |
| AAN[d] | Grade 1: Altered mental status, no LOC, symptoms <15 min <br> Grade 2: Altered mental status, symptoms >15 min <br> Grade 3: LOC of any duration | | | |
| Cantu[e] | Grade 1: no LOC, PTA <30 min, symptoms <24 hours <br> Grade 2: LOC <1 min or PTA >30 min but <24 min but <24 hours or symptoms >24 hours but <7 days <br> Grade 3: LOC >1 min or PTA >24 hours or symptoms >7 days | | | |

*Note.* AAN=American Academy of Neurology; ACRM=American Congress of Rehabilitation Medicine; CDC=Centers for Disease Control and Prevention; GCS=Glasgow Coma Scale; LOC=loss of consciousness; PTA=posttraumatic amnesia; WHO=World Health Organization.

[a]Kay et al. 1993.
[b]Centers for Disease Control and Prevention 2003.
[c]Carroll et al. 2004.
[d]American Academy of Neurology 1997.
[e]Cantu 1986.

fication and management. The pathophysiological mechanisms of concussion are generally thought to center around acceleration-deceleration forces that act on the brain and result in a complex metabolic cascade. Experimental research suggests that the force from concussive blows leads to stretching and shearing of neurons, irregular shifting of ions across cell membranes, and changes in cerebral blood flow, all of which leave neurons temporarily dysfunctional but not destroyed (Giza and Hovda 2001). The metabolic cascade following a concussion is thought to occur in three phases: 1) hyperglycolysis, 2) metabolic depression, and 3) a period of recovery. Computed tomography or magnetic resonance imaging scans are typically normal following mTBI because either the patient's brain has no structural injury or current techniques are not able to detect the damage sustained. Difiori and Giza (2010) describe promising neuroimaging techniques that may be sensitive to the cellular and/or metabolic effects of concussion; however, most of the techniques are currently unavailable, impractical, or not appropriately validated for clinical use in concussion management at the present time.

## Concussion Research in Sports

Concussion is a complex injury that is relatively common, is costly from a public health standpoint, and may have varying characteristics that can make it difficult to detect by traditional clinical methods. Given these challenges, much of the research to better characterize the nature and clinical course of mTBI has focused on sports populations where base rates of concussion are high. Sports-related concussion research has since evolved into methods for the tracking and monitoring of physical and cognitive symptoms in athletes, which has its own unique aspects and challenges.

Mild TBI in sports is quite common. The Centers for Disease Control and Prevention (Giacino and Smart 2007) reported that 200,000 sports-related head injuries are treated in emergency departments annually within the United States and that sports-related concussion accounts for approximately 20% of all TBIs per year. Prevalence estimates have shown that team sports such as ice hockey and football may have the highest rates of concussion (Schulz et al. 2004; Tommasone and McLeod 2006). Barth et al. (2002) report that history of concussion among athletes varies by sport (from highest upper estimates to lowest): equestrian (3%–91%), boxing (1%–70%), rugby

(2%–25%), soccer (4%–22%), and American football (2%–20%). Despite the within-sport variability in concussion rates, the overall incidence rate of such injuries is high. Therefore, sports are in a unique position to serve as a natural laboratory for observing and documenting the clinical features and natural history of concussion.

The use of athletics as a method for tracking and understanding concussion was first described by Barth et al. (2002) in their Sports as a Laboratory Assessment Model (SLAM). This model was originally developed as a method for understanding the nature and mechanisms of mTBI among patients presenting to the emergency department. The SLAM methodology has been useful in characterizing mTBI, and also has revealed differences between sports-related concussions and concussions acquired in other contexts. Relative to a sports-related head injury, injuries from a motor vehicle collision are often associated with substantially higher acceleration forces, result in a higher rate and greater severity of peripheral injuries (which, in turn, lead to increased posttraumatic pain and sleep disorders), and are more likely to result in significant and debilitating anxiety and depression (e.g., posttraumatic stress disorder). Nonathlete populations may also have preexisting risk factors for poor recovery (e.g., substance abuse, psychiatric conditions, poor premorbid cognitive ability, increased age, poor social supports) that are less common among many athletic populations. By contrast, individuals sustaining sports-related concussions tend, on average, to be young, healthy, intelligent, and well educated.

Bailey et al. (2009) provide descriptive statistics for a large sample (*N*=1,109) of collegiate athletes who were administered preinjury baseline neuropsychological testing. The athletes were young adults (mean age of approximately 20 years) with generally above-average college entrance examination test scores (mean SAT score=1,061). A small percentage of individuals (4%–5%) were diagnosed with learning disorders and/or attention-deficit/hyperactivity disorder. Approximately one-third of the athletes reported having experienced previous mTBI, which is relatively consistent with concussion incidence rates in athletic populations. Most importantly, the data showed a level of low symptom report prior to injury, with an average of 5–6 total symptom points (maximum of 120 points) endorsed on a measure of common postconcussion symptoms (20 possible symptoms rated on a Likert scale of 0–6, with 6 being the most severe). This finding suggests that the average athlete reports one severe symptom or, more likely, a small number of mild to moderate symptoms, such as headache, dizziness, depression, or cognitive difficulties. These and other data support the notion that SLAM populations are young, healthy, intelligent, and well educated (Bailey et al. 2006, 2009; Barth et al. 2002; Schulz et al. 2004; Tommasone and McLeod 2006). In general, then, researchers can attribute the cognitive difficulties and symptoms experienced by the participants following a concussion directly to the injury itself as opposed to misattribution of symptoms because of comorbid conditions.

Another difference between athletic populations and the general public is the approach that these groups of individuals take when seeking evaluation and treatment following a concussion. Suboptimal effort in the forensic assessment of mild head injury has been identified as being particularly prevalent, with base rates of poor effort ranging from 20% to 70% (Larrabee 2005). Consistent with this base rate, Belanger et al. (2005) found, in a meta-analytic review of 39 studies, that short-term neuropsychological deficits were fairly common, but that long-term deficits were, for the most part, noted only in forensic cases in which the unusual pattern of "stable or worsening of cognitive functioning over time" (p. 215) was described. In 2005, the National Academy of Neuropsychologists released a policy statement regarding the neuropsychologist's use of symptom validity testing (Bush et al. 2005); the document stated that when a patient is evaluated in a forensic context (many of which cases are associated with mTBI), "any neuropsychological evaluation that does not include careful consideration of the patient's motivation to give their best effort should be considered incomplete" (p. 138).

In contrast to other mTBI populations, athletes do not show a pattern of suspect motivation following concussion. Instead, they often demonstrate the opposite pattern of motivation; that is, poor motivation is a problem at baseline testing rather than at testing conducted postinjury. For example, Bailey et al. (2006) observed greater improvement in neuropsychological scores following a concussion in a subset of athletes. In some cases, improvements of approximately three standard deviations or higher were noted following a concussion (likely due to poor effort at baseline). Not only does this research suggest that an athlete's motivation may have an impact on neuropsychological performance prior to injury (e.g., apathy or disinterest may diminish performance on a preinjury baseline measure) but it also supports strong motivation for performance following the injury, given that the outcome of testing may inform decisions regarding return to play.

From a clinical management perspective, the athlete's approach to postconcussion evaluation and treatment requires a shift in the clinician's treatment strategy. Rather than focusing on whether a patient might be exaggerating or feigning symptoms or whether treatment most effectively targets psychological distress, pain, or sleep disturbance (as is often the case in a standard mTBI evaluation), the clinician's attention is directed to the risk of reinjury associated with return to play. In this context, the problem of concern is not symptom elaboration but rather symptom minimization and/or underreporting. Concerns about risk of additional injury associated with premature return to play inform the emphasis placed on developing and using objective measures of recovery (e.g., neurocognitive testing, postural stability assessment, neuroimaging), rather than self-reported symptoms, in sports concussion research and clinical practice.

## ASSESSMENT AND MANAGEMENT OF SPORTS CONCUSSION

Although concussion is a relatively mild injury by nature, it can be associated with complications and possibly enduring symptoms if it is not managed appropriately. Clinicians need to be knowledgeable about factors that predispose athletes to poorer outcomes after concussion (Carroll et al. 2004). Athletes who have previously sustained a concussion are more than two times more likely to sustain a second concussion (Guskiewicz et al. 2003; Schulz et al. 2004; Zemper 2003) and may be more likely to experience a greater number and perceived severity of postconcussive symptoms (Collins et al. 2002). Evidence suggests that high school and college athletes who sustain concussion may be at greatest vulnerability for repeated concussions within the first 7–10 days, during which time approximately 80% of repeated concussions occur (McCrea et al. 2009).

Multiple concussions over a career in professional football have been shown to lead to an increased likelihood of late-life cognitive impairments, especially memory problems (Guskiewicz et al. 2005) and depression (Guskiewicz et al. 2007). Women may be at greater risk for cognitive symptoms following concussion (Broshek et al. 2005), and children may require longer recovery periods than college athletes (Collins et al. 2006; Field et al. 2003; Lang et al. 1994). Individuals with learning disorders also may have greater cognitive difficulties following mTBI (Collins et al. 1999), although this finding has not been replicated. Rare but catastrophic outcomes related to cerebral edema have also been postulated as occurring from repeated mTBIs (McCrory and Berkovic 1998), particularly if a second injury is sustained before symptom resolution from a first injury. This conjecture is controversial, and some evidence suggests that the cases of "second impact syndrome" may be the result of undiagnosed subdural hemorrhage (Mori et al. 2006). Given these risk factors, Moser et al. (2007) have recommended that an athlete's concussion management be individually tailored, taking into account cognitive and physical postconcussive symptoms.

## Neuropsychological Assessment

Since the seminal work of Barth et al. (1989), neuropsychological assessment has been one of the primary methods of tracking and managing the cognitive symptoms associated with sports-related concussion in athletic populations. Comparison of baseline neuropsychological evaluations of athletes to serial postinjury evaluations is a generally accepted practice in the management of sports concussion (McCrory et al. 2009). Neuropsychological evaluation is sensitive to the residual cognitive effects of concussion in a variety of domains, including attention, working memory, verbal memory, visuospatial memory, verbal learning, information processing speed, reaction time, and executive functions (Bleiberg et al. 2004; Erlanger et al. 2003; Field et al. 2003; Iverson et al. 2006; Lovell et al. 2003; McCrea et al. 2003).

For example, Belanger and Vanderploeg (2005) conducted a meta-analysis of 21 studies involving 790 cases of sports-related concussion in high school, college, and professional athletes and 2,014 control cases. Large effects (Cohen's $d=1.00-1.43$) were noted at 24 hours postinjury in global functioning, memory acquisition, and delayed memory performance, with a moderate overall effect size for neuropsychological performance following sports-related concussion (Cohen's $d=0.49$). However, the effect sizes from the group studies were noted to approach zero after 7 days.

Neuropsychological management of concussion, therefore, occurs in two phases: acute identification of concussion and later identification of return to baseline. The acute assessment of concussion employs standardized measures of physical and cognitive symptoms administered immediately following concussion. One such measure is the Standardized Assessment of Concussion (SAC; McCrea et al. 1998). The SAC is a brief neuropsychological measure designed to be administered by trainers, sports medicine clinicians, and other non-neuropsychologists on the sideline. The SAC requires approximately 5 minutes to administer and includes items that measure an athlete's orientation, immediate memory, concentration, and delayed recall. Decline in SAC performance following concussion has shown good sensitivity (95%) and specificity (76%) for the identification of concussion (McCrea 2001). The SAC is intended for use as a "companion" to more sophisticated neuropsychological assessment of an athlete's cognitive recovery and fitness to return to competition.

Once the athlete has been identified as concussed, a clinician should focus on when the athlete is ready to return to play. Such evaluations generally do not occur on the sidelines, and they are best if a multidimensional team approach is employed in which several professionals trained in sports concussion management track the athlete's reported postconcussive symptoms (e.g., headache, nausea, sensitivity to light and noise), cognitive symptoms, and balance/postural stability. These methods also generally employ the comparative model described earlier in this section, in which athletes undergo a preseason baseline assessment to establish reference points (preinjury postconcussive symptoms, cognitive performance, and balance/postural stability testing). Following a concussion, an athlete engages in serial evaluations to identify when he or she has returned to or exceeded baseline scores.

Several computerized neuropsychological test batteries have been marketed for use in the tracking and management of cognitive repercussions of concussion. These include Immediate Post-concussion Assessment and Cognitive Testing (ImPACT; Lovell et al. 2003), the HeadMinder Concussion Resolution Index (CRI; Erlanger et al. 2003), Automated Neuropsychological Assessment Metrics (ANAM; Bleiberg et al. 2004), and CogSport (Makdissi et al. 2001). There is considerable overlap across these various batteries. Each features a relatively brief administration time (20–30 minutes), automatic development of alternate test forms to minimize practice effect, and a focus on the cognitive domains most susceptible to the effects of concussion (e.g., attention, reaction time, information processing speed, memory). Although these computerized tests are easily administered, interpretation of the data they yield in the postconcussive period is complex, and requires consideration of the psychometric properties of each measure (e.g., effects of serial administration, reliability, effort). Best practice necessitates interpretation of performance on computerized neuropsychological tests by or in consultation with a neuropsychologist with training and experience in their use.

Following concussion, athletes generally are expected to return to baseline levels within a relatively brief period of time. Barth et al. (1989) demonstrated that football players typically returned to baseline performance within 5–10 days (Figure 18–1). This is consistent with subsequent research (McCrea et al. 2003), which showed that symptoms, cognitive performance, and balance testing all returned to baseline within 3–7 days (Figure 18–2). A meta-analysis performed by Belanger and Vanderploeg (2005) demonstrated that the vast majority of concussed athletes return to their previous level within 7–10 days. Some evidence, however, suggests that recovery may be somewhat prolonged in younger athletes (Lovell et al. 2003), but only by a matter of days.

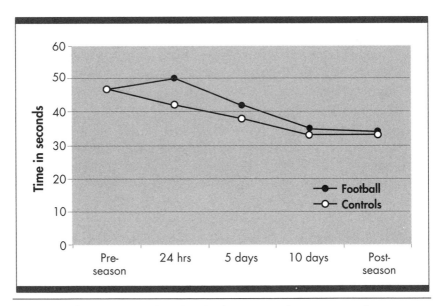

**FIGURE 18–1.** Example of typical recovery from concussion among athletes, using Trail Making Test Part B assessment.

These data are based on the seminal work of Barth et al. (1989) and demonstrate cognitive recovery by 5–10 days in the concussed football players relative to controls.

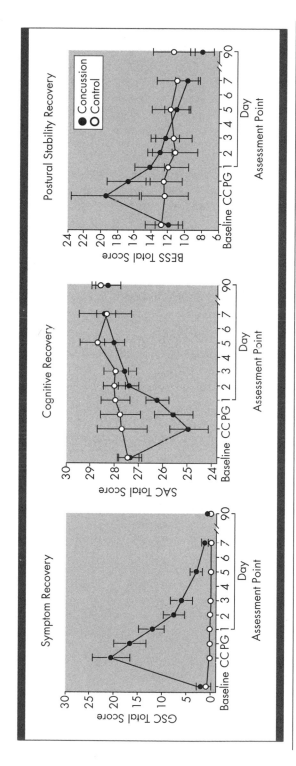

**FIGURE 18–2.** Example of typical recovery curves among concussed athletes.

Generally consistent with Barth et al. (1989), these data from McCrea et al. (2003) demonstrate clinical recovery from sports-related concussion in each of the symptoms, cognitive functioning, and postural stability by 3–7 days postinjury. BESS=Balance Error Scoring System; CC=indicated time of concussion; GSC=Graded Symptom Checklist; PG=postgame/postpractice; SAC=Standardized Assessment of Concussion.

*Source.* Reprinted from McCrea M, Guskiewicz KM, Marshall SW, et al.: "Acute Effects and Recovery Time Following Concussion in Collegiate Football Players: The NCAA Concussion Study." *Journal of the American Medical Association* 290:2556–2563, 2003. Copyright © 2003 American Medical Association. All rights reserved. Used with permission.

Despite clear evidence of the sensitivity of neuropsychological evaluation to cognitive compromise following concussion, some authors have questioned the influence of neuropsychological evaluation in moderating the true risks associated with sports-related concussion (Randolph et al. 2005). The psychometric properties and empirical support for the clinical use of neuropsychological measures in the context of sports concussion, and particularly the reliability, sensitivity, and incremental usefulness of existing measures, are among the most commonly expressed concerns. Despite such concerns, the best overall sensitivity to concussion was achieved in a battery of measures that included neuropsychological testing (89%–95% at day 1), with neuropsychological measures showing the best individual sensitivity to the injury (Broglio et al. 2007). The use of multiple methods, including neuropsychological assessment, is also consistent with the guidelines provided by the current consensus statement on concussion in sports (McCrory et al. 2009) as well as current athletic training guidelines on concussion management (Guskiewicz et al. 2004). Although further research is clearly warranted, continued practice of the multidimensional approach described in this section remains the gold standard in concussion management.

## Treatment Following Concussion

The best initial treatment for anyone who has sustained mTBI is rest and education about the nature and symptoms of the injury and the high likelihood of recovery from it. In nonsports population samples, early intervention with provision of educational materials describing the expected symptoms and the natural course of recovery for concussion has been associated with both a reduced mean symptom duration following concussion (Miller and Mittenberg 1998) and a reduction in distress and number of experienced symptoms (Ponsford et al. 2001). A similar approach with athletes is important, particularly for those individuals whose symptoms may be enduring longer than expected.

Although pharmacotherapy is not considered a first-line treatment for concussion symptoms, it may be useful in the treatment of persistent symptoms, particularly if an athlete has comorbid conditions that may be exacerbating the initial postconcussion symptoms. Treatment for symptoms of persistent headache pain, poor sleep, and/or symptoms of depression or anxiety can be particularly beneficial if an athlete has enduring symptoms. In our experience, these treatments are typically best utilized after a comprehensive neuropsychological evaluation has been performed to better characterize the patient's enduring symptoms and likely exacerbating conditions. It is also important to recognize that an athlete should not be considered ready to return to play when pharmacotherapy, rather than spontaneous recovery, explains remission of postconcussion symptoms.

# Return-to-Play Decision Making

A stepwise increase in activity is the current accepted protocol for returning to play. This method differs from historical approaches in which athletes were kept out of play for predetermined periods on the basis of initial ratings of concussion severity or grade. The most recent consensus statement on concussion in sports (McCrory et al. 2009) lists six steps to return-to-play (Table 18–2), after which recovery from concussion may be presumed with greater confidence. The approach described in this consensus statement holds that an athlete should proceed from one step to the next only if he or she remains asymptomatic at the earlier step for approximately 24 hours. Provided that recovery proceeds without complication, approximately 1 week is required for rehabilitation and to become ready to return to play. If any postconcussion symptoms occur while proceeding through these steps, then the athlete is returned to the highest step at which he or she was consistently asymptomatic, and another attempt is made to progress to the next step after 24 hours.

The National Athletic Trainers' Association's statement on the management of concussion (Guskiewicz et al. 2004) provides guidelines regarding when to disqualify athletes for differing durations. The guidelines suggest that an athlete who has any period of loss of consciousness or persistent concussion symptoms such as headache, dizziness, or amnesia (no matter how mild or transient) should be disqualified from play or practice for the remainder of the day. The National Collegiate Athletic Association's Executive Committee (National Collegiate Athletic Association 2012) has recommended even more stringent guidelines; these require immediate removal of the athlete from competition or practice upon diagnosis of concussion, even when postconcussive symptoms disappear within minutes after injury. Disqualifying an athlete from play for the remainder of a season is appropriate after the athlete's third concussion during that season. However,

**TABLE 18–2.** Sports concussion return-to-play protocol

| STAGE | FUNCTIONAL EXERCISE AT STAGE | OBJECTIVE |
|---|---|---|
| No activity | Complete physical and cognitive rest | Recovery |
| Light aerobic exercise | Walking, swimming, or stationary cycling, keeping intensity at 70% maximum predicted heart rate; no resistance training | Increase heart rate |
| Sport-specific exercise | Drills with no head-impact activities (e.g., skating drills in ice hockey, running drills in soccer) | Add movement |
| Noncontact training drills | Progression to more complex training drills (e.g., passing drills in football and ice hockey); may start progressive resistance training | Exercise, coordination, and cognitive load |
| Full-contact practice | Following medical clearance, participate in normal training activities | Restore confidence and have skills assessed by coaching staff |
| Return to play | Normal game play | |

a variety of factors complicate such decisions, including severity of the injuries and the interval between injuries, among others.

Deciding when to end an athlete's career as a result of concussions is a much more difficult matter. This decision often is made based on the number of concussions sustained, the individual athlete's apparent vulnerability to concussion, and the duration of postconcussive symptoms experienced by the athlete. A single approach will not serve all athletes well, and individual factors must be taken into account when addressing this important issue (McCrory et al. 2009). However, a more conservative approach to these decisions is recommended in the management of high school and youth athletes.

## CONCLUSION

Concussion is one of the most common but most challenging and complex clinical phenomena that sports medicine clinicians are asked to manage. Part of the complexity of this injury is associated with the fact that the basic and clinical science of the injury is still only partially understood. Cantu (2007) notes that more publications on the topic of sports-related concussion have appeared since the year 2000 than the total number of publications on the topic prior to that date. With the high level of recent public interest and this influx of research, great strides in the management of sports concussion and head injury in general have been made. Future research will assist the development of evidence-based diagnoses and treatment recommendations and is likely to reduce further the risk of poor outcome among athletes who sustain concussions.

## *Key Clinical Points*

- Concussion is common in athletic populations, although athletes demonstrate unique characteristics (e.g., drive to return to play) that may complicate the clinical management of concussion.

- Concussion is associated with a complex metabolic cascade that is not observable by conventional neuroimaging.

- Although most individuals who sustain a concussion recover within a relatively brief period of time, complications may arise if recovery is not managed appropriately and/or if repeated injuries are sustained.

- Concussion management employs a multidimensional approach wherein professionals monitor changes in athletes' physical, cognitive, and postural stability symptoms relative to a preseason baseline.

- The best methods of treating postconcussion include educating the patient about the nature and expected recovery curve of the injury and providing support. Pharmacotherapy and behavioral interventions are best reserved for individuals with persistent postconcussive symptoms.

# REFERENCES

American Academy of Neurology: Practice Parameter: The Management of Concussion in Sports. 1997 Available at: http://www.aan.com/professionals/practice/guidelines/pda/Concussion_sports.pdf. Accessed November 6, 2012.

Bailey CM, Echemendia RJ, Arnett PA: The impact of motivation on neuro-psychological performance in sports-related mild traumatic brain injury. J Int Neuropsychol Soc 12:475–484, 2006

Bailey CM, Barth JT, Bender SD: SLAM on the stand: how the sports-related concussion literature can inform the expert witness. J Head Trauma Rehabil 24:123–130, 2009

Barth JT, Alves WM, Ryan TV: Mild head injury in sports: neuropsychological sequelae and recovery of function, in Mild Head Injury. Edited by Levin HS, Eisenberg HM, Benton AL. New York, Oxford University Press, 1989, pp 257–275

Barth JT, Freeman JR, Broshek DK: Mild head injury, in Encyclopedia of the Human Brain, Vol 3. Edited by Ramachandran VS. San Diego, CA, Academic Press, 2002, pp 81–92

Bazarian JJ, McClung J, Shah MN, et al: Mild traumatic brain injury in the United States, 1998–2000. Brain Inj 19:85–91, 2005

Belanger HG, Vanderploeg RD: The neuropsychological impact of sports-related concussion: a meta-analysis. J Int Neuropsychol Soc 11:345–357, 2005

Belanger HG, Curtiss G, Demery JA, et al: Factors moderating neuropsychological outcomes following mild traumatic brain injury: a meta-analysis. J Int Neuropsychol Soc 11:215–227, 2005

Bleiberg J, Cernich AN, Cameron K, et al: Duration of cognitive impairment after sports concussion. Neurosurgery 54:1073–1078, discussion 1078–1080, 2004

Broglio SP, Macciocchi SN, Ferrara MS: Sensitivity of the concussion assessment battery. Neurosurgery 60:1050–1057, discussion 1057–1058, 2007

Broshek DK, Kaushik T, Freeman JR, et al: Sex differences in outcome following sports-related concussion. J Neurosurg 102:856–863, 2005

Bush SS, Ruff RM, Tröster AI, et al: Symptom validity assessment: practice issues and medical necessity NAN policy & planning committee. Arch Clin Neuropsychol 20:419–426, 2005

Cantu RC: Guidelines for return to contact sports after a cerebral concussion. Phys Sportsmed 14(10):75–83, 1986

Cantu RC: Athletic concussion: current understanding as of 2007. Neurosurgery 60:963–964, 2007

Carroll LJ, Cassidy JD, Holm L, et al: Methodological issues and research recommendations for mild traumatic brain injury: the WHO Collaborating Centre Task Force on Mild Traumatic Brain Injury. J Rehabil Med 43(suppl):113–125, 2004

Centers for Disease Control and Prevention: Report to Congress on Mild Traumatic Brain Injury in the United States: Steps to Prevent a Serious Public Health Problem. Atlanta, GA, Centers for Disease Control and Prevention, National Center for Injury Prevention and Control, 2003

Collins M, Grindel SH, Lovell MR, et al: Relationship between concussion and neuropsychological performance in college football players. JAMA 282:964–970, 1999

Collins M, Lovell MR, Iverson GL, et al: Cumulative effects of concussion in high school athletes. Neurosurgery 51:1175–1179, discussion 1180–1181, 2002

Collins M, Lovell MR, Iverson GL, et al: Examining concussion rates and return to play in high school football players wearing newer helmet technology: a three-year prospective cohort study. Neurosurgery 58:275–286, discussion 275–286, 2006

Difiori JP, Giza CC: New techniques in concussion imaging. Curr Sports Med Rep 9:35–39, 2010

Erlanger D, Feldman D, Kutner K, et al: Development and validation of a web-based neuropsychological test protocol for sports-related return-to-play decision-making. Arch Clin Neuropsychol 18:293–316, 2003

Field M, Collins MW, Lovell MR, et al: Does age play a role in recovery from sports-related concussion? A comparison of high school and collegiate athletes. J Pediatr 142:546–553, 2003

Fife D: Head injury with and without hospital admission: comparisons of incidence and short-term disability. Am J Public Health 77:810–812, 1987

Giacino JT, Smart CM: Recent advances in behavioral assessment of individuals with disorders of consciousness. Curr Opin Neurol 20:614–619, 2007

Giza CC, Hovda DA: The neurometabolic cascade of concussion. J Athl Train 36:228–235, 2001

Guskiewicz KM, McCrea M, Marshall SW, et al: Cumulative effects associated with recurrent concussion in collegiate football players: the NCAA Concussion Study. JAMA 290:2549–2555, 2003

Guskiewicz KM, Bruce SL, Cantu RC, et al: National Athletic Trainers' Association position statement: management of sport-related concussion. J Athl Train 39:280–297, 2004

Guskiewicz KM, Marshall SW, Bailes J, et al: Association between recurrent concussion and late-life cognitive impairment in retired professional football players. Neurosurgery 57:719–726, discussion 719–726, 2005

Guskiewicz KM, Marshall SW, Bailes J, et al: Recurrent concussion and risk of depression in retired professional football players. Med Sci Sports Exerc 39:903–909, 2007

Iverson GL, Brooks BL, Collins MW, et al: Tracking neuropsychological recovery following concussion in sport. Brain Inj 20:245–252, 2006

Kay T, Harrington DE, Adams RE, et al: Definition of mild traumatic brain injury: report from Mild Traumatic Brain Injury Committee of the Head Injury Interdisciplinary Special Interest Group of the American Congress of Rehabilitation Medicine. J Head Trauma Rehabil 8:86–87, 1993

Lang DA, Teasdale GM, Macpherson P, et al: Diffuse brain swelling after head injury: more often malignant in adults than children? J Neurosurg 80:675–680, 1994

Larrabee GJ: Assessment of malingering, in Forensic Neuropsychology: A Scientific Approach. Edited by Larrabee GJ. New York, Oxford University Press, 2005, pp 115–158

Lovell MR, Collins MW, Iverson GL, et al: Recovery from mild concussion in high school athletes. J Neurosurg 98:296–301, 2003

Makdissi M, Collie A, Maruff P, et al: Computerised cognitive assessment of concussed Australian Rules footballers. Br J Sports Med 35:354–360, 2001

McCrea M: Standardized mental status assessment of sports concussion. Clin J Sport Med 11:176–181, 2001

McCrea M, Kelly JP, Randolph C, et al: Standardized Assessment of Concussion (SAC): on-site mental status evaluation of the athlete. J Head Trauma Rehabil 13:27–35, 1998

McCrea M, Guskiewicz KM, Marshall SW, et al: Acute effects and recovery time following concussion in collegiate football players: the NCAA Concussion Study. JAMA 290:2556–2563, 2003

McCrea M, Guskiewicz K, Randolph C, et al: Effects of a symptom-free waiting period on clinical outcome and risk of reinjury after sport-related concussion. Neurosurgery 65:876–882, discussion 882–883, 2009

McCrory P, Berkovic SF: Second impact syndrome. Neurology 50:677–683, 1998

McCrory P, Meeuwisse W, Johnston K, et al: Consensus statement on Concussion in Sport 3rd International Conference on Concussion in Sport held in Zurich, November 2008. Clin J Sport Med 19:185–200, 2009

Miller LJ, Mittenberg W: Brief cognitive behavioral interventions in mild traumatic brain injury. Appl Neuropsychol 5:172–183, 1998

Mori T, Katayama Y, Kawamata T: Acute hemispheric swelling associated with thin subdural hematomas: pathophysiology of repetitive head injury in sports. Acta Neurochir Suppl 96:40–43, 2006

Moser RS, Iverson GL, Echemendia RJ, et al: Neuropsychological evaluation in the diagnosis and management of sports-related concussion. Arch Clin Neuropsychol 22:909–916, 2007

National Collegiate Athletic Association: Sports Medicine Handbook, 23rd Edition. Indianapolis, IN, National Collegiate Athletic Association, 2012

Ponsford J, Willmott C, Rothwell A, et al: Impact of early intervention on outcome after mild traumatic brain injury in children. Pediatrics 108:1297–1303, 2001

Randolph C, McCrea M, Barr WB: Is neuropsychological testing useful in the management of sport-related concussion? J Athl Train 40:139–152, 2005

Schulz MR, Marshall SW, Mueller FO, et al: Incidence and risk factors for concussion in high school athletes, North Carolina, 1996–1999. Am J Epidemiol 160:937–944, 2004

Tommasone BA, McLeod TCV: Contact sport concussion incidence. J Athl Train 41:470–472, 2006

Zemper ED: Two-year prospective study of relative risk of a second cerebral concussion. Am J Phys Med Rehabil 82:653–659, 2003

# CHAPTER 19

## Military Personnel and Veterans With Traumatic Brain Injury

*Kimberly Meyer, M.S.N.*
*Michael S. Jaffee, M.D.*

**Military combat** is a well-recognized risk factor for traumatic brain injuries (TBIs), including penetrating brain injuries, blast-related TBIs, and injuries due to motor vehicle accidents, falls, assaults, and other biomechanical force exposures. The vast majority of these injuries are mild TBIs (mTBIs), also referred to as concussions.

Since 2007, increased awareness of combat-related TBI has led to the development of several key TBI programs in the United States. The Defense and Veterans Brain Injury Center (DVBIC), which was founded in 1992 and has a long history in clinical care, education, and research, more recently took responsibility for oversight of military force health protection programs such as TBI surveillance, predeployment neurocognitive testing, and the congressionally mandated Family Caregiver Curriculum. In addition to these programs, DVBIC administers the TBI Care Coordination Program, which tracks all service members with TBI and identifies local resources for individualized treatment. This program has facilitated organization and standardization of TBI care across the service branches and minimized duplicity of services. The approach to TBI care to which DVBIC contributes has influenced the U.S. Department of Defense (DoD) TBI clinical care programs and has been adopted by several North Atlantic Treaty Organization (NATO) allies.

461

# DIFFERENCES BETWEEN MILITARY AND CIVILIAN TBI

Among civilians, TBI is most often caused by blunt trauma mechanisms resulting from acceleration-deceleration or rotational-type forces. By contrast, combat-related TBI often involves blast-related forces. The potential injuries associated with blasts are categorized into four types: primary injuries, which are those resulting from blast energy (e.g., shock waves, complex wave fields) and, by some accounts, electromagnetic energy; secondary injuries, which result from impact by and/or penetration of debris (i.e., biomechanical force) that was set in motion by primary blast forces; tertiary injuries, which result from displacement of the whole body or body parts by blast forces (i.e., acceleration force), subsequent striking of objects or the ground (i.e., biomechanical force), and stopping (deceleration force); and quaternary (or miscellaneous) injuries, which include exposure to heat (e.g., thermal energy), noxious fumes, or other toxins (Warden 2006).

Primary blast forces affect organs with air-fluid interfaces, such as the lungs, gastrointestinal tract, and ears (Mayorga 1997). The effects of primary blast forces on the brain are understood less well (Cernak and Noble-Haeusslein 2010), but recent data suggest that neuropathological differences may exist between blast and blunt brain injuries (Warden et al. 2009). Evidence for this suggestion derives from variations in fractional anisotropy on diffusion tensor imaging of the brain in persons with blast-related TBI, as well as from inflammation observed in patients with experimental blast TBI but not those with blunt neurotrauma (Ling 2010).

In recent years, primary prevention of TBI in the civilian sector has likely contributed to the decreased morbidity and mortality associated with these injuries. The use of helmets in sporting activities, seat belt usage in motor vehicles, and elderly fall prevention programs are examples of preventive measures. Prevention in the military sector is more difficult. Helmets, designed to prevent injury from projectile forces (penetrating injury), may offer less protection against the concussive forces associated with blast injury. Computational models suggest that the addition of a face shield to standard Advanced Combat Helmets may mitigate direct transmission of shock waves to the brain (Nyein et al. 2010), although testing has not been done in vivo. The role of body armor continues to be evaluated. Some investigators have suggested that body armor may increase the interaction between the blast wave and body surface, thereby intensifying the explosive effects (Cernak and Noble-Haeusslein 2010). Other investigators have shown that body armor may protect against lung injuries associated with blast (Ling 2010). Finally, although seat belts minimize injury resulting from acceleration-deceleration or rotational injury in blast-plus mechanisms (i.e., secondary, tertiary, and quaternary mechanisms), they offer no protection against the blast wave associated with roadside explosive devices.

## EPIDEMIOLOGY

From 2000 through the first quarter of 2012, a total of 244,217 service members had been diagnosed with TBIs (Defense and Veterans Brain Injury Center 2012), most of which (80%) were classified as mild or concussive injuries. The annual incidence has been substantially higher since 2006, largely due to increased screening and surveillance efforts within the Military Health System. In the military population, TBI is most likely to affect men (95.5%) under age 30 (55.5%) (Hoge et al. 2008). Compared with service members reporting other types of injuries, those reporting mTBI most often were involved in high-intensity combat maneuvers, had exposure to more than one explosion, and sustained a blast mechanism of injury (Hoge et al. 2008).

Early efforts to triage service members with possible TBI used the Brief Traumatic Brain Injury Screen (Schwab et al. 2007), which included three questions: 1) Did you sustain an injury event during your deployment? 2) Did you sustain a loss of or alteration in consciousness? 3) Do you have any pertinent symptoms following the event? More recently, measures have been instituted to ensure that TBI screening occurs immediately following exposure to a traumatic event, using the Military Acute Concussion Evaluation (MACE). It is available online (www.pdhealth.mil/downloads/MACE.pdf) and may be copied for clinical use. The MACE is used to determine the presence or absence of alteration of consciousness, symptoms, neurological signs, and, when indicated, alteration of cognitive function. The instrument is most useful when administered within 12 hours following injury. Although it usefully identifies those with symptoms that may reflect TBI, it is not diagnostic of this condition.

Additional TBI screening of deployed service members occurs in other contexts as well. When service members are medically evacuated to Landstuhl Regional Medical Center (LRMC) in Germany, they undergo mandatory postdeployment health assessments for any injury or illness. The TBI screening included in the Post Deployment Health Assessment (PDHA; DoD form 2796, January 2008) is based on the Brief Traumatic Brain Injury Screen, which has been modified to include a fourth question designed to delineate the timing of symptoms (i.e., immediate and/or current). Based on self-report given after redeployment, positive responses to question 2 indicate a likely TBI, and affirmative responses to question 3 indicate symptoms of a possibly postconcussive nature. Further clinical evaluation is performed on service members with positive screens to further delineate actual diagnosis.

Of individuals undergoing evaluation at LRMC, approximately 20%–25% screen positive for TBI and are referred for additional clinical examination (Dempsey et al. 2009). Positive screens are followed by detailed clinical evaluations before the formal diagnosis of TBI is made. One study using PDHA found that 22.8% of soldiers in a Brigade Combat Team returning from Iraq had clinician-confirmed TBI (Terrio et al. 2009). Although 33.4% of this sample reported multiple symptoms immediately following the injury, symptom reporting decreased to 7.5% in the postdeployment period. This observation suggests that, like civilians with TBI, most service members with TBI recover within months of injury.

# POPULATION-SPECIFIC CLINICAL ASSESSMENT CONCERNS

Identification of TBI is facilitated by new guidelines that require all service members involved in incidents associated with high risk of concussion to undergo mandatory screening regardless of whether they endorse event-related symptoms. These incidents include being in close proximity to an explosion, in a damaged passenger compartment of a vehicle, or in a building damaged by an explosion. This mandate is intended to maximize screening in those with potential injuries.

Acute evaluations, especially in mTBI, can be hindered by other more life- or limb-threatening injuries. Acute stress reaction and anxiety disorders may complicate the presentation of TBI, thereby impeding the accurate diagnosis of these conditions. When possible, collateral information should be obtained from others in the vicinity of the traumatic event and may clarify the injury history and likelihood of a TBI. Lack of imaging capabilities in the medically austere combat environments often necessitates air or ground evacuation through dangerous territories to trauma care facilities. Injuries requiring more advanced imaging techniques, such as magnetic resonance imaging (MRI), dictate evacuation to the tertiary care facility in Germany (LRMC) or to the continental United States.

Among those service members medically evacuated to LRMC, mandatory postdeployment health assessments for any injury or illness are performed using the Brief Traumatic Brain Injury Screen modified to assess for immediate postinjury and current (i.e., persistent) symptoms. Persistent postconcussive symptoms following combat-related TBI warrant psychological health assessment to ensure that conditions such as depression or stress reactions are not contributing to disability. Other problems such as pain and sleep disturbances may also affect recovery from TBI (Lew et al. 2009b).

The Department of Veterans Affairs (VA) has implemented TBI screening through the clinical reminder system, using a four-question screening assessment for all Veterans of Operation Enduring Freedom (OEF) and Operation Iraqi Freedom (OIF) upon initial presentation to any VA medical center for treatment. Positive screens within the VA system require affirmative responses on all questions, thereby identifying only those service members or Veterans who are still symptomatic.

# TREATMENT

Initial treatment of combat-related TBI involves rest, education about the injury and expected natural history of recovery, and primary symptom management. In uncomplicated cases of mTBI, local medical assets most often suffice. Service members with neurological findings or more severe injuries are evacuated to higher levels of care within the combat theater, where specialty care and additional medical resources are available.

The main priority for management of concussion in the combat theater is safety. The service member is restricted to base to prevent possible exposure to a recurrent concussion before recovering from the initial injury. This is done based on the suggestion of increased brain vulnerability during recovery from concussion. Evaluation and management of concussion are guided by clinical practice guidelines, which incorporate available evidence, expert opinion, and relevant military considerations.

One of the most prevalent symptoms of TBI is headache, occurring in 32%–36% of service members with TBI (Hoge et al. 2008; Schwab et al. 2007). Pharmacological management of headache begins with acetaminophen for the first 48 hours following injury. Nonsteroidal anti-inflammatory drugs (NSAIDs), such as naproxen sodium, may be used after 48 hours in neurologically stable patients. The use of NSAIDs may be considered earlier in patients with negative neuroimaging. For headaches persisting longer than 1 week, prophylactic medications are recommended. Tricyclic antidepressants (nortriptyline or amitriptyline) are instituted at low dosages and titrated to maximum tolerated dosage or headache control. Other agents that are typically used in civilian headache management are less commonly used because many produce unacceptable side effects, require monitoring of drug levels or hepatic function, or are not readily available in the combat theater formulary.

Sleep disturbances are also common complaints. When possible, service members with TBI are encouraged to get 8 hours of uninterrupted sleep. Getting this much sleep, however, is often difficult, especially in times of aggressive operation tempos or in areas where insurgent activity is frequent. Low-dose zolpidem is sometimes prescribed for short-term use. Benzodiazepines are avoided because they may aggravate cognitive difficulties that may follow TBI.

This primary care management protocol is continued for 7 days. Those individuals with severe symptoms can be considered for early evacuation to a higher level of care. Most individuals, however, demonstrate some improvement within the week following injury and remain at their duty station. Those with incomplete recovery undergo a combat stress evaluation. This frequently includes a debriefing regarding the traumatic event and evaluations for acute stress disorder, posttraumatic stress disorder, depression, and other conditions that may cause psychological distress. Early intervention is important because some evidence suggests that persistent symptoms after reasonable treatment may be attributable to emotional distress in patients with mTBI (Belanger et al. 2010). If symptoms persist longer than 3 weeks, transfer to a higher level of care is indicated. This transfer facilitates more detailed assessment and determination of the need for medical care in the continental United States.

A small percentage of service members with chronic problems associated with mTBI, or those with moderate to severe TBI, require prolonged treatment. Treatment may involve chronic headache management (Figure 19–1), using any of a variety of medication classes, including antiepileptic drugs, triptans, β-blockers, and antidepressants. Comparisons of headache types in combat soldiers and civilians suggest that migraine-type headaches are more prevalent following blast-related injury, whereas tension-type headaches are more predominant following blunt trauma (Vargas 2009). Medication selection should be influenced by headache characteristics (see Chapter 13, "Headache"). Some centers report success with less conventional treatment modalities, such as botulinum toxin injections. Difficulties with memory are also common complaints of individuals with persistent postconcussive symptoms. Cognitive rehabilitation may be warranted to treat memory and attention deficits (see Chapter 5, "Cognitive Impairments"); guidelines for the assessment and treatment of service members with cognitive impairment are available and should be used in the management of this population (Helmick 2010).

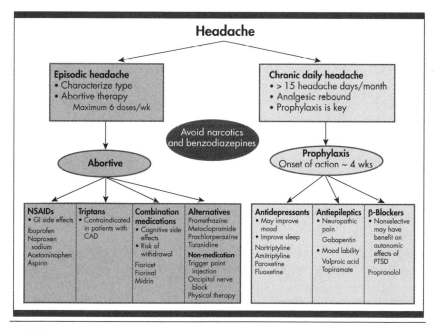

**FIGURE 19–1.** Management of chronic headache.

CAD=coronary artery disease; GI=gastrointestinal; NSAID=nonsteroidal anti-inflammatory drug; PTSD=posttraumatic stress disorder.

Visual and vestibular complaints of OEF/OIF Veterans have drawn increased attention. Goodrich et al. (2007) reported that despite normal or near-normal visual acuity in 50 patients with TBI, significant deficits in convergence, accommodation, and visual-spatial orientation were present. These deficits impair overall binocular vision and, therefore, reading ability. Little difference was found between the blast and nonblast groups. Hoffer et al. (2009), on the other hand, demonstrated differences in objective vestibular testing in patients with blast versus blunt brain injuries. Specifically, variabilities in visual-ocular reflex and vestibular-spinal reflexes have been identified in patients with the two injury patterns. These findings may affect treatment modalities for vestibular dysfunction (Hoffer et al. 2010). Furthermore, emerging evidence suggests that dual sensory impairment may be present in those with persistent postconcussive symptoms, thereby affecting the efficacy of some treatment modalities (Lew et al. 2009a).

# RETURN-TO-DUTY CONSIDERATIONS

Following a waiting period associated with symptom control or resolution, service members undergo exertional testing. This involves a brief period of aerobic exercise and then assessment for return of symptoms and a cognitive evaluation, using an alternate form of the MACE. In most cases, absence of recurrent symptoms and cognitive dysfunction following exercise allows for return to full duty.

Further evaluations, such as computerized neurocognitive assessment batteries, are being used to better inform return-to-duty determinations. To date, 723,981 service members have undergone baseline computerized cognitive assessment with a brief battery that evaluates mathematical processing, processing speeds, attention, and memory; when the battery is repeated following injury, results can be compared to the individual's baseline as part of the return-to-duty evaluation. New cognitive deficits that appear on postinjury computerized cognitive assessment may trigger more detailed neuropsychological testing prior to removal of duty restrictions. Over 5,500 requests have been made for baseline information to aid in postinjury TBI evaluations. The DoD is currently using the Automated Neuropsychological Assessment Metrics (ANAM; US Army Neurocognitive Assessment Branch 2012)) while undertaking objective head-to-head evaluations of available computerized batteries to inform future instrument selection.

Some job classifications may require a functional assessment or a period of supervised work before duty restrictions are removed. Because evidence indicates that multiple concussions may lead to slower recovery or even the development of chronic traumatic encephalopathy (Guskiewicz et al. 2003; McKee et al. 2009), individuals with recurrent concussions are required to wait a longer time before returning to duty than are those with a single concussion. Accordingly, service members with three or more concussions within the same deployment will undergo a more extensive evaluation, including evaluation by a neurologist to assist in return-to-duty determination.

Additional research is required to clarify the usefulness of these approaches to return-to-duty determinations and to identify additional objective metrics that inform such decisions.

# RESOURCES FOR CARE

## Telemedicine

A variety of telemedicine modalities are available to facilitate TBI care within the Military Health System. Electronic consultation via e-mail is available to deployed providers (see www.dvbic.org/concussion-mtbi-information-and-tools-providers). This service offers recommendations for individualized patient care, answers to general TBI questions, and considerations for evacuation. Consults by e-mail are generally answered within 3–4 hours by a TBI subject matter expert. This service has facilitated necessary evacuations and prevented unnecessary transfers by instructing in initial management or connecting direct care providers with other in-theater specialists. Quarterly quality improvement teleconferences are held to facilitate situational awareness of the latest DoD TBI initiatives among the TBI consultants and ensure that appropriate recommendations are provided to the deployed providers.

Interactive video teleconferencing is used to support the transition of patients with moderate or severe injury as they transfer from facilities within the military medical system to VA Polytrauma Rehabilitation Centers. The DVBIC Virtual Traumatic Brain Injury (vTBI) Clinic provides TBI screening, assessment, consultation, and care to patients at remote military medical centers as well as troop-intensive sites where demand for specialized care fluctuates with mass mobilizations. The vTBI Clinic is organized like a traditional clinic with multiple specialties (i.e., neurology, neuropsychology, pain management, rehabilitation) working together to meet the unique needs of each patient. Unlike in traditional TBI clinics, however, direct specialty care is provided at a distance using interactive video teleconferencing. This interaction is made possible with the assistance of local primary care providers who provide on-site testing and therapy.

## Department of Veterans Affairs

Active-duty service members remain in the Military Health System; however, those who medically retire often transition to care within the VA. As mentioned above in "Population-Specific Clinical Assessment Concerns," all OIF/OEF Veterans entering the VA health care system undergo mandatory screening for TBI. Services are available in a variety of settings, including hospitals, outpatient clinics, community living centers, and residential rehabilitation programs. Four Polytrauma Rehabilitation Centers that are equipped with state-of-the-art technology assume care of service members or Veterans with severe or penetrating TBI. The VA also maintains coma emergence programs for patients with disorders of consciousness. VA federal recovery coordinators are assigned to those Veterans with more severe injuries. This program facilitates individualized care across federal health programs and private community resources to optimize recovery from TBI and other potentially devastating injuries.

## DoD and VA Resources

Subject matter experts from the DoD and VA have developed a number of patient and provider resources to facilitate understanding of TBI. An excellent collection of these resources can be found at the Web site of the Defense Centers of Excellence for Psychological Health and Traumatic Brain Injury (www.dcoe.health.mil/ForHealthPros/TBIInformation.aspx); most of these resources are reviewed and updated on a regular basis.

# RESEARCH

The DoD has partnered with other federal agencies, academic centers, and private agencies to further blast-related TBI research. The Center for Neuroscience and Regenerative Medicine (CNRM) focuses on diagnostics/imaging, biomarkers, neuroplasticity, neuroprotection, and rehabilitative medicine. The Preventing Violent

Explosive Neurologic Trauma program seeks to identify causal relationships between blast injury and pathophysiological changes that result in neurological injury. Additionally, Congressionally Directed Medical Research Programs funds a broad range of studies in this area, including protocols addressing pharmacotherapies (e.g., neuroprotectants, antidepressants), hyperbaric oxygen therapy, therapeutic nanotubules, neurodiagnostics (e.g., functional MRI, magnetoencephalography, diffusion tensor imaging), blast models, and blast sensors, among others. These research programs aim to use best scientific research principles and to translate study results to field applications as soon as it is reasonable to do so.

# CONCLUSION

Combat-related TBI remains a complex clinical entity. Aggressive screening and early intervention are thought to decrease the development of chronic symptoms. Clinical practice guidelines and increased provider education initiatives have standardized TBI care across service branches. However, much work is required to fully understand the interaction between blast injury and long-term effects. As knowledge continues to be gained, the clinical practices relevant to the care of service members with TBI will continue to evolve.

## *Key Clinical Points*

- Blast or blast-plus mechanisms are the primary causes of TBI for individuals in the military.

- Factors that influence recovery from combat-related TBI include exposure to multiple blasts with repeated concussions, physiological stress at time of injury (e.g., dehydration, chronic cortisol elevations, sleep deprivation), presence of comorbid psychological distress.

- The diagnosis of concussion may be difficult to make in individuals with life- or limb-threatening conditions such as burns or amputations.

- Aggressive management of postconcussive symptoms is initiated upon identification of TBI.

- Clinical practice guidelines direct the evaluation and management of concussion in various settings, with respect to available resources.

# REFERENCES

Belanger HG, Kretzmer T, Vanderploeg RD, et al: Symptom complaints following combat-related traumatic brain injury: relationship to traumatic brain injury severity and posttraumatic stress disorder. J Int Neuropsychol Soc 16:194–199, 2010

Cernak I, Noble-Haeusslein LJ: Traumatic brain injury: an overview of pathobiology with emphasis on military populations. J Cereb Blood Flow Metab 30:255–266, 2010

Defense and Veterans Brain Injury Center: DOD worldwide numbers for TBI. 2012. Available at: http://www.dvbic.org/dod-worldwide-numbers-tbi. Accessed July 17, 2012.

Dempsey KE, Dorlac WC, Martin K, et al: Landstuhl Regional Medical Center: traumatic brain injury screening program. J Trauma Nurs 16:6–7, 10–12, 2009

Goodrich GL, Kirby J, Cockerham G, et al: Visual function in patients of a polytrauma rehabilitation center: a descriptive study. J Rehabil Res Dev 44:929–936, 2007

Guskiewicz KM, McCrea M, Marshall SW, et al: Cumulative effects associated with recurrent concussion in collegiate football players: the NCAA Concussion Study. JAMA 290:2549–2555, 2003

Helmick K: Cognitive rehabilitation for military personnel with mild traumatic brain injury and chronic post-concussional disorder: results of April 2009 consensus conference. NeuroRehabilitation 26:239–255, 2010

Hoffer ME, Donaldson C, Gottshall KR, et al: Blunt and blast head trauma: different entities. Int Tinnitus J 15:115–118, 2009

Hoffer ME, Balaban C, Gottshall K, et al: Blast exposure: vestibular consequences and associated characteristics. Otol Neurotol 31:232–236, 2010

Hoge CW, McGurk D, Thomas JL, et al: Mild traumatic brain injury in U.S. soldiers returning from Iraq. N Engl J Med 358:453–463, 2008

Lew HL, Garvert DW, Pogoda TK, et al: Auditory and visual impairments in patients with blast-related traumatic brain injury: effect of dual sensory impairment on Functional Independence Measure. J Rehabil Res Dev 46:819–826, 2009a

Lew HL, Otis JD, Tun C, et al: Prevalence of chronic pain, posttraumatic stress disorder, and persistent postconcussive symptoms in OIF/OEF veterans: polytrauma clinical triad. J Rehabil Res Dev 46:697–702, 2009b

Ling G: Preventing Violent Explosive Neurologic Trauma (PREVENT). Arlington, VA, Defense Advanced Research Projects Agency, 2010. Available at: http://www.darpa.mil/Our_Work/DSO/Programs/Preventing_Violent_Explosive_Neurologic_Trauma_(PREVENT).aspx. Accessed December 12, 2010.

Mayorga MA: The pathology of primary blast overpressure injury. Toxicology 121:17–28, 1997

McKee AC, Cantu RC, Nowinski CJ, et al: Chronic traumatic encephalopathy in athletes: progressive tauopathy after repetitive head injury. J Neuropathol Exp Neurol 68:709–735, 2009

Nyein MK, Jason AM, Yu L, et al: In silico investigation of intracranial blast mitigation with relevance to military traumatic brain injury. Proc Natl Acad Sci USA 107:20703–20708, 2010

Schwab KA, Ivins B, Cramer G, et al: Screening for traumatic brain injury in troops returning from deployment in Afghanistan and Iraq: initial investigation of the usefulness of a short screening tool for traumatic brain injury. J Head Trauma Rehabil 22:377–389, 2007

Terrio H, Brenner LA, Ivins BJ, et al: Traumatic brain injury screening: preliminary findings in a US Army Brigade Combat Team. J Head Trauma Rehabil 24:14–23, 2009

US Army Neurocognitive Assessment Branch, Rehabilitation and Reintegration Division, Health Policy and Services Directorate, OTSG/MEDCOM One Staff, San Antonio, TX

Vargas BB: Posttraumatic headache in combat soldiers and civilians: what factors influence the expression of tension-type versus migraine headache? Curr Pain Headache Rep 13:470–473, 2009

Warden D: Military TBI during the Iraq and Afghanistan wars. J Head Trauma Rehabil 21:398–402, 2006

Warden DL, French LM, Shupenko L, et al: Case report of a soldier with primary blast brain injury. Neuroimage 47(suppl):T152–T153, 2009

◆

# Persistent Symptoms After a Concussion

*Jonathan M. Silver, M.D.*
*Thomas Kay, Ph.D.†*

> Since my car accident a year ago, I am a mess. I can't think, I can't re-
> member, and my head hurts all the time. I can't tolerate taking my
> kids to the mall. I can't work, I'm crying and yelling, and my house is
> a wreck. I can't stand being around my friends—and my marriage is
> on the rocks. I need help!

**Although the vast majority** of individuals who have
traumatic brain injuries (TBIs) categorized as "mild" and who have
been diagnosed with "concussion" return to baseline functioning
within several months, a subset of individuals experience persistent
symptoms that affect quality of life. These symptoms may occur in less
than 5% of individuals with mild TBI (mTBI), and are significantly influenced by non-injury-related factors (McCrea et al. 2009). Several
factors are implicated in prolonged symptoms, including the pathophysiology of the injury, preinjury factors (e.g., preexisting psychiat-

---

†Dr. Kay died on August 29, 2012. He was a compassionate and superb clinician who was one of the pioneers in the diagnosis and treatment of individuals with "the unseen injury." He will be missed by patients and colleagues.

ric and substance use problems, previous TBI, intelligence, gender, age, personality style), and postinjury factors (social support, availability of adequate treatment, litigation/compensation) (Carroll et al. 2004; McAllister 2011). This paradigm serves as a guide to the evaluation of the patient with persistent symptoms after a concussion.

What does the psychiatrist or mental health worker do when first confronted with a patient who has persistent symptoms? The first thing *not* to do is to assume that all problems that started after a bump on the head in a motor vehicle accident (or fall, or other injury) are due directly to the mTBI. Acute postconcussion symptoms are fairly consistent in their presentation and, by definition, are time limited. At the initial presentation, several symptoms predominate: problems with thinking, often described as feeling "fuzzy" or "slowed down"; physical problems, including insomnia, fatigue, headache, dizziness, and visual problems; and emotional and behavioral problems, including feeling depressed or tearful, anxious, and irritable.

When symptoms spread into multiple domains, persist for more than a few months, and then begin to coalesce and globally impair— and increasingly erode—functioning, it no longer makes sense to speak of a "postconcussion syndrome." We, along with others, do not believe the term *postconcussion syndrome* is valid or helpful, because symptoms do not represent a single pathophysiological process (McAllister 2011). Similarly, we discourage use of the term *persistent* (or *chronic*) *postconcussion syndrome* (or *symptoms*). We believe that, more accurately, this problem should be referred to as *persistent symptoms that occur after a concussion*. This term, which has diagnostic and therapeutic implications, represents acknowledgment that multiple factors play a role in the persistence of symptoms that may not reflect a continuation of those first evident after the so-called concussion. The constellation of symptoms that resulted directly from the concussion is no longer a unitary force driving dysfunction.

The person who seeks attention for persistent symptoms that occur 6 or more months after TBI is already one who is atypical of most people who suffer concussions. Some combination of factors makes this individual different from those who have recovered typically after mTBI. If the person has been referred into the mental health system, someone likely has already come to this conclusion. Although some patients will present with psychologically uncomplicated neurological abnormalities that have been missed, the vast majority of persons presenting within the mental health system long after a concussion will have a dizzying array of symptoms that need disentangling. These individuals may face psychosocial challenges involving returning to work, relationships with family members, and interactions with the legal and insurance systems. Individual symptoms may amplify and exacerbate each other. The person may have lost confidence in himself or herself, and "secondary" depression may have developed.

Our way of approaching cases of persistent symptoms that occur after a concussion requires a reframing of the core diagnostic question. The question is not whether or not this person has a TBI—a dangerous dichotomizing question that typifies medicolegal quagmires. TBI is an event, not an explanatory diagnosis. Instead, the question is this: If a TBI (mild or severe) did occur in the past, what are its present direct or indirect manifestations, are the persistent symptoms related to it, and what can be done to ameliorate them?

Too often, patients are deemed not to have a "real" TBI and are then dismissed from the rehabilitation system and by other medical specialists. These patients usually have experienced a traumatic event, such as an accident or assault, that has its own emotional ramifications. The challenge to the mental health practitioner is to successfully work with such patients regardless of the etiology of their complex symptoms. Considering the person as a whole—and how the injury may have disrupted his or her sense of self (along neurological, physical, and psychological dimensions)—is more likely to lead to a practical approach to treatment.

In this chapter, we—a neuropsychologist (T.K.) and neuropsychiatrist (J.M.S.)—offer our perspectives on factors that influence the persistence of symptoms after a concussion, and highlight important aspects of evaluation and treatment of such symptoms.

# INTERACTING FACTORS THAT CONTRIBUTE TO FUNCTIONAL DISABILITY

A comprehensive model for understanding functional disability after mTBI emphasizes the interaction of multiple factors. One such model was developed in the early 1990s at the New York University (NYU) Research and Training Center on Head Injury and Stroke (Kay 1993; Kay et al. 1992). In a revision of this model, neurological, psychiatric, physical, psychological, genetic, and legal and insurance factors interact to determine functional disability after mTBI. When a person presents with multiple symptoms long after a concussion, issues to consider include those presented in the following subsections.

## Neurological Factors

In considering neurological factors, the clinician first determines whether a TBI occurred. The question is whether there is evidence—either from loss of consciousness, amnesia, or alteration of consciousness—that disruption of brain functioning occurred at the time of injury. Supportive radiological evidence that injury to the brain occurred should be reviewed; however, subtle brain injury may not show up on all scans.

Next, the clinician explores whether the evolution of symptoms follows the natural course of recovery after a neurological injury, and whether the severity of the symptoms matches the injury severity. Broadly put, neurologically caused deficits will be worst immediately following a TBI and then gradually improve. Symptoms that appear late or that get worse over time are more likely to be influenced by factors other than neurotrauma alone, although this does not mean that they are unrelated to the original injury. There may also be pre-injury neurological factors, such as age; preexisting difficulty with memory, attention, learning, organization, or behavior, or with substance use; or prior concussions (see McAllister 2011 for review).

## Psychiatric Factors

Even in the absence of preexisting vulnerabilities, patients may develop secondary emotional reactions to their trauma, whether or not they experienced a concussion. These symptoms are not specific to concussion. During the acute stage, patients with trauma and no TBI may have similar complaints—and a history of a preinjury anxiety or mood disorder increases the risk of such complaints (Meares et al. 2008). These psychological factors may interfere with the processing of information and masquerade as TBI symptoms.

The presence of psychiatric disorders also is a major factor in impairing ability to function following injury, with or without TBI as a component of that injury. Of a group of 1,084 patients with (40% mTBI) and without TBI who were hospitalized after trauma, 25% of patients with TBI and 20% without TBI had a new psychiatric diagnosis at 12 months. The most common new diagnoses were depression (12%), generalized anxiety disorder (10%), posttraumatic stress disorder (PTSD) (7%), agoraphobia (6%), social phobia (5%), and panic disorder (4%). The prevalence of several disorders (i.e., panic disorder, agoraphobia, and major depression) was similar for patients with and without TBI. After adjustment for injury type and severity, pain, and pretrauma history, the presence of TBI increased the likelihood of PTSD, panic disorder, agoraphobia, or social phobia at 12 months. Psychiatric disorder, not TBI, increased the likelihood of self-reported functional impairment (Bryant et al. 2010).

*Depression and anxiety.* Fann et al. (1995) reported that individuals with TBI and coexistent anxiety and depression had a greater severity of postconcussive symptoms and rated themselves as having a lesser degree of recovery. Satz et al. (1998) found that individuals with depressive symptoms and TBI had poorer outcome as related on the Glasgow Outcome Scale but not on neuropsychological measures. In a group of patients with mTBI, those with depression had greater psychosocial dysfunction and psychological distress, more postconcussive symptoms and neurobehavioral disturbances, and poorer outcome; poorer outcome was not associated with litigation status (Rapoport et al. 2003). Similar findings have been obtained in studies of other neuropsychiatric disorders, such as multiple sclerosis, in which depression and fatigue impaired patients' ability to accurately perceive subjective impairment, including cognitive functioning (Kinsinger et al. 2010).

Depression may impair neuropsychological test performance in some patients with TBI. In a study of 63 consecutive patients who had sustained mild or moderate TBI 6 months earlier, evaluations were conducted to assess subjective cognitive complaints, psychiatric diagnoses, and neuropsychological test performance (Chamelian and Feinstein 2006). In this study, patients with subjective cognitive complaints had significantly milder injury but had significantly worse working memory, visuospatial memory, verbal memory, and perseverative responses. Depression accounted for a significant proportion of both subjective complaints and poor neuropsychological test performance; even after adjustment for depression, several cognitive problems remained significant. Herrmann et al. (2009) examined the influence of depression on postconcussion symptoms in 200 patients with mild to moderate TBI, and reported that the depressed group (96 individuals with major depression or depression-like episodes) had worse self-reported symptoms than the nondepressed group in each symptom cluster (mood/cognition, general somatic, and visual somatic).

*Posttraumatic stress disorder.* Some studies have demonstrated that PTSD is more strongly correlated with "postconcussive" symptoms than is the occurrence of TBI. In a study evaluating soldiers 3–4 months after return from deployment regarding occurrence of TBI, Hoge et al. (2008) gathered data on physical symptoms, depression, and PTSD. Soldiers reporting a concussion were more likely to have PTSD than were those with no injuries. Loss of consciousness or an altered mental state was associated with an increased risk for PTSD. Although soldiers with mTBI had poorer general health, the effect (except for headache) was nonsignificant after controlling for PTSD and depression. In a group of Veterans, PTSD mediated the relationship between mTBI and health and psychosocial outcomes (Pietrzak et al. 2009). Symptoms of PTSD overlap with symptoms following concussion, and PTSD may occur in situations in which a mild brain injury also occurs. It is important but difficult for clinicians to sort out when symptoms are due to PTSD versus the lingering effects of brain injury.

# Physical Factors

Persons who sustain concussions often suffer other physical injuries (as do individuals in accidents who do not have TBI). Many head injuries lead to traditional "postconcussive" symptoms that have nothing to do with brain injury (Meares et al. 2008). These injuries can indirectly lead to brain dysfunction and can mimic the cognitive deficits of TBI. Somatic symptoms such as pain, insomnia, and dizziness produce their own constellation of cognitive, behavioral, and emotional problems. Headaches may involve peripheral nerves, vasculature, and musculoskeletal injury. Inner ear damage can result in vestibular damage and vestibular-visual mismatch, resulting in both imbalance and distress—as well as interference with focus, concentration, communication, and memory—in visually complex situations. Patients with TBI who complain of dizziness experience greater anxiety, depression, and psychosocial dysfunction than those who do not have dizziness (Yang et al. 2007). In addition, dizziness is an independent predictor of returning to work at 6 months after injury (Chamelian and Feinstein 2004). Pain unrelated to a head injury (especially from neck and back injuries sustained concomitantly with a concussion) also can interfere with cognition. When pain becomes chronic, biochemical changes in brain functioning can also interfere with the normal processing of information. Pain produces impairment of cognitive function, attention, processing speed, memory, and executive functions, as well as changes in mood, somatic preoccupation, and sleep disturbances (Zasler et al. 2011). Both pain and emotional distress commonly lead to sleep deprivation, which reduces cognitive functioning. When sleep disturbance combines with pain and secondary depression, it is virtually impossible to distinguish the effects (until treated) from TBI. The brain is in a state of dysfunction, just not for neurological reasons. Concussions can cause seizure disorders or hypothalamic damage resulting in hormonal dysregulation, although these problems are less common after concussions than after more severe TBI.

# Psychological Factors

Psychological factors represent the most complex area of inquiry, but the one for which the mental health practitioner is best prepared. A common error in assessing persons with persistent symptoms is to ignore preexisting personality style. Overt personality disorders will predispose persons to increased psychological distress after any physical injury. However, vulnerable personality styles should also be explored for keys to how physical or cognitive changes may trigger emotional dysfunction. For example, persons who are chronic overachievers (not high achievers) may deteriorate precipitously if they "lose their edge" after a concussion (such persons often have strong obsessive-compulsive, perfectionistic traits). Persons with overly strong dependency needs may become passive and withdrawn after an injury that includes a concussion. High levels of insecurity and anxiety may manifest in unconscious exaggeration of symptoms, as well as avoidance behavior. Those individuals who appear high functioning but have borderline tendencies may become extremely disorganized, with more florid psychiatric symptoms.

A critical part of taking a personal history is inquiring about a history of abuse—sexual, physical, or emotional—and reaching some conclusions as to how the person has integrated that trauma into his or her sense of self. Trauma in adult life has great potential to reactivate trauma from the past. This is especially true in persons who have used dissociative defenses to deal with past abuse. Among persons with a history of sexual or physical abuse, emotional destabilization after relatively mild adult trauma is not uncommon and can masquerade as "brain damage."

The occurrence of adverse or traumatic experiences in childhood and of somatization in the mother increases an individual's risk of developing unexplained somatic symptoms (Craig et al. 2004; Van Ommeren et al. 2001) and may lead to a diagnosis of somatization disorder. One hypothesis of the development of symptom amplification is that there is an attributional bias toward "explanation by disease," with a self-confirmatory pattern of excessive attention to somatic signals that other people would ignore (e.g., after recovering from a herniated lumbar disc, some people become overly aware of any adverse muscle sensation in their back) (Rief and Barsky 2005). Whether due to predisposition, TBI, or some combination of these, some patients may develop abnormalities of filtering of or oversensitivity to somatic signals. In such patients, the automatic, and largely unconscious, processing of bodily signals ("somatic markers") that, under normal circumstances, guide decision making (Damasio 1994) becomes dysfunctional and may lead such patients to misidentify normal body signals as abnormal and to overrespond or respond unusually to those signals.

Expectation of outcome also influences prognosis after concussion. In a group of 73 patients evaluated 3 months after mTBI, 25% had "postconcussion syndrome" (Whittaker et al. 2007). Beliefs about illness duration and consequences significantly predicted symptomatic outcome, above and beyond depression and posttraumatic symptoms. Those who believe that there are more significant problems after a TBI have a worse prognosis (Mittenberg et al. 1992).

Also, when assessing psychological factors, the clinician should evaluate the patient's interpersonal network. The level of support provided by family, friends, and work is a major variable in adjustment after trauma that includes concussion (Cavallo and Kay 2011). Especially when psychological factors outweigh neurological factors in determining a person's level of functioning, intervention in the interpersonal realm may yield the most benefit.

## Genetic Factors

Although we do not evaluate our patients' genetic profiles, several genetic polymorphisms (e.g., interleukins, apolipoprotein E, dopamine receptor genes, brain-derived neurotrophic factor, catechol O-methyltransferase) modulate an individual's response to trauma, neuronal repair, plasticity, and cognitive reserve and capacity (McAllister 2011). These factors independently influence symptoms and recovery after TBI.

# Legal and Insurance Factors (Explanations From Behavioral Economics)

Interaction with the insurance and legal systems is a complicated and adversarial process for a patient with TBI because, unlike patients with other medical illnesses (e.g., chest pain, elevated blood sugar, infection), the patient is assumed not to have the "disorder" and has to "prove" its existence. Insurance companies typically require a series of independent evaluations before approving treatment, because the injury occurred during an accident or at work.

Much has been written about the possible effects of litigation on prolonging disability and symptoms after a concussion (McAllister 2011). Several prospective studies have shown no effects of litigation on the occurrence of depression or PTSD after TBI (Deb et al. 1999; Koren et al. 1999; Rapoport et al. 2003). However, monetary factors influence behavior, and "cheating" is common in a normal population (see Ariely 2009). Potentially, the possibility of monetary rewards could influence symptoms after TBI, just as it could influence the opinions rendered in "independent" evaluations.

Studies in behavioral economics suggest that factors such as loss aversion and the desire for revenge may influence the severity of symptoms (Silver 2012). For this discussion, we need to assume that a relationship exists between monetary rewards and symptoms, although this has not been the direct subject of studies. Studies of loss aversion demonstrate that twice the amount of money is required to emotionally compensate for a loss (i.e., it takes $2 to compensate for a loss of $1) (Kahneman and Tversky 1979). Therefore, when a patient experiences a loss of function, including impairment of cognitive abilities and depression and anxiety, we wonder what amount would be necessary for that individual to feel "compensated" (i.e., what monetary value is equivalent to "twice" the value of the loss). The desire for revenge has its own monetary and brain-behavior effects. In an experimental paradigm, those people whose trust was violated (by not receiving reciprocation in exchange for money) punished the offender. This punishment was correlated with increased activity in the striatum, indicating that the "reward center" was stimulated by revenge (Ariely 2010; de Quervain et al. 2004). Punishment behavior is predicted by right prefrontal cortex baseline activity (Knoch et al. 2010). In many cases of trauma, the offender never acknowledges the injuries that the individual suffered; this is especially interesting given that offering an apology modulates the need for revenge (Ariely 2010).

To the extent that psychological factors are intertwined with neurological and physical factors to determine outcomes after concussion, the adversarial legal process—which often involves challenge and invalidation—may worsen the patient's psychological status, and the process itself can inflate the symptoms and entrench the subjective disability.

# EVALUATION

When symptoms persist after a concussion, several things typically occur: the patient is frustrated with the rate of recovery; the family and employer are puzzled why the individual is not "better," and the insurance and/or legal system is becoming increasingly complicated and adversarial. At this point, a reevaluation of these symptoms is indicated.

## Determining Whether a Mild TBI Occurred

Months or years after the accident, even the diagnosis of TBI may be problematic. Whether or not these symptoms are "unexplained" may be determined by the clinician's "belief" regarding whether a brain injury occurred and cognition remains dysfunctional. Some clinicians believe that the brain injury is the explanation for the physical symptoms and that current modalities (imaging techniques, etc.) have not evolved to be sufficiently sensitive (and specific) to document the injury. Others believe (sincerely) that a concussion cannot result in permanent brain dysfunction and, therefore, that all symptoms that result are "unexplained." When assessing persons with symptoms in the late postinjury period, the clinician must pay close attention to the features of the original event using information derived from both patient self-report and medical records; neither alone is sufficient. Additionally, neuropsychological evaluation and brain imaging may provide useful information.

*Self-report.* The patient should be asked to give an unstructured narrative of the incident, starting with events leading up to the injury.

Patients will most often confuse loss of consciousness with posttraumatic amnesia; a person who is amnestic for an event will not know whether the injury produced a loss of consciousness unless that information has been reported to the patient by a witness to the event. Confusion between posttraumatic amnesia and loss of consciousness based on misinterpreting experience of the former for the latter can lead to misinformation, or the appearance of dissimulation, in the record (e.g., the patient states that he or she was unconscious for several hours, although the patient clearly was awake in the emergency room). If the patient starts glossing over events, or simply reporting what he or she has been told about what happened, the person should be stopped, slowed down, and asked to detail only what he or she remembers. This exploration should continue to the point at which the person has continuous memory—that is, when the posttraumatic amnesia ended—taking into account medical interventions (especially sedation and/or analgesic medication). To fulfill the minimal criteria for mTBI, an individual must have experienced at least an alteration in awareness or a period of confusion (Kay 1993). In addition, a patient's recall of actual events may be inaccurate or even change after multiple iterations, including depositions, viewing of pictures, and so forth (Southwick et al. 1997). As discussed above in "Neurological Factors," establishing the evolution of postconcussional symptoms is also critical. Clinically, consistency in the clinical picture is necessary. Considerations include whether the symptoms changed gradually over time, whether they persisted unchanged, and whether new symptoms have occurred after a long period of time (months).

*Medical records.* Although the examination of medical records is often bypassed in busy clinical settings, failure to examine these records when evaluating patients with TBI can lead to possible misdiagnosis, inappropriate treatment, iatrogenesis, and embarrassment in the courtroom. Attempts should be made to obtain emergency medical service and emergency department records, Glasgow Coma Scale (GCS) scores, behavioral observations, and a record of the time between the ambulance being summoned and the first examination of the patient. The medical facts from the acute time period (e.g., the time required for GCS scores to return to normal), in combination with the results of brain imaging, may be extremely helpful in estimating the neurological severity of the event and, therefore, the neurological basis of postconcussional symptoms. In many cases involving mTBI, no medical records of the event exist, perhaps because emergency services were not sought or patients refused treatment at the time of injury; neither of these occurrences, however, means that mTBI did not occur.

Medical records prior to the injury are useful in establishing the presence or absence of preexisting conditions (which the patient may or may not choose to reveal). Medical records subsequent to the injury may be helpful in documenting when certain symptoms first came to light (which may or may not match the patient's report). Because they evolve in a linear temporal fashion, medical records may reveal a discrete psychological episode, whereas patients' self-reports tend to collapse and intersperse memories from various blocks of time.

Several notes of caution are necessary regarding the veracity of medical records. Summary reports of records (such as independent evaluations) may contain inaccuracies, and even the original records may be wrong by either inclusion or error. Many reports continue to copy prior reports and propagate an error. The following common assumptions are incorrect: that a statement written in any record must be true, and that any effort of the patient to correct errors is based on the need to "revise" the truth. Emergency room records have been demonstrated to fail to document large numbers of brain injuries due to a nonspecific assessment of initial symptoms (e.g., not noting if a patient was dazed or confused, or not testing the patient's memory) (Powell et al. 2008). Additionally, records indicating that a patient was "alert and oriented×3" during emergency medical service or emergency department evaluations are not inconsistent with that patient's experiencing mTBI.

*Neuropsychological testing.* Neuropsychological evaluation may be useful in shedding light on the role of a mild brain injury in functioning. A comprehensive neuropsychological evaluation is more than cognitive testing and should integrate history and psychological issues into its conclusions. However, it is important to realize that neuropsychological test scores are not like an objective cognitive X ray. Test performance is human behavior and is multiply determined by factors attributable to the patient (e.g., level of fatigue), the test administrator (e.g., quality of the interaction), and the process of testing (e.g., duration, testing environment).

Including formal tests of effort is imperative in all neuropsychological evaluations, especially when compensation is at stake. No neuropsychological test results are interpretable without the validation of tests of effort. Substantial evidence indicates that performance on tests of effort contributes significantly to the outcome of cognitive testing (Green 2007). Even when tests of effort are "passed," factors such as depression, anxiety, fatigue, and persistence may affect test performance. Although cognitive complaints are common, they are not always consistent with the measured changes in performance and in fact may be due to the "perceived effort" necessary to complete a task (McAllister et al. 1999). Tests of effort can be failed for reasons other than conscious malingering; these reasons include anger, lack of cooperation, and the need to prove that one is injured (Silver 2012). One possible explanation for poorer than expected results can be found in studies of "stereotype threat," in which expectations of difficulties resulted in impaired performance (Steele 2010), even on neuropsychological tests administered to a nonclinical sample of individuals with a history of concussion (Suhr and Gunstad 2002, 2005).

Campbell et al. (2009) compared neuropsychological performance of groups of Veterans with TBI, PTSD, or both, who were screened for inclusion in the study using an "effort test" (Word Memory Test). Insufficient effort was defined as a score lower than 82.5% on one primary measure of the Word Memory Test. Although only 1 of 26 patients in the TBI-only group and 0 of 16 in the PTSD-only group had insufficient effort, 15 of 34 in the combined TBI/PTSD group "failed" this test. This study highlights the complex interaction between two disorders that commonly coexist and have overlapping symptoms.

*Brain imaging.* The diagnostic and prognostic implications for interpreting newer modalities of brain imaging—including research-quality high–field strength (i.e., 3-tesla, 4-tesla, or higher) magnetic resonance imaging (MRI), functional MRI, magnetic resonance spectroscopy (MRS), diffusion tensor imaging (DTI), positron emission tomography (PET), and single-photon emission computed tomography (SPECT)—are unclear. Many of these modalities are in the early stages of research (Bigler 2011), and for many the information required to distinguish "normal" from "pathological" is not adequately developed. Additionally, the fact that many psychiatric and emotional states are associated with abnormalities on functional imaging makes use of these types of neuroimaging studies to generate "proof" of brain injury problematic.

Not only may neuroimaging results fail to change diagnosis or treatment, but their use carries other implications that need to be considered carefully before neuroimaging studies are performed.

Two important considerations are whether a normal scan will be reassuring (if symptoms continue) and whether an abnormal scan will produce increased anxiety or lead to more intensive but unnecessary therapy. Studies have demonstrated that for patients with low back pain, no relationship exists between findings on MRI and recovery. In fact, more than twice as many of those in whom MRI studies were performed underwent lumbar spine operations than those who received routine lumbar radiographic evaluations, yet outcomes in these groups were similar (Jarvik et al. 2003). Additionally, a finding as "definite" as a lumbar disc bulge or protrusion (but not extrusion) is found in over half of individuals without back pain (Jensen et al. 1994). Similar diagnostic and treatment problems may follow among persons with symptoms in the late period after TBI, because patients may believe that incidental or misinterpreted findings "confirm" their belief that they had a clinically significant TBI.

It is also worth noting that even in severe postconcussion symptom presentations, not only is the severity of symptoms sometimes completely out of line with the possible neurological severity of the injury, but it is possible that a concussion may not have occurred at all. If the person has clear, convincing recall of all details of the events, and sophisticated brain imaging (e.g., DTI) shows absolutely no evidence of damage (given the caveat that advancing technology brings increasingly sophisticated detection of lesions), one cannot attribute the disabling symptoms with any confidence to a mild brain injury. This is not to say that subtle brain injury cannot occur regardless of the inability to detect it in individual cases, or that a small and clinically unapparent strategic lesion in neurologically vulnerable individuals cannot produce significant symptoms. However, the diagnosis of TBI in such circumstances must be regarded as provisional, at best.

## Determining What Factors Are Contributing to Functional Disability

Once the occurrence of a TBI has been established, the mental health clinician needs to carefully evaluate the factors present in the patient's current functioning. These have been detailed above (see "Interacting Factors That Contribute to Functional Disability"), and include depression, anxiety, PTSD, pain, sleep disturbance, fatigue, and a variety of physical factors that can affect mental and emotional functioning (e.g., vestibular disorder, sensory hypersensitivities, seizures).

A thorough neuropsychiatric evaluation should be conducted, including past and family history, developmental and traumatic events, prior brain injuries, and assessment of psychiatric disorders. This also is the point in the clinical evaluation at which alternate or additional diagnoses may be made. It is important to note that concussion does not exclude other psychiatric diagnoses, and that persons with preexisting psychiatric diagnoses may also suffer mTBI with additional consequences, including complication of the presentation and course of pre-TBI conditions.

Traditionally considered, both conscious and unconscious processes may enter into the picture of persistent symptoms. Conscious malingering (or exaggeration of a real injury) is always a concern, especially in compensable situations. In factitious disorder, however, the individual experiences psychological, not external, gain (something that is very difficult to prove). Factitious disorder may exist with or without a real injury, and a real injury may or may not involve a concussion. Unconscious processes include conversion and somatoform disorders. One problem in applying these traditional DSM categories to postconcussion cases is that the diagnostic criteria were not based on studies of individuals with traumatic physical injuries. Especially in situations where the patient has premorbidly shown no tendencies toward conversion or somatization, a clinician should be extremely careful in the application of these diagnoses in situations of real physical trauma. More useful is the idea that some aspects of the symptomatology may have been partly shaped by forces outside the awareness of the individual. In addition, feelings of anger and revenge as well as expectation of poor recovery may be additional factors in increasing symptoms.

# TREATMENT

Treatment of the patient who continues to be symptomatic months after sustaining a concussion requires a thorough evaluation of possible contributing factors and a comprehensive treatment plan that targets these issues. Ameliorating "neurological" symptoms should not be the sole focus of treatment. For persons with TBI, depression worsens all symptoms, whether typical depressive symptoms (e.g., problems with sleep, mood, concentration) or somatic ones (e.g., vision impairments, nausea, headaches, dizziness). The following are examples by analogy: 1) in patients with psychogenic nonepileptic seizures, quality of life is related to depression and somatic symptoms, not sei-zure frequency (LaFrance and Syc 2009), and 2) treatment of depres-sion with cognitive therapy in a group of patients with multiple sclerosis resulted in improvement in subjective cognitive complaints, although objective neuropsychological impairment was unchanged (Kinsinger et al. 2010).

The following are two concepts that are of practical importance for the treatment of persistent symptoms: 1) dysfunctional feedback loops and 2) the idea that certain behavioral dynamics can be acti-vated by a neurological event but then take on a life of their own (even when detached from the neurological cause). Chronic pain serves as a useful example of the application of these concepts: a phys-ical injury occurs and results in pain; that pain triggers psychological factors, including fear and anxiety, which then increase the pain; this increased pain, in turn, fuels the anxiety; and a feedback loop devel-ops that perpetuates the pain.

A similar dysfunctional cognitive feedback loop can develop after concussion. When mTBI occurs, it disrupts cognitive functioning in the short run. In certain individuals, the cognitive slippage and subse-quent change in function may elicit fear and anxiety. Anxiety of suffi-cient magnitude will interfere with cognition in all individuals, and this interference is enhanced when there is a cognitive "weak link" after a concussion. The increased anxiety heightens the postconcussive cogni-tive dysfunction, which increases the anxiety, which further interferes with information processing, and so forth. When depression, sleep dis-turbance, and/or pain enter the picture, the dysfunctional feedback loop gathers sufficient strength that it takes on a life of its own. Even when the neurological effects of the concussion have receded, the pa-tient may continue to exhibit severe cognitive dysfunction. This dy-namic classically evolves and worsens over time. Understanding this dynamic is critical to understanding how the person's sense of self has deteriorated, and is in fact the key to successful intervention.

## Treating Persistent Symptoms as a Disorder of the Self

In clinical reality, a single diagnostic interview is usually inadequate to fully understand the nature of persistent symptoms after concussion in an individual patient, much less to formulate a plan of treatment. For mental health practitioners in particular, starting the process of working with the patient is the only way to really "diagnose"—in the original Greek sense of "seeing through"—the problems. In the following discussion, we organize the treatment of persons with chronic postconcussive symptoms as treatment of a disordered sense of self. The self-system is used loosely to refer to a sense of inner identity, based on experience and self-awareness, that stabilizes one's day-to-day life by providing an intuitive sense of what is possible and what is not. It is that self-system that is hypothesized to break down in the presence of the various neurological, physical, and psychological events that may follow a concussion in vulnerable individuals.

*Validating the self: acceptance of symptoms.* The worst thing a mental health practitioner can do with a patient who has severe, chronic symptoms and who is convinced that he or she has a brain injury (which is usually what the patient believes) is to decide that the patient does not have brain damage and to prematurely communicate this information. Even if it is true, the patient will be driven away and have a deeper need to find someone who will understand and treat his or her brain injury. The second worst thing is to tell such a patient that he or she does in fact have a brain injury that is responsible for all of his or her symptoms. Iatrogenesis, while less prevalent than is usually asserted in court, is a more prominent problem in such cases than is generally acknowledged by most clinicians.

The first stage of treatment of an individual with persistent complaints is to validate that person's sense of self. This task is different from validating that the person has a brain injury, and language must be chosen carefully. As in any sort of therapy, the clinician must first create a trusting relationship with the patient. In validating a person's sense of self, the clinician needs to make sure that the patient understands that the clinician understands that something about the patient's sense of self has been shaken deeply, and that the patient no longer feels like his or her usual self. Until the clinician has the leverage of trust in a relationship, the patient's perceptions will not be able to be adjusted. The recommended approach for the clinician is to accept the patient's symptoms as real but to remain noncommittal about their cause.

*Understanding the self: teasing apart contributing factors.* During the second stage of treatment, the clinician involves the patient in trying to understand the self. Several questions are explored: What deficits are primary, and what are secondary? What is impairment, and what is the patient's reaction to impairment? What is the reaction of the individual's personality style to his or her own experience of the symptoms? At this point, it is essential for the patient with apparent cognitive impairment to bring the problem into the office. Ideally, the patient actually brings work assignments to the office with which he or she is having difficulty outside of the office. This is useful not only as a demonstration of the problem reported by the patient but also because of the potential for direct functional applicability of findings about and solutions to this problem. Alternatively, one can use artificial cognitive tasks or challenges. Whichever approach is used, the objective of the assessment is to stress the patient under performance demands and observe his or her responses. The goal is to sort out the patient's actual performance from his or her beliefs about that performance and the dysfunctional reaction it produces—usually disabling anxiety, avoidance, or disengagement. At the point of stress, the therapist stops the action, focuses on the dysfunctional response, "rewinds the tape," and replays the sequence with intervention.

The goal at this stage of treatment is to focus on cognitive breakdowns: when, why, and where they occur, and how they can be changed. There is no cookbook approach for doing this, and programs of cognitive exercises are essentially useless. The clinician needs to be trusted by the patient, and to quickly and creatively intervene in the moment to short-circuit the dysfunctional response (which is part of the template for more global dysfunction) and deftly replace the response with a more functional one. The goal is for the patient to gain awareness of what he or she can do to break the dysfunctional feedback loops. The patient begins to understand—by experiencing and seeing—how cognitive and emotional factors are related. The in vivo training of self-awareness lays the groundwork for control over symptoms in the next phase.

*Reestablishing an effective self: gaining control over symptoms.* As self-awareness grows, and real-life situations are discussed in subsequent sessions, the patient shifts from complaining about symptoms to being an active problem solver in approaching things differently in the environment. This transition may require the patient to control emotional responses to situations and to consciously adopt compensatory strategies. What may be counterintuitive is that this approach—because it addresses a shaken sense of self—can be effective regardless of the extent of brain injury (including no brain injury at all). When a patient has lost his or her sense of self, the need to reestablish an effective self is primary. When the individual also has neurological limitations due to a brain injury, these obviously need to be taken into account. However, in reality, when a clinician works with a person with persistent symptoms in this manner, the goal is to reduce as much as possible the contribution of psychological factors to subjective dysfunction.

During this and the previous stages of treatment, clinicians need to pay close attention to the language they use, to begin subtly to reframe situations in which their patients believe that brain injury is disabling them. When a patient says, "I can't do this anymore!" the clinician replies, "Well, you're right. You have to figure out a new way of doing this." This response operates at two levels. At the surface level, it works to provide a new approach to solving a problem. At a deeper level, it serves to bolster a shattered sense of self by suggesting, "Yes, you can do this."

*Reintegration of self: role of psychotherapy.* Psychotherapy has two main roles for persons with a history of concussion, regardless of the extent of neurological damage. First, for many patients, factors outside the immediate situation may be fueling persistent symptoms. Factors may include a history of abuse, as discussed above (see "Psychological Factors"), as well as personal factors that are not as dire. A person with low self-esteem who felt external pressure to achieve may become particularly unraveled after a concussion. Conversely, the person who has always been able to succeed, solve all problems, and be in total control in his or her life may be in deep water psychologically after a concussion with physical injury. Deeper, unresolved issues with parents may emerge and complicate recovery from an injury that causes some level of disability. In all of these scenarios, the postconcussive symptoms, as well as a curious failure to recover, may reflect an underlying issue that may require psychotherapy to resolve. The most salient symptoms are not necessarily the most fruitful ones to target in therapy. Patients often remain in therapy to address the older and deeper issues long after their concussion issues have receded.

The second role of psychotherapy is to reestablish a new, acceptable sense of self in persons whose concussion has resulted in a certain degree of permanent neurological impairment. Although this core impairment is usually less serious than it appeared during initial presentation, the presence of extensive psychological overlay does not mean that a core neurological impairment may not exist. Psychotherapy may necessitate anything from limits and adjustments in how the injured person lives, how the person parents his or her children, and how the individual interacts with friends, to restructuring of the work the person does. Separate from the mechanical changes, an important issue involves letting go of an old sense of self, and accepting and embracing a "new self."

## Effect of the Legal and Insurance Systems

The emotional repercussions of interactions with the legal and insurance systems can have a significant adverse impact on well-being. There are adverse psychological consequences to being sent for an independent medical examination in which the veracity of one's experience will be doubted—and the implication made that one is exaggerating one's suffering. The patient's need for "justice" (which cannot be adequately met) increases anger and resentment, which leads to greater depression and anxiety, and further exacerbates symptoms (Silver 2012). The longer the case lasts, the greater its negative emotional costs and the perceived need for compensation. This is a common and self-fulfilling downward spiral. The patients who do the best seem to have the ability to let the case take its course while they go on with their lives—that is, they do not let the case be their lives.

## Calming the Biological Self: Psychopharmacology and Other Interventions

The discussion of treatment of persistent symptoms has up to this point been limited to behavioral interventions within the scope of mental health professionals. A comprehensive discussion of the use of medications for depression, anxiety, irritability, fatigue, sleep disorders, and deficits of attention, concentration, and memory is beyond the scope of this chapter and can be found elsewhere (Silver et al. 2011). However, a comprehensive assessment of neuropsychiatric symptoms is necessary, as is determining whether medications have been effectively prescribed. Because of the common co-occurrence of depression and anxiety and their effects on cognition, disability, and return to work, continued efforts at finding an effective treatment must be pursued (Silver et al. 2009). This effort goes beyond the initial prescribing of a selective serotonin reuptake inhibitor, and includes appropriate augmentation strategies and the possible use of medications such as bupropion or tricyclic antidepressants. Several general principles of psychopharmacology that are important to apply to treatment in this population are described in Table 20–1.

---

**TABLE 20–1.** Principles of psychopharmacology in the setting of traumatic brain injury

---

Dosing of medication shall "start low and go slow, but go."

Employ therapeutic trials of all medications.

Establish a schedule for systematic reassessment of the clinical condition for which treatment is prescribed.

Monitor for the development of drug-drug interactions.

Consider augmentation of partial responses to medications.

Discontinue or lower the dosage of the most recently prescribed medication if there is a worsening of the treated symptom soon after the medication has been initiated or increased.

---

Clinicians need to consider a wide range of potential interventions—both within and outside the field of mental health. Relaxation techniques, slow breathing, and meditation may alleviate anxiety. Cognitive-behavioral therapeutic techniques have been demonstrated to be effective with psychogenic nonepileptic seizures, chronic fatigue syndrome, and somatization disorder (Deale et al. 1997; Goldstein et al. 2010; Hiller et al. 2003). Because many patients become deconditioned after an injury, exercise also may be useful, provided that it is introduced in a manner that does not increase symptoms (Leddy et al. 2010).

The presence of multiple other symptoms affects prognosis, and such symptoms often are overlooked by clinicians unfamiliar with TBI. Headaches caused by neck and shoulder musculoskeletal problems may benefit from physical manipulation, in addition to the use of analgesics (see Chapter 13, "Headache"). Visual problems may result in headaches and exacerbate vestibular symptoms and require specific treatment. Vestibular and vision therapy help with dizziness and balance (see Chapter 16, "Posttraumatic Sensory Impairments"). All of these treatments, at one level, help in restoring a positive sense of self for the injured person.

# Acceptance of Self:
# The Final Common Denominator

> Well, I'm less of a mess. My headaches aren't as bad, and they come less often. I read more slowly and not when I'm tired. I function better because I'm less frantic, and the diary helps when I forget. I'm not so fond of my new job, but it pays the bills. (With the kids being older, it's not as hard on my wife working part time.) We go to the mall right when it opens, and my wife and I eat out at different kinds of places. I'm not so hard on myself, and I've learned to live with this concussion.

Some patients with quite mild neurological deficits never make good recoveries and continue to rage at the changes in their lives, whereas some patients with significant impairments learn to find peace. The ultimate goal—and this is not limited to patients with TBI—is for each patient to find a way to self-acceptance, however that is defined. The primary role of the mental health professional working with a person who comes in overwhelmed by symptoms long after a concussion is to assist, however possible and along as many dimensions as needed, in this process of making peace with a "new self."

## *Key Clinical Points*

- Symptoms that persist long after a concussion may be the result of multiple factors apart from the actual TBI, including neurological, psychiatric, physical, psychological, genetic, legal, and insurance factors.

- Evaluation includes careful review of history, medical records, imaging, and neuropsychological tests. Clinicians should keep in mind that no single test "proves" an injury and that there may be reasons unrelated to brain injury that explain symptoms.

- The presence of psychiatric disorders, such as depression and posttraumatic stress disorder, is often more correlated with continued symptoms than is the actual brain injury.

- Patients may experience dysfunctional feedback loops, as well as certain behavioral dynamics that can be activated by a neurological event but then take on a life of their own (even when detached from the neurological cause).

- Psychological treatment involves multiple stages, which often do not depend on the "brain injury" as the sustaining force behind continued symptoms. These stages include validation and acceptance of symptoms, understanding, gaining control, and reintegration of self. The ultimate goal is to establish an acceptance of self.

- Psychopharmacological and other interventions often are beneficial in the treatment of neuropsychiatric symptoms, including depression, anxiety, fatigue, dizziness, pain, and problems with attention and memory, as well as physical symptoms.

# REFERENCES

Ariely D: Predictably Irrational: The Hidden Forces That Shape Our Decisions, Revised and Expanded Edition. New York, HarperCollins, 2009

Ariely D: The Upside of Irrationality: The Unexpected Benefits of Defying Logic at Work and at Home. New York, Harper, 2010

Bigler ED: Structural imaging, in Textbook of Traumatic Brain Injury, 2nd Edition. Edited by Silver JM, McAllister TW, Yudofsky SC. Washington, DC, American Psychiatric Publishing, 2011, pp 73–90

Bryant RA, O'Donnell ML, Creamer M, et al: The psychiatric sequelae of traumatic injury. Am J Psychiatry 167:312–320, 2010

Campbell TA, Nelson LA, Lumpkin R, et al: Neuropsychological measures of processing speed and executive functioning in combat veterans with PTSD, TBI, and comorbid TBI/PTSD. Psychiatr Ann 39:796–803, 2009

Carroll LJ, Cassidy JD, Peloso PM, et al: Prognosis for mild traumatic brain injury: results of the WHO Collaborating Centre Task Force on Mild Traumatic Brain Injury. J Rehabil Med 43(suppl):84–105, 2004

Cavallo M, Kay T: The family system, in Textbook of Traumatic Brain Injury, 2nd Edition. Edited by Silver JM, McAllister TW, Yudofsky SC. Washington, DC, American Psychiatric Publishing, 2011, pp 483–504

Chamelian L, Feinstein A: Outcome after mild to moderate traumatic brain injury: the role of dizziness. Arch Phys Med Rehabil 85:1662–1666, 2004

Chamelian L, Feinstein A: The effect of major depression on subjective and objective cognitive deficits in mild to moderate traumatic brain injury. J Neuropsychiatry Clin Neurosci 18:33–38, 2006

Craig TK, Bialas I, Hodson S, et al: Intergenerational transmission of somatization behaviour, 2: observations of joint attention and bids for attention. Psychol Med 34:199–209, 2004

Damasio AR: Descartes' Error: Emotion, Reason, and the Human Brain. New York, Putnam, 1994

Deale A, Chalder T, Marks I, et al: Cognitive behavior therapy for chronic fatigue syndrome: a randomized controlled trial. Am J Psychiatry 154:408–414, 1997

de Quervain DJ, Fischbacher U, Treyer V, et al: The neural basis of altruistic punishment. Science 305:1254–1258, 2004

Deb S, Lyons I, Koutzoukis C, et al: Rate of psychiatric illness 1 year after traumatic brain injury. Am J Psychiatry 156:374–378, 1999

Fann JR, Katon WJ, Uomoto JM, et al: Psychiatric disorders and functional disability in outpatients with traumatic brain injuries. Am J Psychiatry 152:1493–1499, 1995

Goldstein LH, Chalder T, Chigwedere C, et al: Cognitive-behavioral therapy for psychogenic nonepileptic seizures: a pilot RCT. Neurology 74:1986–1994, 2010

Green P: The pervasive influence of effort on neuropsychological tests. Phys Med Rehabil Clin N Am 18:43–68, 2007

Herrmann N, Rapoport MJ, Rajaram RD, et al: Factor analysis of the Rivermead Post-Concussion Symptoms Questionnaire in mild-to-moderate traumatic brain injury patients. J Neuropsychiatry Clin Neurosci 21:181–188, 2009

Hiller W, Fichter MM, Rief W: A controlled treatment study of somatoform disorders including analysis of healthcare utilization and cost-effectiveness. J Psychosom Res 54:369–380, 2003

Hoge CW, McGurk D, Thomas JL, et al: Mild traumatic brain injury in U.S. soldiers returning from Iraq. N Engl J Med 358:453–463, 2008

Jarvik JG, Hollingworth W, Martin B, et al: Rapid magnetic resonance imaging vs radiographs for patients with low back pain: a randomized controlled trial. JAMA 289:2810–2818, 2003

Jensen MC, Brant-Zawadzki MN, Obuchowski N, et al: Magnetic resonance imaging of the lumbar spine in people without back pain. N Engl J Med 331:69–73, 1994

Kahneman D, Tversky A: Prospect theory: analysis of decision under risk. Econometrica 47:263–291, 1979

Kay T: Neuropsychological treatment of mild traumatic brain injury. J Head Trauma Rehabil 8:74–85, 1993

Kay T, Newman B, Cavallo M, et al: Toward a neuropsychological model of functional disability after mild traumatic brain injury. Neuropsychology 6:371–384, 1992

Kinsinger SW, Lattie E, Mohr DC: Relationship between depression, fatigue, subjective cognitive impairment, and objective neuropsychological functioning in patients with multiple sclerosis. Neuropsychology 24:573–580, 2010

Knoch D, Gianotti LR, Baumgartner T, et al: A neural marker of costly punishment behavior. Psychol Sci 21:337–342, 2010

Koren D, Arnon I, Klein E: Acute stress response and posttraumatic stress disorder in traffic accident victims: a one-year prospective, follow-up study. Am J Psychiatry 156:367–373, 1999

LaFrance WC Jr, Syc S: Depression and symptoms affect quality of life in psychogenic nonepileptic seizures. Neurology 73:366–371, 2009

Leddy JJ, Kozlowski K, Donnelly JP, et al: A preliminary study of subsymptom threshold exercise training for refractory post-concussion syndrome. Clin J Sport Med 20:21–27, 2010

McAllister TW: Mild brain injury, in Textbook of Traumatic Brain Injury, 2nd Edition. Edited by Silver JM, McAllister TW, Yudofsky SC. Washington, DC, American Psychiatric Publishing, 2011, pp 239–264

McAllister TW, Saykin AJ, Flashman LA, et al: Brain activation during working memory 1 month after mild traumatic brain injury: a functional MRI study. Neurology 53:1300–1308, 1999

McCrea M, Iverson GL, McAllister TW, et al: An integrated review of recovery after mild traumatic brain injury (MTBI): implications for clinical management. Clin Neuropsychol 23:1368–1390, 2009

Meares S, Shores EA, Taylor AJ, et al: Mild traumatic brain injury does not predict acute postconcussion syndrome. J Neurol Neurosurg Psychiatry 79:300–306, 2008

Mittenberg W, DiGiulio DV, Perrin S, et al: Symptoms following mild head injury: expectation as aetiology. J Neurol Neurosurg Psychiatry 55:200–204, 1992

Pietrzak RH, Johnson DC, Goldstein MB, et al: Posttraumatic stress disorder mediates the relationship between mild traumatic brain injury and health and psychosocial functioning in veterans of Operations Enduring Freedom and Iraqi Freedom. J Nerv Ment Dis 197:748–753, 2009

Powell JM, Ferraro JV, Dikmen SS, et al: Accuracy of mild traumatic brain injury diagnosis. Arch Phys Med Rehabil 89:1550–1555, 2008

Rapoport MJ, McCullagh S, Streiner D, et al: The clinical significance of major depression following mild traumatic brain injury. Psychosomatics 44:31–37, 2003

Rief W, Barsky AJ: Psychobiological perspectives on somatoform disorders. Psychoneuroendocrinology 30:996–1002, 2005

Satz P, Forney DL, Zaucha K, et al: Depression, cognition, and functional correlates of recovery outcome after traumatic brain injury. Brain Inj 12:537–553, 1998

Silver JM: Effort, exaggeration and malingering after concussion. J Neurol Neurosurg Psychiatry 83:836–841, 2012

Silver JM, McAllister TW, Arciniegas DB: Depression and cognitive complaints following mild traumatic brain injury. Am J Psychiatry 166:653–661, 2009

Silver JM, McAllister TW, Yudofsky SC (eds): Textbook of Traumatic Brain Injury, 2nd Edition. Washington, DC, American Psychiatric Publishing, 2011

Southwick SM, Morgan CA 3rd, Nicolaou AL, et al: Consistency of memory for combat-related traumatic events in veterans of Operation Desert Storm. Am J Psychiatry 154:173–177, 1997

Steele C: Whistling Vivaldi and Other Clues to How Stereotypes Affect Us. New York, WW Norton, 2010

Suhr JA, Gunstad J: "Diagnosis threat": the effect of negative expectations on cognitive performance in head injury. J Clin Exp Neuropsychol 24:448–457, 2002

Suhr JA, Gunstad J: Further exploration of the effect of "diagnosis threat" on cognitive performance in individuals with mild head injury. J Int Neuropsychol Soc 11:23–29, 2005

Van Ommeren M, Sharma B, Komproe I, et al: Trauma and loss as determinants of medically unexplained epidemic illness in a Bhutanese refugee camp. Psychol Med 31:1259–1267, 2001

Whittaker R, Kemp S, House A: Illness perceptions and outcome in mild head injury: a longitudinal study. J Neurol Neurosurg Psychiatry 78:644–646, 2007

Yang CC, Tu YK, Hua MS, et al: The association between the postconcussion symptoms and clinical outcomes for patients with mild traumatic brain injury. J Trauma 62:657–663, 2007

Zasler ND, Martelli MF, Nicholson K: Chronic pain, in Textbook of Traumatic Brain Injury, 2nd Edition. Edited by Silver JM, McAllister TW, Yudofsky SC. Washington, DC, American Psychiatric Publishing, 2011, pp 375–396

CHAPTER 21

# Forensic Issues and Traumatic Brain Injury

*Robert P. Granacher Jr., M.D., M.B.A.*

**The prior chapters** in this text have focused on assessment and management of persons with traumatic brain injury (TBI). This chapter details the distinctions between the assessment and treatment of persons with TBI and the special issues of forensic examination of persons with TBI. The goals of forensic examinations of litigants (or examinees) are substantially different from those of clinical examinations of patients, although the elements of the assessments performed in both contexts differ substantially across individuals. Moreover, persons with TBI may require legal intervention for guardianship, health care decision making, or disability determination; as noted in Chapter 5, "Cognitive Impairments," these are issues that require specific assessment.

The previous chapters have also provided suggestions for examinations in which a doctor-patient relationship exists. Physicians and other clinicians are ethically required to act as health care advocates for the patients they treat and are mandated to act in the best medical interests of their patients. In most cases, such evaluations do not focus on legal issues such as causation, damages, potential malingering, impairment ratings, or disability. The role of examiners of persons within the context of legal actions or litigation is to focus on such matters and render an expert opinion on them regardless of whether it serves the patient's interests. For these and other reasons, the ethical principles promulgated by the American Academy of Psychiatry and the Law, the professional body that represents forensic psychiatrists, state that in most cases a treating psychiatrist should not be an expert witness in a forensic matter of a patient (American Academy of Psychiatry and the Law 1995).

Physicians and other clinicians have an ethical obligation to assist in the application of the judicial process and to assist courts in carrying out the matters brought to them (Council on Ethical and Judicial Affairs 1997). They have a similar ethical obligation to testify on behalf of patients when asked to do so; however, testimony offered by a treating clinician is that of a fact witness, not an opinion witness. This means that the clinician testifies about the facts of the case, including the examination, clinical findings, treatment plan, and outcomes. As a general rule, a treating clinician examining a person in a legal context should avoid issues of malingering, ratable disability impairment, the patient's truthfulness about his or her health, and other factors that have special importance in a legal forum. Venturing into these areas puts the doctor-patient relationship at risk, which is not permissible.

Conversely, a forensic examiner performing an evaluation within the context of a lawsuit or another form of legal process or legal administration should never state or imply to the examinee that a doctor-patient relationship exists. Because persons with TBI undergoing forensic examinations generally are not familiar with exceptions to the doctor-patient relationship, the examinee is placed in a disadvantageous position. The examinee may assume that the examiner's goal is to provide assistance or treatment for his or her TBI. This is not the case, however, in a forensic examination; the examiner is acting as an agent for the entity or person who hired him or her to perform the examination. The examiner must treat the examinee with compassion and appropriate respect, but the examinee should be left with no doubt about the entity or person employing the examiner—and that it is not the patient. The examinee must be advised of the differences between forensic and clinical examinations and the role of the examiner at the outset of the encounter; ideally, this should be done both verbally and in writing.

It also is prudent for treating clinicians to defer impairment ratings to other, more objective examiners, to avoid potential conflicts of interest and/or blurring of professional roles and boundaries. For instance, a proper forensic evaluation requires a determination of response bias by the examinee, or evaluation and analysis of issues such as symptom magnification and potential malingering. Performing such evaluations in a clinical context can jeopardize the doctor-patient relationship and creates conflicts that must be avoided by treating clinicians. Therefore, treating clinicians are advised to defer disability and impairment examinations to examiners not constrained by the doctor-patient relationship.

# CIVIL PROCEEDINGS

Juries are usually triers of fact for competency proceedings, guardianship and/or conservatorship proceedings, and personal injury trials. Administrative law judges are triers of fact for Social Security disability determinations and Workers' Compensation hearings. Testamentary capacity and undue influence issues are generally tried with juries making fact determinations.

## Competency

The concept of competence is extremely broad and too large in scope to consider in an undifferentiated way. It is best to distinguish between general competence and specific competence. *General competence* is widely accepted to be the ability to handle one's affairs in an adequate manner. *Specific competence,* on the other hand, is defined in relation to a particular act (Appelbaum and Gutheil 2007), such as whether the person with a brain injury can make a will, make a contract, or consent to a medical treatment.

If an individual lacks general competency, a court may need to appoint a guardian or a conservator. Competency examinations of persons with TBI are matters of great social consequence, because findings of incompetency put into abeyance many civil rights. Therefore, the court's standard of proof for incompetency is usually "proof by clear and convincing evidence." Competency usually is decided by a judge rather than by a jury, although some exceptions to this general rule exist, including contentious guardianship and/or conservatorship.

Table 21–1 lists the mental capacities expected to be present in an individual for that person to possess general competency to manage his or her affairs. When any type of competency examination of a person with TBI is performed within a medicolegal framework, the clini-

**TABLE 21–1.**   Mental elements of general competency

Capacity to understand relevant information

Capacity to understand the issues at hand

Capacity to appreciate likely consequences

Capacity to manipulate information and communicate a choice

cian must be aware of the applicable competency standards in the jurisdiction in which that issue will be heard. The clinician may need to obtain legal consultation to determine those standards. A comprehensive mental examination is an essential element of the competency examination, as are supplementary examinations (e.g., psychological testing, behavioral observations).

# Guardianship and Conservatorship

Guardianship proceedings involve application of the *parens patriae* power of the state, and protect the person or property of those unable to act reasonably for themselves (Shuman 2008). *Guardianship* is used to refer to proceedings to protect the person, and *conservatorship* is used to refer to proceedings to protect the person's property. Guardianship is a method of substituted decision making for an individual determined by judicial process to be unable to act on his or her own behalf (Brakel et al. 1985). The mental elements of general competency outlined in Table 21–1 also apply to the evaluation of the need for a guardian or conservator. In some states, assessing these capacities is the work of a multidisciplinary group composed of a physician, a psychologist, and a social worker. In many hospital settings, the social worker testifies to the judge in a mental health court or similar judicial process. The testimony required to meet the "clear and convincing proof" standard is generally that the person is unable to provide for his or her personal safety, obtain necessities such as food and shelter, and see to his or her medical care. If these capacities are lacking, then the person is regarded as being at risk of physical injury, illness, or victimization, and further testimony is usually taken. That testimony may be taken from family members, friends, and colleagues, as well as the individual when that person is capable of testifying.

If legally authorized proxy consent or guardianship can be obtained from a spouse or relative of an individual believed to be incompetent, then it may be possible to avoid complex judicial determinations. Some states permit proxy decision making, the process for which is usually defined in informed consent statutes (Solnick 1985). Unless proxy consent by a relative is authorized by statute or established by case law, relying on the good faith consent of next of kin for treatments provided to a person lacking decisional capacity is not recommended (Klein et al. 1983). Instead, judicial recognition of the family member designated as a substitute decision maker should be sought (Simon 2005). The social and psychological advantages of this designation include maintaining the integrity of the family unit and relying on individuals who are the most likely to act in the person's best interest and to be knowledgeable about his or her wishes or concerns.

## Testamentary Capacity and Vulnerability to Undue Influence

The right of an individual to make a will for the disposition of his or her property is contingent on testamentary capacity. The statutes describing testamentary capacity in every U.S. state are based on the English case of *Banks v. Goodfellow* (1870). The testator must be of "sound mind" at the time that his or her will is executed (Schoenblum 2003); Table 21–2 lists the mental capacities used to make that determination.

---

**TABLE 21–2.** Mental capacities necessary for making a valid will

Testators must know at the time of making their wills that they are making their wills.

They must know the nature and extent of their property.

They must know the natural objects of their bounty.

They must know the manner in which the wills they are making distribute their property to others.

---

Most litigation regarding wills arises after the testator has died and individuals seeking to benefit from the deceased testator's estate attack the will's legitimacy. The examiner of testamentary capacity therefore is usually asked to make a retrospective determination about the mental state of the person at the time the will was made.

Retrospective analysis of the person's mental state is quite complex and has been well delineated by Simon and Shuman (2002). A clinician evaluating testamentary capacity in a deceased person should collect as much information as possible that reflects the elements in Table 21–2. The retrospective examiner of a testator's mental state should always read the will in question to determine the complexity of decisions required and the complexity of the text in the document. Additionally, medical records before and after the date the will was executed require analysis. Work product that may demonstrate the testator's mental capacity at or about the time the will was made, as well as deposition testimony from family and those who knew the testator in life, can be informative. Psychiatric testimony, although not required in determining testamentary capacity, can be highly persuasive. It may be useful in explaining the effects of particular events or conditions on the testator's cognitive capacity. The psychiatrist may provide testimony and explain the effects of a particular mental disorder on the cognitive process, the effects of drugs used to treat the disorder on the cognitive process, or the nature of the emotional ties between the testator and beneficiaries (Shuman 2008).

Rarely, an examiner is asked to evaluate a person's mental state proximate to the time the will is made to verify that person's competency for his or her lawyer. Such evaluations are sometimes undertaken to protect wills from attack after death, particularly those wills made by individuals whose net worth and estates are very large. The examination may be videotaped and preserved as video evidence for use after the person dies.

Undue influence is a strictly legal concept, and the burden of proof is on those claiming undue influence toward the testator. Frolik (2001) and Spar and Garb (1992) have attempted to delineate the indications of undue influence. Many states recognize "badges of undue influence," including the following: 1) the person executing the will is old, physically weak, or mentally weak (e.g., has a TBI); 2) the person signing the paper is in the home of the beneficiary or subject to his or her constant association and supervision; 3) others have little or no opportunity to see the testator or are barred from the presence of the testator; 4) the instrument is different from and revokes a prior instrument; 5) the will is made in favor of one with whom there are no ties of blood; 6) the will disinherits the natural objects of the testator's bounty; and 7) the beneficiary has procured the execution of the will (*In re Will of Turnage* 1935). Four elements must be shown to establish "badges" of undue influence, and these are delineated in Table 21–3. Opportunities for exercising undue influence often arise in confidential relationships such as those between husband and wife, fiancée and fiancé, parent and child, trustee and beneficiary, administrator and legatee, guardian and ward, attorney and client, doctor and patient, and pastor and parishioner. Individuals who aggressively initiate a transaction, insulate a relationship from outside supervision, or discourage the testator from seeking independent advice may be attempting to exercise undue influence. Courts are very wary of testators who make abrupt changes in their last will and testament after being diagnosed with a terminal illness or being declared incompetent, especially if the changes are made at the behest of a beneficiary who stands to benefit from the new or revised testamentary disposition.

---

**TABLE 21–3.** Elements that may establish undue "badges" of influence

The victim must be susceptible to overreaching by the defendant due to mental, psychological, or physical disability or dependency.

There must be an opportunity for the defendant to exercise undue influence.

There must be evidence that the defendant was inclined to exercise undue influence over the testator.

The record must reveal an unnatural or suspicious transaction.

---

The examiner performing an evaluation for undue influence generally requires substantial assistance from a lawyer to gain discovery, to obtain the documents required to understand the nature of the relationship between the testator and the defendant, and to have access to interviews with or information about the plaintiff(s) claiming undue influence in the making of the will. This level of forensic evaluation requires great investigative talents and considerable time and effort. Courts generally accept wills as they are written, and they are very unwilling to overturn them without substantial evidence that sufficient badges of undue influence are present to indicate that fraud occurred in their making.

## Contractual Capacity

Binding legal agreements require the consent of the parties to the agreement. The test for contractual incapacity, based on a mental disorder, is itself a neurocognitive test. If, at the time of the transaction, a mental disorder (such as TBI) renders a party to the contract unable to understand the nature or consequences of the transaction, contractual capacity does not exist (*People v. Cain* 1999). An examiner may be asked to evaluate the contractual capacity of a person with TBI who has signed a mortgage to buy a house, or who has purchased a large life insurance contract, or who has engaged in a banking or other business transaction. If it can be proved that the individual was lucid at the time of the contractual transaction, then contractual capacity exists (*Landmark Medical Center v. Gauthier* 1994). This is a particularly complex issue that requires careful analysis, including assessment for a "lucid interval" among persons with conditions in which capacity may be transiently compromised (e.g., bipolar disorders) (Shuman 2008). It may be suggested that a person with a TBI who develops disinhibition may operate in a fashion similar to a bipolar patient who is manic, resulting in temporary compromise of contractual capacity. Overt secondary mania after TBI also may interfere with contractual capacity (Granacher 2008). The psychiatric assessment for contractual capacity following TBI therefore includes an evaluation for general competency and then an evaluation for the specific competency required to enter into the contract in question.

## Personal Injury

Personal injury litigation is treated as a tort before the law. A tort is a private or civil wrong. A personal tort is one involving an injury to the person, such as a motor vehicle accident producing a TBI. The person bringing the suit to court is the plaintiff. The defendant is the tortfeasor, or the person or entity who (allegedly) committed the tort (i.e., caused the injury). By taking a claim of TBI to court, the injured party is asking the court to provide a remedy in the form of an action for damages. Damages are compensation (usually money) that may be recovered in the courts by a person who has suffered a loss, detriment, or injury to his or her person as a result of TBI. The person with TBI may be compensated for the impairments of brain function and attendant disability. Other causes of action for which damages sometimes are sought in a TBI case include depression, posttraumatic stress disorder, and other psychiatric disorders produced by TBI.

Clinicians who venture into the legal arena in a TBI tort claim must be aware of the fundamental differences between the role of a treating clinician and that of a forensic expert. As noted in the introductory paragraphs of this chapter, treatment and expert roles do not mix (Simon 2005). The treating clinician may be at a distinct disadvantage in court and may not be well equipped to deal with all of the issues in a TBI personal injury case. For example, treating psychiatrists are interested primarily in the patient's perception of his or her difficulties, not necessarily the objective reality. As a result, many treating psychiatrists do not obtain collateral information from third parties or check pertinent nonmedical records required to more comprehensively understand their patients or to corroborate their statements. Moreover, treating psychiatrists generally do not engage in evaluation of response bias or malingering (discussed below in "Population-Specific Clinical Assessment Issues"), which is a requirement for assessing TBI for court (Gutheil and Simon 2002).

The forensic evaluation of causation, damages, outcome, and impairment determination following TBI has been described extensively elsewhere (Granacher 2008). The information the examiner should review in a complete forensic evaluation of personal injury by brain trauma includes the following: police report, photographs of the accident and victim, ambulance or helicopter reports, emergency department records, hospital record, rehabilitation record, outpatient record, school records, and preinjury records such as military and employment records. It is critical that the examiner develop a preinjury baseline of the individual's cognitive capacity in order to determine what changes have occurred as a result of putative TBI. The Test of Premorbid Functioning (TOPF; NCS Pearson 2009) is specifically designed to accomplish this task. With regard to discovering and testifying about damages following TBI, the Centers for Disease Control and Prevention (2003) provided a report to the U.S. Congress outlining the elements of an evaluation of functional status following mild TBI. These include personal care, ambulation, and travel, as well as major activities such as work, school, homemaking, impairment of leisure and recreation abilities, impairment of social integration, and impairment of financial independence.

## Disability

The conduct of a disability evaluation, as well as the elements to be contained therein, is driven by the goal of the examination. For a disability evaluation of a person with TBI, the question to be answered depends on the agency requesting the examination. A disability claim may be raised through any of three major entities: private disability insurance, the Social Security Administration, or state workers' compensation. With private disability insurance, the insurance carrier defines the limits of disability in the examinee's insurance contract and then makes a final determination of disability after the psychiatric examination. For both the Social Security Administration and workers' compensation systems, the disability determination is made by an administrative law judge. The criteria for disability under a private disability insurance policy vary across insurance carriers. The mental criteria for Social Security disability (including Supplemental Security Income) are listed under nine diagnostic categories (Table 21–4). The Social Security Act (42 USC § 423) describes specific criteria for the finding of a mental disorder in each of these categories, and provides three paragraphs (A, B, and C) that describe the actions expected of a psychiatrist examining a person with TBI claiming disability.

Paragraph A requires the examiner to first medically substantiate the presence of a mental disorder. The examination must demonstrate persistent cognitive impairments or affective changes that include at least one of the following: disorientation to time and place; short-term or long-term memory impairment; disturbances of perception or thinking; changes in personality; disturbances in mood; emotional lability; and loss of measured intellectual ability of at least 15 IQ points from premorbid levels. Paragraph B requires at least two of the following to be present: marked restriction of activities of daily living; marked difficulties maintaining social functioning; deficiencies of concentration, persistence, or pace causing failures to complete tasks in a timely manner; and repeated episodes of deterioration or decompensation in work or work-like settings. The evaluation must demonstrate the existence of a medical impairment of the required duration and establish this by medical evidence consisting of clinical signs, symptoms, and/or laboratory or psychological test findings. Paragraph C requires an assessment of additional functional limitations imposed by the impairment (Granacher 2010).

With regard to workers' compensation examinations, the criteria for disability are defined by state statute and administered individually by each of the 50 states. In some states, statutes require the psychiatrist to apply a percentage rating of impairment, regardless of whether the impairment is physical or mental. As a practical matter,

| | |
|---|---|
| **TABLE 21–4.** | Diagnostic categories of mental disorders for Social Security Disability (listing 12.00: mental disorders— adult) |

| | |
|---|---|
| 12.02 | Organic mental disorders |
| 12.03 | Schizophrenic, paranoid, and other psychotic disorders |
| 12.04 | Affective disorders |
| 12.05 | Mental retardation |
| 12.06 | Anxiety-related disorders |
| 12.07 | Somatoform disorders |
| 12.08 | Personality disorders |
| 12.09 | Substance addiction disorders |
| 12.10 | Autistic disorder and other pervasive developmental disorders |

most states use the American Medical Association's (AMA's) *Guides to the Evaluation of Permanent Impairment,* 6th Edition (Rondinelli et al. 2008), for the evaluation of medical impairment within analysis of level of impairment for workers' compensation. Some states, at the time of the writing of this chapter, continue to use the previous edition of this AMA guide. Professionals performing disability examinations of persons with TBI are encouraged to familiarize themselves with Chapter 13 in the AMA guide, which addresses the central and peripheral nervous system examinations that should be performed on persons with TBI (and other brain-based conditions) applying for workers' compensation benefits. The sections of this chapter in the AMA guide most relevant to a psychiatric TBI examination are arousal and sleep disorders (section 13.3c); mental status, cognition, and highest integrated function (section 13.3d); communication impairments: dysphasia and aphasia (section 13.3e); and emotional or behavioral impairments (section 13.3f).

# CRIMINAL PROCEEDINGS

## Competency to Stand Trial

The Sixth Amendment of the U.S. Constitution guarantees a criminal defendant the right to confront opposing witnesses and the right to have the assistance of legal counsel (*United States v. Abuhamra* 2004).

These rights, which are designed to provide the opportunity for fair trial, are of no benefit if the defendant's mental condition impairs his or her recognition of witnesses and/or communication with counsel. Persons with TBI represent a significant challenge to prosecutors, defense counsel, and judges in determining what, if any, retribution is justifiable. In a common scenario, a person with TBI has severe frontal lobe injury and the resulting alterations of impulse control, reasoning, judgment, seeing to the future, and decision-making capacity affect his or her competency to stand trial (CST).

The legal standard for CST was first established by the U.S. Supreme Court in *Dusky v. United States* (1960). As a result of the *Dusky* decision, the court ruled that a minimum constitutional standard for trial competency required that the defendant have "sufficient present ability to consult with his lawyer with a reasonable degree of rational understanding" and "a rational as well as factual understanding of the proceedings against him" (*Dusky v. United States* 1960).

The areas to be evaluated to determine a criminal defendant's ability to assist in his or her defense are delineated by Resnick and Noffsinger (2004) (Table 21–5). Examination of CST must consider the possibility that the defendant is malingering in order to appear incompetent (Gutheil and Simon 2002). Readers are referred to the section on response bias or malingering below for further details about the assessment of potential malingering. It also is critical to evaluate the defendant's reading skill (e.g., assess performance on the Wide Range Achievement Test, 4th Edition [WRAT4; Wilkinson and Robertson 2006]) and to ensure that the defendant is not intellectually disabled (e.g., establish developmental history and test intelligence). The gold standard for measuring test intelligence is the Wechsler Adult Intelligence Scale, 4th Edition (WAIS-IV; Wechsler 2008). Consultation with a psychologist is often required to determine the defendant's reading skill and intellectual capacity. Another necessity is to determine whether the defendant with TBI has dysphasia or aphasia, as occurs in about 2% of persons with TBI (Granacher 2008). The presence of language comprehension and/or communication impairments may compromise CST. If the TBI has been of sufficient severity that the defendant has developed hippocampal damage and/or clinical memory impairment, it may be necessary to ascertain its relevance to CST using psychological consultation and an instrument such as the Wechsler Memory Scale, 4th Edition (WMS-IV; Wechsler 2009).

**TABLE 21–5.** Mental skills necessary for a defendant to assist in his or her defense

Ability to work with defense counsel

Ability to appreciate his or her legal situation as a criminal defendant

Ability to rationally consider a mental illness defense

Ability to appraise evidence and estimate likely outcome of a trial

Ability to have sufficient memory and concentration to understand trial events

Ability to maintain appropriate courtroom behavior

Ability to provide a consistent and organized account of the offense (amnesia for the offense may not prevent a finding of competency by a judge)

Ability to formulate a basic plan of defense

Some jurisdictions may prohibit the evaluator of CST from exploring the defendant's personal account of the crime. Legal concerns about taking a defendant's account of the crime as part of a trial competency evaluation include the possibility that this information will be used against the defendant at a later stage of the trial or will expose likely future defense strategies to the prosecution. To minimize this risk, the evaluation should include only a general statement that the defendant was able to discuss his or her whereabouts on the day of the crime and his or her version of the events surrounding the alleged offense. If the expert is later asked to testify regarding specific information about the crime provided by the defendant, he or she should seek guidance from the court about disclosing any potentially incriminating information before answering the question (Scott 2010).

## Responsibility and the Insanity Defense

Some defendants with TBI who are found competent to stand trial seek acquittal by arguing that they were not criminally responsible for their actions because of insanity at the time of the offense. A psychiatrist evaluating an examinee with TBI who is claiming insanity should carefully review the insanity standard within the jurisdiction in which the case is heard. Some states continue to use only a cognitive standard based on the *M'Naghten* rule (*M'Naghten's Case* 1843), which states that the person is insane if he or she does not know the nature and quality of the alleged act or does not know the act was wrong. Other states follow the American Law Institute insanity defense standard, or a version of it, which includes both cognitive and volitional prongs and provides that "a person is not responsible for criminal conduct if at the time of such conduct as a result of mental disease or defect he lacks substantial capacity either to appreciate the criminality of his conduct or to conform his conduct to the requirements of law." The terms *mental disease* and *mental defect* usually exclude an abnormality that is manifested only by repeated criminal or otherwise antisocial conduct. Therefore, antisocial personality disorder cannot be used as a defense to a crime.

TBI may result in poor impulse control, poor decision making, and other disturbances of executive function, the presence of which may call criminal responsibility into question. Examination for responsibility entails determining the defendant's mental state at or about the time the crime was committed, which requires substantial investigative skill. The defendant's lawyer or the prosecutor (depending on who hired the evaluator) needs to assist with obtaining all evidence regarding the defendant's commission of the crime and incorporating it into the analysis of the mental examination.

When examining a criminal defendant for CST or criminal responsibility, it is essential to make the defendant aware of the nonconfidentiality of the mental examination. Failure to advise a criminal defendant that no doctor-patient relationship exists and that the examination is not confidential and may be known by others is a serious ethical lapse. The evaluation for criminal responsibility also includes the elements of routine clinical examinations of persons with TBI. It also is critically important to read whatever legal documents are available from the prosecutor and/or the defense lawyer, as well as obtain collateral sources of information, including interviews of persons who know the defendant well, hospital records, military records, educational records, witness statements, police reports, any prior medical and psychiatric records, and any prior psychological or neuropsychological evaluation. The defendant's cognitive effort and/or psychological bias must be assessed to determine whether the defendant is malingering insanity. Enlisting the services of a psychologist may be necessary to test for malingering using appropriate instruments, such as the Minnesota Multiphasic Personality Inventory–2 Restructured Form (MMPI-2-RF; Ben-Porath and Tellegen 2008), Personality Assessment Inventory (PAI; Morey 1991), or Structured

Interview of Reported Symptoms (SIRS; Rogers et al. 1992a). Additionally, an MRI of the brain should be obtained if one has not been previously performed.

# POPULATION-SPECIFIC CLINICAL ASSESSMENT ISSUES

## Response Bias or Malingering During Forensic Assessment

Some individuals are motivated to provide false or misleading information during a forensic evaluation. This is particularly true in criminal proceedings in which the defendant wishes to avoid responsibility; child custody cases in which a parent may attempt to "fake good" to enhance the likelihood of obtaining full or partial custody; and civil cases in which appearing more severely injured may enhance a damage award, increase the likelihood of securing a favorable Social Security disability award, or increase workers' compensation benefits.

Psychiatrists are warned that failure to consider malingering during a forensic evaluation is substandard practice (Gutheil and Simon 2002). In *Guides to the Evaluation of Permanent Impairment*, 6th Edition, Rondinelli et al. (2008) explain the importance of determining whether or not malingering is involved in a disability claim. Neuropsychological assessment standards require that an assessment of response bias and/or malingering be part of neuropsychological testing of persons with TBI in compensation-seeking cases where primary or secondary gain may be an issue (Ruff 2009).

Recent research and attention have been given to medical malingering, including in persons with TBI. Malingering can take three forms: 1) cognitive, 2) psychological, and 3) somatic or physical (Granacher and Berry 2008). The evaluator confronted with potential malingering during forensic assessment of a person with TBI will need the assistance of a psychologist or neuropsychologist. Numerous test instruments are available to assist in the measurement of response bias and potential malingering. Methods for determining effort during cognitive evaluation include the Test of Memory Malingering (TOMM; Tombaugh 1996), Victoria Symptom Validity Test (VSVT; Slick et al. 1996, 1997), Word Memory Test (WMT; Green 2000), Validity Indicator Profile (VIP; Frederick 1997), Portland Digit Recognition Test (PDRT; Binder and Willis 1991), and Digit Memory Test (DMT; Hiscock and Hiscock 1989). For determination of psychological response bias or malingering, the MMPI-2-RF (Ben-Porath and Tellegen 2008) is useful. Other instruments for detecting psychological bias or malingering include the PAI (Morey 1991) and the SIRS (Rogers et al. 1992b). Larrabee (2007) and Boone (2007) provide comprehensive reviews of various psychological metrics that are available to aid in the assessment of response bias, symptom validity, or malingering.

# Aphasia

TBI may disturb communication (see Chapter 5, "Cognitive Impairments"), but frank aphasia is a relatively uncommon consequence of TBI (Dikmen et al. 2009; Sarno et al. 1986). When aphasia occurs following TBI, however, it complicates assessment of cognition. Many tests used to examine cognition depend on language function, and aphasia may invalidate results from their administration. Because most psychologists are not trained in the administration of these assessments, the clinician may need to consult with a speech-language pathologist when forensically evaluating patients with suspected aphasia and to request assessment with the Boston Diagnostic Aphasia Examination (BDAE; Goodglass et al. 2000) or Western Aphasia Battery—Revised (WAB-R; Kertesz 2006), which are among the most commonly used instruments for the assessment of language. Cognitive examination of a person with posttraumatic aphasia might include the BDAE plus cognitive tests that rely less heavily on language (e.g., the performance section of the WAIS-IV, the Wisconsin Card Sorting Test [WCST; Grant and Berg 1993], or other similar tests) (Strauss et al. 2006).

# Language Use Other Than English

The forensic evaluation of persons whose first language is not English can be challenging. These challenges are greatest when the examiner and examinee do not speak the same language, and when the standardized cognitive or other psychiatric measures routinely used in the evaluation have not been adapted, validated, and established to be reliable in the language spoken by the examinee. Although an English-speaking examiner can evaluate an individual with TBI who speaks no English, the examiner is ethically required to qualify the examination and to state explicitly in his or her report that language issues limited the examination. A certified interpreter in the primary language of the examinee should be used during the examination. The examiner may find it helpful to use the Test of Nonverbal Intelligence, 4th Edition (TONI-4; Brown et al. 2009), a language-free measure of abstract problem solving normed for persons ranging in age from 5 to 85 years. Another useful intellectual assessment tool is the General Ability Measure for Adults (GAMA; Naglieri and Bardos 2011), which is normed on individuals age 18 years and older. The GAMA is very useful with special populations such as those who speak English as a second language or who read at a low level. It can also be used among persons with severe hearing impairments, individuals with learning disabilities, and persons with TBI. Consultation with a psychologist who is skilled in the assessments of persons whose primary language is not English is recommended.

# Dangerousness

Psychiatrists are often asked to assess dangerousness in a person who may not be charged with a crime and who may not be in any form of litigation. Issues can arise in the workplace when individuals make veiled threats, or can occur in the midst of a contentious child custody or divorce action. For persons with TBI, the question of whether the sequelae of TBI (e.g., executive dysfunction, mood disorders, psychosis, aggression) contribute to the risk of dangerousness may be raised.

An assessment of dangerousness may be undertaken in the context of a criminal proceeding, civil proceeding, employment, and other areas. As with suicide risk assessment, predicting violence risk is limited to the period proximate to the assessment (i.e., within days or a week). A well-trained psychiatrist should be able to assess a person's short-term violence potential with assessment techniques that are analogous to those used in the short-term prediction of suicide potential (Tardiff 2008). The assessment of violence in a person with TBI requires a complete assessment of TBI (see Chapter 2, "Medical Evaluation"). The analysis takes into account factors that may increase the risk of violence in a person with TBI (Table 21–6) (Tardiff 2008). The psychiatrist assessing violence risk uses these factors within the overall risk analysis. Records must be reviewed and collateral information obtained. The type of proceeding and/or the available records dictate the persons with whom the psychiatrist must speak and the type of records reviewed.

| TABLE 21–6. | Factors that must be evaluated in the assessment of short-term violence risks following traumatic brain injury (TBI) |
|---|---|

Appearance of the patient

Presence of violent ideas and the degree to which these ideas are formed and planned

The intent of the person to be violent

The available means to harm and level of access to the potential victim(s)

Past or current history of alcohol or illicit drug use

The presence of active psychosis

The presence of impulsive or sociopathic personality traits

History of noncompliance with psychiatric treatment

Demographic and socioeconomic characteristics associated with violence

History of pre-TBI tendencies to violence and impulsiveness

In some circumstances, a psychiatrist may be asked to make longer-term predictions about violence risk. The best predictor of long-term violence potential following TBI is a pre-TBI history of violence. It is well known that preinjury factors predict outcome of TBI and are often exacerbated or magnified following TBI (Ruff et al. 1996).

## Fitness for Duty

It is not unusual for an employer to require a person with TBI to have a fitness-for-duty evaluation before returning to work. Forensic issues in this context are substantial among individuals working in areas of public safety, such as police, firefighters, school bus drivers, operators of heavy machinery and equipment, health care providers, and airline pilots, among others. Other employers may require fitness-for-duty evaluations among persons with posttraumatic behavioral disturbances and cognitive impairment. The examinations performed in all of these contexts are consistent with those described previously in this section on assessment and in Chapter 3, "Neuropsychological Assessment." Fitness-for-duty examinations, however, also require familiarity with the examinee's specific job description and duties.

Fitness-for-duty examinations are objective assessments of the mental health and mental function of an employee in relation to his or her specific job function. The general purpose of the examination is to determine whether the person with TBI can perform the specific job required and whether the individual presents a hazard to self or others while performing it. The U.S. Department of Health and Human Services (2010) has listed six possible clinical judgments that can be made following a fitness-for-duty examination; these judgments are described in Table 21–7.

**TABLE 21–7.** Categories of fitness-for-duty

| | |
|---|---|
| Fit | The employee is able to perform the job without danger to self or others, and without reservations or restrictions. |
| Temporarily fit | The employee is temporarily able to perform the job without danger to self or others, and without reservations or restrictions. |
| Fit subject to work modifications | The employee could be a hazard to self or others or an impediment to other employees in the workplace if placed back into the job as described. However, the employee would be considered fit to do the job if certain working conditions were modified or certain restrictions were put into place. |
| Temporarily fit subject to work modifications | This means that if the person's condition improves with time, the requirements for work modifications or restrictions may be lifted. |
| Temporarily unfit | This means that the medical condition may improve with time, thus allowing return to work or transfer to some other job. |
| Unfit | This category describes an employee as unable to perform the job without being a hazard to self or others or markedly interfering with the orderly function of the business. If the psychiatrist determines the person is permanently unfit, this usually means that the employee will never be fit for the job and that no modification is reasonably possible. |

# Health Care Decision Making and Informed Consent

Two matters of concern are the ability of persons with TBI to offer informed consent for medical treatment and procedures, and their ability to see independently to their health care needs and treatment. Treatment providers are required to disclose all information about a proposed treatment that a reasonable person in the patient's circumstances would find material to a decision either to undergo or forgo the treatment (*Canterbury v. Spence* 1972). The scope of the treatment provider's duty to disclose information to a person with TBI is determined by the patient's right to decide and not by the custom or practice of either the particular physician or the larger medical profession (Appelbaum et al. 1987).

The capacity to consent to treatment after TBI may or may not be compromised early in the postinjury period; when compromised, this capacity is often restored by spontaneous recovery from TBI. Among persons in the late postinjury period, this decisional capacity may vary with other comorbid problems and medical complications that affect cognition transiently. However, lucid intervals may permit the obtaining of competent consent for health care decisions. In some states, proxy consent by next of kin may not be available for persons with mental impairment, and an increasing number of states require a judicial determination of incompetence and the court's substituted consent before medication such as antipsychotic drugs are administered (Simon 1992).

Demonstrating the capacity for informed consent requires addressing three essential elements: competency, information, and voluntariness. Table 21–8 lists the generally accepted areas of information that are required to be given to a patient to gain his or her consent for a medical procedure or treatment. Offering informed consent requires a level of mental competence sufficient to comprehend and judge the information presented. Individuals with severely compromised mental function after TBI may not meet the minimal requirements for general competency (Table 21–1), in which case they are not able to offer informed consent (a specific competency). The evaluation of this capacity in a person with TBI therefore requires a thorough assessment of cognitive function (see Chapter 5, "Cognitive Impairments"). The objective of such an evaluation is to determine the patient's ability to meet the minimal requirements for consent, as listed in Table 21–1, and then the specific requirements listed in Table 21–8. Except in an emergency, an authorized representative or appointed guardian must make health care decisions on behalf of persons with TBI who lack health care decision-making capacity (*Aponte v. United States* 1984).

**TABLE 21–8.** Reasonable information to be disclosed to obtain informed consent for medical treatment

Description of the medical condition

Nature and purpose of the proposed treatment

Risks and benefits of the treatment or procedure

Possible alternatives to the proposed treatment

# Persistent Vegetative States

Many health care providers today are familiar with the *Cruzan* case (*Cruzan v. Director, Missouri Department of Health* 1990). Nancy Cruzan had been in a persistent vegetative state for 7 years after an apparent hypoxic brain injury. The U.S. Supreme Court ruled that the state of Missouri could refuse to remove a food and water tube surgically implanted into the stomach of Ms. Cruzan without clear and convincing evidence of her wishes. No evidence could be found anywhere in the records that she had made a decision to have life-sustaining measures withheld in a particular circumstance. The *Cruzan* decision carries great importance and weight for physicians who treat or provide consultation to severely impaired persons with TBI who remain in a persistent vegetative state. Such physicians are required to seek clear and competent instructions regarding any foreseeable treatment decisions. In most hospitals, this information will be best provided in the form of a living will, durable power of attorney agreement, or health care proxy agreement. Absent these, a guardianship should be pursued. It is also worth noting that civil liability may now arise from overtreating critically or terminally ill patients (Weir and Gostin 1990).

# Do-Not-Resuscitate Orders

Cardiopulmonary resuscitation (CPR) is a standard medical procedure in all hospitals. In most acute patients, time is not available to think about the consequences of reviving the individual. However, for persons with severe TBI who are critically ill, the physician generally has time to consider whether CPR should be offered based on the patient's prior wishes. Also, it may be possible to consult with a substitute decision maker.

Two key principles are involved concerning do-not-resuscitate decisions: 1) these decisions should be reached by consensus, including the attending physician and the patient or substitute decision maker, and 2)

a do-not-resuscitate order should be written into the chart and the reasoning underlying the order documented by the physician (Schwartz
1987). The basic principles for CPR and emergency cardiac care have
been previously published and should be reviewed by clinicians working with persons with TBI (Council on Ethical and Judicial Affairs 1991;
Emergency Cardiac Care Committee and Subcommittees 1992).

## Advance Directives

Advance directives are generally written in one of three forms: a living will, a health care proxy, or a durable medical power of attorney.
The Patient Self-Determination Act of 1991 requires hospitals, nursing homes, hospices, managed care coordinators, and home health
care agencies to advise patients or family members of their right to accept or refuse medical care and to execute an advance directive (La
Puma et al. 1991). Persons with severe TBI may have such advance directives in place when admitted to a general hospital for medical care
for diseases or emergencies. Such a directive would provide a method
for an individual to have in place proxy health care decisions, assuming that the individual was competent at the time the advance directive was written. A word of caution: ordinary powers of attorney
created for the management of one's business and financial matters
become null and void if the person who created them becomes incompetent at a later time due to TBI or any other reason.

There is no federal input to the right to formulate advance directives. All 50 states and the District of Columbia have developed statu-
tory permission for individuals to create a durable power of attorney.
The durable power of attorney has very important uses and implications because it endures even if the competence of the patient does
not, such as following TBI if the durable power of attorney was written prior to the brain injury. A number of states and the District of
Columbia have durable power of attorney statutes, which expressly
authorize the appointment of proxies for making health care decisions (*Cruzan v. Director, Missouri Department of Health* 1990). A durable
power of attorney has much broader and more flexible specifications
than a living will. The living will generally covers only the period of a
diagnosed terminal illness.

The health care proxy is a legal instrument similar to the durable
power of attorney, but it is created specifically for health care decision
making. If a durable power of attorney or health care proxy is in place

prior to TBI, general or specific instructions will be set forth as to how future decisions should be made in the event that the person becomes unable to make those decisions, such as after a severe TBI. If a person with TBI wishes to put in force a durable power of attorney or health care proxy after injury, because this is a medical question, examination by two physicians is necessary to determine the patient's ability 1) to understand the nature and consequences of the proposed treatment or procedure, 2) to make a choice, and 3) to communicate that choice (Simon 2005).

# Conclusion

Many forensic issues arise during the care and in the lives of persons with TBI. These include civil matters such as competency, guardianship and conservatorship, testamentary and contractual capacity, personal injury litigation, and disability determinations, among others. Criminal issues that may be faced by persons with TBI include competency to stand trial and criminal responsibility, and the sequelae of TBI can bear importantly on these matters. In this chapter, these and other issues were reviewed in the service of providing clinicians with an introduction that may be of practical value in their work with persons with TBI. The difference between the roles of treating clinician and forensic examiner was emphasized, and the general approaches used in the forensic evaluation of persons with TBI were discussed.

## *Key Clinical Points*

- A treating psychiatrist should generally not function as an expert witness for his or her patient in a legal proceeding.

- General competence is widely accepted to be the ability to handle one's affairs in an adequate manner. Specific competence is the ability to perform a particular act adequately.

- The essence of competency to stand trial is the present ability for a defendant to consult with his or her lawyer with a reasonable degree of rational understanding, and to possess a rational as well as a factual understanding of the proceedings against him or her.

- The definition of *insanity* is entirely legal, not medical, and varies from state to state.

- Any psychiatric assessment for legal purposes must contain a determination of response bias and malingering.

# REFERENCES

American Academy of Psychiatry and the Law: Ethical Guidelines for the Practice of Forensic Psychiatry. Bloomfield, CT, American Academy of Psychiatry and the Law, 1995

Aponte v United States, 582 F Supp 555 (1984)

Appelbaum PS, Gutheil TG: Clinical Handbook of Psychiatry and the Law, 4th Edition. Philadelphia, PA, Lippincott Williams & Wilkins, 2007

Appelbaum PS, Lidz CW, Meisel A: Informed Consent: Legal Theory and Clinical Practice. New York, Oxford University Press, 1987

Banks v Goodfellow, LR 5 QB 549 (1870)

Ben-Porath YS, Tellegen A: Minnesota Multiphasic Personality Inventory–2 Restructured Form: Manual for Administration, Scoring, and Interpretation. Minneapolis, University of Minnesota Press, 2008

Binder LM, Willis SC: Assessment of motivation after financially compensable minor head trauma. Psychol Assess 3:175–181, 1991

Boone KB: Assessment of Feigned Cognitive Impairment: A Neuropsychological Perspective. New York, Guilford, 2007

Brakel SJ, Parry J, Weiner BA, et al: The Mentally Disabled and the Law, 3rd Edition. Chicago, IL, American Bar Foundation, 1985

Brown L, Sherbenou RJ, Johnsen SK: Test of Nonverbal Intelligence, 4th Edition. Torrance, CA, Western Psychological Services, 2009

Canterbury v Spence, 464 F2d 772 (D.C. Cir. 1972)

Centers for Disease Control and Prevention: Report to Congress on Mild Traumatic Brain Injury in the United States: Steps to Prevent a Serious Public Health Problem. Atlanta, GA, Centers for Disease Control and Prevention, National Center for Injury Prevention and Control, 2003

Council on Ethical and Judicial Affairs: Guidelines for the appropriate use of do-not-resuscitate orders. JAMA 265:1868–1871, 1991

Council on Ethical and Judicial Affairs: Code of Medical Ethics, Current Opinions and Annotations. Chicago, IL, American Medical Association, 1997

Cruzan v Director, Missouri Department of Health 497 US 261 (1990)

Dikmen SS, Corrigan JD, Levin HS, et al: Cognitive outcome following traumatic brain injury. J Head Trauma Rehabil 24:430–438, 2009

Dusky v United States, 362 US 402 (1960)

Emergency Cardiac Care Committee and Subcommittees: Guidelines for cardiopulmonary resuscitation and emergency cardiac care, part VIII: ethical considerations in resuscitation. JAMA 268:2282–2288, 1992

Frederick RI: Validity Indicator Profile Manual. Minnetonka, MN, NCS Assessments, 1997

Frolik LA: The strange interplay of testamentary capacity and the doctrine of undue influence: are we protecting older testators or overriding individual preferences? Int J Law Psychiatry 24:253–266, 2001

Goodglass H, Kaplan E, Barresi B: Boston Diagnostic Aphasia Examination (BDAE-3), 3rd Edition. Boston, MA, Pearson Education, 2000

Granacher R: Traumatic Brain Injury: Methods for Clinical and Forensic Neuropsychiatric Assessment, 2nd Edition. Boca Raton, FL, CRC Press/ Taylor & Francis Group, 2008

Granacher R: Employment: disability and fitness, in The Psychiatric Report: Principles and Practice of Forensic Writing. Edited by Buchanan A, Norko M. New York, Cambridge University Press, 2010, pp 172–186

Granacher R, Berry D: Feigned medical presentations, in Clinical Assessment of Malingering and Deception, 3rd Edition. Edited by Rogers R. New York, Guilford, 2008, pp 145–156

Grant DA, Berg EA: Wisconsin Card Sorting Test. Lutz, FL, Psychological Assessment Resources, 1993

Green P: Neuropsychological Evaluation of the Older Adult: A Clinician's Guidebook. San Diego, CA, Academic Press, 2000

Gutheil TG, Simon RI: Mastering Forensic Psychiatric Practice: Advanced Strategies for the Expert Witness. Washington, DC, American Psychiatric Publishing, 2002

Hiscock M, Hiscock D: Refining the forced-choice method for the detection of malingering. J Clin Exp Neuropsychol 11, 967–974, 1989

In re Will of Turnage, 208 NC 130, 131–132, 179 S.E. 332, 333 (1935)

Kertesz A: Western Aphasia Battery—Revised. Boston, MA, Pearson Education, 2006

Klein J, Onek J, Macbeth J: Seminar on Law in the Practice of Psychiatry. Washington, DC, 1983

Landmark Medical Center v Gauthier, 635 A2d 1145, 1150 (R.I. 1994)

La Puma J, Orentlicher D, Moss RJ: Advance directives on admission: clinical implications and analysis of the Patient Self-Determination Act of 1990. JAMA 266:402–405, 1991

Larrabee GJ: Assessment of Malingered Neuropsychological Deficits. New York, Oxford University Press, 2007

M'Naghten's Case, 10 Cl. and F. 200, 8 Eng. Rep. 718 (1843)

Morey LC: Personality Assessment Inventory: Professional Manual. Odessa, FL, Psychological Assessment Resources, 1991

Naglieri JA, Bardos AN: General Ability Measure for Adults. San Antonio, TX, Pearson Education, 2011

NCS Pearson: Test of Premorbid Functioning. San Antonio, TX, NCS Pearson, 2009

People v Cain, 238 Mich App 95, 109; 1999 605 NW2d 28 (1999)

Resnick P, Noffsinger S: Competency to stand trial and the insanity defense, in The American Psychiatric Publishing Textbook of Forensic Psychiatry. Edited by Simon RI, Gold LH. Washington, DC, American Psychiatric Publishing, 2004, pp 329–347

Rogers R, Bagby RM, Dickens SE: Structured Interview of Reported Symptoms: Professional Manual. Odessa, FL, Psychological Assessment Resources, 1992a

Rogers R, Kropp PR, Bagby RM, et al: Faking specific disorders: a study of the Structured Interview of Reported Symptoms (SIRS). J Clin Psychol 48:643–648, 1992b

Rondinelli RD, Genovese E, Brigham CR, et al: Guides to the Evaluation of Permanent Impairment, 6th Edition. Chicago, IL, American Medical Association, 2008

Ruff R: Best practice guidelines for forensic neuropsychological examinations of patients with traumatic brain injury. J Head Trauma Rehabil 24:131–140, 2009

Ruff RM, Camenzuli L, Mueller J: Miserable minority: emotional risk factors that influence the outcome of a mild traumatic brain injury. Brain Inj 10:551–565, 1996

Sarno MT, Buonaguro A, Levita E: Characteristics of verbal impairment in closed head injured patients. Arch Phys Med Rehabil 67:400–405, 1986

Schoenblum JA: Page on the Law of Wills: Including Probate, Will Contests, Evidence, Taxation, Conflicts, Estate Planning, Forms, and Statutes Relating to Wills. Cincinnati, OH, Anderson Publishing, 2003

Schwartz H: Do-not-resuscitate orders: the impact of guidelines on clinical practice, in Geriatric Psychiatry and the Law. Edited by Rosner R, Schwartz H. New York, Plenum, 1987, p 91

Scott C: Competency to stand trial and the insanity defense, in The American Psychiatric Publishing Textbook of Forensic Psychiatry, 2nd Edition. Edited by Simon RI, Gold LH. Washington, DC, American Psychiatric Publishing, 2010, pp 327–371

Shuman D: Psychiatric and Psychological Evidence, 3rd Edition. Chicago, IL, Thompson Reuters/West, 2008

Simon RI: Clinical Psychiatry and the Law, 2nd Edition. Washington, DC, American Psychiatric Press, 1992

Simon RI: Ethical and Clinical Legal Issues. Washington, DC, American Psychiatric Publishing, 2005

Simon RI, Shuman DW: Retrospective Assessment of Mental States in Litigation: Predicting the Past. Washington, DC, American Psychiatric Publishing, 2002

Slick DJ, Hopp G, Strauss E, et al: Victoria Symptom Validity Test: efficiency for detecting feigned memory impairment and relationship to neuropsychological tests and MMPI-2 validity scales. J Clin Exp Neuropsychol 18, 911–922, 1996

Slick DJ, Hopp G, Strauss E, et al: Manual for the Victoria Symptom Validity Test. Odessa, FL, Psychological Assessment Resources, 1997

Social Security Act 42 USC § 423

Solnick PB: Proxy consent for incompetent non-terminally ill adult patients. J Leg Med 6:1–49, 1985

Spar JE, Garb AS: Assessing competency to make a will. Am J Psychiatry 149:169–174, 1992

Strauss E, Sherman EMS, Spreen O: A Compendium of Neuropsychological Tests: Administration, Norms, and Commentary, 3rd Edition. New York, Oxford University Press, 2006

Tardiff K: Clinical risk assessment of violence, in Textbook of Violence Assessment and Management. Edited by Simon RI, Tardiff K. Washington, DC, American Psychiatric Publishing, 2008, pp 3–16

Tombaugh TN: Test of Memory Malingering (TOMM). Los Angeles, CA, Western Psychological Services, 1996

United States v Abuhamra, 389 F3d 309, 317 (2d Cir. 2004)

U.S. Department of Health and Human Services: Fitness for Duty. Rockville, MD, U.S. Department of Health and Human Services, 2010. Available at: http://www.guideline.gov. Accessed June 15, 2010.

Wechsler D: Wechsler Adult Intelligence Scale, 4th Edition. San Antonio, TX, Pearson Assessments, 2008

Wechsler D: Wechsler Memory Scale, 4th Edition (WMS-IV). San Antonio, TX, NCS Pearson PsychCorp, 2009

Weir RF, Gostin L: Decisions to abate life-sustaining treatment for nonautonomous patients: ethical standards and legal liability for physicians after *Cruzan*. JAMA 264:1846–1853, 1990

Wilkinson GS, Robertson GJ: WRAT4: Wide Range Achievement Test Professional Manual, 4th Edition. Lutz, FL, Psychological Assessment Resources, 2006

# Appendix A

# SUGGESTED READINGS

Alderfer BS, Arciniegas DB, Silver JM: Treatment of depression following traumatic brain injury. J Head Trauma Rehabil 20:544–562, 2005

Arciniegas DB: Addressing neuropsychiatric disturbances during rehabilitation after traumatic brain injury: current and future methods. Dialogues Clin Neurosci 13:325–345, 2011

Arciniegas DB, Silver JM: Pharmacotherapy of posttraumatic cognitive impairments. Behav Neurol 17:25–42, 2006

Arciniegas DB, Harris SN, Brousseau KM: Psychosis following traumatic brain injury. Int Rev Psychiatry 15:328–340, 2003

Belanger HG, Curtiss G, Demery JA, et al: Factors moderating neuropsychological outcomes following mild traumatic brain injury: a meta-analysis. J Int Neuropsychol Soc 11:215–227, 2005

Berube J, Fins J, Giacino J, et al: The Mohonk Report: A Report to Congress. Disorders of Consciousness: Assessment, Treatment and Research Needs. Charlottesville, VA, National Brain Injury Research, Treatment and Training Foundation, 2006

Bigler ED: Anterior and middle cranial fossa in traumatic brain injury: relevant neuroanatomy and neuropathology in the study of neuropsychological outcome. Neuropsychology 21:515–531, 2007

Carroll LJ, Cassidy JD, Peloso PM, et al: Prognosis for mild traumatic brain injury: results of the WHO Collaborating Centre Task Force on Mild Traumatic Brain Injury. J Rehabil Med:84–105, 2004

Castriotta RJ, Murthy JN: Sleep disorders in patients with traumatic brain injury: a review. CNS Drugs 25:175–185, 2011

Chang BS, Lowenstein DH: Practice parameter: antiepileptic drug prophylaxis in severe traumatic brain injury: report of the Quality Standards Subcommittee of the American Academy of Neurology. Neurology 60:10–16, 2003

Chew E, Zafonte RD: Pharmacological management of neurobehavioral disorders following traumatic brain injury: a state-of-the-art review. J Rehabil Res Dev 46:851–879, 2009

Cicerone KD, Dahlberg C, Kalmar K, et al: Evidence-based cognitive rehabilitation: recommendations for clinical practice. Arch Phys Med Rehabil 81:1596–1615, 2000

Cicerone KD, Dahlberg C, Malec JF, et al: Evidence-based cognitive rehabilitation: updated review of the literature from 1998 through 2002. Arch Phys Med Rehabil 86:1681–1692, 2005

Cicerone KD, Langenbahn DM, Braden C, et al: Evidence-based cognitive rehabilitation: updated review of the literature from 2003 through 2008. Arch Phys Med Rehabil 92:519–530, 2011

Department of Veterans Affairs and Department of Defense: VA/DoD Clinical Practice Guideline for Management of Concussion/Mild Traumatic Brain Injury. J Rehabil Res Dev 46:CP1–CP68, 2009

Dikmen SS, Corrigan JD, Levin HS, et al: Cognitive outcome following traumatic brain injury. J Head Trauma Rehabil 24:430–438, 2009

Frey LC: Epidemiology of posttraumatic epilepsy: a critical review. Epilepsia 44(suppl):11–17, 2003

Granacher RP: Traumatic Brain Injury: Methods for Clinical and Forensic Neuropsychiatric Assessment, 2nd Edition. Boca Raton, FL, CRC Press/Taylor & Francis Group, 2008

Guskiewicz KM, Bruce SL, Cantu RC, et al: National Athletic Trainers' Association position statement: management of sport-related concussion. J Athl Train 39:280–297, 2004

Hoge CW, McGurk D, Thomas JL, et al: Mild traumatic brain injury in U.S. soldiers returning from Iraq. N Engl J Med 358:453–463, 2008

Kay T, Harrington DE, Adams RE, et al: Definition of mild traumatic brain injury: report from Mild Traumatic Brain Injury Committee of the Head Injury Interdisciplinary Special Interest Group of the American Congress of Rehabilitation Medicine. J Head Trauma Rehabil 8:86–87, 1993

Kim E, Lauterbach EC, Reeve A, et al: Neuropsychiatric complications of traumatic brain injury: a critical review of the literature (a report by the ANPA Committee on Research). J Neuropsychiatry Clin Neurosci 19:106–127, 2007

Lane-Brown A, Tate R: Apathy after acquired brain impairment: a systematic review of non-pharmacological interventions. Neuropsychol Rehabil 19:481–516, 2009a

Lane-Brown A, Tate R: Interventions for apathy after traumatic brain injury. Cochrane Database Syst Rev CD006341, 2009b

Linder SL: Post-traumatic headache. Curr Pain Headache Rep 11:396–400, 2007

Marin RS, Wilkosz PA: Disorders of diminished motivation. J Head Trauma Rehabil 20:377–388, 2005

McCrea M: Mild Traumatic Brain Injury and Postconcussion Syndrome: The New Evidence Base for Diagnosis and Treatment. Oxford, United Kingdom, Oxford University Press, 2008

McCrea M, Iverson GL, McAllister TW, et al: An integrated review of recovery after mild traumatic brain injury (MTBI): implications for clinical management. Clin Neuropsychol 23:1368–1390, 2009

McCrory P, Meeuwisse W, Johnston K, et al: Consensus statement on concussion in sport: the 3rd International Conference on Concussion in Sport, held in Zurich, November 2008. J Clin Neurosci 16:755–763, 2009

Menon DK, Schwab K, Wright DW, et al: Position statement: definition of traumatic brain injury. Arch Phys Med Rehabil 91:1637–1640, 2010

Nampiaparampil DE: Prevalence of chronic pain after traumatic brain injury: a systematic review. JAMA 300:711–719, 2008

Orff HJ, Ayalon L, Drummond SP: Traumatic brain injury and sleep disturbance: a review of current research. J Head Trauma Rehabil 24:155–165, 2009

Oster TJ, Anderson CA, Filley CM, et al: Quetiapine for mania due to traumatic brain injury. CNS Spectr 12:764–769, 2007

Parry-Jones BL, Vaughan FL, Miles Cox W: Traumatic brain injury and substance misuse: a systematic review of prevalence and outcomes research (1994–2004). Neuropsychol Rehabil 16:537–560, 2006

Seel RT, Macciocchi S, Kreutzer JS: Clinical considerations for the diagnosis of major depression after moderate to severe TBI. J Head Trauma Rehabil 25:99–112, 2010a

Seel RT, Sherer M, Whyte J, et al: Assessment scales for disorders of consciousness: evidence-based recommendations for clinical practice and research. Arch Phys Med Rehabil 91:1795–813, 2010b

Silver JM, Kramer R, Greenwald S, et al: The association between head injuries and psychiatric disorders: findings from the New Haven NIMH Epidemiologic Catchment Area Study. Brain Inj 15:935–945, 2001

Silver JM, McAllister TW, Yudofsky SC: Textbook of Traumatic Brain Injury, 2nd Edition. Washington, DC, American Psychiatric Publishing, 2011

Stein MB, McAllister TW: Exploring the convergence of posttraumatic stress disorder and mild traumatic brain injury. Am J Psychiatry 166:768–776, 2009

Vanderploeg R: Clinician's Guide to Neuropsychological Assessment. Mahwah, NJ, Erlbaum, 2000

Warden DL, Gordon B, McAllister TW, et al: Guidelines for the pharmacologic treatment of neurobehavioral sequelae of traumatic brain injury. J Neurotrauma 23:1468–1501, 2006

Wheaton P, Mathias JL, Vink R: Impact of pharmacological treatments on cognitive and behavioral outcome in the postacute stages of adult traumatic brain injury: a meta-analysis. J Clin Psychopharmacol 31:745–757, 2011

Wilde EA, Whiteneck GG, Bogner J, et al: Recommendations for the use of common outcome measures in traumatic brain injury research. Arch Phys Med Rehabil 91:1650–1660, 2010

Wortzel HS, Oster TJ, Anderson CA, et al: Pathological laughing and crying: epidemiology, pathophysiology and treatment. CNS Drugs 22:531–545, 2008

Zasler ND, Katz DI, Zafonte RD: Brain Injury Medicine: Principles and Practice. New York, Demos, 2007

# Appendix B

◆

# RELEVANT WEB SITES

| Web site | Web address |
|---|---|
| AfterDeployment.org: Wellness Resources for the Military Community | http://www.afterdeployment.org |
| Anxiety and Depression Association of America (ADAA) | http://www.adaa.org |
| Brain Injury Association of American (BIAA) | http://www.biausa.org |
| BrainLine.org: Preventing, Treating, and Living With Traumatic Brain Injury | http://www.brainline.org |
| Centers for Disease Control and Prevention (CDC), Injury Prevention and Control: Traumatic Brain Injury | http://www.cdc.gov/ traumaticbraininjury |
| Defense Centers of Excellence for Psychological Health and Traumatic Brain Injury: For Families | http://www.dcoe.health.mil/ ForFamilies.aspx |
| Defense Centers of Excellence for Psychological Health and Traumatic Brain Injury: For Warriors | http://www.dcoe.health.mil/ ForWarriors.aspx |
| Defense and Veterans Brain Injury Center (DVBIC) | http://www.dvbic.org |
| Epilepsy Foundation | http:// www.epilepsyfoundation.org |
| Gateway to Post Traumatic Stress Disorder Information: a public service of the Dart Foundation | http://www.ptsdinfo.org |

| National Alliance on Mental Illness (NAMI) | http://www.nami.org |
| National Headache Foundation | http://www.headaches.org |
| National Institute of Mental Health (NIMH): Health Topics | http://www.nimh.nih.gov/health/index.shtml |
| National Institute of Neurological Disorders and Stroke (NINDS) Traumatic Brain Injury Information Page | http://www.ninds.nih.gov/disorders/tbi/tbi.htm |
| Traumatic Brain Injury: The Journey Home (produced by the Center of Excellence for Medical Multimedia and the Defense Health Board) | http://www.traumaticbraininjuryatoz.org |
| U.S. Department of Veterans Affairs Polytrauma/TBI System of Care | http://www.polytrauma.va.gov/index.asp |

## FOR PROFESSIONALS

| Web site | Web address |
| --- | --- |
| American Congress of Rehabilitation Medicine | http://www.acrm.org |
| American Epilepsy Society: Post Traumatic Epilepsy | http://www.aesnet.org/go/patients/post-traumatic-epilepsy/post-traumatic-epilepsy |
| American Psychiatric Association: Clinical Practice Guidelines | http://www.psychiatry.org/practice/clinical-practice-guidelines |
| American Psychiatric Nurses Association: Traumatic Brain Injury Resources | http://www.apna.org/i4a/pages/index.cfm?pageid=4557 |
| Association of Rehabilitation Nurses: Clinical Practice Guidelines: Care of the Patient With Mild Traumatic Brain Injury | http://www.rehabnurse.org/clinical-practice-guidlines/Content/mtbi.html |
| Brain Injury Association of America: Working in Brain Injury | http://www.biausa.org/brain-injury-jobs.htm |

| | |
|---|---|
| Brain Trauma Foundation: BTF Guidelines | http://www.braintrauma.org/ coma-guidelines |
| Defense and Veterans Brain Injury Center (DVBIC) | http://www.dvbic.org |
| Defense Centers of Excellence for Psychological Health and Traumatic Brain Injury: For Health Professionals | http://www.dcoe.health.mil/ ForHealthPros.aspx |
| International Brain Injury Association (IBIA) | http:// www.internationalbrain.org |
| International Headache Society: Classification ICHD-II, Part II: The Secondary Headaches | http://ihs-classification.org/en/ 02_klassifikation/03_teil2 |
| National Institute of Neurological Disorders and Stroke (NINDS): Traumatic Brain Injury Common Data Elements Standards | http:// www.commondataelements.nin ds.nih.gov/TBI.aspx |
| North American Brain Injury Society (NABIS) | http://www.nabis.org |
| Ohio Valley Center for Brain Injury Prevention and Rehabilitation: SynapShots | http://ohiovalley.org/synapshots |
| Traumatic Brain Injury Model Systems: Center for Outcome Measurement in Brain Injury (COMBI) | http://www.tbims.org/combi |
| Traumatic Brain Injury Model Systems Knowledge Translation Center | http://uwmsktc.washington.edu |
| U.S. Department of Veterans Affairs: National Center for PTSD | http://www.ptsd.va.gov/ professional/index.asp |
| U.S. Department of Veterans Affairs: VA/DoD Clinical Practice Guidelines: Management of Concussion–mild Traumatic Brain Injury | http://www.healthquality.va.gov/ management_of_concussion_m tbi.asp |
| World Health Organization: Rehabilitation for Persons With Traumatic Brain Injury | http://whqlibdoc.who.int/hq/ 2004/WHO_DAR_01.9_eng.pdf |

# INDEX

*Page numbers printed in* **boldface** *type refer to tables or figure*

## A

abnormal eye movements 412
abortive treatment for headaches 332
academic history 53
acamprosate, for substance use disorders 315
acceptance-based behavioral therapies, for anxiety disorders 203
accommodative disorders 411
acetaminophen
    headaches 330, 332, **334**
    older population 433
acetylcholinesterase inhibitors
    apathy 294
    cognitive impairments and 157–158
active **372**
acupuncture, for anxiety disorders 203–204
acute posttraumatic encephalopathy 139–143
admissions tests, determining premorbid cognitive function through 90
advance directives 522–523
AES (Apathy Evaluation Scale) 287
ageusia 406–407
aggressive disorders 259–278
    assessment 262–266
    definitions 260
    documentation 266–267, **268, 269**
    epidemiology 260–262
    treatment 267–278
        anticonvulsants 276–277

antidepressants 276
antihypertensives 275–276
antimanics 277
antipsychotics 273–274, 278
anxiolytics 277
    behavioral analysis and environmental interventions 271–273
    benzodiazepines 274
    psychotherapy 270–271
    stimulants 277–278
Agitated Behavior Scale 80
agitation, in older population 434
agnosias, defined 135
agoraphobia
    anxiety disorders 199, 202
    persistent symptoms after concussion 479
akathisias 273
akinetic mutism 105
Alberta Smell Test 407
alcohol abuse and withdrawal
    aggressive disorders 264
    older population 435–436
    posttraumatic epilepsy 349
Alcohol Use Disorders Identification Test (AUDIT) 306
Alcohol, Smoking and Substance Involvement Screening Test (ASSIST) 306
alfuzosin 435
alprazolam, for anxiety disorders **207**
alterations of consciousness (AOC) 44–45, 49, 50

Alzheimer's disease 427
AMA (American Medical
    Association) *Guides to the*
    *Evaluation of Permanent*
    *Impairment*, 6th Edition 511
amantadine
    aggressive disorders 269, 277
    apathy **295**
    cognitive impairments **156**, 157
    fatigue 387
    older population 434
    pathological laughing and
        crying **188**
American Congress of
    Rehabilitation Medicine (ACRM)
        Brain Injury Interdisciplinary
            Special Interest Group
            151
        DOC Task Force 112
        mTBI definition 4, 5
        TBI case definitions 44, **45**
        TBI severity characterization **49**
American Medical Association
    (AMA) *Guides to the Evaluation of*
    *Permanent Impairment*, 6th Edition
    511
American Neuropsychiatric
    Association Committee on
    Research 63
amitriptyline
    aggressive disorders 276
    headaches **334, 335**
    older population 433
    posttraumatic sleep disorders
        **381**
amnesia, defined 136
ANAM (Automated
    Neuropsychological Assessment
    Metrics) 81, 451, 468
anemia 424
anosmia 57, 406–407
anosognosia, defined 139
anterograde amnesia 44, 136
antiepileptic drugs (AEDs) 355–363
    older population 434
    properties of **356**
    prophylactic use of 363–364

side effects and risks of **359**
anxiety disorders 195–208
    assessment 199–201
    epidemiology 197–199
    history of 52
    persistent symptoms after
        concussion 479
    treatment 201–206
        nonpharmacological 201–
            204
        pharmacotherapy 204–206
AOC (alterations of consciousness)
    44–45, **49**, 50
apathy 283–297
    assessment 286–290
        medical and psychiatric
            factors 289–290
        neurobiological substrates
            288–289
        psychosocial factors 290
    definitions 283–285
    depressive disorders versus 171
    epidemiology 285–286
    treatment 290–296
        pharmacological
            interventions
            293–296
        psychological and
            behavioral
            interventions
            291–293
Apathy Evaluation Scale (AES) 287
Apathy Scale (AS) 287
aphasias
    competency to stand trial 512
    defined 137
    forensic evaluation 516
apolipoprotein E ε4 (APOE ε4)
    dementia 426–427
    depressive disorders 168
aprosodias, defined 137
armodafinil, for fatigue 388
arousal
    deficits in older population 434
    defined 133
AS (Apathy Scale) 287
aspirin, for headaches 330

ASSIST (Alcohol, Smoking and
Substance Involvement
Screening Test) 306
attention
deficits in older population 434
defined 134
treating impairments **153**
audiovisual entrainment (AVE), for
sleep disorders 384
AUDIT (Alcohol Use Disorders
Identification Test) 306
Automated Neuropsychological
Assessment Metrics (ANAM) 81,
451, 468
axonal injury 17–19

**B**

BAC (blood alcohol concentration)
306
balance disorders 413–414
balance disturbances 59
Balance Error Scoring System
(BESS) 60, 414
basilar migraines (Bickerstaff's
migraine) 398–399
*BDNF* (brain-derived neurotrophic
factor gene), Val66Met
polymorphism of 169–170
Beck Depression Inventory 172
behavioral assessment and
intervention
aggressive disorders 271–273
anxiety disorders 202
apathy 291–293
disorders of consciousness 110–
113
quantitative individualized
112–113, **114**
standardized 111–112
headache 333–338
posttraumatic epilepsy 364–365
substance use disorders 307–315
behavioral disability, postinjury
levels of 24
benign paroxysmal positional
vertigo (BPPV) 396–397

benzodiazepines
aggressive disorders 274
anxiety disorders 206
military injuries 466
older population 435
posttraumatic sleep disorders
382
BESS (Balance Error Scoring
System) 60, 414
beta-blockers
aggressive disorders 275–276
anxiety disorders 205
headaches 332
Bickerstaff's migraine (basilar
migraines) 398–399
biofeedback, for anxiety disorders
203
bipolar disorder 177–183
assessment 178–181
diagnostic assessment 179–
180
differential diagnosis 178–
179
laboratory and
neurodiagnostic
studies 180–181
epidemiology 177
risk factors 177–178
treatment 181–183
electroconvulsive therapy
183
pharmacotherapy 181–182
psychotherapy 183
bladder function
disorders of consciousness and
118
bladder function, in older
population 431, 435
blast-related TBI
headaches 326
posttraumatic stress disorder
**219**, 221
blood alcohol concentration (BAC)
306
Boston Diagnostic Aphasia
Examination (BDAE) 516
botulinum toxin blocks 119

bowel function
    disorders of consciousness and
        118
bowel function, in older population
    431–432, 435
BPPV (benign paroxysmal
    positional vertigo) 396–397
brain-derived neurotrophic factor
    gene (*BDNF*), Val66Met
    polymorphism of 169–170
Brief Symptom Inventory Anxiety
    subscale 200
Brief Traumatic Brain Injury Screen
    463–465
bromocriptine
    apathy 293, **295**
    cognitive impairments **156**
    fatigue 387
bupropion
    apathy **295**
    depressive disorders **175**, 176
    persistent symptoms after
        concussion 495
burden of adversity hypothesis 222
buspirone, for aggressive disorders
    269, 277
butorphanol, for migraine
    headaches **337**

**C**
CAGE questionnaire **306**
calpains (calcium-dependent
    cysteine proteases), activation of
    19
canalithiasis 396
carbamazepine
    aggressive disorders 276, 277
    manic and mixed mood
        episodes **182**
    posttraumatic epilepsy **358**, 364
    side effects and risks of **361**
carbidopa-levodopa
    apathy **295**
    fatigue 387
    older population 434
cardiopulmonary resuscitation
    (CPR) 521–522

catecholaminergic augmentation,
    for cognitive impairments 158
Cause of Fatigue (COF)
    Questionnaire 385
Center for Epidemiologic Studies
    Depression Scale 173
Center for Neuroscience and
    Regenerative Medicine 471
Center for Outcome Measurement
    in Brain Injury Web site 80
central nodes of Ranvier 18, **20**
cerebrospinal fluid (CSF) 6
cervicogenic headaches 325
    characteristics of **331**
    pharmacotherapy 330–332, **334**
    psychological and behavioral
        interventions 333–334
cervicogenic vertigo 399
chemosensory impairments 406–
    408
chlorpromazine
    aggressive disorders 264
    schizophrenia-like psychosis
        252
choline-magnesium-trisalicylate, for
    headaches **334**
cholinergic augmentation, for
    cognitive impairments 158
cholinesterase inhibitors, for apathy
    295
chronotherapy, for sleep disorders
    379–380
cimetidine, aggressive disorders
    and 264
citalopram
    aggressive disorders 276
    depressive disorders 168, 175,
        **175**
    pathological laughing and
        crying **188**
citicoline (cytidine diphosphate
    choline), for cognitive
    impairments 157, 158
civil proceedings 503–511
    competency **504**
    competency evaluation 503–504
    contractual capacity 507–508

disability evaluation 509–511,
**511**
guardianship and
conservatorship 504–
505
personal injury litigation 508–
509
testamentary capacity 505–506
vulnerability to undue influence
506–507, **507**
clonazepam
aggressive disorders 277
anxiety disorders **207**
headaches **334**
posttraumatic sleep disorders
382
clozapine
apathy 293
schizophrenia-like psychosis
252–253
cochlear hyperacusis 403–404
codeine, aggressive disorders and
264
COF (Cause of Fatigue)
Questionnaire 385
cognition
clinical consequences of mTBI
22–24
clinical consequences of TBI
21–24
defined 132
cognitive impairments 131–159
acute posttraumatic
encephalopathy 139–
143
domains 132–139
arousal 133
attention 134
communication 136–137
executive function 138
insight 138–139
memory 135–136
praxis 137
processing speed 134
recognition 135
visuospatial function 138
working memory 134–135

evaluation 143–147
cognitive 143–144
differential diagnosis 145–
146
functional status 146–147
neuroimaging 145
schizophrenia-like psychosis
249–250
treatment 147–159
cognitive rehabilitation
151–155
education 148–149
environmental and
behavioral 150–
151
pharmacotherapy 155–159
supportive therapy 149–150
cognitive mental status examination
**56**, 62–63
cognitive-behavioral therapy (CBT)
anxiety disorders 202–203
depressive disorders 174
fatigue 386
persistent symptoms after
concussion 495
posttraumatic stress disorder
227–228
sleep disorders 380
CogSport 451
COLDER acronym, headache
history 329
coma
aggressive disorders after 263
definition and differential
diagnosis 104
pathophysiology 107–108
posttraumatic **142, 144**
Coma Recovery Scale–Revised
(CRS-R) 80, 111, 116
communicating hydrocephalus 117
communication
definitions 136–137
headache management in
patients with
impairments of 338–
339
treating impairments **153**

competency
    evaluation of 503–504, **504**
    to stand trial (CST) 511–513
complex partial epilepsy, versus
    pathological laughing and crying
    186
comprehension, defined 137
computed tomography (CT)
    day-of-injury 11, **13**, 51
    disorders of consciousness 115
    medical evaluation 64
    older population 429
    posttraumatic epilepsy 348, 355
    TBI severity characterization
    **49**
computerized neuropsychological
    assessment 88–89
concussions
    anatomy of 8
    mTBI versus 4
conductive hearing loss 405–406
Congressionally Directed Medical
    Research Program 471
conservatorship proceedings 504–
    505
consolidation, defined 135
contractual capacity 507–508
convergence insufficiency 411
cortical blindness 413
cortical spreading depression 328
corticosteroid increases,
    posttraumatic stress disorder and
    217
corticotropin-releasing hormone
    (CRH), posttraumatic stress
    disorder and 217
countertransferences 271
CPR (cardiopulmonary
    resuscitation) 521–522
CRAFFT questionnaire 306
cranial electrotherapy stimulation
    (CES)
    apathy 296
    posttraumatic sleep disorders
    383–384
cranial fossae 5, 8
creatine, for fatigue 388

CRH (corticotropin-releasing
    hormone), posttraumatic stress
    disorder and 217
CRI (HeadMinder Concussion
    Resolution Index) 451
criminal proceedings
    competency to stand trial 511–
    513
    criminal responsibility 513–515
    insanity defense 513–515
criminal responsibility 513–515
CRS-R (Coma Recovery Scale–
    Revised) 80, 111, 116
CSF (cerebrospinal fluid) 6
CST (competency to stand trial)
    511–513
cupulolithiasis 396
CYP450 (cytochrome P450) enzyme
    inhibitors 175
cytidine diphosphate choline
    (citicholine), for cognitive
    impairments **157**, 158

**D**
D-amphetamine, for apathy 293
dangerousness assessment 517–518,
    **518**
declarative memory
    defined 135
    treating impairments 150
deep brain stimulation (DBS), for
    disorders of consciousness 121
Defense and Veterans Brain Injury
    Center (DVBIC) 461
    posttraumatic stress disorder
    225, 227
    Traumatic Brain Injury Clinic
    469
Defense Centers of Excellence for
    Psychological Health and
    Traumatic Brain Injury 470
dementia
    APOPE4 and 426–427
    TBI as factor in onset of 26
Department of Defense (DoD) 470
    TBI case definitions 44
    TBI severity characterization **49**

Department of Veterans Affairs
(VA) 470
TBI assessment 465
TBI case definitions 44
TBI severity characterization
**49**
depressive disorders 168–177
assessment
diagnostic assessment 172–
173
differential diagnosis 170–
172
laboratory and
neurodiagnostic
studies 173
epidemiology 168
history of 52
persistent symptoms after
concussion 478–479
postinjury levels of 24
risk factors 168–170
injury-related
neurobiological
factors 169–170
neurogenetics 168–169
postinjury psychosocial
factors 170
preinjury personal and
psychosocial
factors 169
treatment
electroconvulsive therapy
176–177
pharmacotherapy 174–176
psychotherapy 173–174
described 134
desipramine, for depressive
disorders **175**
detrusor-sphincter dyssynergia 118
dextroamphetamine
apathy **295**
cognitive impairments and **156**
depressive disorders **175**, 176
fatigue 387
dextromethorphan, for
pathological laughing and crying
188, **188**

*Diagnostic and Statistical Manual of
Mental Disorders,* 4th Edition, Text
Revision (DSM-IV-TR)
aggressive disorders 262, **263**,
276
anxiety disorders 200
apathy 284
personality changes **263**
posttraumatic stress disorder
213, **214**, 215, 222
substance use disorders 304,
**305**
diffusion tensor imaging (DTI) 13,
**14**, **15**, **16**
disorders of consciousness 115
medical evaluation 64
Digit Memory Test (DMT) 516
digoxin, aggressive disorders and
264
diminished motivation 26
diplopia 410–411
disability
clinical consequences of TBI 26
economic burden of TBI-
related 26
evaluation of 509–511, **511**
rates of TBI-related 26
disorders of consciousness (DOC)
103–124
assessment 110–117
behavioral 110–113, **114**
electrophysiological 113–
115
neuroimaging 115–116
definitions and differential
diagnosis
coma 104
locked-in syndrome 106
minimally conscious state
105
posttraumatic confusional
state 105–106
vegetative state 104
epidemiology 106–107
pathophysiology 107–108
prognosis 108–110
treatment 117–123

disorders of consciousness (DOC)
(continued)
    environmental 119–120
    family support and care
        planning 121–123
    future of 123
    health maintenance 117–119
    neuromodulation 120–121
    recovery enhancement 119
disorders of mood and affect
    schizophrenia-like psychosis
        248
disorientation 136
disulfiram, for substance use
    disorders 315
divalproex sodium, for migraine
    headaches **335, 337**
divergence paralysis 411
DMT (Digit Memory Test) 516
donepezil
    apathy 294, **295**
    cognitive impairments **157**
do-not-resuscitate (DNR) status
    disorders of consciousness and
        122
    orders 521–522
dopamine decreases, aggressive
    disorders and 274
doxazosin 435
durable medical powers of attorney
    522–523
dysarthria, defined 137
dysautonomia, disorders of
    consciousness and 118
dysfunctional feedback loops 490,
    492
dysgeusia 406–407
dysphagia, in older population
    424
dysphasia, competency to stand trial
    and 512

**E**
early seizures 346
educational contexts,
    neuropsychological assessment in
    76

effort (validity) assessment 82, 90–91
electroconvulsive therapy (ECT)
    depressive disorders 176–177
    mania, mixed mood episodes,
        and bipolar disorder
        183
electroencephalography (EEG) 65–
    66
    depressive disorders 173
    disorders of consciousness 113–
        115
    interictal 65
    manic and mixed mood
        episodes 180
    posttraumatic epilepsy 350–354
    seizures 350–354
electronystagmography (ENG), for
    vestibular disorders 400
electrophysiological assessment 65–
    66
encephalopathy, defined 140
encoding, defined 135
endocrine disturbances and
    dysfunction 26
    disorders of consciousness and
        117
end-of-life care
    advance directives 522–523
    disorders of consciousness and
        122–123
    do-not-resuscitate orders 521–
        522
ENG (electronystagmography), for
    vestibular disorders 400
environmental enrichment, for
    posttraumatic stress disorder 231
epilepsy
    aggressive disorders and 266
    schizophrenia-like psychosis
        and 250–251, 253
EPs (evoked potentials) 65
ergotamines, for migraine
    headaches **336, 337**
ERPs (event-related potentials) 65
escitalopram
    aggressive disorders 276
    depressive disorders **175**

pathological laughing and crying **188**

essential crying, pathological laughing and crying versus 186

eszopiclone, for anxiety disorders **207**

European Federation of Neurological Societies Task Force on Cognitive Rehabilitation 151

event-related disturbances of consciousness 44–46, **47**

event-related potentials (ERPs) 65

evoked potentials (EPs) 65

executive function
    defined 76, 138
    treating impairments **154**

eye movement disturbances 57

**F**

FA (fractional anisotropy) 14

falls, older population 427–428

falx cerebri 6

family support
    aggressive disorders 266
    depressive disorders 174
    disorders of consciousness 121–123
    older population 432

fatigue 371–372, 384–390
    evaluation 385
    nonpharmacological treatment 386
        diet and lifestyle 386, **386**
        education 386
        psychotherapy 386
    pathophysiology 384–385
    pharmacotherapy 387–388
        amantadine 387
        dopamine agonists 387
        modafinil 387–388
        stimulants 387

Fatigue Impact Scale (FIS) 385

Fatigue Severity Scale (FSS) 385

feeding tubes, disorders of consciousness and 118

fitness-for-duty evaluations 518–519, **519**

5HTT (serotonin transporter gene), polymorphisms of 168–170

fixed battery approaches to neuropsychological assessment 82

flexible battery approaches to neuropsychological assessment 82

fluency, defined 136

fluoxetine
    aggressive disorders 276
    anxiety disorders 205
    depressive disorders 175, **175**
    pathological laughing and crying **188**

forensic evaluation 501–523
    advance directives 522–523
    aphasia 516
    civil proceedings 503–511
        competency 503–504, **504**
        contractual capacity 507–508
        disability evaluation 509–511, **511**
        guardianship and conservatorship 504–505
        personal injury litigation 508–509
        testamentary capacity 505–506
        vulnerability to undue influence 506–507, **507**
    criminal proceedings 511–515
        competency to stand trial 511–513
        criminal responsibility 513–515
        insanity defense 513–515
    dangerousness 517–518, **518**
    do-not-resuscitate orders 521–522
    fitness for duty 518–519, **519**

forensic evaluation *(continued)*
    health care decision making
        519–520
    informed consent 519–520,
        **521**
    malingering 515–516
    neuropsychological assessment
        76, 81–82
    persistent vegetative state 521
    response bias 515–516
    when primary language is not
        English 516–517
four-quadrant model, substance use
    disorders 307–314
fractional anisotropy (FA) 14
FRAMES model of intervention
    308, **309**
FSS (Fatigue Severity Scale) 385
functional MRI (fMRI) 64
    disorders of consciousness 115
functional status 43
furosemide, aggressive disorders
    and 264


**G**

gabapentin
    anxiety disorders 205
    posttraumatic epilepsy **357**
    side effects and risks of **360**
GAD-7 (Generalized Anxiety
    Disorder 7-item) scale 200
galantamine, for apathy 294, **295**
Galveston Orientation and Amnesia
    Test (GOAT) 48, 80
gaze paresis 411–412
GCS (Glasgow Coma Scale),
    determining TBI severity 4, **6**, 48,
    **49**
gegenhalten 59
General Ability Measure for Adults
    (GAMA) 517
general competence 503–504, **504**
generalized anxiety disorder (GAD)
    **198**, 199, 202–203
    persistent symptoms after
        concussion 478
    postinjury levels of 24

Generalized Anxiety Disorder 7-
    item (GAD-7) scale 200
generalized cerebral atrophy 12, **14**
Glasgow Coma Scale (GCS),
    determining TBI severity 4, 6, 48,
    49
glucocorticoids, for posttraumatic
    epilepsy 364
GOAT (Galveston Orientation and
    Amnesia Test) 48, 80
guardianship proceedings 504–505
gustatory impairments 406–408, **409**


**H**

haloperidol, for aggressive
    disorders 269, 273
Halstead-Reitan
    Neuropsychological Test Battery
    82
Hamilton Rating Scale for
    Depression 172
headache 323–340
    assessment 328–330
    characteristics of **331**
    definitions 324–325
    epidemiology 325–327
    military injuries 467
    pathophysiology 327–328
    patients with communication
        impairments 338–339
    persistent symptoms after
        concussion 480, 495
    treatment 330–338
        pharmacotherapy 330–
            333, **334, 335, 336,
            337**
        psychological and
            behavioral
            interventions
            333–338
HeadMinder Concussion
    Resolution Index (CRI) 451
health and treatment history **38**,
    51–53
health care decision making 519–
    520
health care proxies 522–523

hearing impairments 404–406
history **36**, 37–46
 health and treatment **38**, 51–53
 injury **38**, 44–46
 of abuse 481–482
 of present illness **38**, 40–44
 social and family **39**, 53–54
 taking 37–40
human immunodeficiency virus
 (HIV) screening
 depressive disorders 173
 manic and mixed mood
   episodes 181
hyperacusis 402–404
hypersomnia 376–377
hypertonia, disorders of
 consciousness and 118
hyposmia 57, 406–407
hypothesis generation 44

**I**
iatrogenesis 491
ibuprofen, for headaches **334**
ICD-10 (*International Statistical
 Classification of Diseases and Related
 Health Problems,* 10th Revision)
 304, **305**
ictal vertigo 398
ICU (intensive care unit), older
 population 430, 437
ideational praxis, defined 137
ideomotor praxis, defined 137
IEDs (interictal epileptiform
 discharges) 350–354
Immediate Post-concussion
 Assessment and Cognitive Testing
 (ImPACT) 451
immediate seizures 346
impairment, defined 63
inattention, defined 134
informants 39, 40
informed consent 519–520, **521**
injury history **36**, **38**, 44–46
innate relative weakness, brain
 impairment versus 91–92
insanity defense 513–515
insight, defined 138–139

insomnia 375–376
intellectual disabilities 24, 53
intelligence tests, determining
 premorbid cognitive function
 through 90
intensive care unit (ICU), older
 population 430, 437
interictal epileptiform discharges
 (IEDs) 350–354
*International Statistical Classification
 of Diseases and Related Health
 Problems,* 10th Revision (ICD-10)
 304, 305
internuclear ophthalmoplegia 411–
 412
interview styles 37–39
intrathecal baclofen, disorders of
 consciousness and 118

**J**
Jastreboff Tinnitus Retraining
 Therapy 401

**K**
ketorolac, for migraine headaches
 **337**
kinesics, defined 137
King-Devick test 57

**L**
laboratory tests 66
labyrinthine concussion 397
lacosamide
 posttraumatic epilepsy **357**
 side effects and risks of **360**
lamotrigine
 aggressive disorders 276
 pathological laughing and
  crying 188, **188**
 posttraumatic epilepsy **356**
 side effects and risks of **359**
language
 defined 136
 when primary language is not
  English 516–517
late seizures 346

legal history 54
legal issues
    effect on self-system 494
    persistent symptoms after
            concussion 483–484
    schizophrenia-like psychosis 253
levetiracetam
    older population 434
    posttraumatic epilepsy **357**
    side effects and risks of **360**
limb-kinetic praxis, defined 137
lithium
    aggressive disorders 277
    manic and mixed mood
            episodes 181–182, **182**
locked-in syndrome (LIS)
    definition and differential
            diagnosis 106
    pathophysiology 108
locomotor disability, postinjury
    levels of 24
lorazepam
    anxiety disorders **207**
    headaches **334**
    posttraumatic sleep disorders
        382
loss aversion 483–484
loss of consciousness (LOC) 44, **49**,
    50
    posttraumatic amnesia versus
        485
loss of smell 57

**M**
M'Naghten rule 513
MACE (Military Acute Concussion
    Evaluation) 463, 468
macroscopic injury 4–8
magnetic resonance imaging (MRI)
    cognitive impairments and 145
    disorders of consciousness 115
    generalized cerebral atrophy
        12, **14**
    medical evaluation 64
    older population 429
    posttraumatic epilepsy 355
    TBI severity characterization **49**

magnetic resonance spectroscopy
    (MRS) 64
magnetoencephalography (MEG) 65
malingering 515–516
    competency to stand trial 512
Management of Concussion–Mild
    Traumatic Brain Injury Working
    Group, Clinical Practice
    Guidelines for Mild TBI 78
mania 177–183
    assessment 178–181
        diagnostic assessment 179–
            181
        differential diagnosis 178–
            179
        laboratory and
            neurodiagnostic
            studies 180–181
    contractual capacity **508**
    epidemiology 177
    risk factors 177–178
    treatment 181–183
        electroconvulsive therapy
            183
        pharmacotherapy 181–182
        psychotherapy 183
medical evaluation 35–67
    examination 55–63
        mental status **56**, 60–63
        neurological 57–60
        physical 55, **56**
    history 37–54
        health and treatment **38**,
            51–53
        injury **38**, 44–46
        of present illness **38**, 40–44
        social and family **39**, 53–54
        taking 37–40
    neurodiagnostic studies **56**, 64–
        66
        electrophysiological
            assessments 65–66
        laboratory tests 66
        neuroimaging 64–65
        neuropsychological
            evaluation 66
    review of systems **39**, 54–55

severity characterization 46–51
  day-of-injury
    neuroimaging 51
  prospective serial
    assessments 47–50
  retrospective assessments
    50–51
medical records, evaluation of 485–486
Medicare 426
medication allergies and
  sensitivities 52
MEG (magnetoencephalography)
  65
melatonin, for posttraumatic sleep
  disorders **381**, 383
memory
  definitions 135–136
  posttraumatic stress disorder
    and 227
  treating impairments **153**
meninges 5
mental flexibility, defined 138
mental status examination **56**, 60–63
  cognitive 62–63
  general 60–62
methylene tetrahydrofolate reductase
  gene (MTHFR), C677T
  polymorphism of 169–170
methylphenidate
  aggressive disorders 269, 277
  apathy 293–294, **295**
  cognitive impairments **156**, 158
  depressive disorders **175**, 176
  disorders of consciousness 120
  fatigue 387
  older population 434
  pathological laughing and
    crying 187, **188**
methysergide, for migraine
  headaches **335**
microscopic injury 17–21
microtubule damage 19
migraine headaches 325
  characteristics of **331**
  pathophysiology 328

pharmacotherapy 332–333,
  **335, 336, 337**
psychological and behavioral
  interventions 334–338
vestibular disorders and 398–399
mild TBI (mTBI)
  attentional, memory, and
    executive functions 76
  cognitive consequences of 22–24
  cognitive impairments 148
  concussions versus 4
  defined 4, 5
  emotional changes 77
  headaches 326
  neuroimaging 24, **25**
  neuropsychological screening
    evaluation 87
  posttraumatic stress disorder
    219, 220–227
  postural instability 413–414
  sleep disorders 374, 375–376
  timing of neuropsychological
    assessment 78–79
Military Acute Concussion
  Evaluation (MACE) 463, 468
military history 53
military personnel and veterans
  461–471
  assessment 464–465
  civilian TBI versus 462–463
  epidemiology 463–464
  headaches 326–327, 338
  neuropsychological assessment
    81
  posttraumatic stress disorder
    199, 220–222, 225–227
  research 470–471
  resources for 469–470
  return-to-duty decision 468–469
  schizophrenia 241
  treatment 465–468
mindfulness (meditation training),
  for anxiety disorders 202
Mini-International
  Neuropsychiatric Interview
  (MINI) 52

minimally conscious state (MCS)
    definition and differential
        diagnosis 105
    epidemiology 106–107
    neuroimaging 116
    neuromodulation treatments
        121
    pathophysiology 108
    prognosis 109
Mini-Mental State Examination
    (MMSE) 63
Minnesota Multiphasic Personality
    Inventory-2–Restructured Form
    (MMPI-2-RF) 514, 516
minocycline, for olfactory
    impairments 408
mirtazapine
    depressive disorders 175
    pathological laughing and
        crying 188
    posttraumatic sleep disorders
        380
mitgehen 59
mixed migraine tension headaches
    325
mixed mood episodes 177–183
    assessment 178–181
        diagnostic assessment
            179–180
        differential diagnosis
            178–179
        laboratory and
            neurodiagnostic
            studies 180–181
    epidemiology 177
    risk factors 177–178
    treatment 181–183
        electroconvulsive therapy
            183
        pharmacotherapy 181–
            182
        psychotherapy 183
MMPI-2–RF (Minnesota
    Multiphasic Personality
    Inventory-2–Restructured Form)
    514, 516

MMSE (Mini-Mental State
    Examination) 63
modafinil
    apathy 295
    cognitive impairments and
        156
    fatigue 387–388
    older population 434
    posttraumatic sleep disorders
        381, 382
monitoring, defined 138
monoamine oxidase inhibitors
    (MAOIs)
    apathy 294
    depressive disorders 176
mood and affect disorders 167–189
    depressive disorders 168–177
        assessment 170–173
        epidemiology 168
        risk factors 168–170
        treatment 173–177
    mania, mixed mood episodes,
        and bipolar disorder
        177–183
        assessment 178–181
        epidemiology 177
        risk factors 177–178
        treatment 181–183
    older population 434–435
    pathological laughing and
        crying 183–189
        assessment 185–187
        epidemiology 183–184
        risk factors 185
        treatment 187–189
morphine sulfate, for migraine
    headaches 337
motor vehicle crashes, older
    population 428
MRS (magnetic resonance
    spectroscopy) 64
MTHFR (methylene
    tetrahydrofolate reductase gene),
    C677T polymorphism of 169–170
Multiple Sleep Latency Test (MSLT)
    374, 376

## N

nadolol, for aggressive disorders 275
naltrexone, for substance use
  disorders 315
naming, defined 136
narcolepsy 376–377, 383
National Athletic Trainers'
  Association 455
National Collegiate Athletic
  Association Concussion
  Committee 455
National Institute of Alcoholism and
  Alcohol Abuse 304, **306**, 315
Nav1.6 Na+ channels 18
Neurobehavioral Functioning
  Inventory Depression Scale 172
Neurobehavioral Rating Scale–
  Revised (NBRS-R) 61, 62
neurodiagnostic studies **56**, 64–66
  electrophysiological
      assessments 65–66
  laboratory tests 66
  neuroimaging 64–65
  neuropsychological evaluation
      66
neurofilament compaction 19
neuroimaging
  apathy 288–289
  cognitive impairments and 145
  day-of-injury 51
  depressive disorders 173
  disorders of consciousness 115–
      116
  headaches 329, 330
  manic and mixed mood
      episodes 180
  medical evaluation 64–65
  military personnel and veterans
      465
  mTBI 24, **25**
  neuropsychological evaluation
      versus 73, 74
  older population 429
  pathological laughing and
      crying 187
  persistent symptoms after
      concussion 487–488

posttraumatic epilepsy 354–355
posttraumatic stress disorder
      219
  schizophrenia-like psychosis 249
  seizures 354–355
  sports-related concussion 446
  structural 11–16
  vestibular disorders 400
neurological examination 57–60
neuromodulation treatments, for
  disorders of consciousness 120–
  121
Neuromonics tinnitus treatment
  protocol 402
neuronal injury 17
Neuropsychiatric Inventory (NPI)
  62, 287
neuropsychological assessment 73–
  93
  common neuropsychological
      impairments 76–78
  methods 82–89
    approaches 82–83
    computerized assessment
        88–89
    domains assessed 83–84, **88**
    screening versus
        comprehensive
        evaluation 84–88
  role of 74–76
  specific contexts 80–82
    forensic 81–82
    military 81
    sports 80–81
  test interpretation 89–93
    comorbidities 92–93
    innate relative weakness or
        brain impairment
        91–92
    premorbid estimation 89–
        90
    validity assessment 90–91
  timing of 78–80
    mild TBI 78–79
    moderate to severe TBI
        79–80
neuropsychological evaluation 66

neuropsychology, defined 73
New York University (NYU)
    functional disability model 477–
    484
        genetic factors 482–483
        insurance and legal factors
            483–484
        neurological factors 478
        physical factors 480–481
        psychiatric factors 478–480
        psychological factors 481–482
        treatment concepts 490
nifedipine, aggressive disorders and
    264
non-rapid eye movement (NREM)
    sleep 373
nonsteroidal anti-inflammatory
    drugs (NSAIDs)
        headaches 330, 332, **334**, **336**
        military injuries 466
        older population 433
nortriptyline
        depressive disorders **175**
        headaches **334**
        older population 433
        pathological laughing and
            crying 187, **188**
NPI (Neuropsychiatric Inventory)
    62, 287
NREM (non-rapid eye movement)
    sleep **373**


**O**
OAS (Overt Aggression Scale) 260,
    267, **268**
OASS (Overt Agitation Severity
    Scale) 260, 267, **269**
obsessive-compulsive disorder
    (OCD) 199, 202, 205
occult seizures 117
occupational history 53
olanzapine
        anxiety disorders 206
        apathy 293
        older population 434
        schizophrenia-like psychosis
            252

older adult (geriatric) population
    423–439
    APOE and dementia 426–427
    assessment 429–432
        bladder function 431
        bowel function 431–432
        medical evaluation 429–430
        medical rehabilitation
            evaluation 430–
            431
        medication review 430
        neuroimaging 429
        social support 432
        swallowing and nutrition
            431
    baseline cognition and
        cognitive recovery
        425–426
    baseline functional status 423–
        424
    epidemiology 427–429
        falls 427–428
        mortality 428
        multiple trauma 429
    functional outcomes 425
    health after TBI 426
    health care funding 426
    medical complications 424–425
    medical rehabilitation 437–438
        intensive care unit 437
        mobility 438
        selection 437
        self-care 438
        sensory health 437–438
    pharmacotherapy 432–435
        agitation 434
        arousal and attention 434
        bladder function 435
        bowel function 435
        mood and sleep alterations
            434–435
        pain 432–433
        seizures 433–434
        venous thromboembolism
            risk 433
    psychological and behavioral
        interventions 435–437

driving 436–437
  recreation and vocation 436
  sexuality 436
  substance abuse 435–436
  sensory health 424
  susceptibility to TBI 424
olfactory impairments 406–408, **409**
optic chiasm trauma 410
optic tract lesions 410
Orientation Log (O-Log) 48
orientation, defined 136
Overt Aggression Scale (OAS) 260, 267, 268
Overt Agitation Severity Scale (OASS) 260, 267, 269
overuse headaches 333
oxcarbazepine
  aggressive disorders 277
  older population 434
  posttraumatic epilepsy **357**
  side effects and risks of **359**
oxygen inhalation, for migraine headaches **336**, 337, **337**

**P**

PAI (Personality Assessment Inventory) 514, 516
panic
  anxiety disorders 199, 202–203
  persistent symptoms after concussion 479
  postinjury levels of 24
parasomnias 377
paratonia 57–60
*parens patriae* power 504
paroxetine
  aggressive disorders 276
  depressive disorders 175, **175**
  older population 433
  pathological laughing and crying **188**
pathological laughing and crying (PLC) 183–189
  assessment 185–187
    diagnostic assessment **184**, 186

differential diagnosis 185–186
  laboratory and neurodiagnostic assessments 187
  epidemiology 183
  risk factors 185
  treatment 187–189 **188**
Pathological Laughter and Crying Scale (PLACS) 186
PCL (PTSD Checklist) 224
PC-PTSD (Primary Care PTSD Screen) 224
PDHA (Post Deployment Health Assessment) 464
PDRT (Portland Digit Recognition Test) 515
pelvic relaxation 431
perilymphatic fistulas (PLFs) 397–398
perinatal accidents, schizophrenia-like psychosis and 251–252
peritraumatic stroke 424
persistent symptoms after concussion 475–496
  evaluation 484–489
    contributing factors 488–489
    medical records 485–486
    neuroimaging 487–488
    neuropsychological testing 486–487
    self-report 484–485
  factors contributing to 477–484
    genetic 482–483
    insurance and legal system 483–484
    neurological 478
    physical 480–481
    psychiatric 478–480
    psychological 481–482
  treatment 489–496
    self-system 490–496
persistent vegetative state (PVS) 104, 109, 521
personal injury litigation 508–509

Personality Assessment Inventory (PAI) 514, 516

personality changes
    aggressive disorders **263**
    anxiety disorders 196

personality disorders, pathological laughing and crying versus 186

PET (positron emission tomography) 64

phenobarbital, for posttraumatic epilepsy 364

phenol nerve and motor point blocks, disorders of consciousness and 119

phenytoin
    disorders of consciousness and 117
    posttraumatic epilepsy **357**, 364
    side effects and risks of **361**

photophobia 412

photosensitivity 412

phototherapy, for posttraumatic sleep disorders 378–379

physical examination 55, **56**

physostigmine, for cognitive impairments 157

pindolol
    aggressive disorders 275
    anxiety disorders 205

Pittsburgh Rehabilitation Participation Scale 200

PLACS (Pathological Laughter and Crying Scale) 186

PLFs (perilymphatic fistulas) 397–398

Portland Digit Recognition Test (PDRT) 515

positron emission tomography (PET) 64

Post Deployment Health Assessment (PDHA) 464

post-injury factors **36**

posttraumatic amnesia (PTA) 44, **49**, 50–51, 79, 139–140, **142**, **144**
    defined 136
    loss of consciousness versus 485
    posttraumatic stress disorder 215, 216, 222

posttraumatic confusional state (PTCS) **142**, **144**
    definition and differential diagnosis 105–106
    depressive disorders 171
    manic and mixed mood episodes 178

posttraumatic dysexecutive syndrome **142**, **144**

posttraumatic encephalopathy (PTE), stages of 142

posttraumatic endolymphatic hydrops (PT-ELH) 397

posttraumatic epilepsy (PTE) 345–367
    assessment 349–355
        differential diagnosis 349–350, **351**
        neurodiagnostic 350–355
    definitions 345–346
    epidemiology 346–349
        genetics 349
        incidence and natural history 346–348
        risk factors 348–349
    manic and mixed mood episodes 179
    tinnitus and 401
    treatment 355–366
        behavioral 364–365
        community resources 366
        complementary 364–365
        pharmacotherapy 355–364
        psychological 364–365
    types of seizures 346

posttraumatic neuroendocrine disturbances 66

posttraumatic psychosis 239–254
    characteristics of TBI 247
    course 248–249
    epidemiology 239–246
        case control studies 242–246
        case reports 240
        cohort studies 241–242
        cross-sectional surveys 240–241

medicolegal considerations 253
psychopathology 247–248
risk factors and
　　　pathophysiology 249–
　　　252
　　age at time of injury 251–
　　　252
　　cognition 249–250
　　epilepsy 250–251
　　neuroanatomical
　　　substrates 249
　　preinjury factors 250
symptoms associated with
　　　mood disturbances
　　　248
treatment 252–253
posttraumatic stress disorder
　(PTSD) 213–233
　anxiety disorders 197, 199
　assessment 223–225
　co-occurrence with TBI 215–
　　　216, **216**
　definitions 213–215
　depressive disorders versus 171
　epidemiology 219–223, **224**
　　civilian populations 222–
　　　223
　　military and veteran
　　　populations 220–
　　　222
　history of 52
　military injuries 199
　neurochemical abnormalities
　　　217
　persistent symptoms after
　　　concussion 478, 480
　postinjury levels of 24
　prevalence of **198**
　structural changes 217–219
　treatment 225–232
　　pharmacotherapy 227–
　　　228, **229**
　　psychological and
　　　behavioral
　　　therapies 228–
　　　231, **231**
postural instability 59, 413–414

praxis
　defined 137
　treating impairments **153**
prazosin, for headaches 332, 338
pregabalin
　anxiety disorders 205
　posttraumatic epilepsy **357**
　side effects and risks of **360**
pre-injury factors **36**
premorbid cognitive function,
　estimation of 89–90
presbycusis 424
present illness, history of **38**, 40–44
　functional status 43
　hypothesis generation 44
　symptoms 40–43, **42**
Preventing Violent Explosive
　Neurologic Trauma program 471
primary axotomy 17, **18**
Primary Care PTSD Screen (PC-
　PTSD) 224
primitive reflexes 59–60
procedural memory, defined 136
processing speed, defined 134
propranolol, for aggressive
　disorders 269, 275–276
prosody, defined 137
prospective serial assessments 47–
　50
prostate hypertrophy 431
protriptyline
　apathy **295**
　older population 433
PTE (posttraumatic
　encephalopathy), stages of **142**
PT-ELH (posttraumatic
　endolymphatic hydrops) 397
PTSD Checklist (PCL) 224
purposive action, defined 138
PVS (persistent vegetative state)
　104, 109, 521

**Q**

qualitative/process-based test
　interpretation 83
Quality of Life in Epilepsy (QOLIE-
　89) inventory 366

quantitative
  electroencephalography (QEEG)
    65–66
    neurofeedback for
      posttraumatic epilepsy
      365
quantitative individualized
  behavioral assessment (QIBA)
  112–113, **114**
quantitative/normative-based test
  interpretation 83
quetiapine
  anxiety disorders 206
  manic and mixed mood
    episodes 182, **182**
  older population 434
  posttraumatic sleep disorders
    383

**R**

ramelteon
  anxiety disorders **207**
  posttraumatic sleep disorders
    383
ranitidine, aggressive disorders and
  264
rapid eye movement (REM) sleep
  **373**
recognition, defined 135
Repeatable Battery for the
  Assessment of
  Neuropsychological Status
  (RBANS) 84–88
repetition, defined 137
rescue treatments for headaches
  332, **337**
resilience, posttraumatic stress
  disorder and 231–232
response bias 515–516
retrieval, defined 135
retrograde amnesia 44
  defined 136
retrospective assessments 50–51
return-to-duty decision 468–469
return-to-play decision 448–449,
  451, 455–456, **456**
revenge 483–484

review of systems **39**, 54–55
rigidity 57
risperidone
  aggressive disorders 274
  apathy 293
  older population 434
  posttraumatic sleep disorders
    383
  schizophrenia-like psychosis
    252
rivastigmine
  apathy **295**
  cognitive impairments and **157**

**S**

SAC (Standardized Assessment of
  Concussion) 451
Schedules for Clinical Assessments
  in Neuropsychiatry (SCAN) 52
schizophrenia
  strength of association between
    TBI and 240–245
schizophrenia-like psychosis 239–
  254
  characteristics of TBI 247
  course 248–249
  epidemiology 239–246
    case control studies 242–
      246
    case reports 240
    cohort studies 241–242
    cross-sectional surveys
      240–241
  medicolegal considerations 253
  psychopathology 247–248
  risk factors and
    pathophysiology 249–
      252
    age at time of injury 251–
      252
    case control studies 245–
      246
    cognition 249–250
    epilepsy 250–251
    neuroanatomical
      substrates 249
    preinjury factors 250

symptoms associated with
mood disturbances
248
treatment 252–253
SCL-90 (Symptom Checklist-90)
205
secondary axotomy 17, **18**
seizures 345–367
assessment 349–355
differential diagnosis 349–
350, **351**
neurodiagnostic 350–355
clinical manifestations of **347**
definitions 345–346
epidemiology 346–349
genetics 349
incidence and natural
history 346–348
risk factors 348–349
older population 433–434
treatment 355–366
behavioral 364–365
community resources 366
complementary 364–365
pharmacotherapy 355–364
psychological 364–365
types of 346
selective serotonin reuptake
inhibitors (SSRIs)
aggressive disorders 269, 276
anxiety disorders 205
apathy 290
depressive disorders 174, 176
manic and mixed mood
episodes 180
older population 435
pathological laughing and
crying 187
selegiline, for apathy 294, **295**
self-report symptom inventories **41**
self-system 490–496
acceptance of self 496
effect of insurance and legal
system 494
interventions 494–495
reestablishing effective self
492–493

reintegration of self 493–494
understanding self 491–492
validating self 491
sensorimotor abnormalities 46, 48
sensorineural hearing loss 405–406
sensory impairments 395–415
chemosensory impairments
406–408, **409**
hearing impairments 404–406
hyperacusis 402–404
older population 437–438
postural instability 413–414
tinnitus 400–402
vestibular disorders 396–400
visual impairments 408–413
sensory stimulation
disorders of consciousness and
119, 120
serotonin transporter gene
(5HTT), polymorphisms of 168–
170
serotonin-norepinephrine reuptake
inhibitors (SNRIs), for depressive
disorders 176
sertraline
aggressive disorders 276
anxiety disorders 205
depressive disorders 175, **175**
pathological laughing and
crying **188**
sexuality, older population 436
sildenafil 436
single-photon emission computed
tomography (SPECT) 64
SIRS (Structured Interview of
Reported Symptoms) 514, 516
skew deviation 411
skin breakdown, disorders of
consciousness and 119
SLAM (Sports as a Laboratory
Assessment Model) 447–448
sleep apnea 376
sleep cycle 372, **373**
sleep disorders 371–384, 388–390
evaluation 378
headache 338
military injuries 466

sleep disorders *(continued)*
  nonpharmacological treatment
      378–380
    chronotherapy 379–380
    diet and lifestyle 378
    phototherapy 378–379
    psychotherapy 380
  normal sleep cycle 372
  older population 434–435
  pathophysiology 374–375
  pharmacotherapy 380–383
    antidepressants 380
    atypical antipsychotics 383
    benzodiazepine sedative-
        hypnotics 382
    melatonin 383
    modafinil 382
    nonbenzodiazepine
        sedative-hypnotics
        381–382
    sodium oxybate 383
  prevalence of 372–374
  types of 375–377
    hypersomnia 376–377
    insomnia 375–376
    parasomnias 377
    sleep-wake cycle
        disturbances 377
sleep disturbances 25
sleep-wake cycle disturbances
  (circadian rhythm disorder) 377,
  378–379
SNRIs (serotonin-norepinephrine
  reuptake inhibitors), for
  depressive disorders 176
social and family history **39**, 53–54
social phobia 199, 202
    persistent symptoms after
        concussion 479
Social Security Disability evaluation
  509–511
sodium oxybate, for posttraumatic
  sleep disorders 383
sodium/calcium exchange 17, 19,
  **20**
somatization disorder 482
sonophobia 403

spasticity 57
specific competence 503
SPECT (single-photon emission
  computed tomography) 64
spectrin, breakdown of 19
speech, defined 137
spinal manipulation, for headaches
  334
Sports as a Laboratory Assessment
  Model (SLAM) 447–448
sports-related concussion 4, 7, 443–
  457
    assessment and management
        449–454
    definition 443–444, **445**
    epidemiology 444
    neuropsychological assessment
        78, 80–81
    pathophysiology 444–446
    recovery from **452**, **453**
    research into 446–449
    return-to-play decision 455–
        456, **456**
    treatment 454–455
Standardized Assessment of
  Concussion (SAC) 451
Structured Interview of Reported
  Symptoms (SIRS) 514, 516
structured interviews 40, **42**
substance abuse and withdrawal
    aggressive disorders 264
    apathy 290
    depressive disorders 171
    history of 52
    manic and mixed mood
        episodes 178
    older population 435–436
substance use disorders 303–316
    assessment 305–307
    definitions 304
    epidemiology 304
    treatment 307–315
        pharmacotherapy 315
        psychological and
            behavioral
            interventions
            307–315

sundowning 434
Symptom Checklist–90 (SCL-90) 205
symptom inventories 40, **41, 42**

**T**
tadalafil 436
tamulosin 435
telemedicine, for military personnel and veterans 469–470
temazepam
  anxiety disorders **207**
  posttraumatic sleep disorders 382
tension headaches 324–325
  characteristics of **331**
  pharmacotherapy 330–332, **334**
  psychological and behavioral interventions 333–334
tentorium cerebelli 6
terazosin 435
Test of Memory Malingering (TOMM) 515
Test of Nonverbal Intelligence, 4th Edition (TONI-4) 517
Test of Premorbid Functioning (TOPF) 90, 509
testamentary capacity 505–506
thalamic volume loss 12
theophylline, aggressive disorders and 264
thioridazine, aggressive disorders and 264, 276
thrombophlebitis, disorders of consciousness and 119
thyroid dysfunction screening
  depressive disorders 173
  manic and mixed mood episodes 180
timolol, for migraine headaches **335**
tinnitus 400–402
TOMM (Test of Memory Malingering) 515
TON (traumatic optic neuropathy) 409–410

TONI-4 (Test of Nonverbal Intelligence, 4th Edition) 517
TOPF (Test of Premorbid Functioning) 90, 509
topiramate
  headaches 332, **334, 335**
  posttraumatic epilepsy **356**
  side effects and risks of **359**
  substance use disorders 315
torts 508
tractography 13, **16**
  disorders of consciousness 115
tramadol, for migraine headaches **336, 337**
transferences 271
Trauma Symptom Inventory (TSI) 224
traumatic brain injury (TBI) 3–27
  anatomy of 4–21
    macroscopic injury 4–8
    microscopic injury 17–21
    structural neuroimaging 11–16
  biomechanics and regional differences in 7, 9
  clinical consequences of 21–26
    cognition 21–24
    disability 26
    noncognitive neuropsychiatric functions 24–26
  defined 4
  incidence of 3
  severity characterization 46–51
    day-of-injury neuroimaging 51
    prospective serial assessments 47–50
    retrospective assessments 50–51
traumatic optic neuropathy (TON) 409–410
trazodone
  aggressive disorders 276
  anxiety disorders **207**
  posttraumatic sleep disorders 380

tricyclic antidepressants (TCAs)
  aggressive disorders 264
  anxiety disorders 205
  depressive disorders 174
  headaches 332, **334**
  military injuries 466
  older population 433
  pathological laughing and
    crying 187
  persistent symptoms after
    concussion 495
  posttraumatic sleep disorders
    380
triptans, for migraine headaches
  **336**, **337**
TSI (Trauma Symptom Inventory)
  224

**U**

undue influence, vulnerability to
  506–507, **507**
University of Pennsylvania Smell
  Identification Test (UPSIT) 407

**V**

vagus nerve stimulator (VNS), for
  posttraumatic epilepsy 365–366
validity (effort) assessment 82, 90–91
Validity Indicator Profile (VIP) 515
valproate
  headaches **334**
  manic and mixed mood
    episodes 181–182
  schizophrenia-like psychosis 252
valproic acid
  aggressive disorders 276, 277
  anxiety disorders 205
  posttraumatic epilepsy **358**, 364
  side effects and risks of **361**
vardenafil 436
vegetative state (VS)
  definitions and differential
    diagnosis 104
  epidemiology 106–107
  neuroimaging 116
  neuromodulation treatments
    120, 121

pathophysiology 107–108
  prognosis 109
  recovery enhancement 119
venlafaxine
  anxiety disorders 205
  apathy **295**
  depressive disorders **175**
  pathological laughing and
    crying **188**
venous thromboembolism, in older
  population 433
vestibular disorders 396–400
vestibular hyperacusis 403–404
vestibular impairments
  military injuries 468
  persistent symptoms after
    concussion 480, 495
Victoria Symptom Validity Test
  (VSVT) 515
VIP (Validity Indicator Profile) 515
virtual reality systems, for
  posttraumatic stress disorder 232
visual impairments 408–413
  military injuries 468
  persistent symptoms after
    concussion 495
visuospatial function
  defined 138
  persistent symptoms after
    concussion 479
  treating impairments **154**
vitreous disorders 412
VNS (vagus nerve stimulator), for
  posttraumatic epilepsy 365–366
voice, defined 137
volition, defined 138
VSVT (Victoria Symptom Validity
  Test) 515

**W**

Wechsler Adult Intelligence Scale–
  4th Edition (WAIS-IV) 82, 90,
  512, 516
Wechsler Adult Intelligence Scale–
  3rd Edition (WAIS-III) 90
Wechsler Memory Scale, 4th
  Edition (WMS-IV) 83, **512**

Wechsler Test of Adult Reading
(WTAR) 90
Western Aphasia Battery–Revised
(WAB-R) 516
Wide Range Achievement Test–4th
Edition (WRAT4) 512
Wisconsin Card Sorting Test
(WCST) 516
Word Memory Test (WMT) 487, 515
working memory (immediate
memory, registration)
defined 134–135
persistent symptoms after
concussion 479
treating impairments 150

**Y**
Yale-Brown Obsessive Compulsive
Scale (Y-BOCS) 205

Young Mania Rating Scale 180

**Z**
zaleplon
anxiety disorders **207**
posttraumatic sleep disorders
381
zolpidem
anxiety disorders **207**
disorders of consciousness and
121
military injuries 466
posttraumatic sleep disorders
381
zonisamide
posttraumatic epilepsy **356**
side effects and risks of **359**
Zurich consensus statement 4, 7